Cancer: Clinical and Translational Research

Cancer: Clinical and Translational Research

Editor: Lydia Doyle

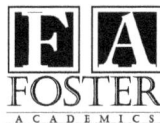

FA
FOSTER
ACADEMICS

www.fosteracademics.com

www.fosteracademics.com

FA
FOSTER
ACADEMICS

Cataloging-in-Publication Data

Cancer : clinical and translational research / edited by Lydia Doyle.
    p. cm.
Includes bibliographical references and index.
ISBN 978-1-63242-883-7
1. Cancer. 2. Cancer--Research. 3. Clinical medicine. 4. Cancer cells. 5. Cancer--Treatment. I. Doyle, Lydia.
RC261 .C36 2020
616.994--dc23

Foster Academics,
118-35 Queens Blvd., Suite 400,
Forest Hills, NY 11375, USA

ISBN 978-1-63242-883-7 (Hardback)

Contents

Permissions

List of Contributors

Index

Preface

Cancer refers to a family of diseases, which involves an abnormal growth of cells that can invade or spread to other parts of the body. Survival rates in people suffering from cancer vary according to the cancer type and stage in which it is diagnosed. The prognosis is worse for cancers that have metastasized. Cancer survivors often develop a second primary cancer. Cancer research strives to identify possible causes and strategies for the prevention, diagnosis and treatment of cancer. It involves various aspects of molecular bioscience, cancer epidemiology and clinical trials for evaluating and comparing outcomes of different cancer therapies. Translational research in cancer seeks to understand the mechanisms of cancer development and progression, and translate such scientific findings into formulating approaches in the treatment and prevention of cancer. Clinical cancer research is devoted to the development of surgical procedures, pharmaceutical agents and medical technologies for the treatment of cancer. This book is a compilation of chapters that discuss the most vital concepts and emerging trends in the field of cancer management. The topics covered herein deal with the clinical and translational research in the field of oncology. For all readers who are interested in this field, the case studies included herein will serve as an excellent guide to develop a comprehensive understanding.

Significant researches are present in this book. Intensive efforts have been employed by authors to make this book an outstanding discourse. This book contains the enlightening chapters which have been written on the basis of significant researches done by the experts.

Finally, I would also like to thank all the members involved in this book for being a team and meeting all the deadlines for the submission of their respective works. I would also like to thank my friends and family for being supportive in my efforts.

Editor

Interactions between life expectancy and the incidence and mortality rates of cancer

Xiuying Gu[1], Rongshou Zheng[2], Changfa Xia[2], Hongmei Zeng[2], Siwei Zhang[2], Xiaonong Zou[2], Zhixun Yang[2], He Li[2] and Wanqing Chen[2*]

Abstract

Background: The relationship between cancer and life expectancy is well established in both developed and developing countries. China is a vast country with significant geographical differences in population structure and healthcare, and thus provides a unique opportunity to analyze the complex relationship between life expectancy and cancer incidence and mortality rates.

Methods: Cancer data were extracted for a total of 255 units (cities or counties) from the 2013 National Central Cancer Registry. Life expectancy data at the unit level were obtained from the National Centers for Disease Control and Prevention. Linear regression analysis was used to analyze the relationship between life expectancy and crude incidence and mortality rates of cancer. In a separate analysis, life expectancy was rated as low (< 76.0 years), middle (76–80 years), or high (> 80 years).

Results: Overall, the cancer incidence and mortality rates positively correlated with life expectancy in both sexes (R at 0.37 and 0.50, $P < 0.001$). The correlation was significant for the following cancers: lung, colorectal, prostate, bladder and pancreas, as well as for lymphoma in men (R 0.36–0.58, $P < 0.001$), lung, breast, colorectal, thyroid, uterus, and ovary in women (R 0.18–0.51, $P < 0.001$). We failed to observe an association between upper gastrointestinal cancer and life expectancy. The number of cities/counties with low, middle and high life expectancy levels were 110, 101 and 44, respectively. The highest age-standardized cancer incidence rate was observed in areas with a high life expectancy level (192.83/100,000). The highest age-standardized mortality rate was in areas with the lowest life expectancy (118.44/100,000). Cancers of the stomach, liver and esophagus are major cancer types in areas with low and middle life expectancy. In contrast, areas with high life expectancy had high incidence and mortality rates of colorectal cancer, breast cancer in women and prostate cancer in men.

Conclusions: Longer life expectancy is associated with higher overall cancer incidence and mortality in China. The cancer pattern also varies substantially across areas with different life expectancy levels. Life expectancy levels must be considered when developing strategies to prevent and treat cancers.

Keywords: Cancer, Incidence, Mortality, Life expectancy, China

*Correspondence: chenwq@cicams.ac.cn
[2] National Office for Cancer Prevention and Control, National Cancer Center/Cancer Hospital, Chinese Academy of Medical Sciences and Peking Union Medical College, Beijing 100021, P. R. China
Full list of author information is available at the end of the article

Introduction

Cancer is a major public health problem worldwide [1, 2]. The majority of cancer types are more common in elderly populations. The relationship between cancer and life expectancy in the general population has been extensively studied [3–6]. The results provided consistent evidence for differing cancer profiles across life expectancy levels. In particular, cancer is associated with an aging population and socioeconomic development. Aging populations have led to major changes in the structure of the global population and in the scale of the cancer problem worldwide [7]. The United Nations Development Program (UNDP) has now incorporated life expectancy as a component of the Human Development Index (HDI) to evaluate the influence of social development on health issues (including cardiovascular diseases and cancer) across different countries [8–10].

Global life expectancy has increased by 5 years since 2000, with an increasingly narrower gap between high- and low-income countries [8]. In China, the average life expectancy in 2015 was 76.34 years (73.64 for men and 79.43 for women); up 5 years from 2000 [11]. Despite the rapidly increasing life expectancy, overall cancer incidence has been relatively stable, with decreasing age-standardized mortality rates in both men and women [2, 12–14]. The cancer pattern in China, however, is rather different from developed countries [15]. Also, China is a vast country with significant differences in population structure and healthcare, and thus provides a unique opportunity to analyze the complex relationship between cancer incidence, mortality and life expectancy, with potential relevance on a global scale.

Materials and methods

Data source

Cancer data were retrieved from the National Central Cancer Registry (NCCR). A total of 255 units (cities or counties) were included in the analysis, that covered 31 provinces, 88 cities and 167 counties. The total population covered by NCCR was 226,494,490 (114,860,339 men and 111,634,151 women) and accounted for 16.65% of the national population at the end of 2013. Life expectancy data were obtained from the National Centers for Disease Control and Prevention (NCDC). Life expectancy was low (<76 years) in 110 units, 101 units in the middle (76–80 years) and high (>80 years) in 44 units. Life expectancy levels, based on geographical location, are shown in Fig. 1.

Quality control

Cancer data were collected, audited and maintained by the NCCR according to the standards set forward by the "*Guideline for Chinese Cancer Registration*", "Cancer

Incidence in Five Continents Volume IX", as well as relevant data quality criteria by the International Agency for Research on Cancer/International Association of Cancer Registries (IARC/IACR) [16]. The assessments of quality measures include, but are not limited to, the proportion of morphologic verification (MV%), the percentage of cancer cases identified with death certification only (DCO%), the mortality (M) to incidence (I) ratio (M/I), the percentage of uncertified cancers (UB%). The MV%, DCO%, and M/I ratio of overall indicators in this analysis were 68.04%, 1.74% and 0.62%, respectively.

Statistical analysis

For descriptive analysis, the 255 units (cities/counties) were divided into three categories and based on the average life expectancy based on the 2009 report by the National Population Census [11]: low, middle, and high using 76 and 80 years of age as the cutoff points. A linear regression model (considering life expectancy as a continuous variable) was used to estimate the relationship between crude incidence and mortality rates of cancer and life expectancy using the data for each city/county. A sex-stratified analysis was conducted. A separate set of correlation analyses were conducted to analyze the relationship between each of the top 10 cancers with life expectancy. The Chinese population in 2000 and the World Segi's population were used to calculate age-standardized rates. Softwares for data checking and evaluation included MS-Excel, IARCcrgTools2.05 issued by International Agency for Research on Cancer (IARC) and International Association of Cancer Registries (IACR) [17]. All statistical analyses were conducted using SAS (SAS Institute Inc.; Cary, NC, USA).

Results

Linear regression analysis between cancer data and life expectancy

In both men and women, life expectancy correlated positively with both overall cancer incidence ($R_{male\ incidence} = 0.45$, $R_{female\ incidence} = 0.50$, $P < 0.001$ for both men and women) and mortality ($R_{male\ mortality} = 0.42$, $R_{female\ mortality} = 0.37$, $P < 0.001$ for both men and women) (Fig. 2).

The correlation between life expectancy and the incidence of the top 10 cancers are shown in Fig. 3. In men, life expectancy correlated positively with the incidence of cancers in the lungs ($R = 0.36$, $P < 0.001$), colorectum ($R = 0.54$, $P < 0.001$), prostate ($R = 0.58$, $P < 0.001$), bladder ($R = 0.43$, $P < 0.001$), pancreas ($R = 0.50$, $P < 0.001$) and lymphoma ($R = 0.43$, $P < 0.001$). The correlation was most robust for prostate cancer ($R = 0.58$, $P < 0.001$). Life expectancy did not correlate with cancers of the stomach, liver, esophagus, brain and central nervous system (CNS). In women, life expectancy correlated positively

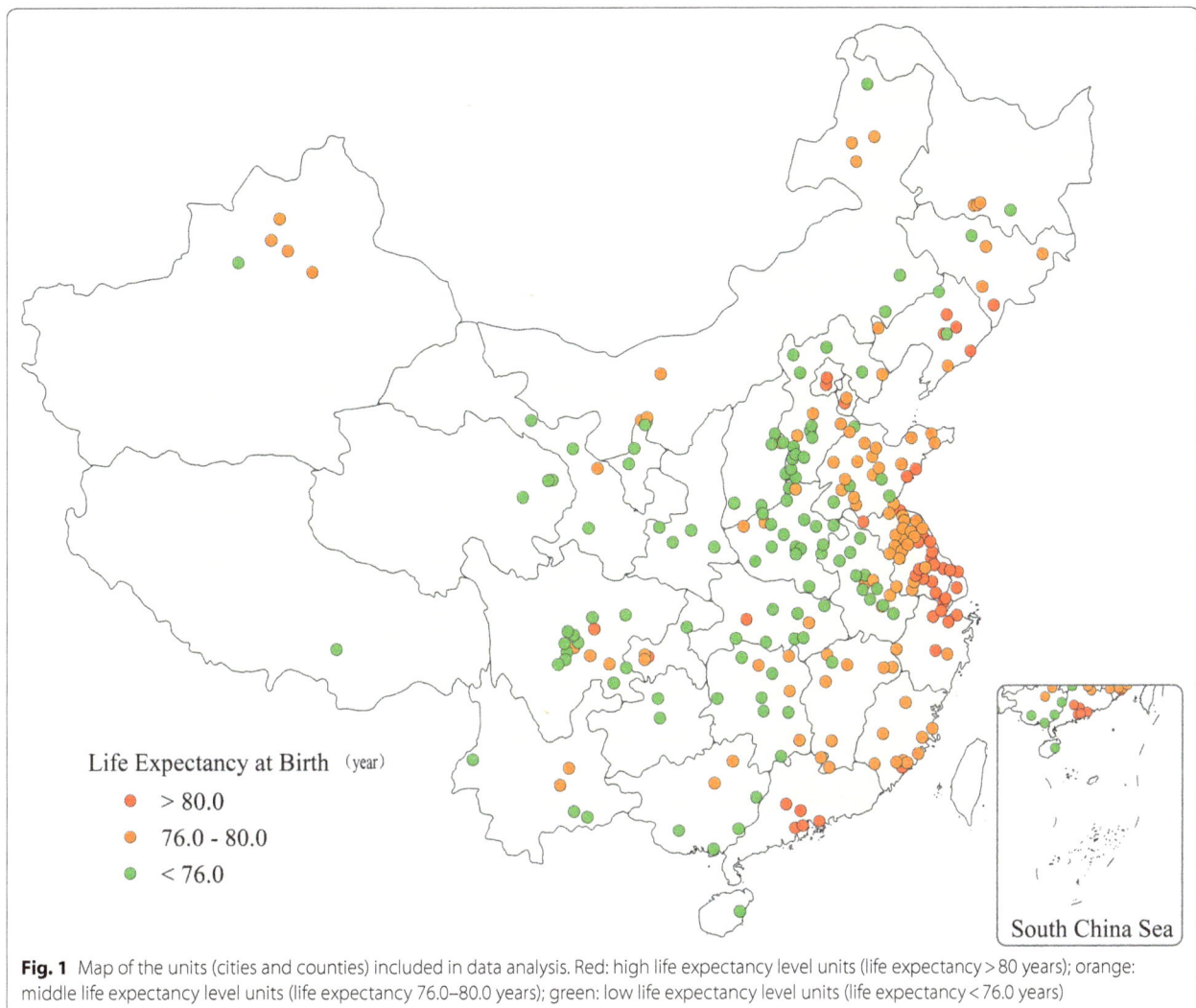

Fig. 1 Map of the units (cities and counties) included in data analysis. Red: high life expectancy level units (life expectancy > 80 years); orange: middle life expectancy level units (life expectancy 76.0–80.0 years); green: low life expectancy level units (life expectancy < 76.0 years)

with the incidence of cancers in the lungs, breast, colorectum, thyroid, uterus and ovary (R from 0.18 to 0.51, all $P<0.01$). The correlation was most robust for colorectal cancer ($R=0.51$, $P<0.001$).

The correlation between life expectancy and cancer mortality of the top 10 cancers are shown in Fig. 4. In men, life expectancy was correlated positively with the mortality in cancers of the lungs, liver, colorectum, pancreas, prostate, leukemia, and lymphoma (R from 0.16 to 0.55, all $P<0.05$), but not cancers of the upper gastrointestinal tract ($R=0.01$, $P=0.419$). The correlation was most robust for pancreatic cancer ($R=0.55$, $P<0.001$). In women, life expectancy correlated positively with the mortality in cancers of the lungs, colorectum, breast, pancreas and leukemia (R from 0.23 to 0.53, all $P<0.05$), but not cancers of the liver, stomach, esophagus, brain and CNS and cervix. The association between life

expectancy and less common types of cancer varied substantially. Such as, in both sexes, life expectancy correlated positively with the incidence of oral, nasopharynx, gallbladder, kidney and melanoma of the skin cancers (R from 0.07 to 0.52, all $P<0.05$). And there were the same associations between life expectancy and mortality in those cancers (R from 0.05 to 0.45, all $P<0.05$) (Figs. 5, 6).

Incidence

Overall incidence

Overall cancer incidence rates in the areas with different life expectancy levels are shown in Table 1. Areas with high life expectancy (>80 years) had a high crude incidence rate, followed by areas with middle (76–80 years) and low (<76 years) life expectancy levels. There was a U-shaped association between age-standardized incidence rates and life expectancy levels: areas with a middle

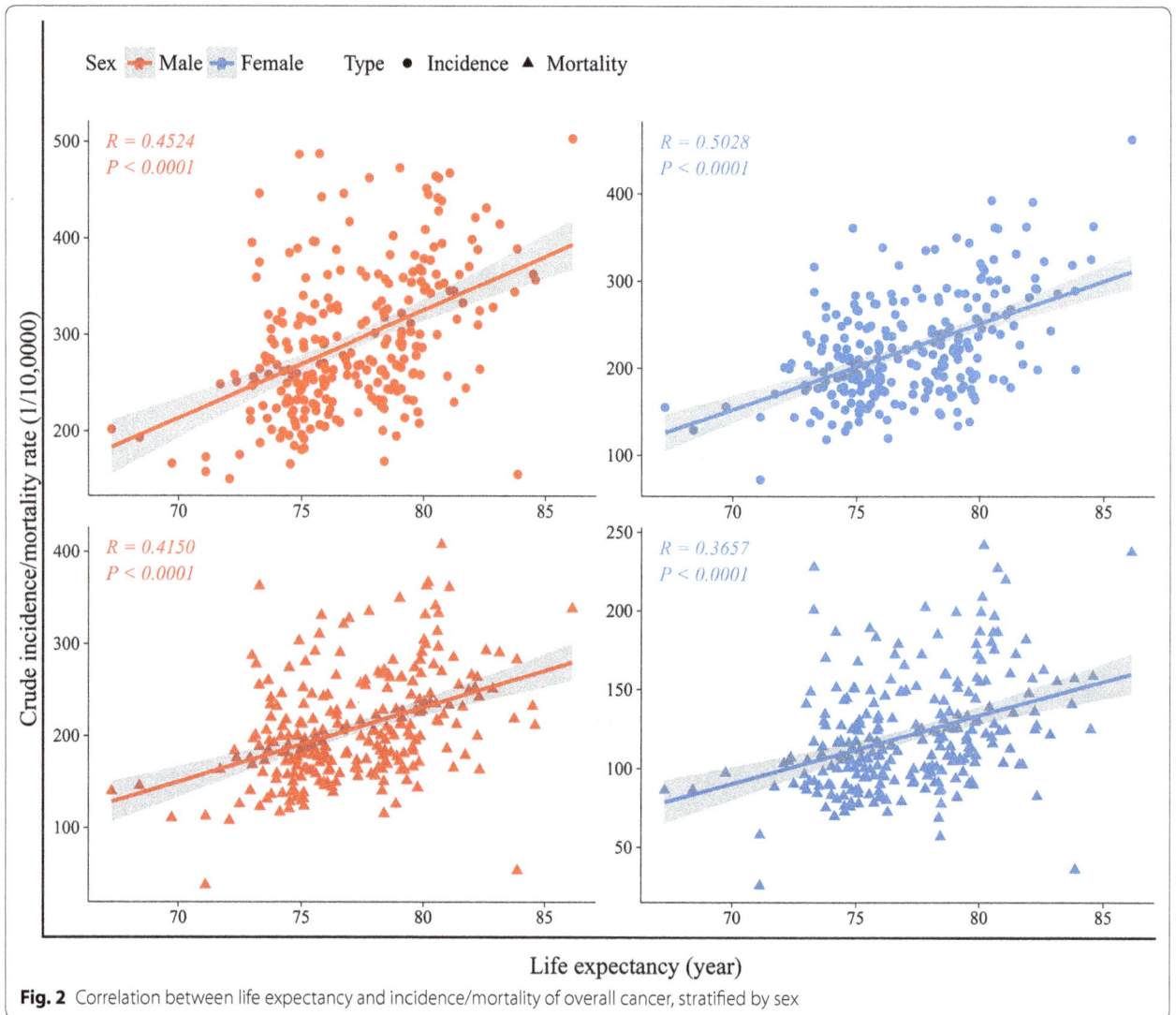

Fig. 2 Correlation between life expectancy and incidence/mortality of overall cancer, stratified by sex

life expectancy level had the lowest age-standardized incidence rate by world standard population (ASIRW). The patterns of crude incidence rates in men and women were similar to the overall sample that included both sexes. However, after adjusting for age, cancer incidence rates in men in low life expectancy level areas was higher than that in high and middle level areas. In women, the adjusted incidence rate was much higher in high life expectancy level areas than that of low and middle life expectancy level areas.

Top ten leading cancer types
Incidence rates for the top 10 cancers in the areas with different life expectancy levels are shown in Table 1. The overall analysis showed that lung cancer is the most common cancer in both sexes. ASIRW was significantly higher in low life expectancy areas (37.41/100,000)

than in high life expectancy level areas (34.90/100,000). Cancers of the stomach, liver, and esophagus were all in the top 5 list in both low and middle life expectancy level areas. Similar to that of lung cancer, the ASIRW in middle life expectancy areas were lower than in low life expectancy areas (21.66 vs. 28.76/10,000, 18.56 vs. 22.25/10,000, and 16.27 vs. 20.58/10,000) for the three types of cancers, respectively. In high life expectancy level areas, colorectal cancer ranked second which was higher than middle and low life expectancy areas. And incidence rates of breast and thyroid cancers in women increased stepwise from low to high expectancy level areas.

Cancer types varied significantly among areas with different life expectancy. In low and middle life expectancy level areas, the most common cancers in men were the cancers of the lung, stomach, liver and esophagus. In

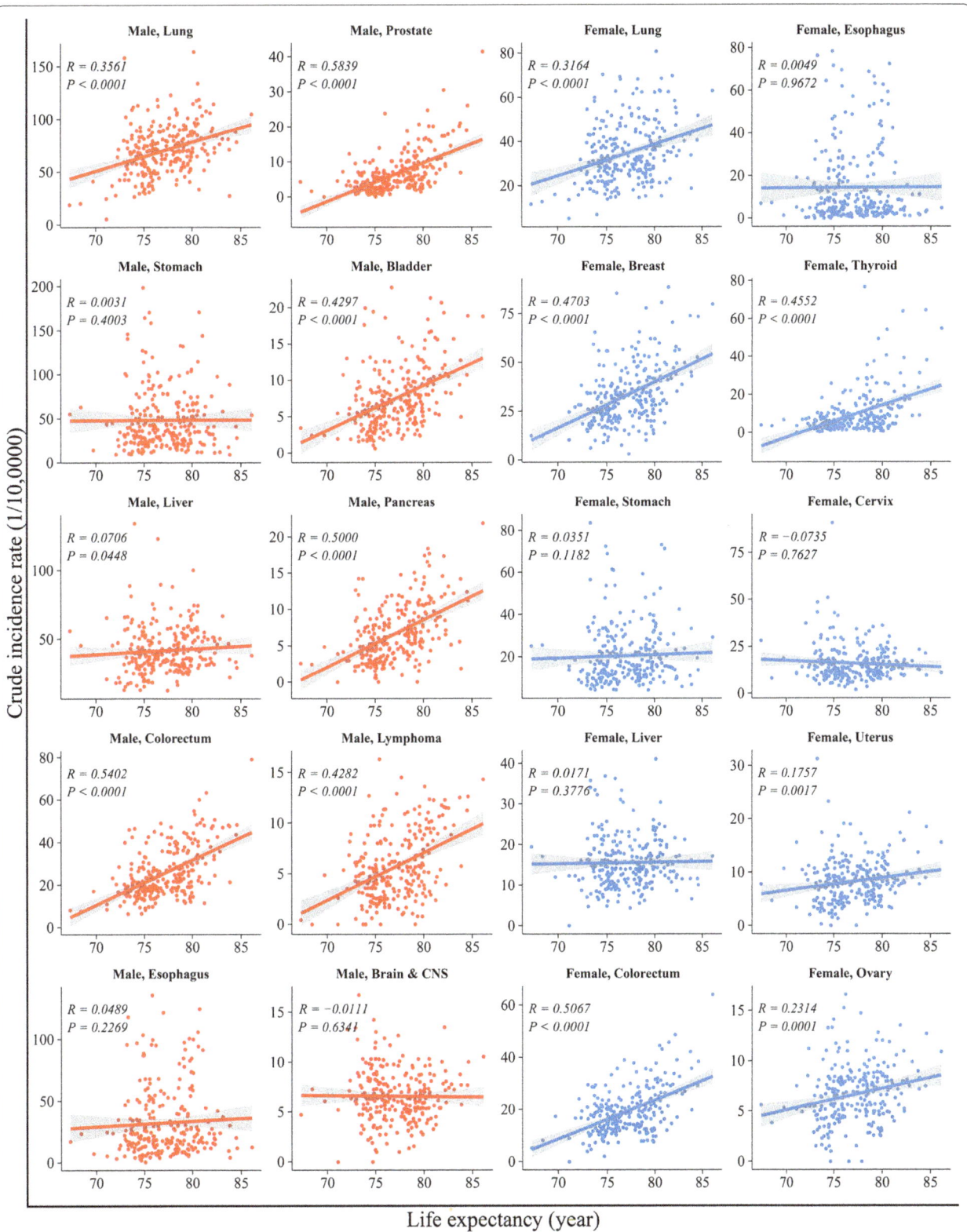

Fig. 3 Correlation between life expectancy and incidence rates for the top ten leading types of cancers, stratified by sex. The top ten leading types of cancer incidence were published by overall cancer registration data in 2013 and published previously on *Cancer Letters* (Chen W, Zheng R, Zhang S, et al. Cancer incidence and mortality in china, 2013 [12]. Cancer Lett. 2017;401:63–71)

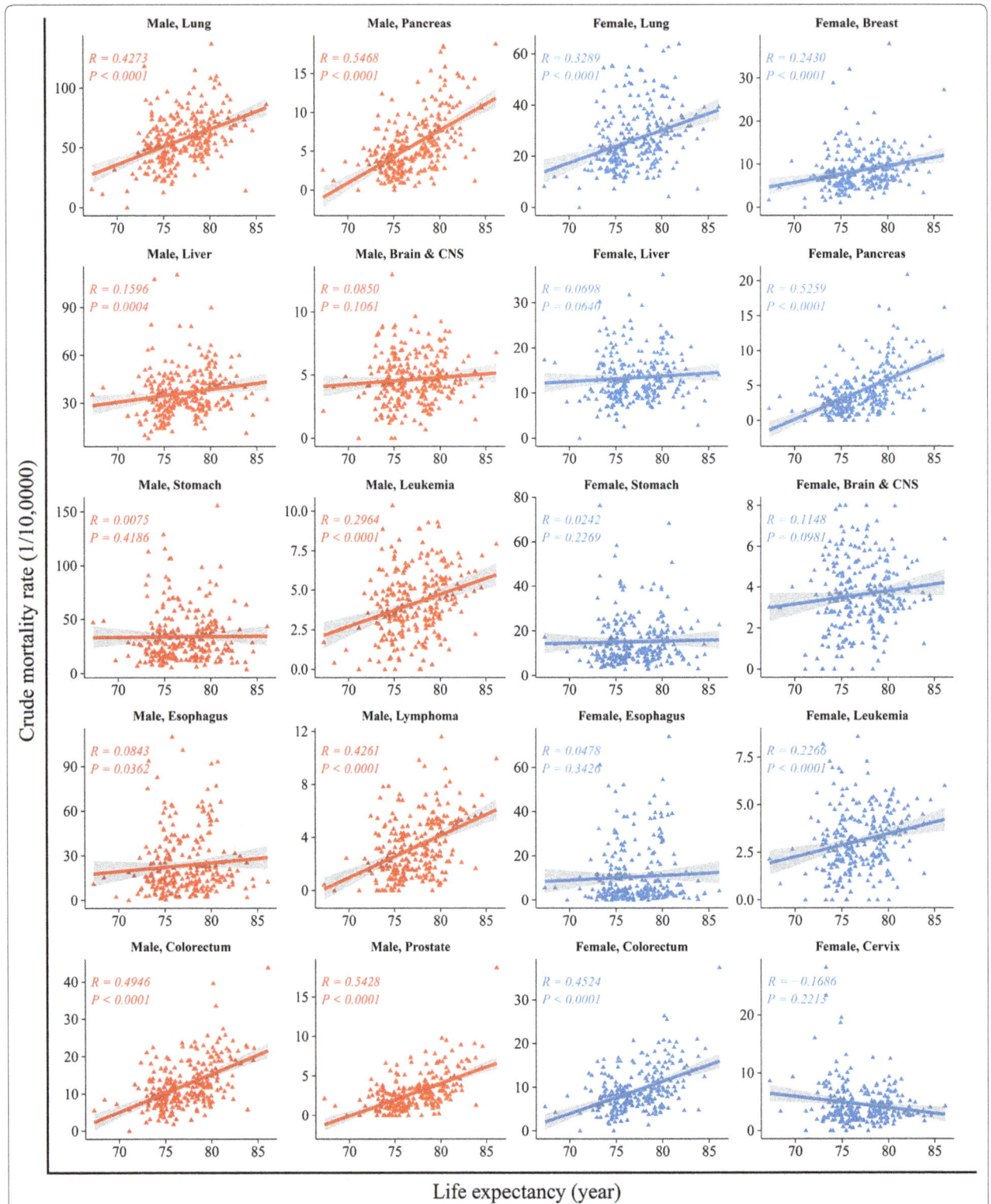

Fig. 4 Correlation between life expectancy and mortality rates for the top ten leading types of cancers, stratified by sex. The top ten leading types of cancer death were published by overall cancer registration data in 2013 and published previously on *Cancer Letters* (Chen W, Zheng R, Zhang S, et al. Cancer incidence and mortality in china, 2013 [J]. Cancer Lett. 2017;401:63–71)

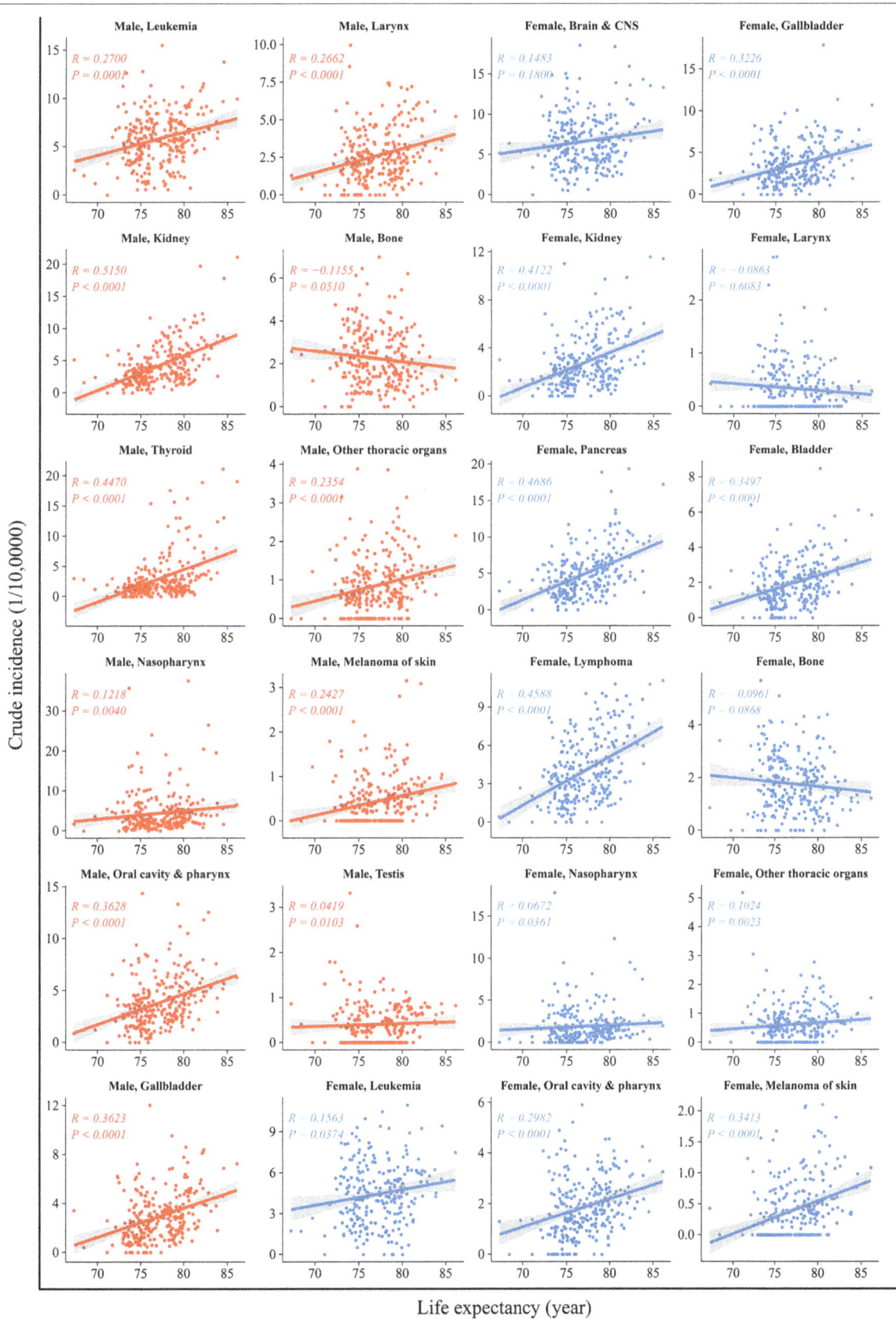

Fig. 5 Correlation between life expectancy and incidence rates in others cancers, stratified by sex

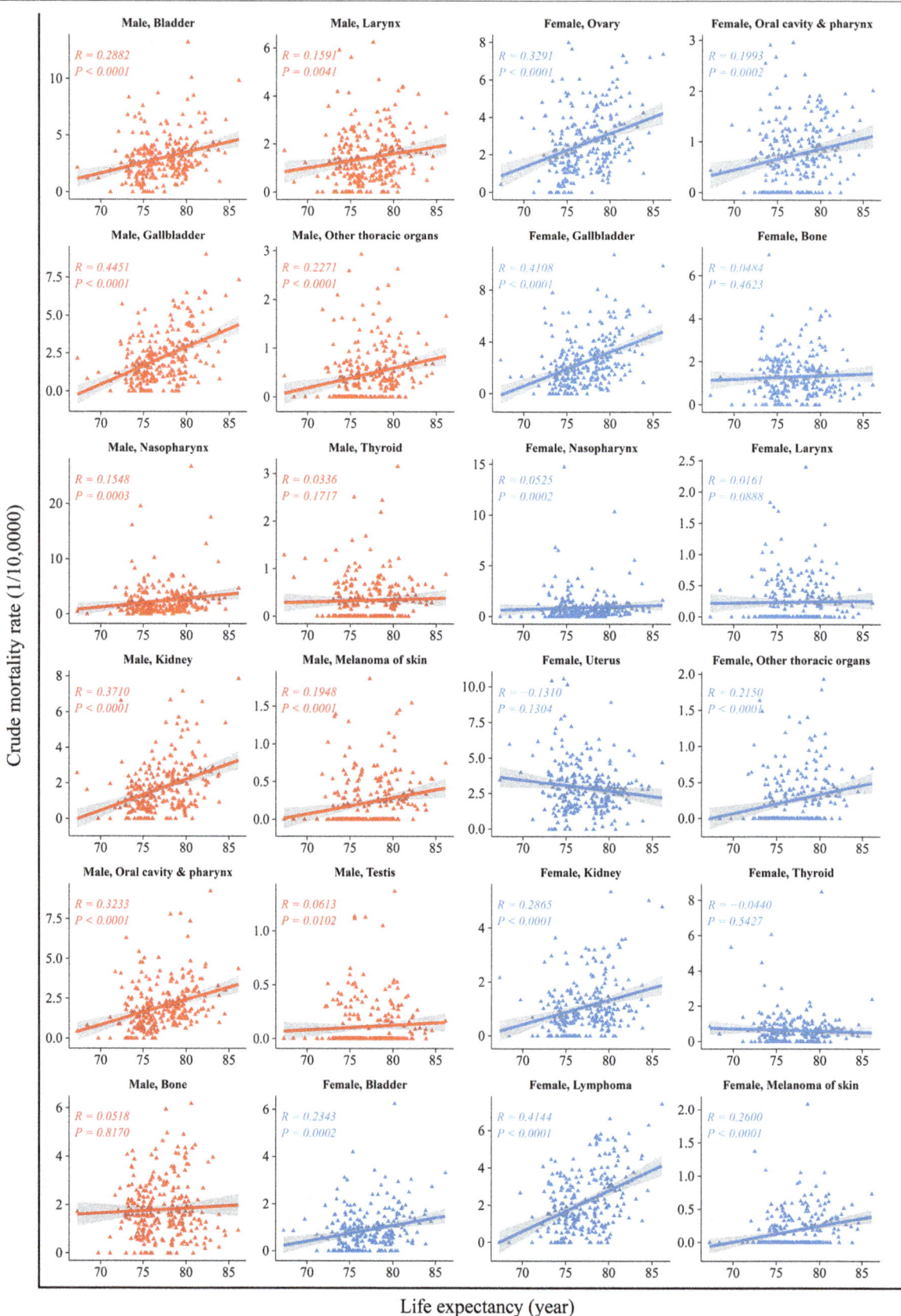

Fig. 6 Correlation between life expectancy and mortality rates in others cancers, stratified by sex

Table 1 Top 10 cancer incidence in three life expectancy levels areas of China, 2013

Rank	Gender	Low life expectancy level areas				Middle life expectancy level areas				High life expectancy level areas			
		Site	Incidence (1/10⁵)	Proportion (%)	ASRª (1/10⁵)	Site	Incidence (1/10⁵)	Proportion (%)	ASRª (1/10⁵)	Site	Incidence (1/10⁵)	Proportion (%)	ASRª (1/10⁵)
0	Both	All sites	242.77	100.00	186.91	All sites	262.81	100.00	179.00	All sites	339.61	100.00	192.83
1		Lung	49.39	20.34	37.41	Lung	55.64	21.17	36.88	Lung	66.44	19.56	34.90
2		Stomach	37.50	15.45	28.76	Stomach	32.36	12.31	21.66	Colorectum	38.42	11.31	20.57
3		Liver	29.17	12.01	22.25	Liver	27.42	10.43	18.56	Stomach	31.83	9.37	17.08
4		Esophagus	26.87	11.07	20.58	Esophagus	24.42	9.29	16.27	Breast	56.75	8.35	34.59
5		Colorectum	17.85	7.35	13.60	Colorectum	22.61	8.60	15.12	Liver	28.08	8.27	15.83
6		Breast	28.36	5.67	21.26	Breast	37.05	6.94	25.18	Thyroid	17.54	5.16	12.19
7		Cervix	16.24	3.25	12.19	Thyroid	8.17	3.11	5.89	Esophagus	16.14	4.75	8.55
8		Brain, CNS	6.79	2.80	5.53	Cervix	14.21	2.66	9.71	Pancreas	10.16	2.99	5.21
9		Leukemia	4.83	1.99	4.46	Brain, CNS	6.21	2.36	4.63	Brain, CNS	8.81	2.59	5.82
10		Pancreas	4.03	1.66	3.06	Pancreas	6.10	2.32	4.04	Lymphoma	8.74	2.57	5.21
0	Men	All sites	276.05	100.00	220.73	All sites	294.24	100.00	207.57	All sites	365.39	100.00	209.60
1		Lung	65.90	23.87	52.32	Lung	73.76	25.07	51.26	Lung	86.09	23.56	47.22
2		Stomach	51.72	18.74	41.26	Stomach	44.90	15.26	31.41	Colorectum	43.61	11.94	24.27
3		Liver	41.18	14.92	32.42	Liver	39.91	13.56	27.97	Stomach	43.53	11.91	24.21
4		Esophagus	35.64	12.91	28.47	Esophagus	33.74	11.47	23.61	Liver	41.14	11.26	24.16
5		Colorectum	19.84	7.19	15.75	Colorectum	25.67	8.72	17.87	Esophagus	23.95	6.55	13.38
6		Brain, CNS	6.97	2.52	5.79	Bladder	7.81	2.66	5.36	Prostate	16.80	4.60	8.51
7		Bladder	5.37	1.94	4.21	Pancreas	6.95	2.36	4.83	Bladder	13.24	3.62	7.08
8		Leukemia	5.29	1.92	4.97	Prostate	6.72	2.28	4.48	Pancreas	11.26	3.08	6.13
9		Lymphoma	4.72	1.71	3.89	Lymphoma	6.17	2.10	4.53	Kidney	10.23	2.80	6.04
10		Pancreas	4.56	1.65	3.61	Leukemia	6.00	2.04	5.24	Lymphoma	9.96	2.72	6.12

Table 1 (continued)

Rank	Gender	Low life expectancy level areas				Middle life expectancy level areas				High life expectancy level areas			
		Site	Incidence (1/10^5)	Proportion (%)	ASR^a (1/10^5)	Site	Incidence (1/10^5)	Proportion (%)	ASR^a (1/10^5)	Site	Incidence (1/10^5)	Proportion (%)	ASR^a (1/10^5)
0	Women	All sites	207.45	100.00	154.66	All sites	230.36	100.00	152.91	All sites	313.81	100.00	178.58
1		Lung	31.86	15.36	22.94	Breast	37.05	16.08	25.18	Breast	56.75	18.08	34.59
2		Breast	28.36	13.67	21.26	Lung	36.93	16.03	23.28	Lung	46.78	14.91	23.36
3		Stomach	22.41	10.80	16.31	Colorectum	19.46	8.45	12.51	Colorectum	33.24	10.59	17.10
4		Esophagus	17.58	8.47	12.79	Stomach	19.42	8.43	12.32	Thyroid	26.34	8.39	18.22
5		Liver	16.42	7.91	11.98	Esophagus	14.81	6.43	9.18	Stomach	20.13	6.41	10.37
6		Cervix	16.24	7.83	12.19	Liver	14.54	6.31	9.27	Cervix	15.25	4.86	9.74
7		Colorectum	15.73	7.58	11.50	Cervix	14.21	6.17	9.71	Liver	15.02	4.79	7.67
8		Uterus	7.75	3.74	5.84	Thyroid	12.74	5.53	9.12	Uterus	12.02	3.83	7.14
9		Brain, CNS	6.60	3.18	5.28	Uterus	8.31	3.61	5.66	Brain, CNS	9.71	3.09	6.18
10		Ovary	6.12	2.95	4.78	Ovary	7.26	3.15	5.11	Ovary	9.17	2.92	5.77

^{a} ASR: age-standardized incidence rate (Segi's Standard Population)

high life expectancy level areas, colorectal cancer was also very common; the ASIRW of prostate and bladder cancers was also higher than in low and middle level areas. In women, cancers of the lung, breast, stomach, esophagus and liver were the most common types in low life expectancy level areas. In middle life expectancy level areas, cancers of the breast, lung, colorectum, stomach, and esophagus were the most common cancers in women. In high life expectancy level areas, cancers of the breast, lung, colorectum, thyroid and stomach were the most common cancers.

Mortality
Overall mortality
Cancer mortality rates in areas with different life expectancy levels are shown in Table 2. High life expectancy level areas had higher crude mortality rates, followed by middle and then low life expectancy level areas. Stratified analysis based on sex produced similar findings: the crude cancer mortality rate in high life expectancy level areas was higher than that in middle and low-level areas. However, the age-standardized mortality rate correlated negatively with life expectancy, with the low life expectancy level areas having the highest age-standardized mortality rate by world standard population (ASMRW). The patterns of ASMRW in men and women were similar to the overall analysis that included both men and women.

Top ten leading cancer types
Mortality rates for the top 10 leading cancers in areas with different life expectancy levels are shown in Table 2. Lung cancer was the leading cause of cancer death regardless of life expectancy levels in both men and women. Other cancer types with high mortality rates included cancers of the stomach, liver, esophagus and colorectum. The ASMRW of colorectal and pancreatic cancers in high life expectancy level areas was significantly higher than that in low and middle level areas.

The pattern of ASMRW in men was similar to that in the overall analysis that included both sexes. In low and middle life expectancy level areas, stomach cancer ranked second in cancer mortality in women, followed by liver and esophageal cancers. The mortality of cervical cancer in low life expectancy level areas was higher than that in other areas. The ASMRW of colorectal and breast cancers in women was higher in high life expectancy level areas than that in low and middle level areas.

Discussion
Life expectancy was adopted by the United Nations General Assembly as an important domain of the Sustainable Development Goals (SDGs) in 2015 [8]. It provides an estimate of the average expected life span under certain conditions, based on current mortality rates. It is the most representative and comprehensive index to judge the social economy and healthcare development of a country or region. Differences in life expectancy were significant across different levels of socioeconomic status, including income [18], education [19] and health services [20].

In the present study, 255 geographical units (cities or counties) were divided into 3 levels based on life expectancy: high, middle and low. The analysis showed the highest crude cancer incidence and mortality rate in high life expectancy level areas, whereas the low life expectancy level areas had the lowest crude cancer incidence and mortality. Areas with higher life expectancy typically have higher incidence and relatively lower mortality [21]. In the present study, the high crude cancer incidence in high life expectancy level areas could be mainly attributed to the high incidence of breast and colorectal cancers (Table 1). The incidence of these cancers is relatively low in less developed and developing countries, but is expected to rise with increasing life expectancy, urbanization, and the adoption of a western lifestyle [22, 23].

Consistent with previous studies [24–26], longer life expectancy was associated with a variety of cancers in the present study, including colorectal, breast, thyroid, prostate and bladder cancers. Coinciding with the transforming cancer trends, these cancers constitute a large burden of disease with the aging population in China [12]. China has undergone rapid demographic and epidemiological changes in the past few decades, including striking declines in fertility and increases in life expectancy at birth [27]. The increase in life expectancy is a key driver of years of life lost (YLLs) and the increases of future burden of cancer [28]. The WHO reported that high income countries (e.g., Japan, Switzerland, Singapore and the US) had an average life expectancy of 80 years or more, but low-middle income countries have greater annual increases in life expectancy [8]. The residents of countries with high living standards have lower mortality rates [1]. In the US, overall cancer death rates have decreased by 25% over the past 2 decades [29]. In China, overall cancer mortality continues to decline while cancer incidence remains relatively stable [2, 28]. In this study, we found highest the ASIRW and the lowest ASMRW in high life expectancy level areas. In contrast, low life expectancy level areas had the highest ASMRW.

Lung cancer remains the most commonly diagnosed cancer and the leading cause of cancer deaths. The incidence of lung cancer was positively associated with life expectancy. Underlying risk factors remain unknown, but could include factors other than ageing itself, including cigarette smoking, air pollution and radon exposure,

Table 2 Top 10 cancer mortality in three life expectancy levels areas of China, 2013

Rank	Gender	Low life expectancy level areas				Middle life expectancy level areas				High life expectancy level areas			
		Site	Mortality (1/10⁵)	Proportion (%)	ASR[a] (1/10⁵)	Site	Mortality (1/10⁵)	Proportion (%)	ASR[a] (1/10⁵)	Site	Mortality (1/10⁵)	Proportion (%)	ASR[a] (1/10⁵)
0	Both	All sites	156.51	100.00	118.44	All sites	167.98	100.00	110.99	All sites	200.41	100.00	103.08
1		Lung	38.07	24.32	28.45	Lung	46.05	27.41	29.90	Lung	54.93	27.41	27.43
2		Stomach	26.56	16.97	19.93	Liver	24.56	14.62	16.44	Liver	24.85	12.4	13.61
3		Liver	24.70	15.78	18.73	Stomach	23.32	13.88	15.15	Stomach	22.91	11.43	11.42
4		Esophagus	19.21	12.28	14.38	Esophagus	18.21	10.84	11.77	Colorectum	18.53	9.25	8.94
5		Colorectum	8.75	5.59	6.46	Colorectum	10.94	6.51	7.04	Esophagus	13.02	6.50	6.53
6		Brain, CNS	4.14	2.64	3.35	Pancreas	5.36	3.19	3.51	Pancreas	9.69	4.83	4.86
7		Breast	8.48	2.63	6.30	Breast	9.12	2.67	5.99	Breast	12.26	3.06	6.54
8		Leukemia	3.22	2.06	2.92	Brain, CNS	4.19	2.49	3.09	Leukemia	4.87	2.43	3.20
9		Pancreas	3.18	2.03	2.38	Leukemia	3.86	2.30	3.09	Lymphoma	4.85	2.42	2.61
10		Cervix	4.93	1.53	3.69	Lymphoma	3.00	1.79	2.06	Gallbladder	4.67	2.33	2.24
0	Men	All sites	194.79	100.00	154.68	All sites	210.95	100.00	146.69	All sites	247.26	100.00	134.05
1		Lung	51.47	26.43	40.63	Lung	61.67	29.23	42.34	Lung	73.50	29.73	38.95
2		Stomach	36.02	18.49	28.50	Liver	35.78	16.96	24.93	Liver	36.47	14.75	20.98
3		Liver	35.08	18.01	27.63	Stomach	32.11	15.22	22.16	Stomach	30.98	12.53	16.33
4		Esophagus	25.50	13.09	20.26	Esophagus	24.98	11.84	17.23	Colorectum	20.80	8.41	10.76
5		Colorectum	9.85	5.05	7.73	Colorectum	12.40	5.88	8.51	Esophagus	19.05	7.70	10.26
6		Brain, CNS	4.60	2.36	3.84	Pancreas	6.01	2.85	4.16	Pancreas	10.72	4.33	5.77
7		Pancreas	3.67	1.89	2.91	Brain, CNS	4.53	2.15	3.45	Prostate	6.69	2.71	3.09
8		Leukemia	3.63	1.86	3.31	Leukemia	4.34	2.06	3.55	Lymphoma	5.69	2.30	3.22
9		Lymphoma	2.53	1.30	2.06	Lymphoma	3.62	1.72	2.58	Leukemia	5.62	2.27	3.74
10		Bladder	2.50	1.28	1.95	Bladder	3.10	1.47	2.09	Brain, CNS	4.92	1.99	3.28
0	Women	All sites	115.89	100.00	83.64	All sites	123.62	100.00	77.46	All sites	153.53	100.00	74.37
1		Lung	23.84	20.57	16.78	Lung	29.92	24.21	18.28	Lung	36.35	23.68	16.76
2		Stomach	16.53	14.26	11.6	Stomach	14.24	11.52	8.57	Colorectum	16.26	10.59	7.28
3		Liver	13.69	11.81	9.81	Liver	12.97	10.49	8.10	Stomach	14.83	9.66	6.91
4		Esophagus	12.54	10.82	8.71	Esophagus	11.23	9.09	6.57	Liver	13.22	8.61	6.43
5		Breast	8.48	7.31	6.30	Colorectum	9.43	7.63	5.68	Breast	12.26	7.99	6.54
6		Colorectum	7.58	6.54	5.29	Breast	9.12	7.38	5.99	Pancreas	8.65	5.64	3.98
7		Cervix	4.93	4.25	3.69	Pancreas	4.69	3.80	2.89	Esophagus	6.99	4.55	2.99
8		Brain, CNS	3.64	3.14	2.87	Brain, CNS	3.84	3.11	2.71	Gallbladder	4.97	3.24	2.20
9		Uterus	3.22	2.78	2.38	Cervix	3.65	2.96	2.38	Ovary	4.62	3.01	2.51
10		Leukemia	2.80	2.41	2.53	Leukemia	3.36	2.71	2.64	Leukemia	4.13	2.69	2.70

[a] ASR: age-standardized mortality rate (Segi's Standard Population)

as previously suggested by epidemiological studies [30, 31]. With the tobacco epidemic shifting to less developed areas, lung cancer incidence is also increasing in developing regions. Cigarette smoking in China has increased substantially since the 1980s [32]. Smoking is the most important risk factor associated with rising death risks, with 50% of the five million smoking-related deaths worldwide occurring in low- and middle-income countries, and 80% of which are men [33]. In China, the higher rate of smoking was not only in men, but also especially in rural residents [34]. Household air pollution may be another main reason for lung cancer in China, especially in rural areas with the use solid fuels [35].

Breast cancer is the most commonly diagnosed cancer in Chinese women and the disease burden has experienced a rapid growth over the last decade [2, 36]. There is a direct, strong, and meaningful correlation between life expectancy and standardized breast cancer incidence and mortality rates [4]. The age-standardized incidence rate of breast cancer in high life expectancy level areas was 1.6 times as much as that in low life expectancy level areas. Such difference could possibly be attributed to westernization and differences in age at menarche, number of completed births, and other reproductive and hormonal factors [3, 37].

In a previous study, the incidence of colorectal cancer was 6–7 times higher in regions with very high versus low HDI in both sexes [6]. It has been considered one of the clearest markers of transition, as increases in colorectal cancer incidence have generally paralleled increases in human development across most countries [12, 38]. In China, the ASIR of colorectal cancer in urban areas has been reported to be 52% higher than in rural areas [39]. We also observed a positive correlation between life expectancy and the incidence rates of prostate, and pancreatic cancers, but the significance of such association is obscure due to the relatively low incidence rates of these cancers in China [29, 40, 41]. Besides, the incidence of thyroid cancer in high life expectancy level areas was also higher than that in low and middle level areas, likely reflecting improved diagnosis and treatment. Overdiagnosis of thyroid cancer, however, could have also contributed to the association [42, 43]. A finding distinct from that reported in western countries is the fact that cancers of the stomach and liver were major causes of death regardless of life expectancy levels. In contrast to a positive correlation between life expectancy and stomach cancer incidence rate reported by others [25], we did not find any significant correlation between life expectancy and either the incidence or mortality rates of the cancers of the stomach or liver.

The highest ASIR occurred in low life expectancy regions in men, but in high life expectancy regions in women. Such difference could be partially attributed to the higher incidence rates of most common cancers (such as lung, stomach, liver and esophageal cancers) in men in low life expectancy areas (versus in the high life expectancy areas). Factors that influence life expectancy, including health-related behaviors (smoking, obesity, and exercise) and local area characteristics (education, income and government expenditure levels), produce robust impact on the development of cancers [18]. In women, the incidence of breast cancer significantly increased from low life expectancy level areas to high level areas. Ghoncheh's study showed that the incidence of breast cancer increases with increasing life expectancy, increasing urbanization, and the adoption of a western lifestyle [4]. However, earlier detection may have contributed to the observed increase of incidence for both breast and thyroid cancers [33]. Evidently, the major burden of over diagnosis or overtreatment occurs in women [44]. It is noteworthy that cervical cancer incidence was much higher in low life expectancy level areas in the present study, most likely due to disparities in socioeconomic status and access to high-quality health care [45]. In the 2013 report by the NCCR, the highest mortality rate of cervical cancer was in the northwest and southern rural areas (4.4 per 100,000), with the lowest mortality in eastern urban and northeast rural areas (2.1 per 100,000) [12]. Such geographical distribution pattern is consistent with life expectancy differences across the country [46].

The strength of the present study is its wide coverage of geographical locations and socioeconomic status. The study included data from a total of 255 cities and counties across 31 provinces of China and represented a population of 226.5 million people. However, the sampling was not random. Also, the areas covered by the registry probably had disproportionately high levels of economic development levels, and thus longer life expectancy levels than the national average. Nevertheless, the cancer data used in this study represents the best available nationwide data in China. Moreover, we used the same methods to compare cancer incidence and mortality in three urbanization [47] and GDP [48] levels. These findings may provide an important basis for the next phase of HDI research.

Conclusions

Longer life expectancy is associated with overall rising cancer incidence and mortality in China. However, there is a complex relationship between cancer patterns (incidence, mortality and types) and life expectancy. Ongoing trends, as reflected by differences among cities/counties with varying life expectancy, include a reduction in infection-related cancers (for example, stomach, liver and cervical cancers) and an increase in cancers linked to a western lifestyle (for example, breast and colorectal cancers). Strategic planning at the governmental level, including the appropriation of resources and programs must be a priority when considering these changes.

Abbreviations

NCCR: National Central Cancer Registry; ASIR: age-standardized incidence rate; ASMR: age-standardized mortality rate; HDI: Human Development Index; UNDP: United Nations Development Program; NCDC: National Centers for Disease Control and Prevention; IARC/IACR: International Agency for Research on Cancer/International Association of Cancer Registries; CI5: Cancer Incidence in Five Continents.

Authors' contributions

CWQ contributed to the conception and design of the study proposal. ZRS cleared up the data and performed data analysis. GXY and XCF wrote the initial version of the manuscript. CWQ revised the manuscript and assisted with formatting and language editing. All authors read and approved the final manuscript.

Author details

[1] Cancer Research Institute, Cancer Hospital, Xinjiang Medical University, Urumqi 830011, P. R. China. [2] National Office for Cancer Prevention and Control, National Cancer Center/Cancer Hospital, Chinese Academy of Medical Sciences and Peking Union Medical College, Beijing 100021, P. R. China.

Acknowledgements

We acknowledged the contribution of the National Central Cancer Registry and its local branches in providing cancer statistics, data collection, sorting, verification and database creation. The authors assume full responsibility for data analyses and interpretation.

Competing interests

The authors declare that they have no competing interests.

Funding

This study was supported by CAMS Innovation Fund for Medical Sciences (2016-12M-2-004), and Ministry of Science and Technology of China (2014FY121100).

References

1. Torre LA, Bray F, Siegel RL, Ferlay J, Lortet-Tieulent J, Jemal A. Global cancer statistics, 2012. CA Cancer J Clin. 2015;65(2):87–108. https://doi.org/10.3322/caac.21262.
2. Chen W, Zheng R, Baade PD, Zhang S, Zeng H, Bray F, et al. Cancer statistics in China, 2015. CA Cancer J Clin. 2016;66(2):115–32. https://doi.org/10.3322/caac.21338.
3. Fidler MM, Soerjomataram I, Bray F. A global view on cancer incidence and national levels of the Human Development Index. Int J Cancer. 2016;139(11):2436–46.
4. Ghoncheh M, Mirzaei M, Salehiniya H. Incidence and Mortality of Breast Cancer and their Relationship with the Human Development Index (HDI) in the World in 2012. Asian Pac J Cancer Prev. 2016;16(18):8439–43. https://doi.org/10.7314/apjcp.2015.16.18.8439.
5. Rafiemanesh H, Mehtarpour M, Khani F, Hesami SM, Shamlou R, Towhidi F, et al. Epidemiology, incidence and mortality of lung cancer and their relationship with the development index in the world. Asian Pac J Cancer Prev (Apjcp). 2016;17(1):381.
6. Rafiemanesh H, Mohammadianhafshejani A, Ghoncheh M, Sepehri Z, Shamlou R, Salehiniya H, et al. Incidence and mortality of colorectal cancer and relationships with the Human Development Index across the world. Asian Pac J Cancer Prev (Apjcp). 2016;17(5):2465.
7. Horton S, Gauvreau CL. Cancer in low- and middle-income countries: an economic overview. In: Gelband H, Jha P, Sankaranarayanan R, Horton S, editors. Cancer: disease control priorities. 3rd ed. Washington (DC): The International Bank for Reconstruction and Development; 2015.
8. World Health Organization. World health statistics. Monitoring health for the SDGs Sustainable Development Goals. 41st ed. Geneva: World Health Organization; 2016. p. 293–328.
9. Koh HK, Blakey CR, Roper AY. Healthy People 2020. JAMA. 2014;311(24):2475–6.
10. Pe Ntilde la, oacute pez. Human Development Index. Chapters. 2010;8707:3012-3.
11. China NBoSo. Statistical communiqué of the People's Republic of China on the 2016 National Economic and Social http://www.stats.gov.cn/english/PressRelease/201702/t20170228_1467503.html. Accessed 28 Feb 2017.
12. Chen W, Zheng R, Zhang S, Zeng H, Xia C, Zuo T, et al. Cancer incidence and mortality in China, 2013. Cancer Lett. 2017;401:63–71. https://doi.org/10.1016/j.canlet.2017.04.024.
13. Chen W, Zheng R, Zuo T, Zeng H, Zhang S, He J. National cancer incidence and mortality in China, 2012. Chin J Cancer Res. 2016;28(1):1–11. https://doi.org/10.3978/j.issn.1000-9604.2016.02.08.
14. Chen W, Zheng R, Zhang S, Zhao P, Zeng H, Zou X. Report of cancer incidence and mortality in China, 2010. Ann Transl Med. 2014;2(7):61. https://doi.org/10.3978/j.issn.2305-5839.2014.04.05.
15. Siegel RL, Miller KD, Jemal A. Cancer statistics, 2016. CA Cancer J Clin. 2016;66(1):7–30. https://doi.org/10.3322/caac.21332.
16. Curado MP, Edwards B, Shin HR, Storm H, Ferlay J, Heanue M, Boyle P. Cancer Incidence in Five Continents, vol. IX. Lyon: IARC Scientific Publications; 2008.
17. Cancer IAfRo. IARCcrgTools. 2008. http://iarccrgtools.software.informer.com/. Accessed 8 May 2018.
18. Chetty R, Stepner M, Abraham S, Lin S, Scuderi B, Turner N, et al. The association between income and life expectancy in the United States, 2001–2014. JAMA. 2016;315(16):1750–66.
19. Hendi AS. Trends in US life expectancy gradients: the role of changing educational composition. Int J Epidemiol. 2015;44(3):946–55.
20. Stenberg K, Hanssen O, Edejer TT, Bertram M, Brindley C, Meshreky A, et al. Financing transformative health systems towards achievement of the health Sustainable Development Goals: a model for projected resource needs in 67 low-income and middle-income countries. Lancet Glob Health. 2017;5(9):e875.
21. Zhou M, Wang H, Zhu J, Chen W, Wang L, Liu S, et al. Cause-specific mortality for 240 causes in China during 1990–2013: a systematic subnational analysis for the Global Burden of Disease Study 2013. Lancet. 2016;387(10015):251–72.
22. Hajmanoochehri F, Asefzadeh S, Kazemifar AM, Ebtehaj M. Clinicopathological features of colon adenocarcinoma in Qazvin, Iran: a 16 year study. Asian Pac J Cancer Prev (Apjcp). 2014;15(2):951.
23. World Health Organization. Breast cancer: prevention and control. World Health Stat Ann. 2012;41(7):697–700.
24. Khazaei S, Rezaeian S, Khazaei S, Mansori K, Sanjari MA, Ayubi E. Effects of human development index and its components on colorectal cancer incidence and mortality: a global ecological study. Asian Pac J Cancer Prev (Apjcp). 2016;17:253.
25. Khazaei S, Rezaeian S, Soheylizad M, Khazaei S, Biderafsh A. Global incidence and mortality rates of stomach cancer and the Human Development Index: an ecological study. Asian Pac J Cancer Prev. 2016;17(4):1701–4.
26. Greiman AK, Rosoff JS, Prasad SM. Association of Human Development Index with global bladder, kidney, prostate and testis cancer incidence and mortality. BJU Int. 2017;120:799–807.
27. Yang G, Wang Y, Zeng Y, Gao GF, Liang X, Zhou M, et al. Rapid health transition in China, 1990–2010: findings from the Global Burden of Disease Study 2010. Lancet. 2013;381(9882):1987–2015.

28. Fitzmaurice C, Dicker D, Pain A, Hamavid H, Moradilakeh M, Macintyre MF, et al. The global burden of cancer 2013. Jama Oncol. 2015;1(4):505.

29. Siegel RL, Miller KD, Jemal A. Cancer Statistics, 2017. CA Cancer J Clin. 2017;67(1):5.

30. Ridge CA, Mcerlean AM, Ginsberg MS. Epidemiology of lung cancer. Chest. 1996;32(1):133.

31. Guo Y, Zeng H, Zheng R, Li S, Barnett AG, Zhang S, et al. The association between lung cancer incidence and ambient air pollution in China: a spatiotemporal analysis. Environ Res. 2016;144(Pt A):60–5.

32. Chen ZM, Peto R, Iona A, Guo Y, Chen YP, Bian Z, et al. Emerging tobacco-related cancer risks in China: a nationwide, prospective study of 0.5 million adults. Cancer. 2015;121(S17):3097–106.

33. Freddie Bray SI. The changing global burden of cancer: transitions in human development and implications for cancer prevention and control. In: Gelband H, Jha P, Sankaranarayanan R, Horton S, editors. Cancer: disease control priorities, vol. 9. 3rd ed. Washington (DC): The World Bank; 2015. p. 363.

34. Li Q, Hsia J, Yang G. Prevalence of smoking in China in 2010. N Engl J Med. 2011;364(25):2469–70.

35. Wei JS, Hu W, Vermeulen R, Hosgood HD, Downward GS, Chapman RS, et al. Household air pollution and lung cancer in China: a review of studies in Xuanwei. Chin J Cancer. 2014;33(10):471–5.

36. Jia M, Zheng R, Zhang S, Zeng H, Zou X, Chen W. Female breast cancer incidence and mortality in 2011, China. J Thorac Dis. 2015;7(7):1221.

37. Bray F, Mccarron P, Parkin DM. The changing global patterns of female breast cancer incidence and mortality. Breast Cancer Res. 2004;6(6):229.

38. Arnold M, Sierra MS, Laversanne M, Soerjomataram I, Jemal A, Bray F. Global patterns and trends in colorectal cancer incidence and mortality. Gut. 2017;66(4):683–91.

39. Liu S, Zheng R, Zhang M, Zhang S, Sun X, Chen W. Incidence and mortality of colorectal cancer in China, 2011. Chin J Cancer Res. 2015;27(1):22.

40. Wong MC, Goggins WB, Wang HH, Fung FD, Leung C, Wong SY, et al. global incidence and mortality for prostate cancer: analysis of temporal patterns and trends in 36 countries. Eur Urol. 2016;70(5):862–74.

41. Tominaga S. Epidemiology of pancreatic cancer. Semin Surg Oncol. 2016;15(44):3–7.

42. La VC, Malvezzi M, Bosetti C, Garavello W, Bertuccio P, Levi F, et al. Thyroid cancer mortality and incidence: a global overview. Int J Cancer. 2015;136(9):2187.

43. Baker SR, Bhatti WA. The thyroid cancer epidemic: is it the dark side of the CT revolution? Eur J Radiol. 2006;60(1):67–9.

44. Davies L, Welch HG. Current thyroid cancer trends in the United States. Jama Otolaryngol Head Neck Surg. 2014;140(4):317–22.

45. Du P-L, Wu K-S, Fang J-Y, Zeng Y, Xu Z-X, Tang W-R, et al. Cervical cancer mortality trends in China, 1991–2013, and predictions for the future. Asian Pac J Cancer Prev. 2015;16(15):6391–6. https://doi.org/10.7314/apjcp.2015.16.15.6391.

46. Xia C, Ding C, Zheng R, Zhang S, Zeng H, Wang J, et al. Trends in geographical disparities for cervical cancer mortality in China from 1973 to 2013: a subnational spatio-temporal study. Chin J Cancer Res. 2017;29(6):487–95.

47. Chen W, Zheng R, Zhang S, Zeng H, Zuo T, Xia C, et al. Cancer incidence and mortality in China in 2013: an analysis based on urbanization level. Chin J Cancer Res. 2017;29(1):1–10. https://doi.org/10.21147/j.issn.1000-9604.2017.01.01.

48. Yang Z, Zheng R, Zhang S, Zeng H, Xia C, Li H, et al. Comparison of cancer incidence and mortality in three GDP per capita levels in China, 2013. Chin J Cancer Res (Chung-kuo yen cheng yen chiu). 2017;29(5):385.

2

Transcriptomic but not genomic variability confers phenotype of breast cancer stem cells

Mengying Tong[1†], Ziqian Deng[1,2†], Mengying Yang[1], Chang Xu[1], Xiaolong Zhang[1], Qingzheng Zhang[1], Yuwei Liao[1], Xiaodi Deng[1], Dekang Lv[1], Xuehong Zhang[1], Yu Zhang[1], Peiying Li[1], Luyao Song[1], Bicheng Wang[2,3], Aisha Al-Dherasi[1], Zhiguang Li[1*] and Quentin Liu[1,2*]

Abstract

Background: Breast cancer stem cells (BCSCs) are considered responsible for cancer relapse and drug resistance. Understanding the identity of BCSCs may open new avenues in breast cancer therapy. Although several discoveries have been made on BCSC characterization, the factors critical to the origination of BCSCs are largely unclear. This study aimed to determine whether genomic mutations contribute to the acquisition of cancer stem-like phenotype and to investigate the genetic and transcriptional features of BCSCs.

Methods: We detected potential BCSC phenotype-associated mutation hotspot regions by using whole-genome sequencing on parental cancer cells and derived serial-generation spheres in increasing order of BCSC frequency, and then performed target deep DNA sequencing at bulk-cell and single-cell levels. To identify the transcriptional program associated with BCSCs, bulk-cell and single-cell RNA sequencing was performed.

Results: By using whole-genome sequencing of bulk cells, potential BCSC phenotype-associated mutation hotspot regions were detected. Validation by target deep DNA sequencing, at both bulk-cell and single-cell levels, revealed no genetic changes specifically associated with BCSC phenotype. Moreover, single-cell RNA sequencing showed profound transcriptomic variability in cancer cells at the single-cell level that predicted BCSC features. Notably, this transcriptomic variability was enriched during the transcription of 74 genes, revealed as BCSC markers. Breast cancer patients with a high risk of relapse exhibited higher expression levels of these BCSC markers than those with a low risk of relapse, thereby highlighting the clinical significance of predicting breast cancer prognosis with these BCSC markers.

Conclusions: Transcriptomic variability, not genetic mutations, distinguishes BCSCs from non-BCSCs. The identified 74 BCSC markers have the potential of becoming novel targets for breast cancer therapy.

Keywords: Breast cancer, Cancer stem cell, Genomics, Sequencing, Transcriptomics

Background

Traditional breast cancer therapies that target bulk cell populations often have substantial short-term effects, and the existence of breast cancer stem cells (BCSCs) is a major barrier for achieving curability. BCSCs are cells that have the ability to self-renew, and they are considered responsible for key aspects of tumors, such as tumor

initiation, progression, and drug resistance [1–5]. Therefore, approaches targeting BCSCs have important clinical implications [6]. Although several discoveries have been made on BCSC characterization [7–9], the origin of BCSCs is still unclear. Currently, two models are usually proposed to explain BCSCs. The first model [10, 11] is clonal evolution, in which tumor cells progressively accumulate mutations, some of which confer the ability of self-renewal and allow tumor cells with these mutations to become BCSCs and out-compete other tumor cells. This model is a canonical hardwired BCSC hierarchy, and BCSC dedication is largely defined by intrinsic

*Correspondence: zhiguangli2013@126.com; liuq9@mail.sysu.edu.cn
†Mengying Tong and Ziqian Deng contributed equally to this work
[1] Center of Genome and Personalized Medicine, Institute of Cancer Stem Cell, Dalian Medical University, Dalian 116044, Liaoning, P. R. China
Full list of author information is available at the end of the article

genetic properties. In the second model [12, 13], BCSCs do not necessarily acquire mutations and are instructed by dedicated niche signals following competition dynamics. Breast cancer cells can be reprogrammed into BCSCs through plasticity in tumor microenvironment.

To determine the factors critical to the origination of BCSCs, we assumed that genetic mutations contributes to the acquisition of cancer stem-like phenotypes, e.g., BCSCs specifically carry heritable genetic changes. We then tested this hypothesis using next-generation sequencing (NGS) analysis, including whole-genome sequencing (WGS), target deep DNA sequencing, and transcriptome sequencing at both bulk-cell and single-cell levels.

Materials and methods

Cell culture

The human breast cancer cell line MDA-MB-231 was obtained from the American Type Culture Collection (ATCC). The cell line was authenticated at ATCC before purchase by the standard short tandem repeat DNA typing and cultured in its standard medium as recommended by ATCC.

Sphere formation assay

The single-cell suspension was obtained by trypsinization. Clumped cells were excluded with a 40-μm sieve. Single cells were plated in ultra-low attachment 6-well plates (Corning, NY, USA) at a low density (1000 cells/well). The cells were maintained in serum-free Dulbecco's modified eagle medium/nutrient mixture F12 (DMEM/F12, Gibco, Waltham, MA, USA) supplemented with B27 (Invitrogen, Waltham, MA, USA), 20 ng/mL epidermal growth factor (EGF, Sigma, Darmstadt, Germany), and 20 ng/mL basic fibroblast growth factor (bFGF, BD Biosciences, Franklin Lakes, NJ, USA) for 7–10 days. For sphere passage, the spheres were collected by centrifugation (1000 rpm, 5 min), dissociated with trypsin-ethylene diamine tetraacetic acid (EDTA), and mechanically dispersed. The resulting single cells were then centrifuged (1000 rpm, 5 min) to remove the enzyme and re-suspended in serum-free medium. The spheres were passed every 7–10 days, and only spheres bigger than 50 μm in diameter were included in the analyses.

Serial sphere formation assay

The single-cell suspension of MDA-MB-231 cells was obtained by trypsinization. Cells were seeded in an ultra-low attachment 96-well plate (1 cell/well). The cells were maintained in serum-free DMEM/F12 supplemented with B27, and 20 ng/mL EGF, 20 ng/mL bFGF. Only wells that initially contained a single cell were used for subsequent studies. For sphere passage, the single cell-derived

sphere was sucked up by a micro-pipette, dissociated with a small amount of trypsin-EDTA, and mechanically dispersed. The resulting single cells were then re-suspended in serum-free medium. The spheres were passed every 7–10 days, and only spheres bigger than 50 μm in diameter were included in the analyses.

ALDEFLUOR assay by fluorescence activated cell sorting (FACS)

The ALDEFLUOR kit (STEMCELL, Vancouver, British Columbia, Canada, Cat. 01700) was used for isolating the cell population with high aldehyde dehydrogenase (ALDH) enzymatic activity. Cells were suspended in an ALDEFLUOR assay buffer containing ALDH substrate bodipy aminoacetaldehyde (BAAA, 1 mol/L per 1×10^6 cells) and incubated for 45 min at 37 °C. As negative controls, for each example of cells, an aliquot was treated with 50 mmol/L diethylaminobenzaldehyde (DEAB), a specific ALDH inhibitor. The ALDH-positive subpopulation was isolated by FACS.

Transwell invasion assay

Parental cells (MDA-MB-231) were obtained by trypsinization and resuspended in pure DMEM. Spheres bigger than 50 μm were obtained through a 40-μm cell strainer (Meilun Biotechnology, Dalian, Liaoning, China). Then the spheres were centrifuged (1000 rpm, 5 min), dissociated with trypsin-EDTA, and mechanically dispersed in pure DMEM. For every chamber, 30,000 cells were placed onto 1% matrigel (BD Biosciences)-coated membrane in the upper chamber (24-well insert, 8 μm, Corning, Cat. 3422). Medium with 10% fetal bovine serum (FBS, Gibco) was used as an attractant in the lower chamber. After being incubated for 24 h, cells that invaded through the membrane were fixed with 4% paraformaldehyde and stained with 0.1% crystal violet. The stained cell images were captured under a microscope (Olympus, Tokyo, Japan), and cells were counted for five random fields at ×10 magnification. Results are presented as mean ± standard deviation from at least three independent experiments.

RNA extraction, reverse transcription-PCR, and quantitative real-time PCR

Total RNA was extracted by using TRIzol reagent (Life Technologies, Waltham, MA, USA). cDNA was generated by reverse transcription-PCR using EasyScript One-Step gDNA Removal and cDNA Synthesis SuperMix Kit (TransGen Biotech, Beijing, China) according to the manufacturer's instructions. Quantitative real-time polymerase chain reaction (qRT-PCR) was performed by using the chamQ Universal SYBR qPCR Master Mix (Vazyme, Najing, Jiangsu, China) in a MX3000p cycler

(Stratagene, La Jolla, CA, USA). Changes of mRNA levels were detected by the $2^{-\Delta\Delta CT}$ method using Actin for internal crossing normalization. Detailed primer sequences for qRT-PCR are listed in Additional file 1: Table S1.

Western blot analysis

Samples were lysed on ice in RIPA buffer (50 mmol/L Tris [pH 8.0], 150 mmol/L sodium chloride, 0.5% sodium deoxycholate, 0.1% sodium dodecyl sulfate, and 1% NP-40) supplemented with protease inhibitors [1 mmol/L Na_3VO_4, 1 µg/mL leupeptin, and 1 mmol/L phenylmethanesulfonyl fluoride (PMSF)]. The protein concentration was detected by the Coomassie brilliant blue dye method. In all, equal amounts of protein per lane were run in 10% sodium dodecyl sulfate-polyacrylamide electrophoresis gels and subsequently transferred to a nitrocellulose membrane (Millipore, Darmstadt, Germany) via submerged transfer. After blocking the membrane with 5% milk at room temperature for 1 h, the membrane was incubated overnight at 4 °C with various primary antibodies. After incubation with peroxidase-conjugated secondary antibodies (Thermo Scientific, Waltham, MA, USA) for 1 h at room temperature, the signals were visualized using an enhanced chemiluminescence western blot detection kit (K-12045-D50; Apgbio, Beijing, China) according to the manufacturer's instructions. The blots were developed using the Bio-Rad Molecular Imager instrument (Bio-Rad, Berkeley, CA, USA). The information regarding the antibodies used are listed as follows: mouse anti-human monoclonal ACTB antibody (Proteintech, Chicago, IL, USA, 66009-1-Ig), rabbit anti-human monoclonal NANOG antibody (Abcam, Cambridge, England, ab109250), mouse anti-human monoclonal SOX2 antibody (Santa Cruz Biotechnology, Santa Cruz, CA, USA, sc-365823).

Whole-genome sequencing and data processing in bulk cells

DNA extraction, library preparation, and sequencing

The genomic DNA of bulk cells (1×10^6 cells) was extracted using the ALLPrep DNA/RNA Mini Kit (Qiagen, Hilden, Germany, Cat. 80204) according to the manufacturer's manual. Quantified 50 ng genomic DNA was used to prepare the paired-end library using the TruePrep DNA library Prep Kit V2 for Illumina (Vazyme, Cat. TD-501). The quality and concentration of DNA fragments in the DNA libraries generated were assessed using High-Sensitivity Bioanalyzer (Agilent, Santa Clara, CA, USA). The prepared library was then subjected to Illumina HiSeqXten Sequencer (San Diego, CA, USA) with the paired-end 150 bp read option.

Reads mapping and variants calling

The Feb. 2009 human reference sequence (GRCh37) was used in this study, and it was produced by the Genome Reference Consortium. BWA MEM (version 0.7.12) was used to align all paired-end reads to the Hg 19 reference genome with default parameters. We performed base quality score recalibration and local realignment using the Genome Analysis Toolkit (GATK, version 3.6). The duplicated reads were marked using the function "MarkDuplicates" of Picard Tools (version 1.126) and then removed. Following this, variants were called using SAMtools mpileup with the following parameters: -Q 30 −q 10. The variants [single nucleotide variant (SNV) and indel] were identified by VarScan (version 2.3.7) mpileup2cns with the following parameters: --min-coverage 2 --min-reads2 1 --variants 1 --P value 0.05 --min-var-freq 0.1.

Variant filtering

In each sample [the parental cells (2D) and derived spheres of the first generation (SP1) and fourth generation (SP4)], putative SNVs and indels were filtered with the following criteria: (1) calls falling on the mitochondria genome, Y chromosome, unknown chromosome, genomic SuperDups, and RepeatMasker regions (available on the download page at the University of California Santa Cruz website (http://www.genome.ucsc.edu/) were removed and (2) depth range from 10 to 200. Finally, we obtained 1,628,063 variant sites, including SNV and indel, existing in at least one sample.

Further variant selection for hotspot calling

We assumed that sample 2D possess the lowest proportion of BCSCs, while SP4 the highest; then, the proportion of the cell population carrying variants were increased from 2D to SP4, which was quantified by variant allele frequency (VAF). Thus, to select significantly increased sites based on VAF between 2D and SP4, we performed the Fisher's exact test on the read counts supporting the reference and variation in each site. A total of 30,797 sites were considered significantly increased from 2D to SP4 and were selected for calling hotspots following the two conditions: P value less than 0.1 and the VAF of 2D less than the VAF of SP4.

Target deep DNA sequencing and data processing in bulk cells

Amplicon primer design

We selected 54 hotspots for the multi-PCR target validation design. ION AmpliSeq Designer (http://www.ampliseq.com) was able to successfully design amplicon primers for 97% of the targets. For hotspots with a length less than 500 bp, amplicon primers were designed to cover the whole regions, otherwise, amplicon primers were designed covering the SNV sites in the hotspots. According to this principle, we designed 128 amplicons to target these 54 hotspots (Additional file 2: Table S2).

Library preparation and sequencing for amplicons

The detailed protocol of target deep DNA sequencing was as follows:

A. Multiplex PCR amplification: The 128 amplicons were amplified by multiplex PCR on Veriti 96-well Thermal Cycler (Applied Biosystems, Waltham, MA, USA), which was performed using 30 ng genomic DNA, 15 μL Primer mix/pool (2 pools in total), 10 μL Q5 reaction buffer (NEB, Ipswich, MA, USA, Cat. B9027S), 10 μL Q5 high GC enhancer (NEB, Cat. B9028A), 1.5 μL dNTPs mix (NEB, Cat. N0447S), 0.5 μL Q5 high-fidelity DNA polymerase (NEB, Cat. M0491L), and ddH$_2$O to make the final reaction volume to 50 μL. The reaction system was incubated initially at 98 °C for 30 s. Fifteen cycles of PCR were performed at 98 °C for 10 s and 62 °C for 4 min. Then, the reaction was held at 4 °C.

B. Column purification of PCR product: All PCR products were purified using DNA Purification Kit (TIANGEN, Beijing, China, Cat. DP214-03).

C. End repair and A-tailing of DNA fragments: The mixture of 37.5 μL DNA, 5 μL Cut Smart (NEB, Cat. B7204S), 5 μL Adenosine 5′-Triphosphate (NEB, Cat. P0756L), 0.5 μL of 100 mmol/L dATP solution (NEB, Cat. N0440S), 1 μL T4 Polynucleotide Kinase (NEB, Cat. M0201L) and 1 μL 5 units Klenow exo-DNA polymerase (NEB, Cat. M0212L) was incubated at 37 °C for 1 h on Veriti 96-well Thermal Cycler.

D. Column purification: The PCR products were purified with Universal DNA Purification Kit (TIANGEN, Cat. DP214-03).

E. Adapter ligation: The mixture of 25 μL A-tailed DNA, 1 μL of 50 μmol/L multiplexing adapter, 3 μL of 10× T4 DNA ligase buffer (NEB, Cat. B0202), and 1 μL of 400 units/μL T4 DNA ligase (NEB, Cat. M0202L) was used in adapter ligation step followed by incubation at 16 °C overnight.

F. Ampure cleanup of adapter-ligated reaction: We added 1 × volume (30 μL) of Agencourt AMPure XP DNA beads (BECKMAN, Brea, CA, USA, Cat. 15604000) and incubated at room temperature for 5–10 min and then placed on magnetic stand. We discarded the supernatant which contained primer dimers. Beads were washed twice with 200 μL of 80% ethanol for 30 s at room temperature and dried at room temperature for 5–10 min. Then, 25 μL Buffer EB was added to the beads, mixed up and down for ten times, incubated for 2 min at room temperature, and put on magnetic stand at room temperature for about 5 min. After that, 22 μL of supernatant was transferred to a new PCR tube.

G. PCR amplification: PCR enrichment was conducted by using 22 μL Adapter-ligated DNA, 25 μL of 2 × NEB Next high-fidelity PCR master buffer (NEB, Cat. M0541L), 1.5 μL of 10 μmol/L MUP primer, 1.5 μL of 10 μmol/L barcode primer. The reaction was incubated initially at 98 °C for 3 min. Fifteen cycles of PCR were performed at 98 °C for 20 s, 65 °C for 15 s, and 72 °C for 20 s. The reaction was then held at 4 °C.

H. Extraction and purification of the final library: electrophoresis was conducted in agarose gel with the PCR products from the last step and then extracting and purifying DNA from agarose gel using the gel extraction kit (TIANGEN, Cat. DP214-03).

I. Quality control and sequencing of the final library: The quality and concentration of DNA fragments in the DNA libraries generated were assessed using High-Sensitivity Bioanalyzer. The prepared library was then subjected to Illumina HiSeqXten with the paired-end 150 bp read option.

Data processing

The sequence of primer regions was first trimmed off from the fastq data by PrimerTrim. (available at http://github.com/DMU-lilab). BWA MEM (version 0.7.12) was then used to align primer-removed reads to the Hg 19 reference genome with default parameters. We removed secondary alignments and alternative hits by SAMtools with the following parameters: x XA –F 0x100. Then, variants were called using SAMtools mpileup with the following parameters: -Q 30 -q 10. The variants (SNV and indel) were identified by VarScan (version 2.3.7) mpileup2cns with the following parameters: --min-coverage 60 --min-reads2 1 --variants 1 --P value 0.05 --min-var-freq 0.1.

Single-cell target deep DNA sequencing
Characterization of the cancer hotspot mutation (CHM) panel and amplicon design

The targeted genes and mutations are listed in Additional file 3: Table S3, including the whole exonic region of 48 cancer hotspot genes (from 50 cancer hotspot genes identified by the Mayo Clinic) and 1513 mutations. Of the 1513 mutations, 224 were identified from The Cancer Genome Atlas (TCGA, https://cancergenome.nih.gov/) data, and 1286 were identified from the Catalogue Of Somatic Mutations In Cancer (COSMIC, https://cancer.sanger.ac.uk/cosmic/) data, and 3 were identified from both databases. ION AmpliSeq Designer (Thermo Fisher, http://www.ampliseq.com) was used to design 128 amplicons covering the WGS hotspot mutation (WHM) panel (Additional file 2: Table S2) and 3124 amplicons covering the hotspots in the CHM panel (Additional file 4: Table S4).

Single-cell isolation, genomic DNA extraction, and multiple displacement amplification (MDA)

Single cells or single spheres were sucked up by a micropipette. Whole genome amplification (WGA) was performed to these cells using the Discover-sc Single Cell Kit (Vazyme, Cat. N601-01) according to the manufacturer's manual, and a reaction of human tissue genomic DNA was marked as a positive control. The amplified DNA products were then stored at $-20\,^{\circ}\text{C}$.

Quantification and genome-integrity assessment of WGA products

The DNA concentration of the WGA products was measured using the Qubit Quantitation platform (Life Technologies, Invitrogen, Waltham, MA, USA). Ten housekeeping genes located on different chromosomes were selected to check the coverage of amplified products. WGA products of best performance in relation to housekeeping PCR ($>8/10$) and Qubit assays (>60 ng/μL) were selected for downstream experiments. All of the above steps were performed with a sample of genomic DNA from human tissue as a positive control.

Library preparation and sequencing for amplicons

Target regions were amplified by multiplex PCR in WGA products. Choosing the correct number of cycles for the multiplex PCR is critical based on the starting amount and coverage of WGA products. The quality and concentration of the DNA libraries generated was assessed using High-Sensitivity Bioanalyzer. The prepared target libraries were then subjected to Illumina HiseqXten with the paired-end 150 bp read option.

Single-cell RNA sequencing (scRNA-seq)
Generation of scRNA-seq libraries

The generation of single-cell cDNA libraries was implemented by the Discover-sc WTA Kit (Vazyme, Cat. N711-01) according to the manufacturer's manual for single cell-derived spheres and single cells. Quantified 1 ng amplified cDNA was then used to prepare the paired-end library using TruePrep DNA library Prep Kit V2 for Illumina (Vazyme, Cat. TD-503). The quality and concentration of DNA fragments in the cDNA libraries generated was assessed using High-Sensitivity Bioanalyzer. Massively parallel RNA sequencing (RNA-seq) was performed on the Illumina HiSeqXten platform with

paired-end 150-bp read-length by Berry Genomic Corporation (Beijing, China).

Data analysis

TopHat2 was used to align reads according to the University of California Santa Cruz hg19 reference genome, and the corresponding gene annotation format file from GENCODE was fed to the TopHat2 for defining transcript coordinates. Gene-level expression abundance (fragments per kilobase of exon per million fragments mapped) and the results of differential gene expression analysis were obtained from the Cufflinks package. By the comparison between BCSCs and non-BCSCs, we identified the differentially expressed gene set according to the fold change (FC) and false discovery rate (FDR). Genes with FDR < 0.05 and log2-transformed FC > 1 were considered to be highly expressed in BCSCs.

Gene set enrichment analysis

The gene expression dataset containing gene symbols and gene expression values of 8 single-cell RNA-seq samples were submitted to gene set enrichment analysis (GSEA) (version v2.2.1) software [14] according to the GSEA user guide. GSEA was performed with the gene set of MSigDB: Gene Ontology Biological Process. The nominal P value < 0.01 and FDR < 0.25 were used to investigate significantly enriched gene sets.

Kaplan–Meier (KM) survival analysis

To investigate the association between BCSC highly expressed genes and patient survival, we evaluated the relapse-free survival after surgery in all patients available in the Kaplan–Meier plotter online database [15] (http://kmplot.com/analysis/index.php?p=background). A user-selected probe set was chosen, and patients were grouped according to the optimized cut-off.

Interaction analysis in the STRING database

A newly identified BCSC marker gene set was submitted to the STRING database [16] (https://string-db.org/cgi) to identify associated genes and pathways. Interactions including curated databases and experimentally determined gene neighborhoods, gene fusions, gene co-occurrence, text mining, co-expression, and protein homology were investigated.

Survival analysis in pan-cancer

The table of survival z scores collapsed by cancer/cancer subtype was downloaded from the PREdiction of Clinical Outcomes from Genomic Profiles (PRECOG) database (https://precog.stanford.edu/index.php) [17]. For the z scores of the BCSC marker gene set in pan-cancer, we made a hierarchical clustering analysis in R (version

3.3.2) using the hclust function (https://stat.ethz.ch/R-manual/R-devel/library/stats/html/hclust.html).

Biomarker validation by SurvExpress

Nine breast cancer relapse datasets were analyzed for the BCSC marker gene set in the SurvExpress online database [18] (http://bioinformatica.mty.itesm.mx:8080/Biomatec/SurvivaX.jsp). A Cox regression model was used to generate 2 risk groups by splitting the samples at the median after ranking by their prognostic index, which were estimated using beta coefficients multiplied by gene expression values. The box plot obtained as the results of SurvExpress visualized the expression levels of each gene in the risk groups generated. The P value was obtained from a t test for two groups.

Analysis of differential gene expression between cancer and normal tissues from the TCGA dataset

Gene expression data of 38 cancer types were downloaded from FireBrowse (http://firebrowse.org). To ensure sufficient statistical power, the number of either normal or cancer samples was at least 5, and 22 of 38 cancer types meet the requirement and were used for the following analysis. Differential gene expression between normal and cancer samples were evaluated by t test.

Statistical analyses
Hotspot calling

After potential BCSC-associated SNV sites were identified by WGS in bulk cells, a statistical model was established to call hotspot regions where variants (30,797 variants in all) were densely distributed. When the mutations in a given length of DNA were considered as Poisson distributed, and the distance between two adjacent mutations followed an exponential distribution (Additional file 7: Fig. S1a). Then, the probability of a given distance could be calculated as follows:

$$P(x) = 1 - e^{-\lambda x} \left(\lambda = \frac{1}{\bar{x}}, x > 0 \right)$$

where x refers to the distance between two adjacent SNV sites and $\bar{x}$ refers to the average distance of all two adjacent SNV sites in the genome.

Thereafter, hotspot regions were detected using Run-length encoding (RLE) algorithm (Additional file 7: Fig. S1b). Hotspots with length longer than 100,000 bp were removed, and 54 hotspots were obtained (Additional file 5: Table S5). Specifically, the median length of the hotspots was 318 bp, and most hotspots overlapped with intronic and intergenic regions (Additional file 7: Fig. S1c and S1d). Subsequently, we calculated the P value evaluating the significance of the hotspot regions as follows:

$$P(X \geq m) = 1 - P(X < m)$$

$$= 1 - \sum_{i=0}^{m-1} \frac{\binom{b}{i} \times \binom{a-b}{n+m-i}}{\binom{a}{n+m}}$$

where a stands for the total number of distances of two adjacent SNV sites, b stands for the number of distances whose exponential distribution P value (P_{exp}) < 0.01 (in our case a = 30,774, b = 4003), n stands for the number of distances allowed within a hotspot whose $P_{exp} \geq 0.01$, and m stands for the number of distances whose $P_{exp} < 0.01$. X is the random variable representing the number of distances with $P_{exp} < 0.01$ in a region. Under the minimum requirement ($m = 5$, $n = 1$) of our hotspot-calling algorithm, P was equal to 1.988×10^{-4}.

Computation of the genetic distance between every two samples (single cells)

At a given position, the genetic distance between C1 and C2 was exemplified as follows. We defined C1 = (C_1W_A, C_1W_T, C_1W_G, C_1W_C) and C2 = (C_2W_A, C_2W_T, C_2W_G, C_2W_C), where C_1W_A refers to the weight (i.e., proportion) of read counts supporting base "A" of sample C1, and C_2W_T refers to the weight of read counts supporting base "T" of sample C2, as an analogy). Then, the genetic distance (d) between C1 and C2 was calculated by the Pythagorean formula:

$$d(C1, C2) = \sqrt{\left(\sum_{n=A,T,G,C} (C_1W_n - C_2W_n) \right)^2}$$

Analysis of base-position differences between BCSCs and non-BCSCs (single cells)

Step 1. Acquiring for binary alignment (BAM) files.

BAM files were generated using the pipeline identical to the target deep DNA sequencing of bulk cells, as described under "Data processing" in the subsection "Target deep DNA sequencing and data processing in bulk cells".

Step 2. Count data.

Nucleotides were counted from recalibrated BAM files using Rsamtools (http://bioconductor.org/packages/release/bioc/html/Rsamtools.html). Only positions in the target regions and covered by all samples were kept for further analysis. Here, the following was denoted for the considered position:

Total count (TC) = sum of A, T, C, and G counts

Major count (MC) = the highest nucleotide count

Background count (BC) = TC − MC

Subscript $c =$ BCSCs

Subscript $n =$ non-BCSCs

Step 3. Position error rate [19] (PER) of non-BCSCs (the two single cells).

At each position, we estimated the PER of non-BCSCs as follows:

$$PER_n = \frac{\sum BC_n}{\sum TC_n}$$

Step 4. Binomial analysis of BCSCs (the three spheres).

At each base position, we calculated the probability of BC_c (PBC) from a binomial distribution with the parameter PER (corrected). PBC represents the statistical probability to observe the specific number of background allele at a position. PER was obtained as in Step 3 from the two non-BCSC single cells. The following is the PBC calculation formula:

$$P = \text{binom.test}\left(\frac{\sum BC_c}{3}, \frac{\sum TC_c}{3}, PER_n \right.$$
$$\left. +c\sqrt{\frac{PER_n}{TC_n}}, \text{alternative} = \text{"greater"}\right)$$

where c represents the quantile of order 1-alpha of the standard Gaussian, with c equaling to 1.64 (quantile of order 95% for the Gaussian) Binomial test was the R function to obtain an exact test of a simple null hypothesis about the probability of success in a Bernoulli experiment (https://www.rdocumentation.org/packages/stats/versions/3.4.3/topics/binom.test).

Step 5. Permutation.

The case group denoted the group of 3 BCSCs versus 2 non-BCSCs, and the other 9 (i.e., $C_5^2 - 1$) random arrangements were defined as permutation groups (Additional file 6: Table S6). The general approach for calculating the P values of permutation groups was the same as in Step 4.

Step 6. Case-permutation ratio (CPR).

After the computation of the P value of each position in each group, we counted the number of positions (NP) with P value less than the specific P value threshold (ranging from 0 to 0.1) in each group. To assess the difference in NP between the case group and each permutation group, we defined CPR as follows:

$$CPR = \frac{NP_{case}}{NP_{permutation} + NP_{case}}$$

Pearson correlation analysis, Fisher's exact test, and Student's t test

Pearson correlation analysis and Fisher's exact test were performed in R-2.3.2 using "cor()" and "fisher.test()" command, respectively. Student's t test was performed in GraphPad Prism 5.0 (GraphPad Software, La Jolla, CA, USA).

Results

Bulk-cell target deep DNA sequencing revealed no evidence for BCSC phenotype-associated genetic variants

Serial sphere formation assay was performed to enrich BCSCs of the breast cancer cell line MDA-MB-231. Then, an ALDEFLUOR assay was performed to investigate the proportion of BCSCs. Compared with the parental cells grown in a monolayer culture, spheres displayed gradually increased percentage of ALDH-positive cells, with almost half of the spheres of the fourth generation being composed of BCSCs (Fig. 1a; Additional file 7: Figs. S2a, S2b). In addition, compared with parental cells, spheres exhibited an obviously increased invasive capacity and higher expression of cancer stem cell markers (Fig. 1b, 1c, Additional file 7: Fig. S2c). Then, we collected the parental cells (2D) and derived spheres of the first generation (SP1) and fourth generation (SP4) for the WGS analysis. We assumed that if BCSCs were to be associated with particular genetic alterations, then the proportion of SNVs which BCSC population specifically carried would increase from 2D to SP4, leading to an increased VAF of these SNVs. Therefore, the SNVs with increased VAF from 2D to SP4 should be the genetic basis of BCSCs. However, the VAF of most SNV sites in the whole genome were similar in both 2D and SP4 (Fig. 1d).

To determine the SNV sites with significantly increased VAF, we performed Fisher's exact test on the read counts supporting the variant in each SNV site between 2D and SP4. To find out whether these SNVs were evenly distributed or spatially clustered, we developed a hotspot-calling algorithm based on the fact that the distances between every two adjacent potential SNV sites follow exponential distribution (Additional file 7: Fig. S1a). Hotspots were defined as the regions with SNV sites more densely distributed than statistically expected (Fig. 1e; Additional file 7: Fig. S1b), representing the most likely regions harboring genetic variants associated with BCSCs.

To determine whether genomic alteration contributed to the BCSC phenotype and to investigate the genetic basis associated with BCSCs, we performed target deep DNA sequencing in bulk cells on 2D, SP1, and SP4.

Target deep DNA sequencing covering all the hotspots yielded a median of 4500-fold coverage per site (Additional file 7: Fig. S3); however, no difference was found in the VAF from 2D to SP4 (Fig. 1f), making the hypothesis of heritable genetic changes contributing to the BCSC phenotype unlikely.

Single-cell target deep DNA sequencing confirmed the absence of significant genetic difference between BCSCs and non-BCSCs

To understand BCSC at a single-cell level, we turned to single-cell sequencing on non-BCSCs and BCSCs, with non-BCSC denoted as a single cell that cannot give rise to spheres and BCSC denoted as the sphere derived from a single cell (Additional file 7: Fig. S4). Single-cell target deep DNA sequencing was performed on both the hotspots we identified in the WHM panel (Additional file 5: Table S5) and the CHM panel (Additional file 2: Table S2).

The landscape and general approach for the single-cell DNA sequencing analysis was exemplified by the WHM panel (Fig. 2a). Target deep DNA sequencing of the WHM panel in 5 samples yielded a median of 4000-fold coverage per site (Additional file 7: Fig. S5). On the basis of the extremely high correlation coefficient of the base weight between every two samples and the lack of a significant difference ($P = 0.379$) between the inter-group (BCSC versus non-BCSC) and intra-group (BCSC versus BCSC or non-BCSC versus non-BCSC) (Fig. 2b; Additional file 7: Fig. S6), we inferred the identical genetic spectrum across the 5 samples. On the other hand, all the genetic distances, a metric to measure nucleotide composition pattern differences between two samples, were extremely small with an average of approximately 0.001 for both inter-group

and intra-group samples (Fig. 2c), further indicating the reliability of the result.

To systematically compare the genomic program between BCSCs and non-BCSCs and distinguish the genuine variants from sequencing artifacts, we developed a method based on quantification of the error rate for each base position. This approach assessed PBC in the 3 BCSCs from a binomial distribution with PER determined by 2 non-BCSCs. It indicated whether it was possible to observe the amount of variant alleles at a genomic position where no genuine variant exist. Thereafter, 764 positions of all 13,855 WHM sites were flagged as potential mutation sites with a P value less than 7.218×10^{-8} ($0.001/13,855$). To quantify the amount of false positives, a permutation analysis was performed on the 5 samples. For each permutation, we randomly chose 2 samples to calculate PER, and the rest 3 samples were used to calculate PBC. The numbers of potential mutation sites of each permutation were similar. Furthermore, with the threshold P value varying from 0 to 0.1, the numbers of mutation sites in both permutation group and case group were evenly reduced, leading to a consistent and constant trend of CPR (Fig. 2d). Therefore, we concluded that the dissimilarity between the genome of BCSCs and non-BCSCs was due to technical noise, predicting no evidence for genomic changes in BCSCs. The conclusion was also supported by the target deep DNA sequencing of the CHM panel (Additional file 7: Figs. S7–9).

scRNA-seq showed that self-renewal capability was marked by a distinct profile of gene expression

We then wondered whether BCSCs possess characteristic differences in single-cell gene expression. Multiple single cells (approximately 1000) isolated from the

---

(See figure on next page.)

Fig. 1 Identification and investigation of potential breast cancer stem cell (BCSC)-associated mutation hotspots. **a** Ascending trend of the percentage of the aldehyde dehydrogenase (ALDH)-positive cell population across the samples from the breast cancer cell line MDA-MB-231. **b** The invasion ability of enriched spheres was analyzed by transwell invasion assay. ***$P < 0.001$, two-tailed Student's t tests. Error bars represent mean ± standard deviation (SD). **c** Expression levels of markers related to cancer stem cells [nanog homeobox (NANOG) and SRY (sex determining region Y)-box 2 (SOX2)] were assessed by real-time quantitative PCR in both enriched spheres (SP) and monolayer parental cells (2D). ***$P < 0.001$, two-tailed Student's t-tests. Error bars represent mean ± SD. **d** Histogram 2D plots, conducted by the R package "plotly", show the comparison of variant allele frequency (VAF) between every two samples. The VAF of most single nucleotide variant (SNV) sites in the whole genome is observed as being similar. **e** One hotspot region in chromosome 7 highlighted with a yellow bar is displayed as an example. First, potential SNV sites along the genome were ordered from the first to the last variant on chromosome 7 and colored according to P values. The distance between each mutation and the one prior to it (the inter-SNV distance) is plotted on the vertical axis (rainfall plot). P values were determined by an exponential distribution formula. Additionally, the number of potential SNV sites of each bin was visualized by University of California Santa Cruz Genome Browser (GB), with the whole chromosome divided into 10,000 equal bins. Next, hotspots of parental cells (2D), and derived spheres of the fourth generation (SP4) hotspot was displayed by GB using the sliding window approach, which was performed by shifting one base each time along the chromosome from start to end and calculating the SNV density and VAF level in each 1000 bp window. **f** Target deep DNA sequencing of comparison of VAF between every two samples revealed no difference from 2D to SP4 (left and middle). R^2 was determined by regression analysis. Cor denotes the Pearson correlation coefficient. The dotted line represents the diagonal line. Sanger sequencing validated part of the results of target deep DNA sequencing (right)

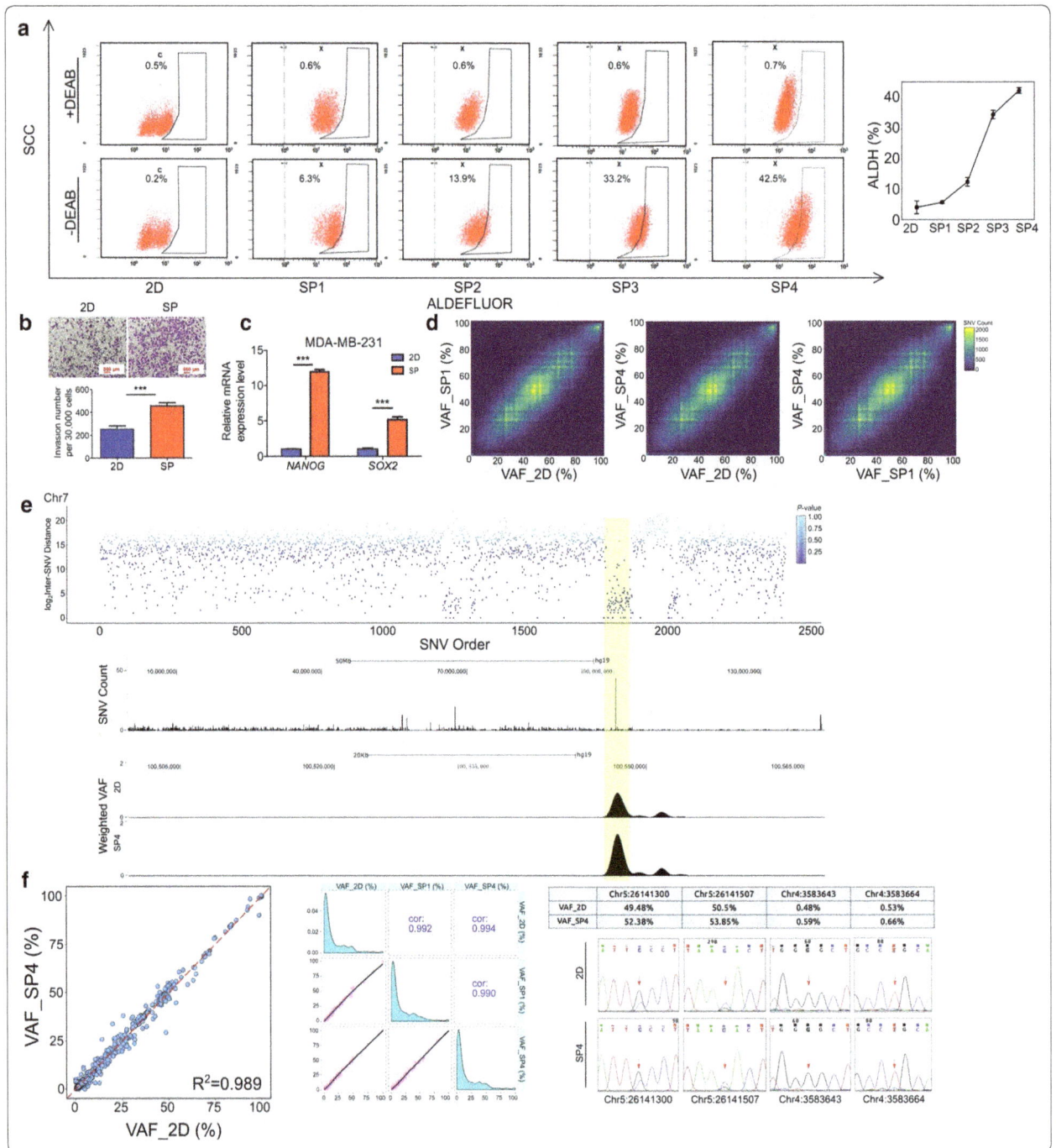

MDA-MB-231 cell line were cultured in a sphere condition of 1 cell/well, with a very small proportion of the single cells giving rise to spheres (Fig. 3a), indicating that sporadic cells had a BCSC property characterized by a distinct profile of gene expression. To identify the transcriptional program associated with BCSCs, 5 single cell-derived spheres (BCSCs) and 3 single cells that could not give rise to sphere (non-BCSCs) were subjected to scRNA-seq. Notably, as revealed by GSEA associated with biological processes (MSigDB: Gene Ontology Biological Process), the "regulation of stem cell proliferation" and other sets were strongly enriched for the group of spheres (Fig. 3b), illustrating that the difference in single-cell gene expression was associated with BCSCs.

Next, 74 genes with significantly higher expression in BCSCs (BCSC highly expressed genes) than in

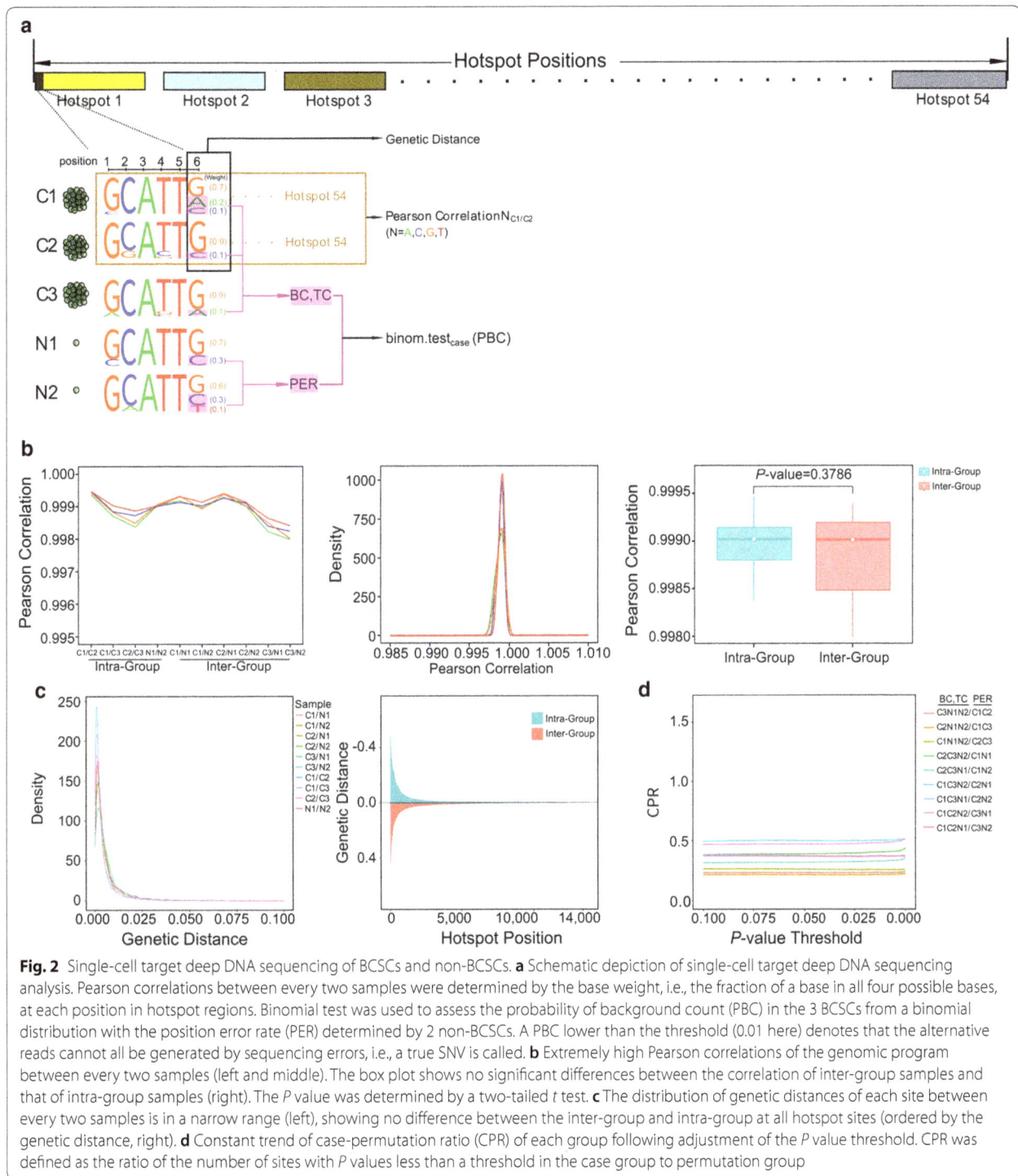

Fig. 2 Single-cell target deep DNA sequencing of BCSCs and non-BCSCs. **a** Schematic depiction of single-cell target deep DNA sequencing analysis. Pearson correlations between every two samples were determined by the base weight, i.e., the fraction of a base in all four possible bases, at each position in hotspot regions. Binomial test was used to assess the probability of background count (PBC) in the 3 BCSCs from a binomial distribution with the position error rate (PER) determined by 2 non-BCSCs. A PBC lower than the threshold (0.01 here) denotes that the alternative reads cannot all be generated by sequencing errors, i.e., a true SNV is called. **b** Extremely high Pearson correlations of the genomic program between every two samples (left and middle). The box plot shows no significant differences between the correlation of inter-group samples and that of intra-group samples (right). The P value was determined by a two-tailed t test. **c** The distribution of genetic distances of each site between every two samples is in a narrow range (left), showing no difference between the inter-group and intra-group at all hotspot sites (ordered by the genetic distance, right). **d** Constant trend of case-permutation ratio (CPR) of each group following adjustment of the P value threshold. CPR was defined as the ratio of the number of sites with P values less than a threshold in the case group to permutation group

non-BCSCs were identified (Fig. 3c). Notably, most of the 74 genes showed similar expression pattern as in multiple bulk-cell RNA-seq results, and the correlation of scRNA-seq and bulk-cell RNA seq results was high, illustrating the reliability of the 74 genes identified by scRNA-seq (Fig. 3a, d). Among them, we recovered well-known markers and related genes of cancer stem cells, including activated leukocyte cell adhesion molecule (*ALCAM*) [20–40], pyruvate kinase (*PKM*) [41], fatty acid synthase (*FASN*) [42], vascular endothelial growth factor (*VEGFA*) [43–45], a disintegrin and metalloproteinase domain-containing protein

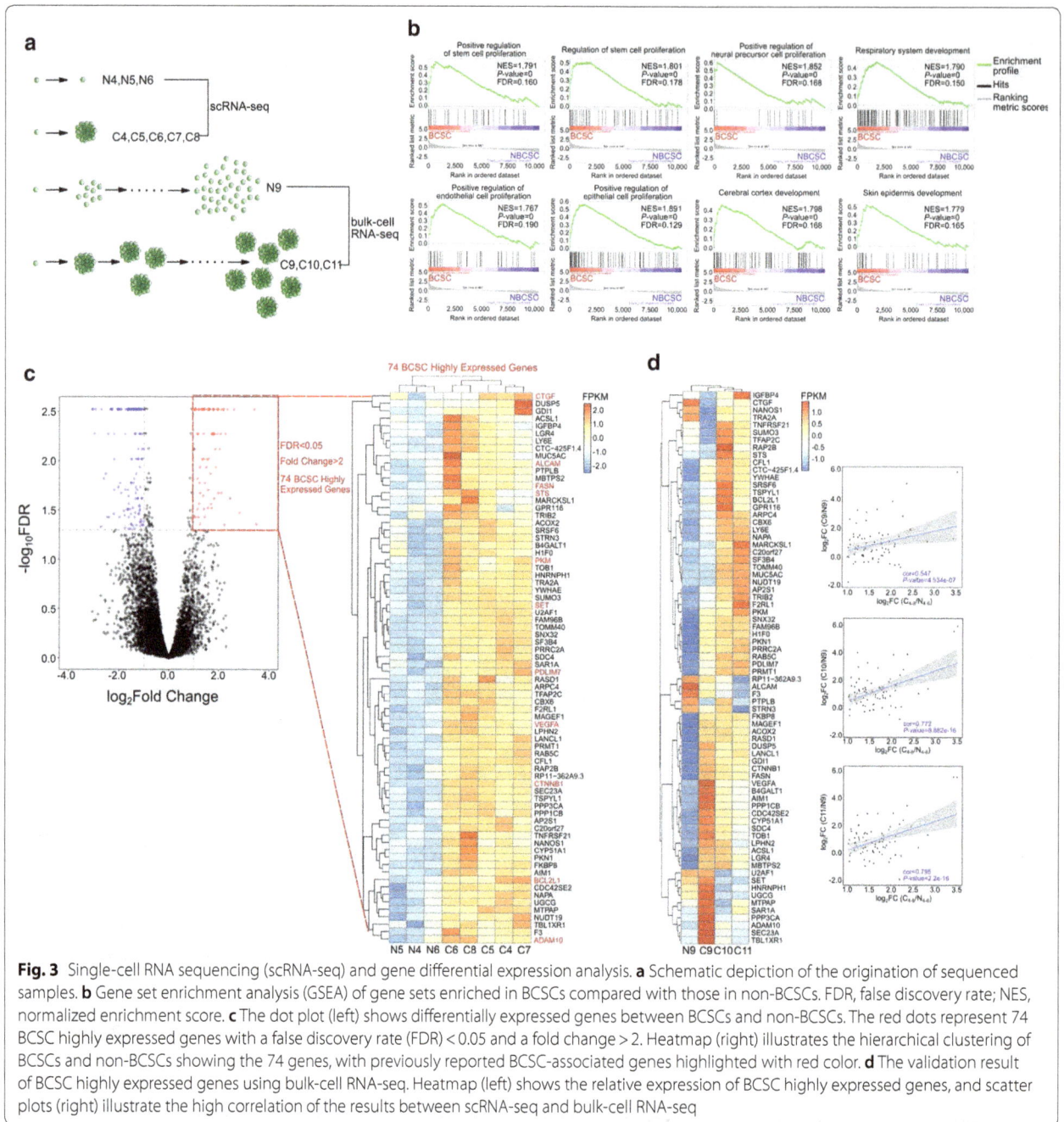

Fig. 3 Single-cell RNA sequencing (scRNA-seq) and gene differential expression analysis. **a** Schematic depiction of the origination of sequenced samples. **b** Gene set enrichment analysis (GSEA) of gene sets enriched in BCSCs compared with those in non-BCSCs. FDR, false discovery rate; NES, normalized enrichment score. **c** The dot plot (left) shows differentially expressed genes between BCSCs and non-BCSCs. The red dots represent 74 BCSC highly expressed genes with a false discovery rate (FDR) < 0.05 and a fold change > 2. Heatmap (right) illustrates the hierarchical clustering of BCSCs and non-BCSCs showing the 74 genes, with previously reported BCSC-associated genes highlighted with red color. **d** The validation result of BCSC highly expressed genes using bulk-cell RNA-seq. Heatmap (left) shows the relative expression of BCSC highly expressed genes, and scatter plots (right) illustrate the high correlation of the results between scRNA-seq and bulk-cell RNA-seq

10 (*ADAM10*) [46], B cell lymphoma 2 like 1 (*BCL2L1*) [47–50], connective tissue growth factor (*CTGF*) [51], catenin beta 1 (*CTNNB1*) [52, 53], PDZ and LIM domain protein 7 (*PDLIM7*) [54–59], steroid sulfatase (*STS*) [60–64], and SET nuclear proto-oncogene (*SET*) [65–67].

Exploring BCSC highly expressed genes for BCSC markers
Functionally, Gene Ontology (GO) analysis indicated that the 74 BCSC highly expressed genes were associated

with embryonic development, epithelial cell migration, and positive regulation of cell migration, as expected from BCSCs (Fig. 4a). Additionally, the functional networks involved in the 74 genes were determined (protein–protein interaction enrichment P value = 0.004) in STRING datasets, indicating that the genes were biologically connected and coordinated and revealing the core functional networks underlying positive regulation of the cellular process (FDR = 0.003) and cell surface receptor signaling pathway (FDR = 0.003) (Fig. 4b), suggesting the

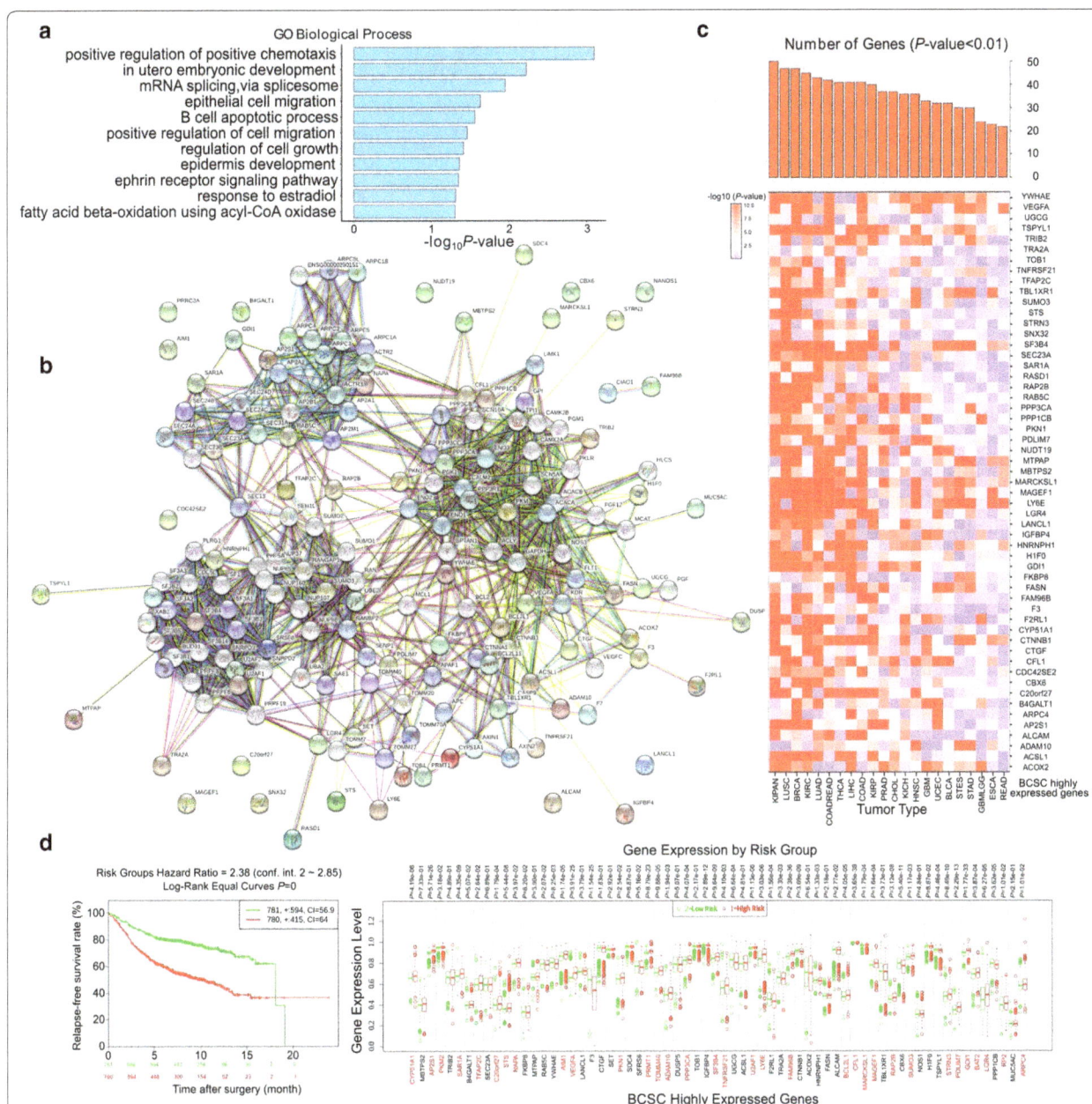

Fig. 4 Biological and clinical significance of the BCSC highly expressed genes. **a** Gene Ontology (GO) analysis of the BCSC highly expressed genes in biological process. *P* values (one-tail Fisher exact *P* values used for gene enrichment analysis) were calculated in the DAVID database (https://david.ncifcrf.gov/tools.jsp). **b** Interaction network of BCSC highly expressed genes integrated from the STRING database. Network nodes represent genes, and edges represent gene–gene associations. A detailed legend is available at https://string-db.org. **c** Investigation of the clinical relevance of BCSC highly expressed genes in 22 cancer types. The expression of each gene in cancer and corresponding normal tissues was analyzed by a two-tailed *t* test. Heatmap was horizontally sorted by the number of genes with *P* < 0.01 in a particular cancer type, shown as red columns on the top. **d** Kaplan–Meier relapse-free survival curve (left) of patients with low (green) and high (red) risk grouped by BCSC highly expressed genes in SurvExpress (dataset: Breast cancer relapse data). The total number of each group was shown in the top right corner, and the number of censoring samples are marked with a "+" symbol. The concordance index (CI) per curve was also included. The *P* value was determined by a log-rank test. The x axis represents the years of the study. In rows and corresponding colors, the numbers of samples not presenting the event at the matching time are shown. The box plot (right) shows the comparison of the gene expression between the low- and high-risk groups. Genes significantly (*P* < 0.05) highly expressed in the high-risk group are highlighted in red. *P* values were calculated using two-tailed *t* test

possibility of these genes being BCSC markers. Further-more, to evaluate whether BCSC highly expressed genes generated from the in vitro model had clinical relevance, we queried TCGA datasets across multiple cancer types. Most of the genes manifested significant differential expression between cancer and normal tissues, further suggesting the feasibility of them being BCSC markers (Fig. 4c; Additional file 7: Fig. S10a).

To systematically assess the prognostic significance of the BCSC markers we identified, we performed survival analysis of breast cancer patients using the SurvExpress database. A significant prognostic association was observed, and most of the genes were expressed at higher levels in the high-risk relapse group than in the low-risk relapse group, indicating their value in predicting adverse prognosis (Fig. 4d). Additionally, individual inspection of these genes further confirmed their prognostic significance in breast cancer (Additional file 7: Fig. S11). More-over, the clustering of PRECOG z scores [17] revealed prognostic specificity across distinct cancer types and subtypes, with neuroblastoma being the most affected (Additional file 7: Fig. S10b). Taken together, our results highlight the clinical significance of these BCSC markers, suggesting novel targets for anticancer therapy.

Discussion

Cancer stem cells can result from cancer cells by acquiring mutations [68, 69], but in other cases there is no clear genetic cause, raising the possibility of non-genetic cell transcriptomic variability [70–72]. The present work aimed at a better understanding of cancer stem cells. Breast cancer, which often relapses and metastasizes, is a paradigmatic example for studying cancer stem cells. Serial sphere formation assay, a widely used in vitro technique for assessing self-renewal capacity [73, 74], was performed to enrich BCSCs. Recent works have demonstrated that there were no significant tumorigenicity differences between $ALDH^+CD44^+CD24^-$ cell population and $ALDH^+CD44^-CD24^-$ cell population [75] and that $ALDH^-$ cells bearing the $CD44^+CD24^-/lin^-$ phenotype was not tumorigenic. By contrast, the $ALDH^+$ population that did not display the $CD44^+/CD24^-/lin^-$ phenotype was capable of generating tumors [76]. Taken together, it is suggestive that high ALDH activity can be considered as an identifier of the tumorigenic cell fraction, capable of self-renewal and generating tumors. In the present study, we used ALDH in FACS assay to investigate the proportion of BCSCs in spheres. To investigate the genetic basis of BCSCs origination, we determined the potential mutation hotspot regions using WGS, and performed target deep DNA sequencing on parental cancer cells and derived serial-generation spheres in

increasing order of BCSC frequency, which revealed no validated genetic changes specifically associated with BCSCs. With respect to the different VAF provided by WGS and target deep DNA sequencing, we suggest that the latter quantifies VAF more precisely by generating deeper genome coverage. Previous studies also applied target deep DNA sequencing to examine clonal evolution through its unequivocal evidence of defining VAF [77, 78].

Population-based sequencing indicated no clear genetic cause contributing to BCSC. To understand BCSCs at the single-cell level, single-cell DNA sequencing was performed on non-BCSCs and BCSCs. All cells of one sphere were derived from the originally seeded single cell, leading to a homogenous genome within one sphere. Thus, sequencing of the sphere increased the accuracy in identifying variants without the disturbances of genomic heterogeneity. Nevertheless, single-cell DNA sequencing also have some limitations, for instance, a fraction of stochastic allele-alterations could be introduced by the process of whole genome amplification [79]. Concerned with this issue, we performed single-cell target deep DNA sequencing for the WHM and CHM panels. The generation of high-depth sequencing data allowed us to accurately quantify the allele frequency in all samples, permitting the calculation of a base weight for each site in a hotspot region. On the basis of base weight of each site, we obtained the correlation coefficients and genetic distances to globally assess the genomic program across all samples. Moreover, a method based on quantification of error rate of each base position was developed, allowing us to systematically analyze the genomic program. Taken together, single-cell target deep DNA sequencing confirmed the absence of significant genetic difference between BCSCs and non-BCSCs.

The emergence of self-renewal capability is a complex process involving transcriptomic variability. Profiling the transcriptomes of individual cells via scRNA-seq allowed the functional role of heterogeneity in gene expression levels between cells to be investigated [80]. Bioinformatics analysis identified 74 candidate BCSC highly expressed genes through single-cell transcriptome sequencing. These 74 genes overlapped with some genes identified by other studies [41–47], and many extend beyond breast cancer, suggesting the existence of a general expression program co-opted in the cancer stem cell phenotype. Overall, the present study explored the identity of BCSC and provided a framework for understanding BCSC.

Here, we documented proof of the concept that a non-genetic cause leads to BCSCs, suggestive of common, shared epigenetic regulation that contributes to the BCSC phenotype. Further elucidation of the reprogramming and plasticity of switching between BCSC and non-BCSC states at an epigenetic level may open new avenues for therapeutic targeting. For instance, epigenetic activation of twist family bHLH transcription factor 1 (TWIST1) by metadherin (MTDH) promotes cancer stem-like cell traits in breast cancer [12]. MTDH activates TWIST1 expression indirectly by facilitating histone H3 acetylation on the TWIST1 promoter, a process mediated by the histone acetyltransferase cAMP-response element binding protein (CREB)-binding protein (CBP). Similarly, poised chromatin at the zinc finger E-box binding homeobox 1 (ZEB1) promoter enables breast cancer cell plasticity and enhances tumorigenicity [13], supporting a dynamic model in which interconversions between low and high tumorigenic states occur frequently, thereby increasing tumorigenic and malignant potential. Therefore, the roles of the epigenetics are being increasingly required for phenotypic plasticity, specifically in a context where genome sequences are not altered. In addition, epigenetic and genetic causes of BCSC are not mutually exclusive. Epigenetic effects may provide the initial BCSC state, allowing a small subpopulation of tumor cells to potentially self-renew until some acquire secondary mutations that drive cancer progression to relapse. The unification of in vivo studies will allow for a more comprehensive description of BCSCs.

Conclusions

The present study demonstrated that no genetic changes contributed to the BCSC identity. Breast cancer cells displayed transcriptomic variability at the single-cell level and determined BCSC phenotype. The single-cell transcriptomic variability involved coordinated transcription of a number of BCSC markers and was found to be significantly associated with clinical prognosis.

Additional files

Additional file 1: Table S1. Primer sequences for real-time quantitative PCR.

Additional file 2: Table S2. Amplicon primers designed for the WGS hotspot mutation (WHM) panel.

Additional file 3: Table S3. Targeted genes and mutations in the cancer hotspot mutation (CHM) panel.

Additional file 4: Table S4. Amplicon primers designed for the CHM panel.

Additional file 5: Table S5. The WHM panel of hotspots identified by whole-genome sequencing (WGS).

Additional file 6: Table S6. Definition of case groups and permutation groups.

Additional file 7: Fig. S1. Potential mutation hotspots associated with breast cancer stem cells (BCSCs) are identified by bulk-cell whole-genome sequencing (WGS). **a,** Distances of potential single nucleotide variations (SNV) sites follow an exponential distribution. **b,** Two hotspots in chromosome 6 highlighted with a yellow bar are displayed as an example. **c and d,** Distribution of length (C) and proportion of functional annotations (D) for hotspots. **Fig. S2.** This figure related to Figure 1A. Serial sphere formation assay. **a,** Serial sphere formation assay from the first to fourth generation was performed in MDA-MB-231 cells. The spheres were photographed using an inverted microscope (Olympus). Scale bar, 200 μm. **b,** Cell number of spheres from the first to fourth generation. **c,** Expression levels of markers related to cancer stem cells [nanog homeobox (NANOG) and SRY (sex determining region Y)-box 2(SOX2)] was assessed by western blot assay in both enriched spheres (SP) and monolayer parental cells (2D). **Fig. S3.** Bulk-cell target deep DNA sequencing data evaluation. The violin plot (A) illustrates the distribution of depth in the target deep DNA sequencing, and the reads coverage distribution of each hotspot are shown by the pile-up bar plots (B). **Fig. S4.** Single-cell sphere formation assay. Images of single cell-derived spheres (red, BCSCs) and single cells that could not form spheres (green, non-BCSCs). The spheres and single cells were photographed using an inverted microscope (Olympus). Scale bar, 50 μm. **Fig. S5.** Data evaluation of single-cell target deep DNA sequencing of the hotspot region panel. **a and b,** Depth distribution of target deep DNA sequencing of hotspots from 5 samples. **c and d,** Reads coverage distribution of hotspots. **Fig. S6.** Pearson correlations of the genomic program (the hotspot region panel) between every two samples. **Fig. S7.** Data evaluation of single-cell target deep DNA sequencing of the cancer hotspot mutation (CHM) panel. **a and b,** Depth distribution of target deep DNA sequencing of hotspots from 5 samples. **c,** Reads coverage distribution of hotspots. **Fig. S8.** Pearson correlations of the genomic program (the CHM panel) between every two samples. **Fig. S9.** Single-cell target deep DNA sequencing of the CHM panel confirms no significant difference between BCSCs and NBCSCs. **Fig. S10.** Clinical significance of the BCSC highly expressed genes in pan-cancer. **a,** The expression of each gene in cancer and corresponding normal tissues was analyzed by a two-tailed Student's t test. The heatmap is vertically sorted by the number of cancer types with fold change (FC) < -2 or FC > 2 shown as red columns in the right. **b,** Hierarchical clustering of PRECOG z scores is shown by heatmap. **Fig. S11.** Prognosis significance of the BCSC highly expressed genes in breast cancer. Kaplan-Meier curves of estimated relapse-free survival (RFS) for breast cancer patients with low (black) and high (red) expression of BCSC highly expressed genes in the Kaplan-Meier database. HR, hazard ratio. P values were determined by log-rank test.

Abbreviations

BCSCs: breast cancer stem cells; NGS: next-generation sequencing; WGS: whole-genome sequencing; DEAB: diethylaminobenzaldehyde; RLE: run-length encoding; MDA: multiple displacement amplification; WGA: whole genome amplification; TC: total count; MC: major count; BC: background count; PER: position error rate; PBC: probability of background count; CPR: case-permutation ratio; NP: number of positions; DEG: differentially expressed gene; FC: fold change; FDR: false discovery rate; SNVs: single nucleotide variations; VAF: variant allele frequency; GSEA: gene set enrichment analysis; GO: gene Ontology; GB: genome Browser; NES: normalized enrichment score; CI: concordance Index.

Authors' contributions

MT and ZD performed experiments, analyzed the data and wrote the paper; XD, DL, XZ (Xuehong Zhang), and AD were involved in drafting the manuscript and revising for substantial intellectual content; MY, CX, and BW made substantial contribution to spheres culturing, RNA extraction, reverse transcription-PCR, quantitative real-time PCR, Western blot analysis, and fluorescence activated cell sorting; PL designed the CHM panel; YZ, QZ, YL, XZ (Xiaolong Zhang), and LS made substantial contribution to statistical analyses; ZL and QL jointly designed, oversaw, and directed the study. All authors read and approved the final manuscript.

Author details

[1] Center of Genome and Personalized Medicine, Institute of Cancer Stem Cell, Dalian Medical University, Dalian 116044, Liaoning, P. R. China. [2] State Key Laboratory of Oncology in South China, Collaborative Innovation Center of Cancer Medicine, Sun Yat-sen University Cancer Center, Guangzhou, Guangdong 510060, P. R. China. [3] Cancer Center, Union Hospital, Tongji Medical

College, Huazhong University of Science and Technology, Wuhan, Hubei 430022, P. R. China.

Acknowledgements
Not applicable.

Competing interests
The authors declare that they have no competing interests.

Funding
This research work was supported by Program for Changjiang Scholars and Innovative Research Team in University of Ministry of Education of China (No. IRT_17R15), National Natural Science Foundation of China (Nos. 81630005 to QL, 81573025 to QL, 81472637 to ZL, 81672784 to ZL, and 81602200 to DL), Innovative Research Team in University of Liaoning (No. LT2017001 to QL), The program for climbing Scholars of Liaoning, Dalian High-level Talent Innovation Program (2016RD12 to QL) and International Scientific and Technological Cooperation of Dalian (2015F11GH095 to QL).

References

1. Geng SQ, Alexandrou AT, Li JJ. Breast cancer stem cells: multiple capacities in tumor metastasis. Cancer Lett. 2014;349(1):1–7.
2. Kotiyal S, Bhattacharya S. Breast cancer stem cells, emt and therapeutic targets. Biochem Biophys Res Commun. 2014;453(1):112–6.
3. Liu S, Wicha MS. Targeting breast cancer stem cells. J Clin Oncol. 2010;28(25):4006–12.
4. Cicalese A, Bonizzi G, Pasi CE, et al. The tumor suppressor p53 regulates polarity of self-renewing divisions in mammary stem cells. Cell. 2009;138(6):1083–95.
5. Spike BT, Engle DD, Lin JC, et al. A mammary stem cell population identified and characterized in late embryogenesis reveals similarities to human breast cancer. Cell Stem Cell. 2012;10(2):183–97.
6. Brooks MD, Burness ML, Wicha MS. Therapeutic implications of cellular heterogeneity and plasticity in breast cancer. Cell Stem Cell. 2015;17(3):260–71.
7. Sansone P, Ceccarelli C, Berishaj M, et al. Self-renewal of cd133(hi) cells by il6/notch3 signalling regulates endocrine resistance in metastatic breast cancer. Nat Commun. 2016;7:10442.
8. Boo L, Ho WY, Ali NM, et al. Mirna transcriptome profiling of spheroid-enriched cells with cancer stem cell properties in human breast mcf-7 cell line. Int J Biol Sci. 2016;12(4):427–45.
9. Okuda H, Kobayashi A, Xia B, et al. Hyaluronan synthase has2 promotes tumor progression in bone by stimulating the interaction of breast cancer stem-like cells with macrophages and stromal cells. Cancer Res. 2012;72(2):537–47.
10. Dave B, Migliaccio I, Gutierrez MC, et al. Loss of phosphatase and tensin homolog or phosphoinositol-3 kinase activation and response to trastuzumab or lapatinib in human epidermal growth factor receptor 2-overexpressing locally advanced breast cancers. J Clin Oncol. 2011;29(2):166–73.
11. Foulkes WD, Stefansson IM, Chappuis PO, et al. Germline brca1 mutations and a basal epithelial phenotype in breast cancer. J Natl Cancer Inst. 2003;95(19):1482–5.
12. Liang Y, Hu J, Li J, et al. Epigenetic activation of twist1 by mtdh promotes cancer stem-like cell traits in breast cancer. Cancer Res. 2015;75(17):3672–80.
13. Chaffer CL, Marjanovic ND, Lee T, et al. Poised chromatin at the zeb1 promoter enables breast cancer cell plasticity and enhances tumorigenicity. Cell. 2013;154(1):61–74.
14. Subramanian A, Tamayo P, Mootha VK, et al. Gene set enrichment analysis: a knowledge-based approach for interpreting genome-wide expression profiles. Proc Natl Acad Sci USA. 2005;102(43):15545–50.
15. Lanczky A, Nagy A, Bottai G, et al. Mirpower: a web-tool to validate survival-associated mirnas utilizing expression data from 2178 breast cancer patients. Breast Cancer Res Treat. 2016;160(3):439–46.
16. Brohee S, van Helden J. Evaluation of clustering algorithms for protein protein interaction networks. BMC Bioinform. 2006;7:488.
17. Gentles AJ, Newman AM, Liu CL, et al. The prognostic landscape of genes and infiltrating immune cells across human cancers. Nat Med. 2015;21(8):938–45.
18. Aguirre-Gamboa R, Gomez-Rueda H, Martinez-Ledesma E, et al. Survexpress: an online biomarker validation tool and database for cancer gene expression data using survival analysis. PLoS ONE. 2013;8(9):e74250.
19. Pecuchet N, Rozenholc Y, Zonta E, et al. Analysis of base-position error rate of next-generation sequencing to detect tumor mutations in circulating DNA. Clin Chem. 2016;62(11):1492–503.
20. Botchkina GI, Zuniga ES, Das M, et al. New-generation taxoid sb-t-1214 inhibits stem cell-related gene expression in 3d cancer spheroids induced by purified colon tumor-initiating cells. Mol Cancer. 2010;9:192.
21. Botchkina IL, Rowehl RA, Rivadeneira DE, et al. Phenotypic subpopulations of metastatic colon cancer stem cells: genomic analysis. Cancer Genom Proteom. 2009;6(1):19–29.
22. Giampieri R, Scartozzi M, Loretelli C, et al. Cancer stem cell gene profile as predictor of relapse in high risk stage ii and stage iii, radically resected colon cancer patients. PLoS ONE. 2013;8(9):e72843.
23. Haraguchi N, Ishii H, Mimori K, et al. Cd49f-positive cell population efficiently enriches colon cancer-initiating cells. Int J Oncol. 2013;43(2):425–30.
24. Hostettler L, Zlobec I, Terracciano L, et al. Abcg5-positivity in tumor buds is an indicator of poor prognosis in node-negative colorectal cancer patients. World J Gastroenterol. 2010;16(6):732–9.
25. Hwang WL, Yang MH, Tsai ML, et al. Snail regulates interleukin-8 expression, stem cell-like activity, and tumorigenicity of human colorectal carcinoma cells. Gastroenterology. 2011;141(1):279–291, 291 e271–275.
26. King JB, von Furstenberg RJ, Smith BJ, et al. Cd24 can be used to isolate lgr5 + putative colonic epithelial stem cells in mice. Am J Physiol Gastrointest Liver Physiol. 2012;303(4):G443–52.
27. Leng Z, Tao K, Xia Q, et al. Kruppel-like factor 4 acts as an oncogene in colon cancer stem cell-enriched spheroid cells. PLoS ONE. 2013;8(2):e56082.
28. Levi E, Sochacki P, Khoury N, et al. Cancer stem cells in helicobacter pylori infection and aging: implications for gastric carcinogenesis. World J Gastrointest Pathophysiol. 2014;5(3):366–72.
29. Lin JJ, Huang CS, Yu J, et al. Malignant phyllodes tumors display mesenchymal stem cell features and aldehyde dehydrogenase/disialoganglioside identify their tumor stem cells. Breast Cancer Res. 2014;16(2):R29.
30. Lugli A, Iezzi G, Hostettler I, et al. Prognostic impact of the expression of putative cancer stem cell markers cd133, cd166, cd44s, epcam, and aldh1 in colorectal cancer. Br J Cancer. 2010;103(3):382–90.
31. Margaritescu C, Pirici D, Cherciu I, et al. Cd133/cd166/ki-67 triple immunofluorescence assessment for putative cancer stem cells in colon carcinoma. J Gastrointestin Liver Dis. 2014;23(2):161–70.
32. Moon BS, Jeong WJ, Park J, et al. Role of oncogenic k-ras in cancer stem cell activation by aberrant wnt/beta-catenin signaling. J Natl Cancer Inst. 2014;106(2):djt373.
33. Nautiyal J, Kanwar SS, Yu Y, et al. Combination of dasatinib and curcumin eliminates chemo-resistant colon cancer cells. J Mol Signal. 2011;6:7.
34. Oh PS, Patel VB, Sanders MA, et al. Schlafen-3 decreases cancer stem cell marker expression and autocrine/juxtacrine signaling in folfox-resistant colon cancer cells. Am J Physiol Gastrointest Liver Physiol. 2011;301(2):G347–55.
35. Piscuoglio S, Lehmann FS, Zlobec I, et al. Effect of epcam, cd44, cd133 and cd166 expression on patient survival in tumours of the ampulla of vater. J Clin Pathol. 2012;65(2):140–5.
36. Tachezy M, Zander H, Gebauer F, et al. Activated leukocyte cell adhesion molecule (cd166)—its prognostic power for colorectal cancer patients. J Surg Res. 2012;177(1):e15–20.
37. Tachezy M, Zander H, Wolters-Eisfeld G, et al. Activated leukocyte cell adhesion molecule (cd166): an "inert" cancer stem cell marker for non-small cell lung cancer? Stem Cells. 2014;32(6):1429–36.
38. Yan M, Yang X, Wang L, et al. Plasma membrane proteomics of tumor spheres identify cd166 as a novel marker for cancer stem-like cells in head and neck squamous cell carcinoma. Mol Cell Proteom. 2013;12(11):3271–84.
39. Yang L, Levi E, Zhu S, et al. Cancer stem cells biomarkers in gastric carcinogenesis. J Gastrointest Cancer. 2013;44(4):428–35.
40. Zhou J, Li P, Xue X, et al. Salinomycin induces apoptosis in cisplatin-resistant colorectal cancer cells by accumulation of reactive oxygen species. Toxicol Lett. 2013;222(2):139–45.

41. Morfouace M, Lalier L, Oliver L, et al. Control of glioma cell death and differentiation by pkm2-oct4 interaction. Cell Death Dis. 2014;5:e1036.

42. Wahdan-Alaswad RS, Cochrane DR, Spoelstra NS, et al. Metformin-induced killing of triple-negative breast cancer cells is mediated by reduction in fatty acid synthase via mirna-193b. Horm Cancer. 2014;5(6):374–89.

43. Gokmen-Polar Y, Goswami CP, Toroni RA, et al. Gene expression analysis reveals distinct pathways of resistance to bevacizumab in xenograft models of human er-positive breast cancer. J Cancer. 2014;5(8):633–45.

44. Yamanouchi K, Ohta T, Liu Z, et al. The wilms' tumor gene wt1—17aa/—kts splice variant increases tumorigenic activity through up-regulation of vascular endothelial growth factor in an in vivo ovarian cancer model. Transl Oncol. 2014;7(5):580–9.

45. Zhao D, Pan C, Sun J, et al. Vegf drives cancer-initiating stem cells through vegfr-2/stat3 signaling to upregulate myc and sox2. Oncogene. 2015;34(24):3107–19.

46. Rappa G, Mercapide J, Anzanello F, et al. Biochemical and biological characterization of exosomes containing prominin-1/cd133. Mol Cancer. 2013;12:62.

47. Aldinucci D, Poletto D, Nanni P, et al. Cd40l induces proliferation, self-renewal, rescue from apoptosis, and production of cytokines by cd40-expressing aml blasts. Exp Hematol. 2002;30(11):1283–92.

48. Faderl S, Harris D, Van Q, et al. Granulocyte-macrophage colony-stimulating factor (gm-csf) induces antiapoptotic and proapoptotic signals in acute myeloid leukemia. Blood. 2003;102(2):630–7.

49. Moretti L, Li B, Kim KW, et al. At-101, a pan-bcl-2 inhibitor, leads to radiosensitization of non-small cell lung cancer. J Thorac Oncol. 2010;5(5):680–7.

50. Nanta R, Kumar D, Meeker D, et al. Nvp-lde-225 (erismodegib) inhibits epithelial-mesenchymal transition and human prostate cancer stem cell growth in nod/scid il2rgamma null mice by regulating bmi-1 and microrna-128. Oncogenesis. 2013;2:e42.

51. Edwards LA, Woolard K, Son MJ, et al. Effect of brain- and tumor-derived connective tissue growth factor on glioma invasion. J Natl Cancer Inst. 2011;103(15):1162–78.

52. Bauer L, Langer R, Becker K, et al. Expression profiling of stem cell-related genes in neoadjuvant-treated gastric cancer: a notch2, gsk3b and beta-catenin gene signature predicts survival. PLoS ONE. 2012;7(9):e44566.

53. Chan TA, Wang Z, Dang LH, et al. Targeted inactivation of ctnnb1 reveals unexpected effects of beta-catenin mutation. Proc Natl Acad Sci USA. 2002;99(12):8265–70.

54. Abdulkarim B, Sabri S, Zelenika D, et al. Antiviral agent cidofovir decreases epstein-barr virus (ebv) oncoproteins and enhances the radiosensitivity in ebv-related malignancies. Oncogene. 2003;22(15):2260–71.

55. Du C, Wen B, Li D, et al. Downregulation of epstein-barr virus-encoded latent membrane protein-1 by arsenic trioxide in nasopharyngeal carcinoma cells. Tumori. 2006;92(2):140–8.

56. Kondo S, Wakisaka N, Muramatsu M, et al. Epstein-barr virus latent membrane protein 1 induces cancer stem/progenitor-like cells in nasopharyngeal epithelial cell lines. J Virol. 2011;85(21):11255–64.

57. Yang CF, Peng LX, Huang TJ, et al. Cancer stem-like cell characteristics induced by eb virus-encoded lmp1 contribute to radioresistance in nasopharyngeal carcinoma by suppressing the p53-mediated apoptosis pathway. Cancer Lett. 2014;344(2):260–71.

58. Yoshizaki T, Kondo S, Wakisaka N, et al. Pathogenic role of epstein-barr virus latent membrane protein-1 in the development of nasopharyngeal carcinoma. Cancer Lett. 2013;337(1):1–7.

59. Zhang Q, Zhang Z, Wang C, et al. Proteome analysis of the transformation potential of the epstein-barr virus-encoded latent membrane protein 1 in nasopharyngeal epithelial cells np69. Mol Cell Biochem. 2008;314(1–2):73–83.

60. Fujii T, Saito D, Yoshida S, et al. the influence of sodium thiosulfate on the antitumor effect of cisplatin in human gastric cancer cell lines. Gan To Kagaku Ryoho. 1988;15(12):3227–32.

61. Kehlen A, Greither T, Wach S, et al. High coexpression of ccl2 and cx3cl1 is gender-specifically associated with good prognosis in soft tissue sarcoma patients. Int J Cancer. 2014;135(9):2096–106.

62. MacIsaac ZM, Shang H, Agrawal H, et al. Long-term in vivo tumorigenic assessment of human culture-expanded adipose stromal/stem cells. Exp Cell Res. 2012;318(4):416–23.

63. Mohrin M, Chen D. Sirtuins, tissue maintenance, and tumorigenesis. Genes Cancer. 2013;4(3–4):76–81.

64. Taubert H, Wurl P, Greither T, et al. Stem cell-associated genes are extremely poor prognostic factors for soft-tissue sarcoma patients. Oncogene. 2007;26(50):7170–4.

65. Abelson S, Shamai Y, Berger L, et al. Niche-dependent gene expression profile of intratumoral heterogeneous ovarian cancer stem cell populations. PLoS ONE. 2013;8(12):e83651.

66. Mezencev R, Wang L, McDonald JF. Identification of inhibitors of ovarian cancer stem-like cells by high-throughput screening. J Ovarian Res. 2012;5(1):30.

67. Perumal D, Singh S, Yoder SJ, et al. A novel five gene signature derived from stem-like side population cells predicts overall and recurrence-free survival in nsclc. PLoS ONE. 2012;7(8):e43589.

68. Li C, Wu S, Yang Z, et al. Single-cell exome sequencing identifies mutations in kcp, loc440040, and loc440563 as drivers in renal cell carcinoma stem cells. Cell Res. 2017;27(4):590–3.

69. Yang Z, Li C, Fan Z, et al. Single-cell sequencing reveals variants in arid1a, gprc5a and mll2 driving self-renewal of human bladder cancer stem cells. Eur Urol. 2017;71(1):8–12.

70. Wang Y, Cardenas H, Fang F, et al. Epigenetic targeting of ovarian cancer stem cells. Cancer Res. 2014;74(17):4922–36.

71. Shah M, Allegrucci C. Stem cell plasticity in development and cancer: epigenetic origin of cancer stem cells. Subcell Biochem. 2013;61:545–65.

72. Bapat SA. Epigenetic regulation of cancer stem cell gene expression. Subcell Biochem. 2013;61:419–34.

73. Beck B, Blanpain C. Unravelling cancer stem cell potential. Nat Rev Cancer. 2013;13(10):727–38.

74. Pastrana E, Silva-Vargas V, Doetsch F. Eyes wide open: a critical review of sphere-formation as an assay for stem cells. Cell Stem Cell. 2011;8(5):486–98.

75. Liu M, Liu Y, Deng L, et al. Transcriptional profiles of different states of cancer stem cells in triple-negative breast cancer. Mol Cancer. 2018;17(1):65.

76. Ginestier C, Hur MH, Charafe-Jauffret E, et al. Aldh1 is a marker of normal and malignant human mammary stem cells and a predictor of poor clinical outcome. Cell Stem Cell. 2007;1(5):555–67.

77. Ding L, Ley TJ, Larson DE, et al. Clonal evolution in relapsed acute myeloid leukaemia revealed by whole-genome sequencing. Nature. 2012;481(7382):506–10.

78. Ley TJ, Mardis ER, Ding L, et al. DNA sequencing of a cytogenetically normal acute myeloid leukaemia genome. Nature. 2008;456(7218):66–72.

79. Borgstrom E, Paterlini M, Mold JE, et al. Comparison of whole genome amplification techniques for human single cell exome sequencing. PLoS ONE. 2017;12(2):e0171566.

80. Kim JK, Kolodziejczyk AA, Ilicic T, et al. Characterizing noise structure in single-cell rna-seq distinguishes genuine from technical stochastic allelic expression. Nat Commun. 2015;6:8687.

3

Role of (myo) fibroblasts in the development of vascular and connective tissue structure of the C38 colorectal cancer in mice

Edina Bugyik[1], Vanessza Szabó[1], Katalin Dezső[1], András Rókusz[1], Armanda Szücs[1], Péter Nagy[1], József Tóvári[2], Viktória László[4,5], Balázs Döme[3,4,5,6*] and Sándor Paku[1,7*]

Abstract

Background: It remains unclear if the vascular and connective tissue structures of primary and metastatic tumors are intrinsically determined or whether these characteristics are defined by the host tissue. Therefore we examined the microanatomical steps of vasculature and connective tissue development of C38 colon carcinoma in different tissues.

Methods: Tumors produced in mice at five different locations (the cecal wall, skin, liver, lung, and brain) were analyzed using fluorescent immunohistochemistry, electron microscopy and quantitative real-time polymerase chain reaction.

Results: We found that in the cecal wall, skin, liver, and lung, resident fibroblasts differentiate into collagenous matrix-producing myofibroblasts at the tumor periphery. These activated fibroblasts together with the produced matrix were incorporated by the tumor. The connective tissue development culminated in the appearance of intratumoral tissue columns (centrally located single microvessels embedded in connective tissue and smooth muscle actin-expressing myofibroblasts surrounded by basement membrane). Conversely, in the brain (which lacks fibroblasts), C38 metastases only induced the development of vascularized desmoplastic tissue columns when the growing tumor reached the fibroblast-containing meninges.

Conclusions: Our data suggest that the desmoplastic host tissue response is induced by tumor-derived fibrogenic molecules acting on host tissue fibroblasts. We concluded that not only the host tissue characteristics but also the tumor-derived fibrogenic signals determine the vascular and connective tissue structure of tumors.

Keywords: Metastasis, Vasculature, Myofibroblasts, Incorporation

Introduction

The mechanism of vascularization in primary and metastatic tumors has long been debated. The tumor vascular pattern has been proposed to be indicative of the histologic type of the tumor [1]. Konerding et al. [2] examined the vascular structure of subcutaneous tumors using four tumor cell lines of different origins. They found that the vascular structure is characteristic of the individual tumor and showed that the vascular structure does not depend on the size and/or the rate of lesion growth but rather on the tumor type. In contrast, Solesvik et al. [3] investigated human malignant melanoma xenografts, and despite the identical histological type, different vascular patterns were found. They also observed that slow-growing melanomas had higher necrotic fractions and lower vessel volume per intact tumor volume than rapidly growing tumors.

*Correspondence: balazs.dome@meduniwien.ac.at; paku@korb1.sote.hu
[1] First Department of Pathology and Experimental Cancer Research, Semmelweis University, Budapest, Üllői út 26, 1085, Hungary
[4] Department of Thoracic Surgery, Medical University of Vienna, Waehringer Guertel 18-20, 1090 Vienna, Austria
Full list of author information is available at the end of the article

In addition to tumor type, the extracellular matrix (collagen and basement membrane) structure of the host tissue can also have an influence on the vascular and connective tissue structure of the tumor. It was demonstrated that in brain metastases, the capillary basement membrane (BM) is the primary substrate for adhesion, migration and growth of the extravasated cells [4–6]. It was shown that the highly metastatic Lewis lung carcinoma (3LL-HH) tumor cell line uses the cellular side of the BM as a substrate for spreading during invasion of muscle, peripheral nerve and adipose tissue [7]. During this process, host cells are detached from their BM and become degraded; however, their BM remains intact. Tumor cell migration on the cellular side of the BM also plays an important role in the vascularization of 3LL-HH liver metastases [8].

In liver [9, 10], brain [11] and lung [12] metastases, it was shown that the differentiation grade of the tumor can also have an impact on the histologic structure of the metastases. Three different growth patterns were described in liver metastases of colorectal adenocarcinomas [9]. In the replacement growth pattern (high grade), the structure of the liver is preserved. However, in desmoplastic and pushing growth patterns, the structure of the liver is disturbed. In the pushing growth pattern, liver plates are pushed aside. As a result, compressed liver parenchyma surrounds the metastases. In the desmoplastic growth, a robust fibrous capsule separates the liver parenchyma from the tumor tissue.

Earlier, we described the development of the vasculature in a "pushing-type" experimental colorectal carcinoma model (C38) in the liver [13]. During the growth of metastases, smooth muscle actin (SMA)-positive cells appeared at the tumor-parenchyma interface, while hepatocytes disappeared from this region. This process resulted in the appearance of vascular lakes formed by the fusion of hepatic sinusoids at the border of the metastases. Fused sinusoids and collagenous matrix-producing SMA-positive myofibroblasts became incorporated into the growing tumor. The deepest part of the invagination was separated from the surrounding host tissue, and the process culminated in the formation of connective tissue columns with a centrally located, functional vessel. We believe that the formation of these columns is a characteristic feature of the C38 tumor. However, in experimental brain metastases, these structures were not present. Instead, the brain microvessels were directly surrounded by the tumor cells. This raises the question of whether the appearance of vessel-containing columns is a consequence of the host tissue's microenvironmental effects on the tumor or, alternatively, whether these structures are intrinsic characteristic features of certain tumor types. Thus, their presence is independent from the target host

tissue microenvironment. The main goal of the present study was to clarify whether the vascular and connective tissue structure of tumors are intrinsically determined by the tumor type or, alternatively, if these features are defined by the host tissue. We generated experimental tumors (C38 colon cancer) at five different locations (skin, cecal wall, liver, brain and lung) and analyzed their vascular and connective tissue structures. As the formation and remodeling of myofibroblast-containing connective tissue columns require active fibrogenesis, we also investigated the possible role of fibrogenic growth factors during column formation.

Materials and methods
Animals and tumor cell line
Eight-week-old male C57Bl/6 mice were obtained from the animal facility of the First Department of Pathology and Experimental Cancer Research of Semmelweis University (Budapest, Hungary). The animal study protocols were conducted according to National Institute of Health (NIH) guidelines for animal care and were approved by the Animal Care and Use Committee of Semmelweis University (PEI/001/2457-6/2015). The C38 colorectal carcinoma cell line was maintained in vivo by serial subcutaneous transplantations, as described previously [13]. Subcutaneous tumors were removed and cut into small pieces (~ 0.5 cm^3) and were implanted under the skin of C57Bl/6 mice.

In vivo experiments
To generate experimental tumors (subcutaneous tissue, cecal wall, brain, liver, and lung), subcutaneously growing C38 tumor tissue was removed, cut into small pieces (~ 2 mm^3), and digested in RPMI-1640 medium (Cat. No.: R8758, Sigma-Aldrich, St Louis, MO, USA) supplemented with 0.7 mg/mL collagenase (Cat. No.: C5138, Sigma-Aldrich) at 37 °C, for 45 min. After filtration through fourfold sterile gauze, cells were centrifuged (800 rpm, 10 min, 4 °C). The pellet was resuspended in 10 mL of RPMI-1640 medium without any supplement, and the number of viable tumor cells was counted using the trypan blue exclusion test. Mice were anesthetized with an intraperitoneal injection of ketamine–xylazine (Cat. No.: K113, 80:12 mg/kg; Sigma-Aldrich).

In the orthotopic primary tumor model, a midline incision was made in the abdomen, and the cecum was gently exteriorized onto gauze impregnated with saline. Cells were injected into the cecal wall of mice with a 30-gauge needle (Braun, Melsungen, Germany) in ~ 5 µL volume ($\sim 2 \times 10^4$ cells). The cecum was returned to the abdominal cavity, and the incision was closed.

Cells were injected heterotopically into the brain, spleen, and footpad of the mice. Brain tumors were produced as described previously [11]. Briefly, the right parietal bone was drilled with a 21-gauge needle (Braun) 2 mm posterior to the coronal suture and 1 mm lateral to the sagittal suture. Ten thousand cells in a volume of 2 μL were slowly injected using a 10 μL Hamilton syringe. Liver metastases were produced by injecting tumor cells (2×10^5 cells in a volume of 50 μL) into the spleen of mice as described previously [13]. To produce lung metastases, cell suspension (5×10^4 cells in a volume of 20 μL) was injected into the footpads of the hind legs of the mice. The legs were amputated 18–28 days following tumor cell injection.

Subcutaneous tumors were generated by implanting 0.5 cm³ tumor pieces under the skin of the mice.

Animals were sacrificed 7–10 days after intracranial injection, 15–18 days after intrasplenic injection, 15–21 days after subcutaneous transplantation, 21 days after orthotopic injection, and 5–8 weeks after hind leg amputation.

Immunofluorescence analysis

Tumors from the five different locations were removed and frozen in isopentane (Sigma-Aldrich) chilled with liquid nitrogen. Frozen sections (15 μm) were fixed in methanol (-20 °C) for 10 min and incubated at room temperature (1 h) with a mixture of primary antibodies (Table 1). After washing, sections were incubated (30 min) with appropriate secondary antibodies (Life Technologies, Carlsbad, CA, USA) (Table 1). Samples were analyzed by confocal laser scanning microscopy using a Bio-Rad MRC-1024 system (Bio-Rad, Richmond, CA, USA).

Morphometric analysis

Frozen sections of tumor samples from all locations were stained for CD31 and laminin. Sections were scanned using Pannoramic Scanner (3D-Histech Ltd., Budapest, Hungary), and a morphometric analysis was performed using Pannoramic Viewer software (3D-Histech Ltd.). Only the columns containing one individual vessel were used during measurements. The distance between the

basement membrane (BM) of the central vessel and the laminin deposited by the tumor cells around the column was measured at two sides of the vessel. The orientation of the columns in the tumor tissues was random, resulting in cut profiles of different ovality. Therefore, we always determined the smallest distance between the central vessel and the column edge. At least 5 mice/ tumor location and three slides from each tumor were used. Ten to twenty vessels/slide were measured.

Electron microscopy

Tumor-bearing mice were anesthetized and perfused via the left ventricle with $1\times$ phosphate-buffered saline (PBS) for 10 min and with a mixture of 4% paraformaldehyde and 1% glutaraldehyde in PBS (pH 7.2) for 15 min at room temperature. Tissues containing tumors (cecal wall, brain, liver, lung, and subcutaneous tissue) were removed, cut into 1–2 mm pieces, and immersed in the same fixative for an additional 2 h. Pieces were postfixed in 1% OsO_4 and 0.5% K-ferrocyanide in PBS for 2 h, dehydrated in a graded series of acetone, and embedded in Spurr's mixture. Semi-thin sections of samples stained by 0.5% toluidine blue (pH 8.5) were analyzed. Ultrathin sections cut by an RMC MT-7 ultramicrotome (Research and Manufacturing Co, Tucson, AZ) were contrasted with uranyl-acetate and lead citrate and analyzed using a Philips CM10 electron microscope (Philips, Eindhoven, The Netherlands).

Cell lines

B16 mouse melanoma cells were cultured in RPMI-1640 supplemented with 10% fetal bovine serum (Sigma-Aldrich), and 1×10^6 tumor cells were collected in lysis buffer.

To obtain a cell culture from the dissociated C38 tumor, 2.5×10^5 viable tumor cells were seeded into T-25 flasks containing 5 ml of complete media and incubated at 37 °C in 5% CO_2. The cells were subcultured every 3 days by a conventional trypsinization method, and 1×10^6 tumor cells were collected in lysis buffer.

Table 1 Antibodies and fluorescent dye used for immunofluorescence

Antibody	Species	Manufacturer	Catalog number	Dilution
CD31	Rat monoclonal	BD Pharmingen, Franklin Lakes, NJ, USA	550275	1:50
Laminin	Rabbit polyclonal	DAKO, Glostrup, Denmark	Z0097	1:200
Collagen I	Rabbit polyclonal	Chemicon, Billerica, MA, USA	AB765P	1:100
SMA	Mouse monoclonal	DAKO, Glostrup, Denmark	M0851	1:200
panCK-FITC	Mouse monoclonal	DAKO, Glostrup, Denmark	F0859	1:100
TOTO-3		Invitrogen, Carlsbad, CA, USA	T3604	1:500

(See figure on next page.)
Fig. 1 Accumulation and incorporation of vessels and connective tissue at the tumor surface. **A**, **B** Subcutaneously growing C38 tumor. The accumulation of collagen I (*red*)- and smooth muscle actin (SMA)-expressing myofibroblasts (*blue*) is present at the tumor surface (*arrows*). Black areas represent viable tumor mass (*T*) beneath the tumor surface. For clarity, **B** shows the blue (SMA) channel separately. Numerous vessels (CD31, *green*) are being incorporated (together with connective tissue) by the tumor (*large arrowheads*). Smaller connective tissue columns separated from the incorporated connective tissue are visible within the tumor tissue (*small arrowheads*). *N* necrosis. **C**, **D** C38 tumor (*T*) growing in the liver. In the left upper part of **c**, the peritumoral liver parenchyma—with the dense CD31-positive network of sinusoids (green)—is visible. The tumor-parenchyma interface is indicated by arrows. Here, accumulation of SMA-positive cells can be observed (see also **D**, for the separate blue channel). These cells are also present in the invaginations (*large arrowheads*) and in the incorporated host connective tissue deep within the tumor (*small arrowheads*). The invaginations and the incorporated host tissue pieces are delineated by the laminin (*red*) deposited by the tumor cells. Inset: high-power micrograph of the surface of a C38 liver metastasis, demonstrating the accumulation of SMA-positive cells (*blue*). Tumor tissue is present on the left side (*black area*). On the right side, pan-cytokeratin-expressing hepatocytes (*green*) and CD31-positive vessels (*red*) are visible. Between the hepatocytes and the tumor tissue, SMA-positive cells (*blue*) can be observed. **E**, **F** A C38 brain metastasis (**E**) is highlighted and bordered by laminin (*red*), which is deposited by tumor cells. CD31-positive vessels (*green*) appear yellowish because of their close proximity of the basement membrane (*red*) (**E**). No SMA accumulation is present at the periphery of the tumor, as can be seen on the separate blue (SMA) channel (**F**). The peritumoral vessels are smaller than the intratumoral vessels, which are surrounded by SMA-positive pericytes (*blue*). SMA-positive cells are not found around the peritumoral vessels, excluding the arterioles. *N* necrosis, *T* tumor tissue

Gene expression analysis
Total RNA was isolated with Trizol (Cat. No.: 15596–018, Life Technologies, Waltham, MA, USA). RNA concentration was measured by a NanoDrop 1000 Spectrophotometer (Thermo Fisher Scientific, Wilmington, DE), and 1 µg RNA per sample was converted into cDNA.

A high capacity cDNA reverse transcription kit (Cat. No.: 4368814, Thermo Fisher Scientific) was used for cDNA synthesis as recommended by the supplier. Quantitative real-time polymerase chain reaction. (qRT-PCR) was performed by the ABI Quant Studio3 (Thermo Fisher Scientific) sequence detection system using Thermo Fisher Scientific TaqMan gene expression assays (connective tissue growth factor (Ctgf): Mm01192931_g1; Fibroblast growth factor 2 (Fgf2): Mm00433287_m1; Transforming growth factor-β 1 (Tgfb1): Mm01178820_m1; Transforming growth factor-β2 (Tgfb2): Mm00436955_m1; Transforming growth factor-β3 (Tgfb3): Mm00436960_m1; Platelet-derived growth factor-β Pdgfb: Mm01298578_m1) according to the manufacturer's instructions. Glyceraldehyde-3-phosphate dehydrogenase (GAPDH, Thermo Fischer Scientific, Cat No.: 4352932E) was used as an endogenous control. All samples were run in triplicate in a 20 µL reaction volume. The results were obtained as threshold cycle (CT) values. Expression levels were calculated using the ΔCT method. The values were calculated as the mean values of three independent measurements, and the expression levels of mRNA in all samples were defined as ratios to GAPDH expression (%).

Statistical analysis
Data are represented as the mean $\pm$ SD of at least three independent experiments. The statistical significance of differences between groups was analyzed with Student's *t* test. Values of $P < 0.05$ were considered statistically significant (GraphPad Software, La Jolla, CA).

Results
Incorporation of vessels and connective tissue at the tumor surface
At the periphery of C38 tumors growing in subcutaneous tissue, liver, colon, and lung, we found smooth muscle actin (SMA)-expressing activated fibroblasts (myofibroblasts) and the consequently accumulated collagen (Fig. 1A–D). However, there was no myofibroblast or collagen accumulation around tumors growing in the brain, as only the pericytes of the intratumoral vessels were SMA-positive (Fig. 1E, F). Accordingly, although C38 tumors acquired their vasculature by the incorporation of the peritumoral host tissue at all tumor sites, the incorporation process in the brain was different from the incorporation process in the skin, colon, liver, and lung. For the latter organs, where SMA-positive cells and collagen accumulated around the tumors, invaginations of different sizes were formed at the surface of the tumors containing vessels and perivascular connective tissue (Figs. 1A, C, 2A–C). BM deposited by the tumor delineated the invaginations (Fig. 2A).

The situation was slightly different in the lung tissue, where the tumor mass advanced through the alveoli, thereby incorporating the alveolar walls (with all of its components). This process resulted in invagination-like structures in the tumor (Fig. 3D).

In contrast, in tumors growing in the brain, the parenchyma (astrocytes) was completely separated from the vessels and excluded from the tumor (Fig. 2D). However, pericytes maintained their original position, and invaginations did not develop in the brain. Instead, the tumor tissue engulfed the cerebral capillaries one by one at the advancing margin. The tumor cells attached tightly to the capillary BM, and no deposited collagen could be observed between the vessels and the tumor cells (Fig. 2E).

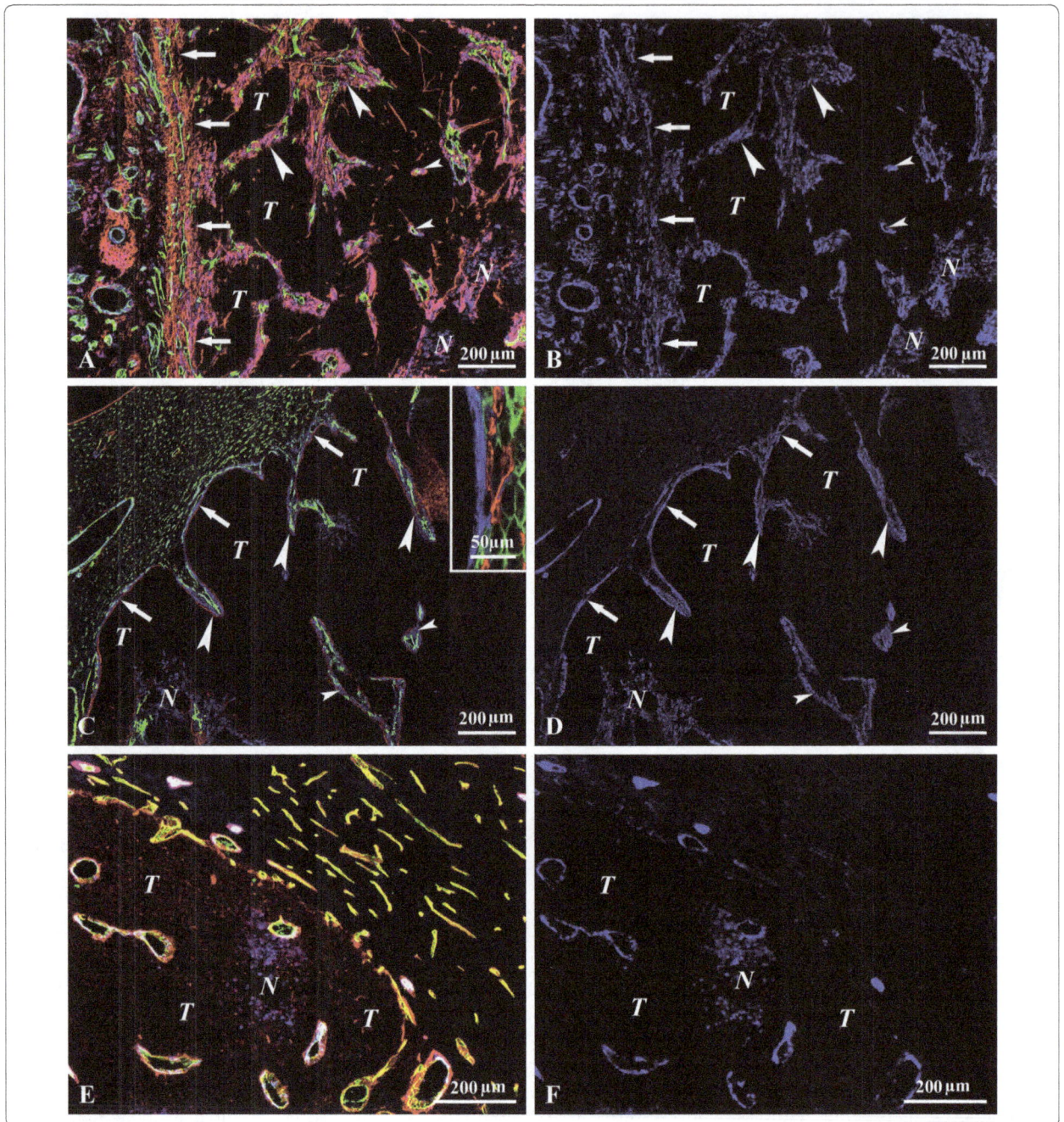

Maturation of the columns

In early invaginations, the number of incorporated vessels and the amount of connective tissue were dependent on the size of the vessels and the invaginations (Figs. 1A, C, 3A–D, 4A). As invaginations with multiple capillaries moved deeper into the tumor tissue, tumor cells separated the microvessels from each other. This "maturation" process culminated in the appearance of connective tissue columns with a single central vessel (Figs. 3A–D, 4A–E). In detail, the cross-sectional view of the columns showed the following structural elements from inside out: endothelial layer, capillary BM, SMA-positive cells embedded in collagen-containing matrix, and BM of the tumor (Fig. 4B–F). We observed that both the size of the connective tissue columns and the amount of deposited perivascular BM material increased from the peritumoral host tissue towards the tumor center (Fig. 4A). We found the thickest connective tissue columns in subcutaneous tumors (18.9±1.9 μm,) whereas the diameter of the columns at other locations (liver: 15.5±1.7 μm*, lung: 12.2±2.3 μm*,

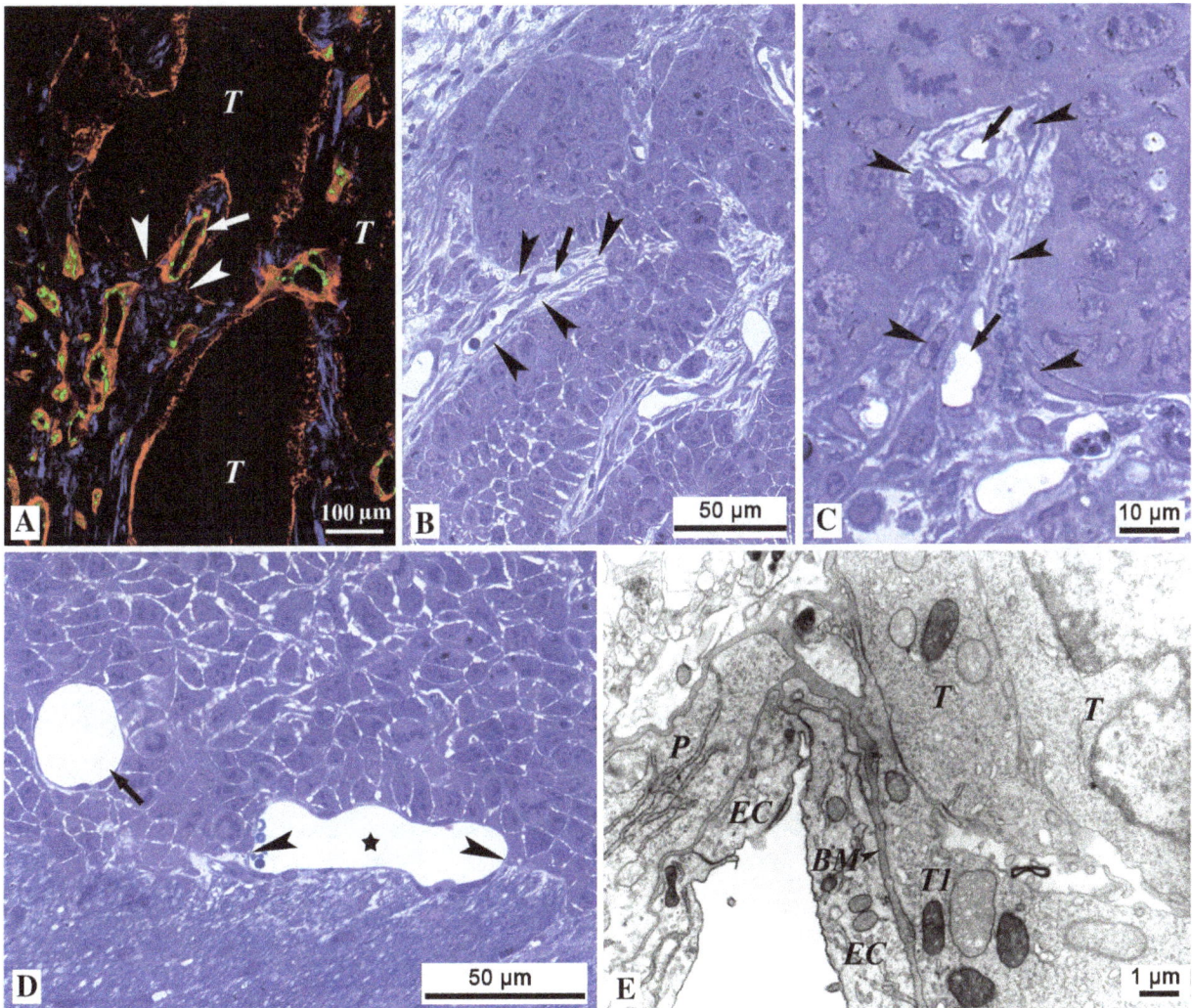

Fig. 2 The process of vessel incorporation. **A** Frozen section of a subcutaneous C38 tumor stained for laminin (*red*), CD31 (*green*) and SMA (*blue*). The tumor tissue (*T*) appears black and is surrounded by laminin (*red*) deposited by the tumor cells. A large vessel (*arrow*) is being incorporated together with SMA-positive cells (*blue*) in an invagination. The outer part of the invagination, in contrast to the inner part, is delineated by a thinner and more fragmented basement membrane (*arrowheads*). **B, C** Semi-thin sections of C38 tumors growing in the subcutaneous tissue (**B**) and in the cecal wall (**C**). Blood vessels (*arrows*) and the surrounding connective tissue with cellular elements (*arrowheads*) are being incorporated by the tumor. **D** Semi-thin section of a C38 brain metastasis. A vessel (*asterisk*) is partially engulfed by the tumor mass (*arrowheads*). During this process, the brain parenchyma (located in the lower part of the picture) is excluded from the tumor (located in the upper part of the picture). The tumor cells are in close vicinity to the wall of the fully incorporated vessel (*arrow*). **E** An electron micrograph of a partially incorporated brain capillary at the surface of the tumor (*T*). A tumor cell (*T1*) is in touch with the basement membrane (*BM*) of the capillary. Collagen fibers cannot be observed between the tumor cell (*T1*) and the capillary basement membrane. *EC* endothelial cell, *P* pericyte

cecal wall: 13.2 ± 2.1 µm*) were significantly smaller (*t test, $P \leq 0.05$). The final consequence of the maturation process was that at all locations (where collagen and SMA-positive cells accumulated around the tumors), the same connective tissue and vascular structure developed.

As the brain parenchyma lacks fibroblasts, no connective tissue columns were produced in this location. However, we occasionally observed connective tissue columns also in the C38 cerebral metastases when the growing tumor reached the meningeal fibroblasts (Fig. 4F).

However, we could only minimally detect columns that reached the single-vessel stage during their development.

Relative gene expression analysis of fibrogenic growth factors

In our earlier work, we analyzed in detail the vascularization of primary (intracutaneous) and metastatic (lung) B16 melanoma and found no accumulation of collagen at the tumor periphery or around the incorporated vessels (i.e., we did not observe intratumoral tissue columns

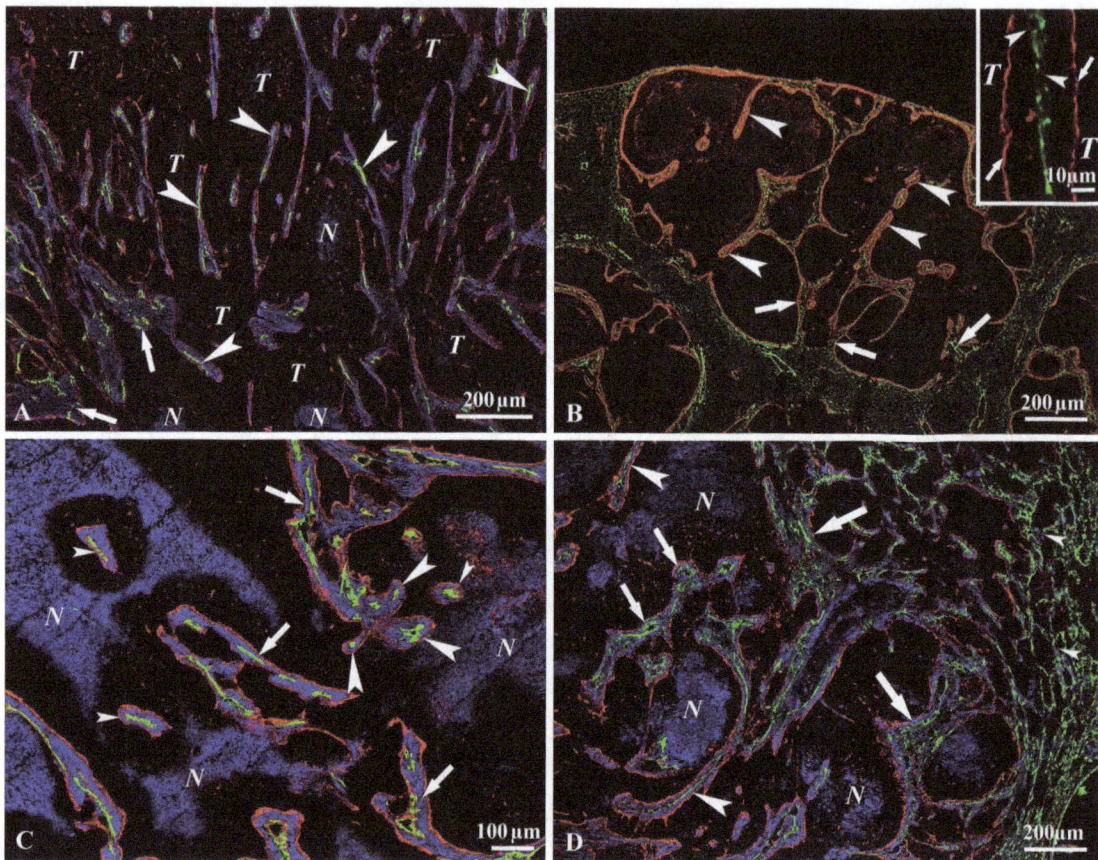

Fig. 3 "Processing" of the invaginations. **A** A C38 tumor growing in the cecal wall. Incorporated connective tissue, which contains myofibroblasts (SMA, blue) and numerous vessels (CD31, green) (arrows) is visible throughout the tumor mass. All blue areas represent the columns, excluding necrotic areas (marked by N). Necrotic tissue is also highlighted by the nonspecific binding of the anti-mouse secondary antibody (used to detect the mouse monoclonal primary antibody against SMA) to these areas. Note the high number of advanced-stage connective tissue columns that contain only one single vessel (*arrowheads*). The columns are delineated by laminin (red) containing basement membrane produced by the tumor (T). **B** C38 metastasis in the liver. The early-stage incorporations contain numerous vessels (CD31, green) (*arrows*). Advanced-stage connective tissue columns, which contain single central vessels, are present intratumorally (*arrowheads*). Laminin (*red*) deposited by the tumor cells borders the incorporated tissue and the columns. The inset shows the fine structure of a longitudinally sectioned column containing a single central vessel (CD31, green). The basement membrane of the vessel is marked by small arrowheads. The basement membrane marked by small arrows is deposited by the tumor (T) at the surface of the column. **C** Subcutaneous C38 tumor. In addition to columns filled with myofibroblasts (SMA, *blue*) (*small arrowheads*) and containing a single central vessel (CD31, *green*), there are areas containing connective tissue columns with numerous vessels (*arrows*). Note the columns (*large arrowheads*) separated only partially from a larger connective tissue mass during the final steps of the maturation process. The incorporated connective tissue and the columns are bordered by laminin (*red*) deposited by the tumor cells. N marks areas of necrotic tissue that also appear blue, although this staining is due to the nonspecific binding of the anti-mouse secondary antibody used to detect the anti-SMA antibody. **D** C38 lung metastasis. The section is labeled with anti-CD31 (*green*), anti-laminin (*red*) and anti-SMA antibodies (*blue*). There are no SMA-positive cells (*blue*) in the alveolar walls of the normal lung tissue far from the metastasis (right edge of the micrograph). SMA-positive cells begin to appear in the peritumoral lung tissue (*small arrowheads*), but the number of these cells only notably increases intratumorally. Large early-stage connective tissue columns are present at the tumor periphery (*large arrows*), from which smaller tissue pieces containing different numbers of vessels are detaching (*small arrows*). *Large arrowheads* indicate mature columns with single vessels. N marks areas of necrotic tissue that also appear blue, although this staining is due to the nonspecific binding of the anti-mouse secondary antibody used to detect the anti-SMA antibody

in B16 tumors) [12, 14, 15]. Therefore, we used the B16 cell line as a control to compare the expression levels of fibrogenic factors with those of the column-inducing C38 tumor line. We found that the relative expression levels of Pdgfb, Fgf2, Ctgf (Fig. 5a) and Tgf-β (Fig. 5b) mRNAs were significantly higher in C38 cells.

Discussion

In the present study, we analyzed the vascular and connective tissue structures of C38 colon carcinoma growing in different host tissues. The cecal wall represents the primary tumor site, whereas the skin, liver, lung, and brain tissues can be considered metastatic locations.

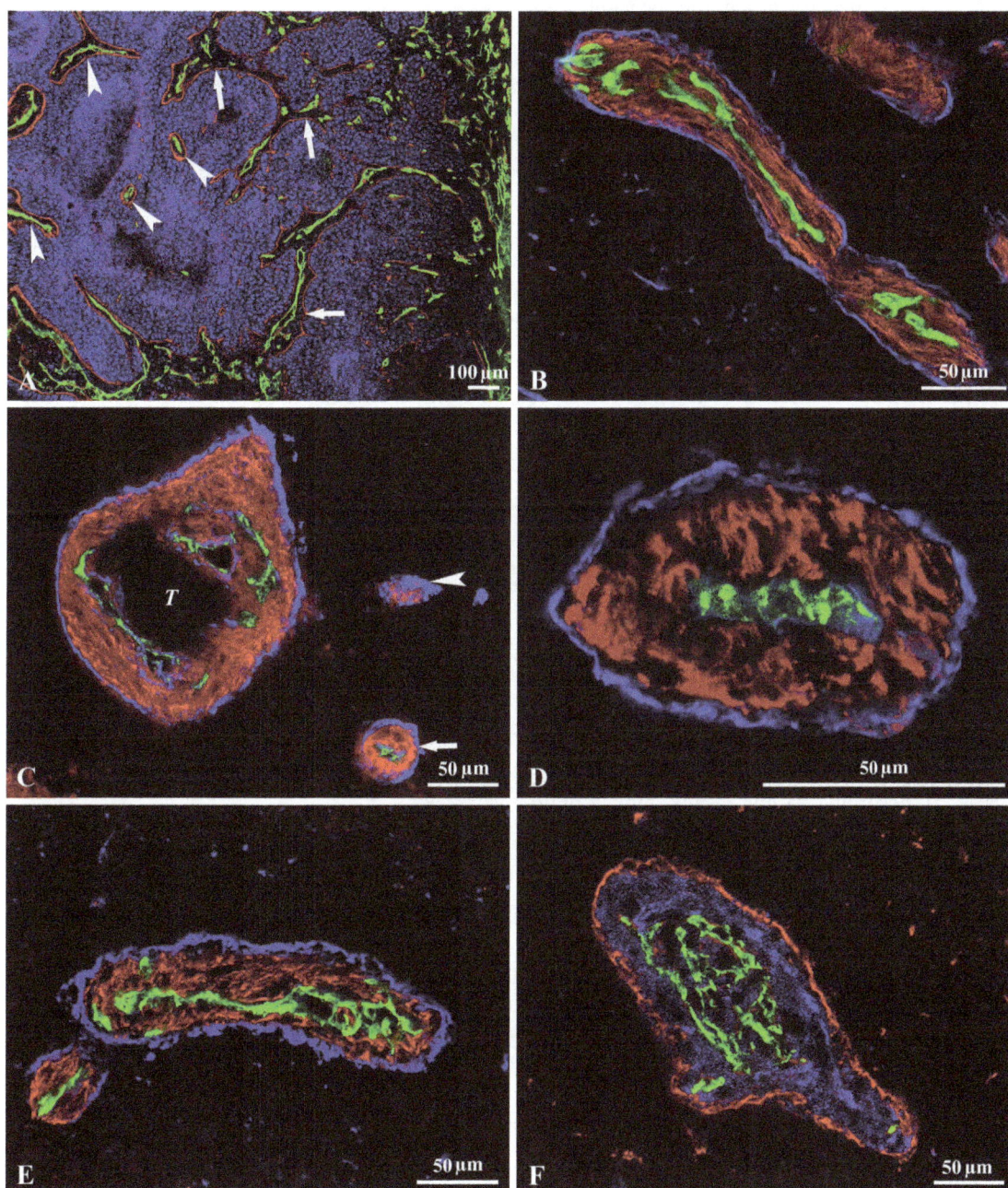

Fig. 4 Maturation and final form of the columns. **A** Frozen section of a subcutaneous C38 tumor labeled for laminin (*red*), CD31 (*green*) and cell nuclei (TOTO-3, *blue*). The maturation process of the columns can be observed as we move from the peritumoral host tissue (right side of the picture) towards the center of the tumor (left side): the size of the columns and the amount of the deposited laminin increase from the periphery towards the tumor center. The newly incorporated connective tissue columns contain more vessels (*arrows*). After "processing" by tumor cells, they contain only a single vessel (*arrowheads*). **B** Tissue column in an orthotopically growing C38 tumor (black areas). The centrally located vessel (CD31, *green*) is surrounded by SMA-positive myofibroblasts (*red*) and enclosed by laminin (*blue*). **C** The frozen section of a C38 liver metastasis labeled with CD31 (*green*), SMA (*red*) and laminin (*blue*). Black areas represent tumor tissue. As maturation of the tissue columns progresses, the central part of the large column containing multiple vessels is invaded by the tumor (*T*). The tumor mass present within the column is not delineated by laminin, which indicates an early phase of invasion. At the lower right, a mature column is visible (*arrow*) containing a single vessel located centrally. Note the presence of a "misprocessed" column (*arrowhead*) that contains no vessels. **D** Connective tissue column in a subcutaneous C38 tumor (tumor cells fill the outer black area). The completely matured column contains a single central vessel (CD31, green) surrounded by connective tissue, which contains collagen I (*red*) and laminin deposited by the tumor cells (blue). **E** C38 lung metastasis. The black area represents tumor tissue. The column shows the same structure as in other locations. A central vessel can be seen (CD31, *green*), surrounded by SMA-positive cells (*red*) and laminin (*blue*). **F** C38 metastasis (black areas) reaching the brain surface. A connective tissue column that contains numerous vessels (CD31, *green*) surrounded by SMA-positive cells (*blue*) and laminin (*red*) produced by the tumor can be observed at this location

Tumor structure is dependent on the availability of tumor-derived fibrogenic factors and host tissue fibroblasts. Subcutaneous, cecal, hepatic, and pulmonary fibroblasts were peritumorally transformed into collagen-producing myofibroblasts. The evolution of tumorous connective tissue in these organs culminated in the appearance of intratumoral connective tissue columns with central vessels. The structure of these columns was identical in all of the aforementioned locations, resulting in a similar histological appearance of the tumors independent of the host organ. Therefore, it can be concluded that the tumor cells activate the peritumoral host tissue fibroblasts, which then participate in the formation of connective tissue columns. The activation of fibroblasts may be stimulated by the synthesis and secretion of tumor cell-derived "fibrogenic" factors. This concept, although requiring further studies, is supported by our observation that column-inducing C38 cells express higher levels of fibrogenic factors (e.g., Tgf-betas, Fgf2, Pdgfb, and Ctgf) [16–18] than B16 cells, which do not form tissue column-containing tumors in any locations [12, 14, 15]. In further support of our aforementioned findings, we observed that no intratumoral connective tissue columns developed in the brain (which lacks fibroblasts); instead, the capillaries of C38 cerebral metastasis were surrounded exclusively by tumor cells. Although previous studies suggest that pericytes can play an active role in connective tissue production [19–21], according to our results, mouse brain capillary pericytes did not produce connective tissue in the experimental conditions we used. It is also important to mention that intratumoral tissue columns were detected in cerebral C38 tumors when the metastatic tissue reached the meninges, where fibroblasts are located. In summary, the presence of the appropriate cell type (i.e., fibroblasts) in the tumor microenvironment and the synthesis of fibrogenic factors by the tumor cells can result in the same histological appearance of the tumor, regardless of the origin of the host tissue.

The early invaginations inevitably produced at the surface of the growing tumor spheres generally contain numerous incorporated vessels. Deeper in the tumor, the invaginations are "processed" (the tumor tissue pinches off connective tissue pieces, including vessels) down to the single-vessel stage (i.e., the connective tissue column produced contains only a single vessel). Although the size of these columns was fairly uniform in the different organs, we found significantly larger tissue columns in the skin compared with other organs. We cannot provide a reasonable explanation for this difference, as one would expect the diameter of the columns to be determined by the diffusion of oxygen and nutrients. However, tissue columns with the largest diameter can provide sufficient blood supply for several rows of tumor cells around the

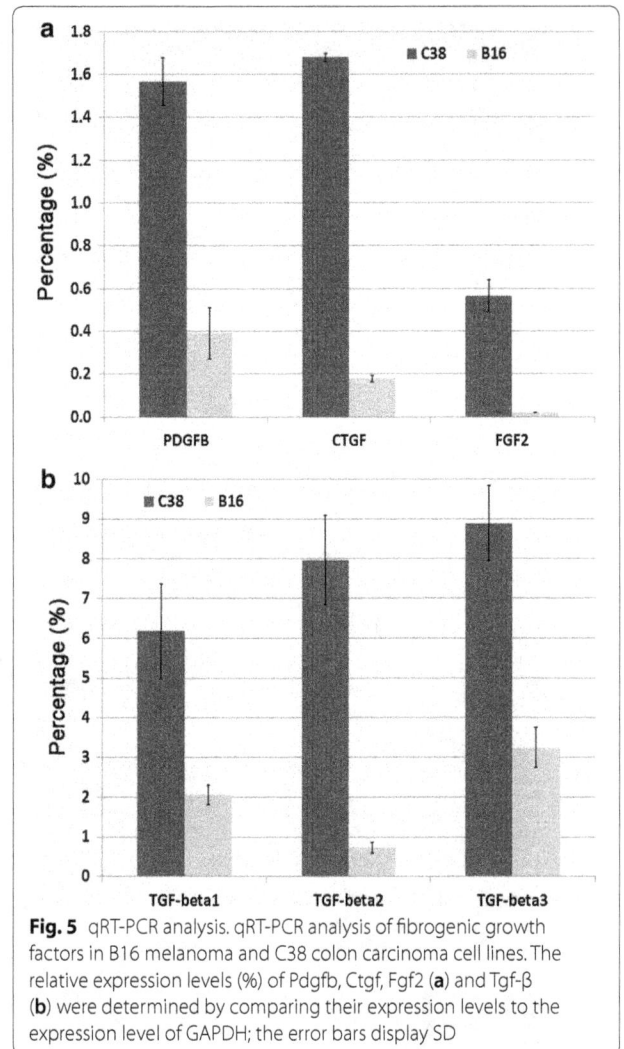

Fig. 5 qRT-PCR analysis. qRT-PCR analysis of fibrogenic growth factors in B16 melanoma and C38 colon carcinoma cell lines. The relative expression levels (%) of Pdgfb, Ctgf, Fgf2 (**a**) and Tgf-β (**b**) were determined by comparing their expression levels to the expression level of GAPDH; the error bars display SD

columns. It is also worth noting that the generation of intratumoral columns with such a regular structure is a unique characteristic of C38 tumors. Nevertheless, other tumor types also incorporate and process connective tissue (including the blood vessels) into rather irregular networks that are still able to provide tumors with oxygen and nutrients (unpublished data).

We found that the amount of connective tissue present in the columns and the integrity and thickness of the BM deposited by the tumor increased towards the tumor center, suggesting that the structures in the center of the tumor are older than those at the periphery. This finding is in line with the notion that "for tumor survival the edge is the future and the center is history" [22] and, moreover, provides additional proof that vascularization occurs by vessel incorporation, not vessel ingrowth [11–13, 23–31].

In conclusion, in the current study, we examined the microanatomy and the vascularization process of C38 colon carcinoma in five different organs using confocal and electron microscopy. Our results suggest that the vascular and connective tissue structures of tumors are determined by both the primary tumor type (i.e., the production of tumor-derived fibrogenic factors) and the host tissue microenvironment (i.e., the availability of suitable connective tissue elements).

Authors' contributions
SP, BD, JT, PN, and EB wrote the manuscript. EB, VS, and KD performed the animal experiments and immunofluorescence analysis. EB performed the morphometric analysis. SP performed the electron microscopic studies. AS was responsible for the in vitro cell cultures. AR, AS, and VL performed the gene expression analysis and the statistics. All authors read and approved the final manuscript.

Author details
[1] First Department of Pathology and Experimental Cancer Research, Semmelweis University, Budapest, Üllői út 26, 1085, Hungary. [2] Department of Experimental Pharmacology, National Institute of Oncology, Budapest 1122, Hungary. [3] Department of Thoracic Surgery, Semmelweis University-National Institute of Oncology, Budapest 1122, Hungary. [4] Department of Thoracic Surgery, Medical University of Vienna, Waehringer Guertel 18-20, 1090 Vienna, Austria. [5] Department of Biomedical Imaging and Image-guided Therapy, Medical University of Vienna, 1090 Vienna, Austria. [6] National Koranyi Institute of Pulmonology, Budapest 1122, Hungary. [7] Tumor Progression Research Group, Hungarian Academy of Sciences-Semmelweis University, Budapest 1085, Hungary.

Competing interests
The authors declare that they have no competing interests.

Funding
KD is the recipient of the Bolyai fellowship of the Hungarian Academy of Sciences and received support from the National Excellence Program (TÁMOP 4.2.4. A/1-11-1-2012-0001). BD acknowledges support from the Hungarian NRDI Office (K109626, K108465, KNN121510 and SNN114490). SP and VL acknowledge support from the Hungarian NRDI Office (ANN125583). JT acknowledges support from the National Research, Development and Innovation Office (NKFIH116295). EB is the recipient of postdoctoral fellowship from the Hungarian Academy of Sciences.

References
1. Milne EN, Margulis AR, Noonan CD, Stoughton JT. Histologic type-specific vascular patterns in rat tumors. Cancer. 1967;20(10):1635–46.
2. Konerding MA, Malkusch W, Klapthor B, van Ackern C, Fait E, Hill SA, et al. Evidence for characteristic vascular patterns in solid tumours: quantitative studies using corrosion casts. Br J Cancer. 1999;80(5–6):724–32.
3. Solesvik OV, Rofstad EK, Brustad T. Vascular structure of five human malignant melanomas grown in athymic nude mice. Br J Cancer. 1982;46(4):557–67.
4. Kienast Y, von Baumgarten L, Fuhrmann M, Klinkert WE, Goldbrunner R, Herms J, et al. Real-time imaging reveals the single steps of brain metastasis formation. Nat Med. 2010;16(1):116–22.
5. Dome B, Timar J, Paku S. A novel concept of glomeruloid body formation in experimental cerebral metastases. J Neuropathol Exp Neurol. 2003;62(6):655–61.
6. Carbonell WS, Ansorge O, Sibson N, Muschel R. The vascular basement membrane as "soil" in brain metastasis. PLoS ONE. 2009;4(6):e5857.
7. Paku S, Timar J, Lapis K. Ultrastructure of invasion in different tissue types by Lewis lung tumour variants. Virchows Archiv A Pathol Anat Histopathol. 1990;417(5):435–42.
8. Paku S, Lapis K. Morphological aspects of angiogenesis in experimental liver metastases. Am J Pathol. 1993;143(3):926–36.
9. Vermeulen PB, Colpaert C, Salgado R, Royers R, Hellemans H, Van Den Heuvel E, et al. Liver metastases from colorectal adenocarcinomas grow in three patterns with different angiogenesis and desmoplasia. J Pathol. 2001;195(3):336–42.
10. Stessels F, Van den Eynden G, Van der Auwera I, Salgado R, Van den Heuvel E, Harris AL, et al. Breast adenocarcinoma liver metastases, in contrast to colorectal cancer liver metastases, display a non-angiogenic growth pattern that preserves the stroma and lacks hypoxia. Br J Cancer. 2004;90(7):1429–36.
11. Bugyik E, Dezso K, Reiniger L, Laszlo V, Tovari J, Timar J, et al. Lack of angiogenesis in experimental brain metastases. J Neuropathol Exp Neurol. 2011;70(11):979–91.
12. Szabo V, Bugyik E, Dezso K, Ecker N, Nagy P, Timar J, et al. Mechanism of tumour vascularization in experimental lung metastases. J Pathol. 2015;235(3):384–96.
13. Paku S, Kopper L, Nagy P. Development of the vasculature in "pushing-type" liver metastases of an experimental colorectal cancer. Int J Cancer. 2005;115(6):893–902.
14. Alino SF, Hilario E. Nodular organization and differential intrametastatic distribution of the fluorescent dye Hoechst 33342 in B16 melanoma liver metastasis. Exp Cell Biol. 1989;57(5):246–56.
15. Dome B, Paku S, Somlai B, Timar J. Vascularization of cutaneous melanoma involves vessel co-option and has clinical significance. J Pathol. 2002;197(3):355–62.
16. Anderberg C, Li H, Fredriksson L, Andrae J, Betsholtz C, Li X, et al. Paracrine signaling by platelet-derived growth factor-CC promotes tumor growth by recruitment of cancer-associated fibroblasts. Can Res. 2009;69(1):369–78.
17. Meng XM, Nikolic-Paterson DJ, Lan HY. TGF-beta: the master regulator of fibrosis. Nat Rev Nephrol. 2016;12(6):325–38.
18. Darby IA, Zakuan N, Billet F, Desmouliere A. The myofibroblast, a key cell in normal and pathological tissue repair. Cell Mol Life Sci. 2016;73(6):1145–57.
19. Goritz C, Dias DO, Tomilin N, Barbacid M, Shupliakov O, Frisen J. A pericyte origin of spinal cord scar tissue. Science. 2011;333(6039):238–42.
20. Soderblom C, Luo X, Blumenthal E, Bray E, Lyapichev K, Ramos J, et al. Perivascular fibroblasts form the fibrotic scar after contusive spinal cord injury. J Neurosci. 2013;33(34):13882–7.
21. Makihara N, Arimura K, Ago T, Tachibana M, Nishimura A, Nakamura K, et al. Involvement of platelet-derived growth factor receptor beta in fibrosis through extracellular matrix protein production after ischemic stroke. Exp Neurol. 2015;264:127–34.
22. Thompson WD. Tumour versus patient: vascular and tumour survival versus prognosis. J Pathol. 2001;193(4):425–6.
23. Thompson WD, Shiach KJ, Fraser RA, McIntosh LC, Simpson JG. Tumours acquire their vasculature by vessel incorporation, not vessel ingrowth. J Pathol. 1987;151(4):323–32.
24. Pezzella F, Pastorino U, Tagliabue E, Andreola S, Sozzi G, Gasparini G, et al. Non-small-cell lung carcinoma tumor growth without morphological evidence of neo-angiogenesis. Am J Pathol. 1997;151(5):1417–23.
25. Pezzella F, Di Bacco A, Andreola S, Nicholson AG, Pastorino U, Harris AL. Angiogenesis in primary lung cancer and lung secondaries. Eur J Cancer. 1996;32A(14):2494–500.
26. Adighibe O, Micklem K, Campo L, Ferguson M, Harris A, Pozos R, et al. Is nonangiogenesis a novel pathway for cancer progression? A study using 3-dimensional tumour reconstructions. Br J Cancer. 2006;94(8):1176–9.
27. Pezzella F, Manzotti M, Di Bacco A, Viale G, Nicholson AG, Price R, Ratcliffe C, Pastorino U, Gatter KC, Harris AL, Altman DG. Evidence for novel non-angiogenic pathway in breast-cancer metastasis. Breast cancer progression working party. Lancet. 2000;355(9217):1787–8.
28. Yousem SA. Peripheral squamous cell carcinoma of lung: patterns of growth with particular focus on airspace filling. Hum Pathol. 2009;40(6):861–7.
29. Sardari Nia P, Hendriks J, Friedel G, Van Schil P, Van Marck E. Distinct angiogenic and non-angiogenic growth patterns of lung metastases from renal cell carcinoma. Histopathology. 2007;51(3):354–61.
30. Frentzas S, Simoneau E, Bridgeman VL, Vermeulen PB, Foo S, Kostaras E, et al. Vessel co-option mediates resistance to anti-angiogenic therapy in liver metastases. Nat Med. 2016;22(11):1294–302.

Phenformin alone or combined with gefitinib inhibits bladder cancer via AMPK and EGFR pathways

Yanjun Huang[1], Sichun Zhou[1], Caimei He[1], Jun Deng[1], Ting Tao[1], Qiongli Su[1], Kwame Oteng Darko[1], Mei Peng[1,2] and Xiaoping Yang[1]*

Abstract

Background: In previous studies, we have shown that the combination of metformin and gefitinib inhibits the growth of bladder cancer cells. Here we examined whether the metformin analogue phenformin, either used alone or in combination with gefitinib, could inhibit growth of bladder cancer cells.

Methods: The growth-inhibitory effects of phenformin and gefitinib were tested in one murine and two human bladder cancer cell lines using MTT and clonogenic assays. Effects on cell migration were assessed in a wound healing assay. Synergistic action between the two drugs was assessed using CompuSyn software. The potential involvement of AMPK and EGFR pathways in the effects of phenformin and gefitinib was explored using Western blotting.

Results: In MTT and clonogenic assays, phenformin was > 10-fold more potent than metformin in inhibiting bladder cancer cell growth. Phenformin also potently inhibited cell migration in wound healing assays, and promoted apoptosis. AMPK signaling was activated; EGFR signaling was inhibited. Phenformin was synergistic with gefitinib, with the combination of drugs showing much stronger anticancer activity and apoptotic activation than phenformin alone.

Conclusions: Phenformin shows potential as an effective drug against bladder cancer, either alone or in combination with gefitinib.

Keywords: Phenformin, Gefitinib, Bladder cancer, AMPK, EGFR

Introduction

The biguanide metformin is widely used as a first-line oral hypoglycemic drug against diabetes [1]. It is well tolerated and safe, with well-characterized pharmacokinetics [2, 3]. Accumulating evidence suggest that metformin could also improve the survival of patients with colorectal, breast cancer, or prostate cancer [4–6]. In fact, it may lower the risk of certain types of cancer [7]. However, obtaining approval from regulatory authorities such as the US Food and Drug Administration to use metformin as an anticancer drug has proven challenging because effective drug concentrations are much higher than antidiabetic doses. Such high concentrations in the blood are not achievable via conventional oral administration [8, 9].

Phenformin is a derivative of metformin, with higher anticancer potency at lower doses [10–12]. Phenformin is more lipophilic than metformin, and does not require cell-surface transporters such as Oct1 to enter cells. This feature makes phenformin potentially more versatile than metformin for targeting cancer tissues, since Oct1 is not expressed in all tissues [13, 14]. Here we examined whether phenformin shows efficacy against bladder cancer [15–17]. In a previous study, we showed that the combination of metformin and the epidermal growth factor receptor (EGFR) inhibitor gefitinib produces cytotoxic effects in bladder cancer cells [9]. Gefitinib is effective as adjuvant treatment of primary bladder cancer [18]. Metformin is synergistic with gefitinib [19]. In the present

*Correspondence: Xiaoping.Yang@hunnu.edu.cn
[1] Key Laboratory of Study and Discovery of Targeted Small Molecules of Hunan Province and Department of Pharmacy in the School of Medicine and Laboratory of Animal Nutrition and Human Health, Hunan Normal University, Changsha 410013, Hunan, P. R. China
Full list of author information is available at the end of the article

study, we examined the anticancer effects of phenformin alone and in combination with gefitinib. Our goal was to determine whether phenformin could inhibit bladder cancer cell growth effectively at lower doses than metformin. Since metformin produces antitumor effects by activating adenosine monophosphate (AMP)-activated protein kinase (AMPK) and subsequent inhibition of the mTOR signaling [20–22], we also examined whether phenformin could inhibit cancer growth by activating AMPK [2, 23].

Materials and methods

Reagents
Phenformin (Aladdin Chemistry, Shanghai, China) was prepared in a range of concentrations in culture medium. Gefitinib (Selleck-Biotool, Shanghai, China) was prepared as a stock solution of 5 mmol/L in DMSO. Antibodies against the following target proteins were obtained from Cell Signaling (Beverly, MA, USA): total p70 S6 kinase, phospho-p70 S6 kinase (Thr389), total AMPKα, phospho-AMPKα (Thr172), total mTOR, phospho-mTOR (Ser2448), total 4E-BP1, phospho-4EBP1, total EGFR, phospho-EGFR and β-actin.

Cell lines and culture conditions
The mouse bladder cancer cell line MB49 and the human bladder cancer cell lines T24 and UMUC3 were generously provided by Dr. P. Guo of the Institute of Urology at Xi'an Jiaotong University (Xi'an, Shaanxi, China) [9]. All cell lines were cultured in DMEM (Hyclone, Logan, UT, USA) supplemented with 10% fetal bovine serum (FBS; Hyclone) and 1% penicillin–streptomycin. Cultures were incubated at 37 °C in humidified air containing 5% CO_2.

Cell viability assay
Cell viability was assessed using a tetrazolium-based assay. Briefly, cells were seeded at 8×10^3 per well in 96-well culture plates and incubated in medium containing 10% FBS. At 24 h later, cells were treated for 48 h with different concentrations of phenformin alone or in combination with gefitinib. The tetrazolium salt of MTT (50 μL; Sigma) was dissolved in Hank's balanced salt solution to a concentration of 2 mg/mL, and added to each well. The plates were incubated another 5 h. The medium was aspirated from each well, DMSO (150 μL; Sigma) was added to dissolve formazan crystals, and absorbance was measured using a microplate reader (Biotek, SYNERGY HTX, VT, USA) at 490 nm (against reference absorbance at 630 nm). Dose–response curves were generated and used to calculate the half-maximal inhibitory concentration (IC_{50}) using SPSS 16.0 (IBM, Chicago, IL, USA).

Clonogenic assay
Briefly, 8×10^3 cells were seeded into 24-well dishes in 0.5 mL of medium. At 24 h, cells were treated with different concentrations of phenformin alone or combined with gefitinib for a further 6–8 day period in medium containing 10% FBS. Cells were fixed with 10% formaldehyde, stained with 0.1% crystal violet. Absorbance was measured using a microplate reader (Biotek) at 550 nm wavelength. Colony formation images were captured under a microscope (DFC450C; Leica, Wetzlar, Germany).

Cell migration
Cells (5×10^3) were seeded into 6-well plates and allowed to reach confluence. The monolayer was scratched using a cocktail stick. Cells were incubated with serum-free DMEM medium for different time periods before capturing the digital images with a DFC450C microscope (Leica). Wound closure was determined by measuring the migrated distance of cells from the 0 h using Image J (US National Institutes of Health, Bethesda, MD, USA). Experiments were repeated three times.

Apoptosis
In one set of experiments, apoptosis was assessed using fluorescence microscopy. Cells (1.2×10^4) were seeded into 96-well plates. After 24 h, cells were treated with phenformin alone or with gefitinib for 24 h. Then the cells were incubated at room temperature in the dark for 15 min with 100 μL binding buffer, 1 μL FITC-conjugated Annexin V (MultiSciences Biotech, Hangzhou, China) and 1 μL of propidium iodide (MultiSciences Biotech). Cells were observed under a DFC450C fluorescence microscope (Leica).

Apoptosis was assessed using flow cytometry in a separate experiment. Briefly, cells treated with the different drug combinations were harvested with trypsinization, washed twice with phosphate-buffered saline (PBS), and resuspended in binding buffer to 1×10^6 cells/mL. Then 5 μL of Annexin V-FITC and 10 μL of propidium iodide were added to 100 μL of cell suspension, incubated for 30 min at room temperature in the dark, and then mixed with 400 μL of binding buffer. Within 30 min, labeled cells were counted by flow cytometry on a FACS Calibur flow cytometer [excitation wavelength, 488 nm; emission wavelengths, 530 nm (FL-1 channel, FITC) and 670 nm (FL-3 c3 channel, propidium iodide)]. Data were analyzed using Cell Quest software (Becton–Dickinson). Non-apoptotic cells were defined as those negative for Annexin-V and propidium iodide; necrotic/late apoptotic cells as those positive for both labels; and early apoptotic cells as those positive for Annexin V but negative for propidium iodide.

Western blotting

Proteins were fractionated by SDS-PAGE, transferred to membranes, and then incubated overnight at 4 °C with different primary antibodies described in Reagents section above (Cell Signaling, Beverly, MA, USA) in buffer containing bovine serum albumin (BSA). Membranes were washed with TBS containing 0.05% Tween-20, blotted with secondary antibody for 1 h at room temperature, then washed again three times. Pierce Super Signal chemiluminescent substrate (Rockford, IL, USA) was added, and the blot was imaged immediately on a Chemi Doc system (Bio-Rad, Hercules, CA, USA) and a Perfection V500 camera (Epson). Band intensities were quantified using Image J.

Statistical analyses

All data are presented as mean ± SD. Statistical analysis was performed using SPSS 16.0. Differences between groups were assessed for significance using Student's t test for experiments involving only two groups and using ANOVA and the least significant difference (LSD) test for experiments involving more than two groups. Graphs were generated using GraphPad Prism 6.0. Two levels of statistical significance were considered: $*P < 0.05$ and $\#P < 0.01$.

Results

Phenformin inhibits bladder cancer cell proliferation

Phenformin inhibited cell proliferation within a concentration range of 0.02–8 mmol/L in a concentration-dependent manner (Fig. 1). The most sensitive cell line

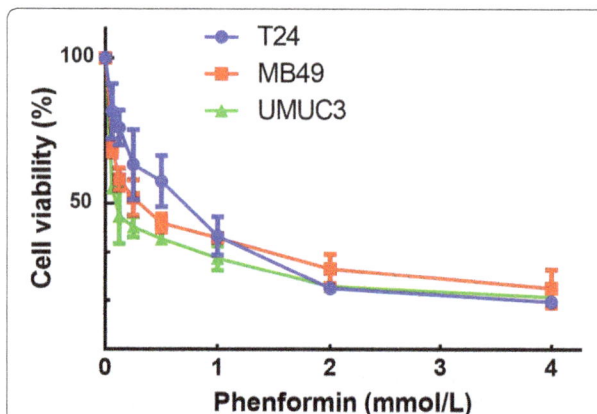

Fig. 1 Effect of phenformin on bladder cancer cell proliferation. Viability of T24, UMUC3 and MB49 cells was assessed after 48-h exposure to phenformin at concentrations ranging from 0 to 8 mmol/L using a tetrazolium-based assay. Results are the mean ± SD of three independent experiments

Table 1 IC$_{50}$ values for phenformin against bladder cancer cell lines

	Bladder cancer cell line		
	MB49	T24	UMUC3
IC$_{50}$ (mmol/L)	0.57	0.97	0.25

was UMUC3 (IC$_{50}$, 0.25 mmol/L); the most resistant cell line was T24 ((IC$_{50}$, 0.87 mmol/L; Table 1).

Phenformin synergistically potentiates the anti-proliferative effects of gefitinib

Consistent with our previous study [9], gefitinib did not affect the growth of the cell lines (Fig. 2, Table 2), but interacted synergistically with phenformin to inhibit cancer cell growth (Fig. 3).

Phenformin alone or combined with gefitinib suppresses colony formation

Phenformin alone inhibited colony formation in all three cell lines at concentrations of 0–0.5 mmol/L (Fig. 4). At a concentration as low as 0.125 mmol/L, phenformin significantly reduced the numbers of T24 and MB49 colonies. The most sensitive cell line was UMUC3. Combining phenformin with gefitinib led to an even greater inhibition (Fig. 5).

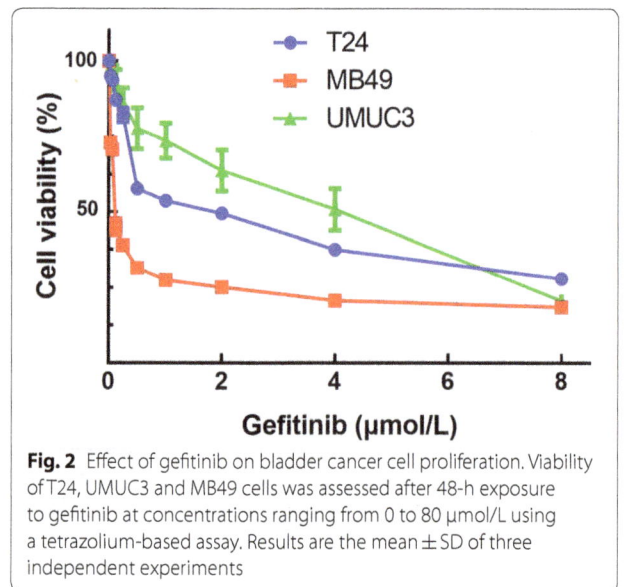

Fig. 2 Effect of gefitinib on bladder cancer cell proliferation. Viability of T24, UMUC3 and MB49 cells was assessed after 48-h exposure to gefitinib at concentrations ranging from 0 to 80 μmol/L using a tetrazolium-based assay. Results are the mean ± SD of three independent experiments

Table 2 IC$_{50}$ values for gefitinib against bladder cancer cell lines

	Bladder cancer cell line		
	MB49	T24	UMUC3
IC$_{50}$ (μmol/L)	1.6	30.1	17

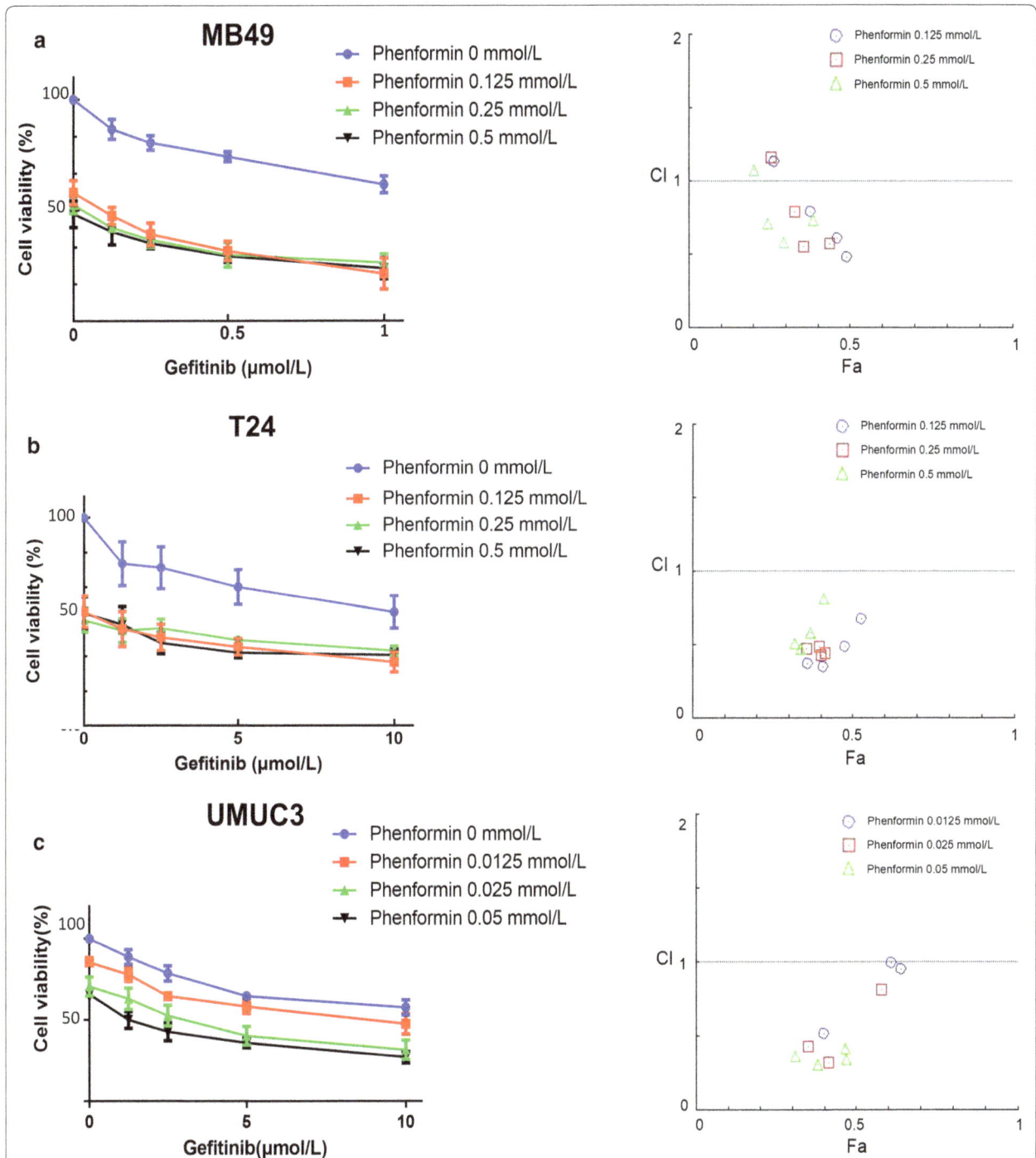

Fig. 3 Effect of gefitinib combined with phenformin on bladder cancer cell proliferation. **a** Gefitinib combined with phenformin inhibited MB49 proliferation synergistically. Above: Cell viability was assessed after 48-h treatment with gefitinib (0, 0.125, 0.25, 0.5, or 1 μmol/L) alone or combined with phenformin (0.125, 0.25, or 0.5 mmol/L). Below: The combination index (CI) assessing synergy between the two drugs was calculated. **b** Gefitinib combined with phenformin inhibited T24 proliferation synergistically. Above: Cell viability was assessed after 48-h treatment with gefitinib (0, 1.25, 2.5, 5, or 10 μM) alone or combined with phenformin (0.125, 0.25, or 0.5 mmol/L). Below: The combination index (CI) assessing synergy between the two drugs was calculated. CI = 1 denotes additivity; CI > 1, antagonism; CI < 1, synergism. CI values in nearly all combinations were less than 0.5, indicating moderately strong synergism. **c** Gefitinib combined with phenformin inhibited UMUC3 proliferation synergistically. Above: Cell viability was assessed after 48-h treatment with gefitinib (0, 1.25, 2.5, 5, or 10 μmol/L) alone or combined with phenformin (0.0125, 0.025, or 0.05 mmol/L). Below: The combination index (CI) assessing synergy between the two drugs was calculated. Results are the median of five independent experiments

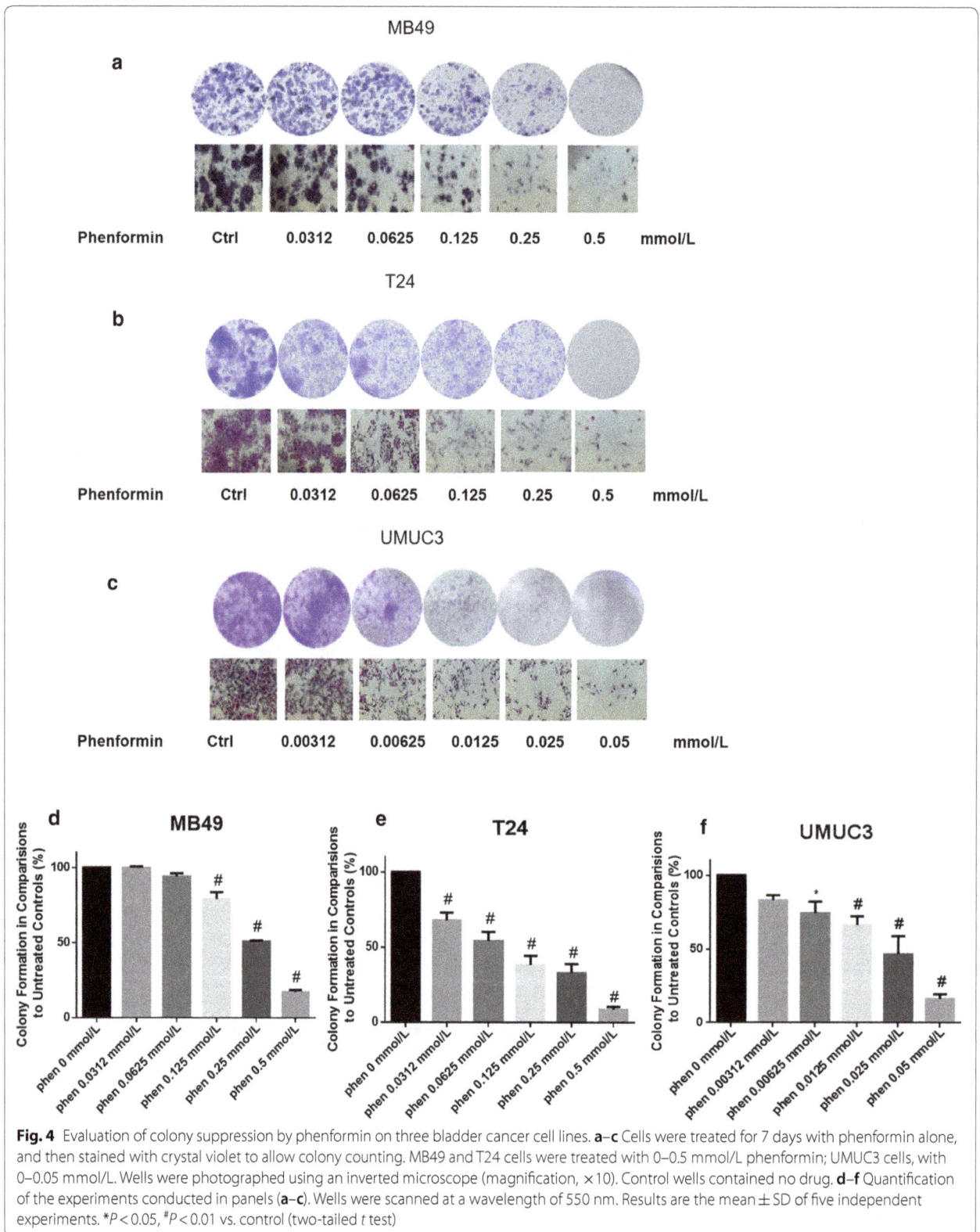

Fig. 4 Evaluation of colony suppression by phenformin on three bladder cancer cell lines. **a–c** Cells were treated for 7 days with phenformin alone, and then stained with crystal violet to allow colony counting. MB49 and T24 cells were treated with 0–0.5 mmol/L phenformin; UMUC3 cells, with 0–0.05 mmol/L. Wells were photographed using an inverted microscope (magnification, ×10). Control wells contained no drug. **d–f** Quantification of the experiments conducted in panels (**a–c**). Wells were scanned at a wavelength of 550 nm. Results are the mean ± SD of five independent experiments. *$P<0.05$, #$P<0.01$ vs. control (two-tailed t test)

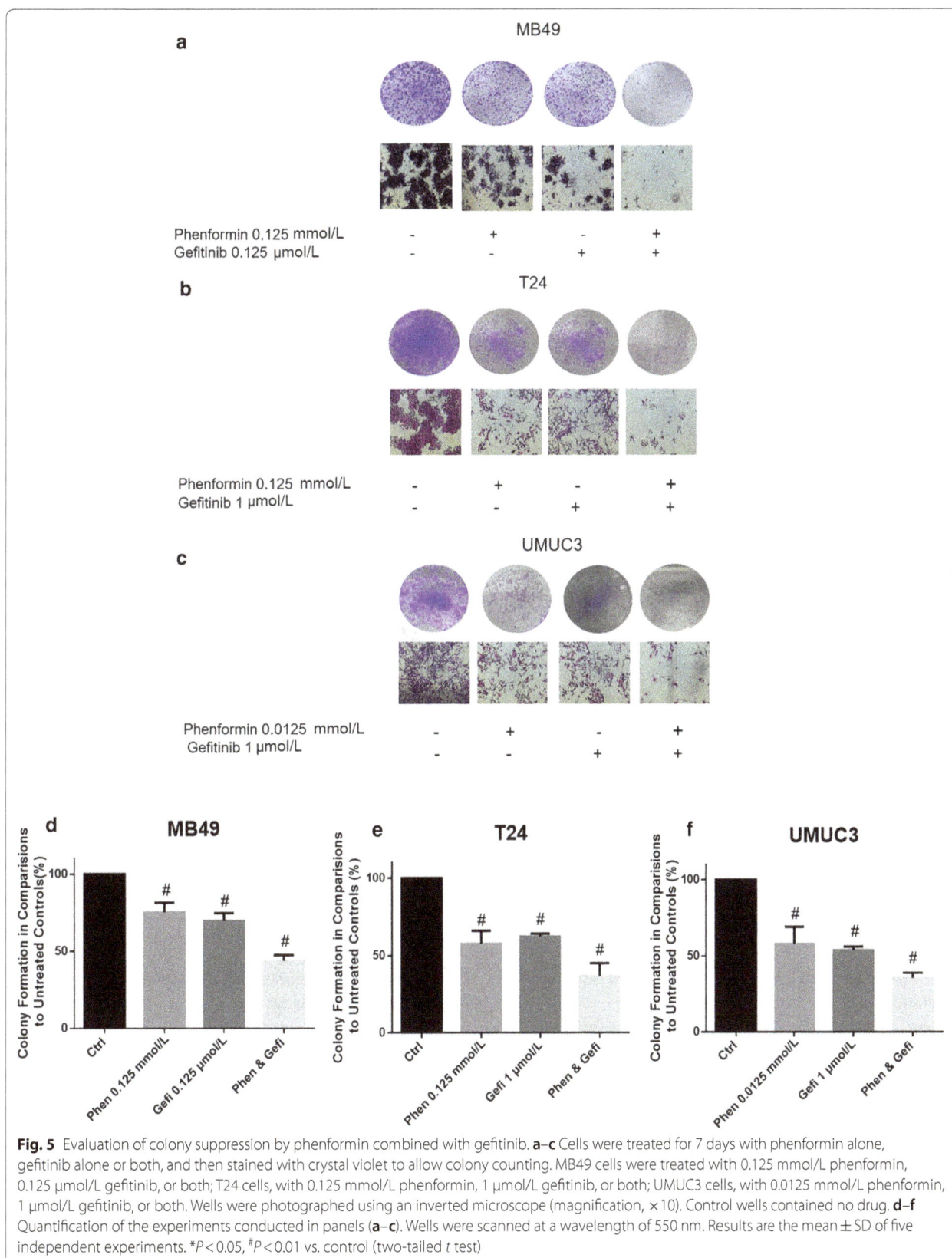

Fig. 5 Evaluation of colony suppression by phenformin combined with gefitinib. **a–c** Cells were treated for 7 days with phenformin alone, gefitinib alone or both, and then stained with crystal violet to allow colony counting. MB49 cells were treated with 0.125 mmol/L phenformin, 0.125 μmol/L gefitinib, or both; T24 cells, with 0.125 mmol/L phenformin, 1 μmol/L gefitinib, or both; UMUC3 cells, with 0.0125 mmol/L phenformin, 1 μmol/L gefitinib, or both. Wells were photographed using an inverted microscope (magnification, ×10). Control wells contained no drug. **d–f** Quantification of the experiments conducted in panels (**a–c**). Wells were scanned at a wavelength of 550 nm. Results are the mean ± SD of five independent experiments. *$P < 0.05$, #$P < 0.01$ vs. control (two-tailed t test)

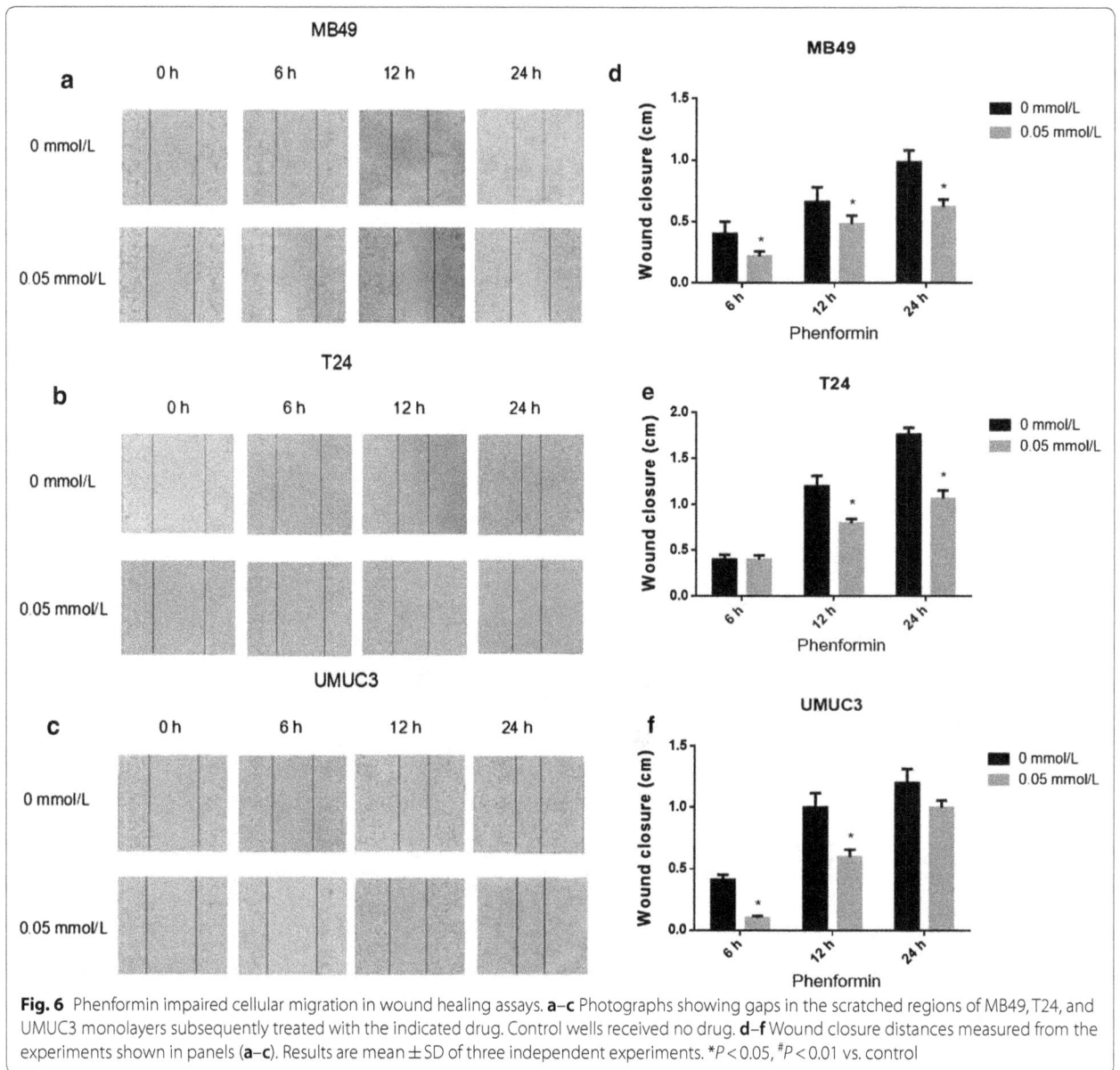

Fig. 6 Phenformin impaired cellular migration in wound healing assays. **a–c** Photographs showing gaps in the scratched regions of MB49, T24, and UMUC3 monolayers subsequently treated with the indicated drug. Control wells received no drug. **d–f** Wound closure distances measured from the experiments shown in panels (**a–c**). Results are mean ± SD of three independent experiments. *$P < 0.05$, #$P < 0.01$ vs. control

Phenformin alone or combined with gefitinib inhibits cell migration

In the scratch assay, phenformin significantly increased the cell-free area at 24 h ($P < 0.05$ vs. control, Fig. 6). The assay was repeated by treating MB49 cells with 0.05 mmol/L phenformin alone, 1.25 µmol/L gefitinib alone or their combination. In addition, the assay was repeated by treating T24 and UMUC3 cells with 0.05 mmol/L phenformin alone, 10 µmol/L gefitinib alone or their combination. The combination of drugs inhibited migration to a greater extent than either drug alone (Fig. 7).

Phenformin alone or combined with gefitinib activates AMPK signaling pathways

All three cell lines were treated with phenformin at doses of 0–0.5 mmol/L for 36 h, and cell lysates were analyzed by Western blotting for levels of p-AMPK (T172), p-mTOR (S2448) and the mTOR downstream effectors p70S6K and p4EBP1 (Fig. 8). Phenformin activated AMPK and led to lower levels of phosphorylated 4EBP1 and p70S6K. In our previous work, we observed similar effects with metformin but only at much higher concentrations [9].

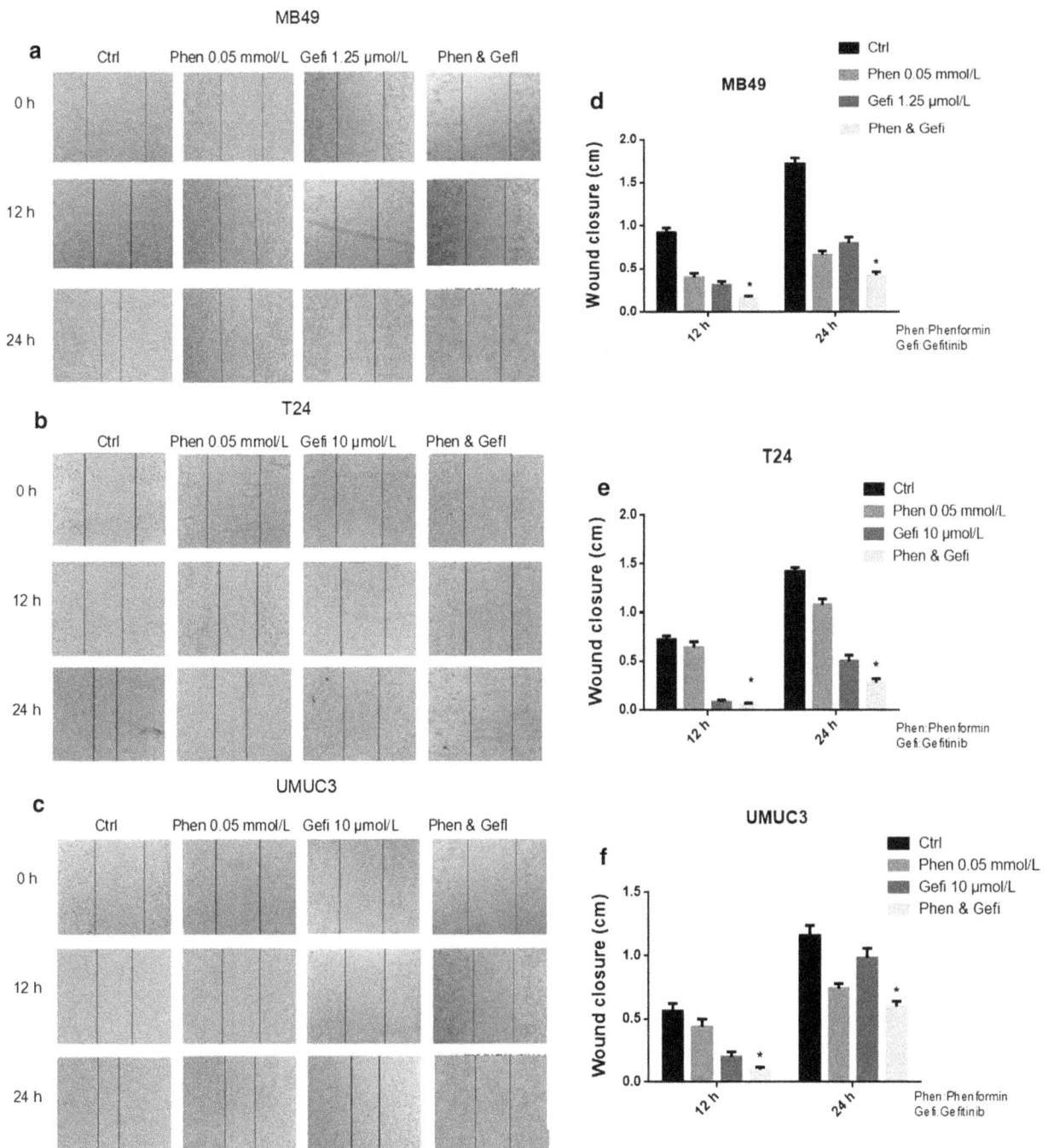

Fig. 7 Phenformin treatment combined with gefitinib impaired cellular migration in wound healing assays. **a–c** Photographs showing gaps in the scratched regions of MB49, T24, and UMUC3 monolayers subsequently treated with the indicated drug alone or combination. Control wells received no drug. **d–f** Wound closure distances measured from the experiments shown in panels (**a–c**). Results are mean ± SD of three independent experiments. *$P < 0.05$, #$P < 0.01$ vs. control

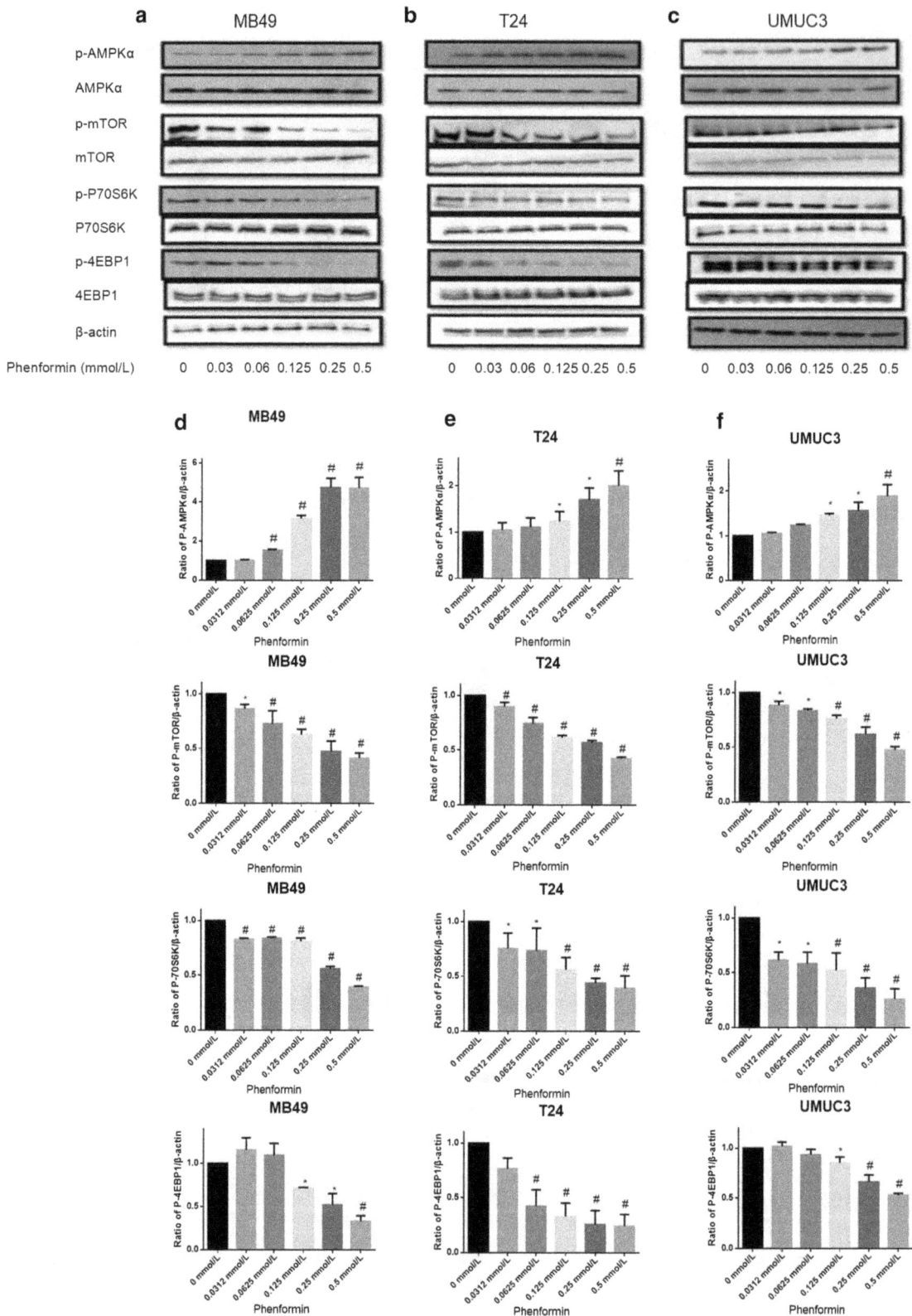

Fig. 8 Effects of phenformin on AMPK intracellular signaling pathways. Western blot analysis was used to examine the levels of total (t) and phosphorylated (p) forms of various signaling proteins in MB49, T24, and UMUC3 cells treated with phenformin at various concentrations. Control cells received no drugs. **a–c** Western blots of p-AMPK, p-mTOR, p-p70S6K, p-4EBP1, t-AMPK, t-mTOR, t-p70S6K and t-4EBP1. β-actin was included as a loading control. **d–f** Relative levels of various proteins. Results are mean ± SD. *$P < 0.05$, #$P < 0.01$ vs. control

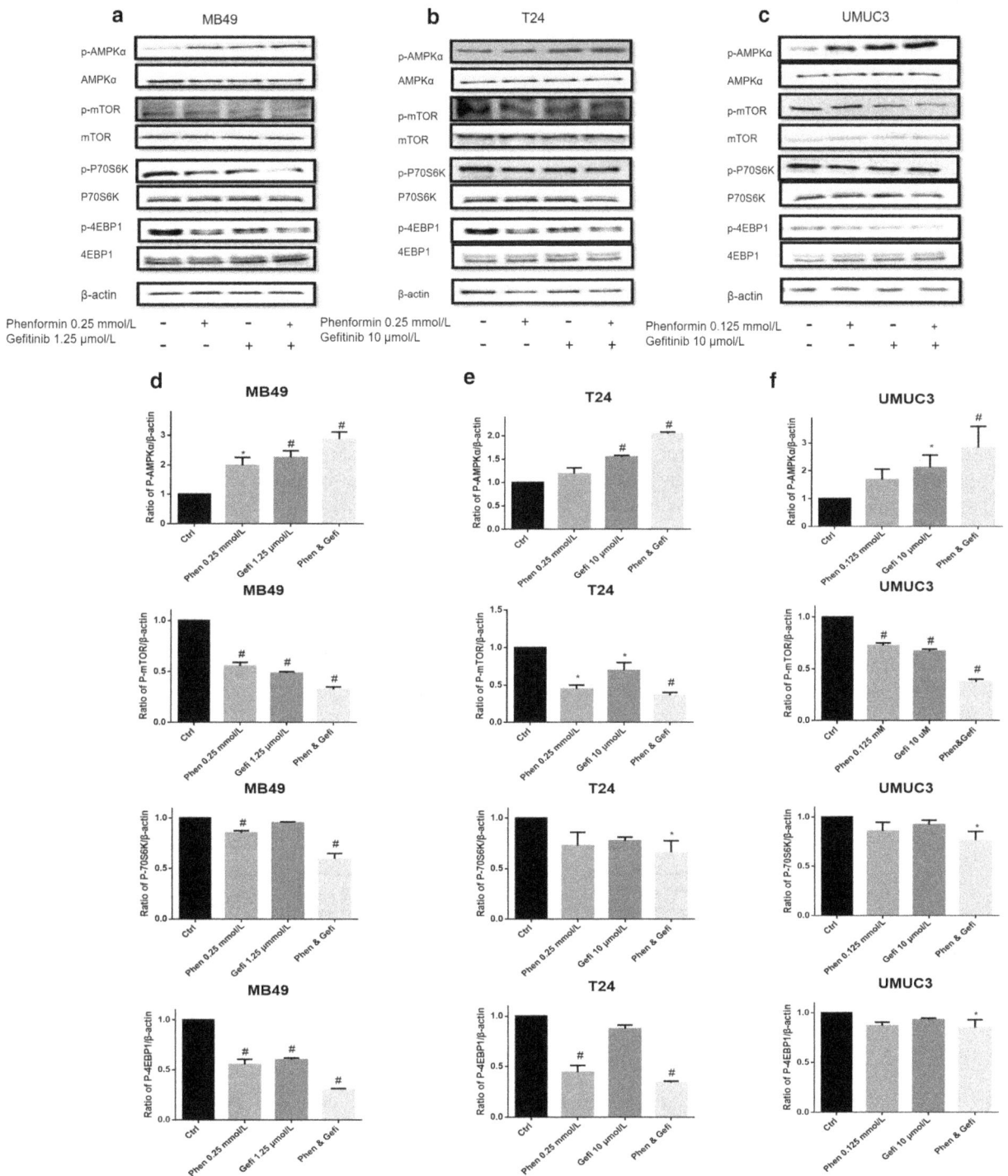

Fig. 9 Effects of the combination of gefitinib with phenformin on AMPK signaling pathways. Western blot analysis was used to examine total (t) and phosphorylated (p) forms of various signaling proteins in MB49, T24, and UMUC3 cells treated with phenformin, gefitinib or their combination. Control cells received no drugs. **a–c** Western blots of p-AMPK, p-mTOR, p-p70S6K, p-4EBP1, t-AMPK, t-mTOR, t-p70S6K and t-4EBP1. β-actin was included as a loading control. **d–f** Relative levels of various proteins. Results are mean ± SD. *$P < 0.05$, #$P < 0.01$ vs. control

AMPK signaling pathway activation was much higher upon treatment with phenformin in combination with gefitinib than with either drug alone (Fig. 9). In our previous work [9], we achieved strong synergy with the combination of metformin and gefitinib, but at a metformin concentration eightfold higher than the phenformin concentration in the present work. The synergy between phenformin and gefitinib was greatest for the UMUC3 cell line.

Phenformin alone or combined with gefitinib inhibits the EGFR signaling pathways

In our previous work [19], we showed that metformin and gefitinib cooperatively inhibited bladder cancer growth by inhibiting EGFR signaling. Here we examined whether the same was true for the combination of phenformin and gefitinib (Figs. 10 and 11). We found that phenformin alone or together with gefitinib inhibited EGFR signaling at concentrations eightfold lower than used in our previous work.

Phenformin alone or combined with gefitinib promotes apoptosis

Either phenformin or gefitinib alone substantially increased the proportion of apoptotic cells in all three cell lines (Fig. 12). The combination of the two drugs

led to a much higher proportion of apoptotic cells than either drug alone.

Discussion

The results from the current study showed that phenformin, either alone or in combination with gefitinib, could produce antitumor effects in bladder cancer cells. Phenformin may be better suited for this purpose than its parent compound metformin. Metformin has been shown to inhibit bladder cancer cell proliferation in vitro and in vivo [9], but only at concentrations that are difficult or impossible to achieve in human subjects. In addition, a trial in patients with type 2 diabetes failed to find an association between the use of metformin and decreased incidence of bladder cancer [24].

Our results in the present study suggest that phenformin can substantially inhibit bladder cancer cell proliferation, colony formation and migration at much lower concentrations than metformin. For example, phenformin inhibited colony formation in the most sensitive UMUC3 cell line by > 100-fold greater than metformin at tenfold lower concentrations. These cellular effects at much lower phenformin concentrations were associated with the activation of AMPK signaling and inhibition of EGFR signaling. Our findings extended the literature of

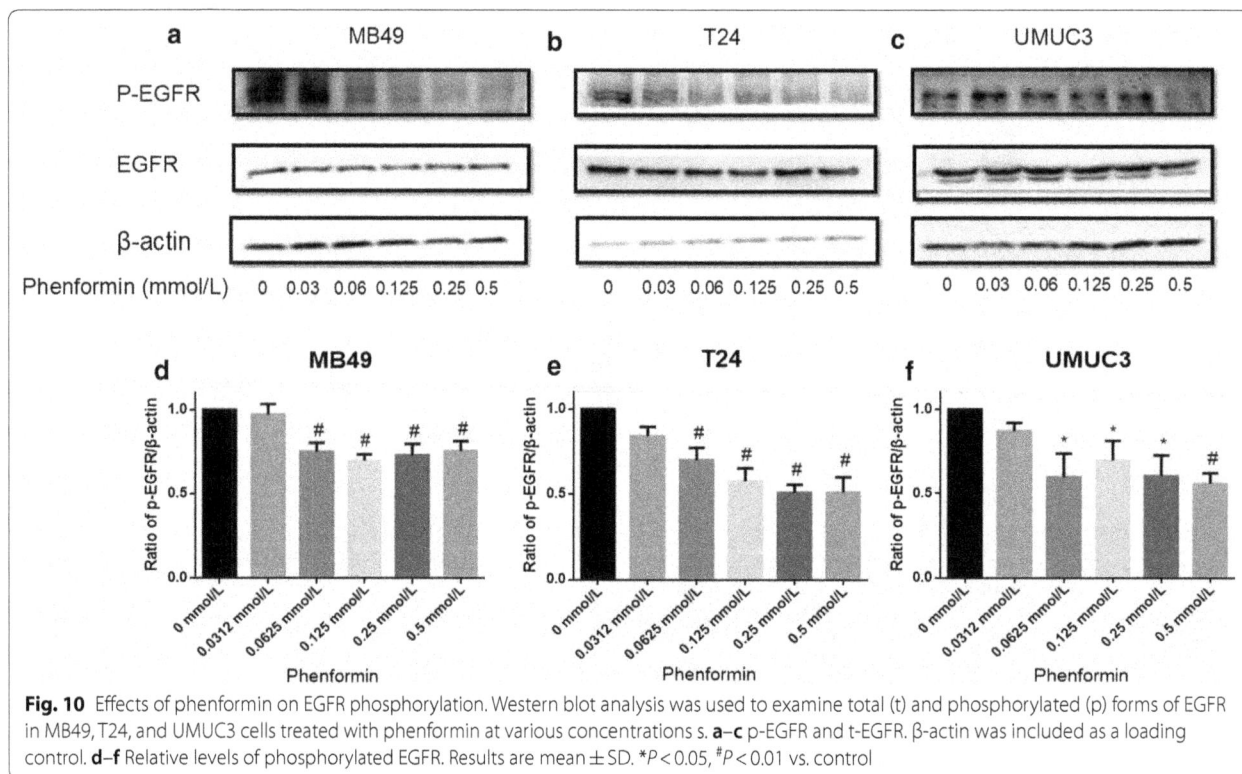

Fig. 10 Effects of phenformin on EGFR phosphorylation. Western blot analysis was used to examine total (t) and phosphorylated (p) forms of EGFR in MB49, T24, and UMUC3 cells treated with phenformin at various concentrations s. **a–c** p-EGFR and t-EGFR. β-actin was included as a loading control. **d–f** Relative levels of phosphorylated EGFR. Results are mean ± SD. *$P < 0.05$, #$P < 0.01$ vs. control

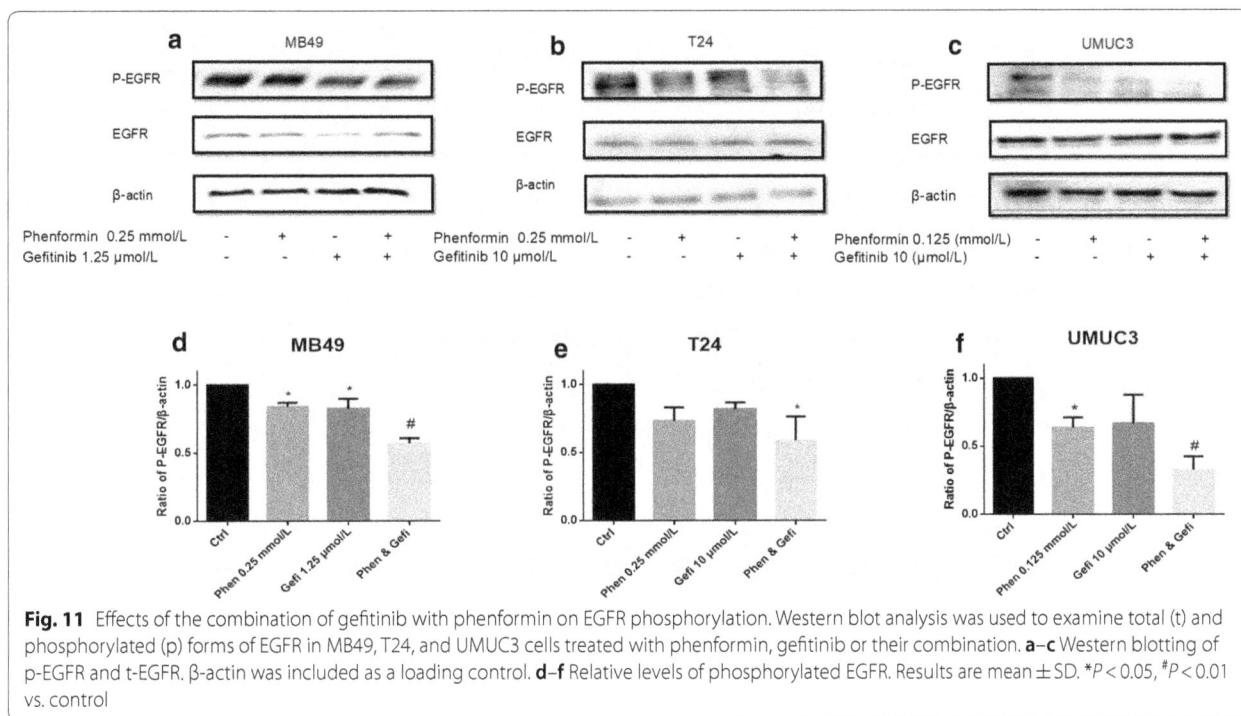

Fig. 11 Effects of the combination of gefitinib with phenformin on EGFR phosphorylation. Western blot analysis was used to examine total (t) and phosphorylated (p) forms of EGFR in MB49, T24, and UMUC3 cells treated with phenformin, gefitinib or their combination. **a–c** Western blotting of p-EGFR and t-EGFR. β-actin was included as a loading control. **d–f** Relative levels of phosphorylated EGFR. Results are mean ± SD. *$P < 0.05$, #$P < 0.01$ vs. control

phenformin antitumor activities from breast cancer cells and other cell types to bladder cancer [25].

Based on previous work [19, 26], we speculate that the much higher therapeutic efficiency of phenformin over metformin can be attributed to higher lipophilicity of phenformin and the fact that phenformin does not require organic cation transporters to enter cells [27]. Such transporters are not expressed in all tissues. As a result, phenformin can readily enter a broader range of cell types.

Metformin and phenformin increase AMPK activity without increasing the AMP/ATP ratio [28], which is important for the anti-cancer mechanism of both biguanides [9]. Tumorigenesis is a multistep process and tumor cells often undergo metabolic re-programming to support the rapid growth [29]. Targeting metabolic re-programming using biguanides represents a promising therapeutic strategy in cancer. In the present study, we showed that phenformin activates AMPK phosphorylation in bladder cancer cells. We also demonstrated that phenformin inactivates two proteins that act downstream of AMPK, namely 4EBP1 and p70S6K. These results suggest that phenformin may induce apoptosis

in bladder cancer cells via the AMPK/mTOR/p70S6K axis.

Targeting multiple sites, such as with phenformin and gefitinib is generally superior to single-target anticancer therapy. The synergistic action observed in the current study probably reflects mechanistic "crossover": we showed here that phenformin inhibits EGFR signaling in a dose-dependent manner, and we previously showed that gefitinib can activate AMPK signaling [19]. As a result of this synergy, the combination of the two drugs inhibited bladder cancer cell proliferation and colony formation while stimulating apoptosis to a much greater extent than either drug alone.

Our in vitro findings here should be verified and extended in preclinical animal studies. In addition to efficacy, whether the combination therapy is associated with toxic effects in vivo should be examined. Despite these limitations, the present work provides evidence that phenformin can effectively inhibit bladder cancer growth by activating AMPK signaling and inhibiting EGFR signaling. The results also encourage future studies to explore phenformin on its own and combined with gefitinib as multi-targeted anticancer therapy.

(See figure on next page.)
Fig. 12 Effect of gefitinib combined with phenformin on apoptosis. **a–c** Fluorescence micrographs to assess FITC and propidium iodide staining of MB49, T24, and UMUC3 cell lines treated with the indicated drugs. Control cells received no drugs. **d–f** Representative flow cytometry scatter plots showing propidium iodide (y axis) and Annexin V-FITC (x axis) staining. Quantitation of flow cytometry experiments. Results are the mean ± SD of three independent experiments. *$P < 0.05$, #$P < 0.01$ vs. control

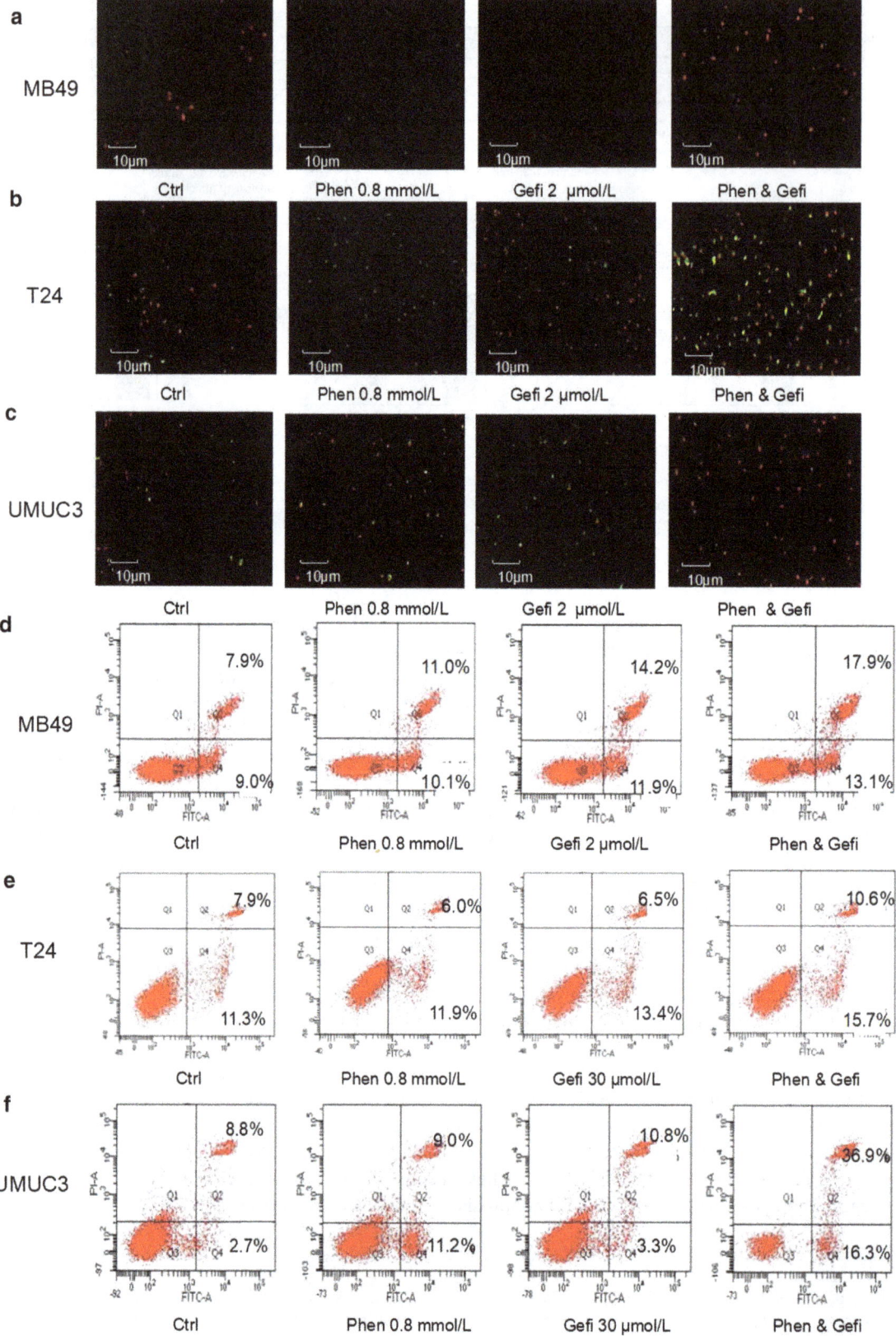

Authors' contributions

YH analyzed the data and wrote the paper. YH, SZ and TT prepared and calculated the data. QS and CH participated in sample and data collection. KOD, JD, MP processed and analyzed the data. XY contributed to study design and manuscript review. All authors read and approved the final manuscript.

Author details

[1] Key Laboratory of Study and Discovery of Targeted Small Molecules of Hunan Province and Department of Pharmacy in the School of Medicine and Laboratory of Animal Nutrition and Human Health, Hunan Normal University, Changsha 410013, Hunan, P. R. China. [2] Department of Pharmacy, Xiangya Hospital, Central South University, Changsha 410008, Hunan, P. R. China.

Acknowledgements

We deeply appreciate the help of our colleagues at Hunan Normal University.

Competing interests

The authors declare that they have no competing interests.

Funding

This work was supported by grants to X.Y. from the Hunan Natural Science Foundation (2016JJ2187), the Key Project of Hunan Province 2016 (2016JC2036) and Start-up Funds of the Key Laboratory of Study and Discovery of Targeted Small Molecules of Hunan Province (2017TP1020); and by a grant to M.P. from the Chinese National Science Foundation (81703008).

References

1. Nathan DM, Buse JB, Davidson MB, Ferrannini E, Holman RR, Sherwin R, et al. Medical management of hyperglycemia in type 2 diabetes: a consensus algorithm for the initiation and adjustment of therapy a consensus statement of the American Diabetes Association and the European Association for the Study of Diabetes. Diabetes Care. 2009;32:193–203.
2. Shaw RJ, Lamia KA, Vasquez D, Koo SH, Bardeesy N, DePinho RA, et al. The kinase LKB1 mediates glucose homeostasis in liver and therapeutic effects of metformin. Science. 2005;310:1642–6.
3. Sui X, Xu Y, Wang X, Han W, Pan H, Xiao M. Metformin: a novel but controversial drug in cancer prevention and treatment. Mol Pharm. 2015;12:3783–91.
4. Bansal M, Siegel E, Govindarajan R. The effect of metformin (M) on overall survival (OS) of patients (Pts) with colorectal cancer (CRC) treated with chemotherapy (CTX). J Clin Oncol. 2011;29:2608.
5. Chlebowski RT, McTiernan A, Aragaki AK, Rohan T, Wactawski-Wende J, Ipp E, et al. Metformin and breast cancer incidence in postmenopausal diabetic women in the Women's Health Initiative (WHI). J Clin Oncol. 2011;29:1503.
6. Mayer MJ, Klotz LH, Venkateswaran V. The effect of metformin use during docetaxel chemotherapy on prostate cancer specific and overall survival of diabetic patients with castration resistant prostate cancer. J Urol. 2017;197:1068–74.
7. Fan C, Wang Y, Liu Z, Sun Y, Wang X, Wei G, et al. Metformin exerts anticancer effects through the inhibition of the Sonic hedgehog signaling pathway in breast cancer. Int J Mol Med. 2015;36:204–14.
8. Menendez JA, Quirantes-Pine R, Rodriguez-Gallego E, Cufi S, Corominas-Faja B, Cuyas E, et al. Oncobiguanides: paracelsus' law and nonconventional routes for administering diabetobiguanides for cancer treatment. Oncotarget. 2014;5:2344–8.
9. Peng M, Su Q, Zeng Q, Li L, Liu Z, Xue L, et al. High efficacy of intravesical treatment of metformin on bladder cancer in preclinical model. Oncotarget. 2016;7:9102–17.
10. Wang ZD, Wei SQ, Wang QY. Targeting oncogenic KRAS in non-small cell lung cancer cells by phenformin inhibits growth and angiogenesis. Am J Cancer Res. 2015;5:3339.
11. Lea MA, Chacko J, Bolikal S, Hong JY, Chung R, Ortega A, et al. Addition of 2-deoxyglucose enhances growth inhibition but reverses acidification in colon cancer cells treated with phenformin. Anticancer Res. 2011;31:421–6.
12. Yuan P, Ito K, Perez-Lorenzo R, Del Guzzo C, Lee JH, Shen C-H, et al. Phenformin enhances the therapeutic benefit of BRAF(V600E) inhibition in melanoma. Proc Natl Acad Sci USA. 2013;110:18226–31.
13. Hawley SA, Ross FA, Chevtzoff C, Green KA, Evans A, Fogarty S, et al. Use of cells expressing gamma subunit variants to identify diverse mechanisms of AMPK activation. Cell Metab. 2010;11:554–65.
14. Weinberg SE, Chandel NS. Targeting mitochondria metabolism for cancer therapy. Nat Chem Biol. 2015;11:9–15.
15. Blaveri E, Simko JP, Korkola JE, Brewer JL, Baehner F, Mehta K, et al. Bladder cancer outcome and subtype classification by gene expression. Clin Cancer Res. 2005;11:4044–55.
16. Dyrskjot L, Zieger K, Real FX, Malats N, Carrato A, Hurst C, et al. Gene expression signatures predict outcome in non-muscle invasive bladder carcinoma: a multicenter validation study. Clin Cancer Res. 2007;13:3545–51.
17. Kim W-J, Kim S-K, Jeong P, Yun S-J, Cho I-C, Kim IY, et al. A four-gene signature predicts disease progression in muscle invasive bladder cancer. Mol Med. 2011;17:478–85.
18. Lu Y, Liu P, Van den Bergh F, Zellmer V, James M, Wen W, et al. Modulation of gene expression and cell-cycle signaling pathways by the EGFR inhibitor gefitinib (Iressa) in rat urinary bladder cancer. Cancer Prev Res. 2012;5:248–59.
19. Peng M, Huang Y, Tao T, Peng C-Y, Su Q, Xu W, et al. Metformin and gefitinib cooperate to inhibit bladder cancer growth via both AMPK and EGFR pathways joining at Akt and Erk. Sci Rep. 2016;6:28611.
20. Busada JT, Niedenberger BA, Velte EK, Keiper BD, Geyer CB. Mammalian target of rapamycin complex 1 (mTORC1) Is required for mouse spermatogonial differentiation in vivo. Dev Biol. 2015;407:90–102.
21. Churchward-Venne TA, Burd NA, Phillips SM. Nutritional regulation of muscle protein synthesis with resistance exercise: strategies to enhance anabolism. Nutr Metab. 2012;9:40.
22. Proud CG. Signalling to translation: how signal transduction pathways control the protein synthetic machinery. Biochem J. 2007;403:217–34.
23. Yamaguchi O, Otsu K. Role of autophagy in aging. J Cardiovasc Pharmacol. 2012;60:242–7.
24. Mamtani R, Pfanzelter N, Haynes K, Finkelman BS, Wang X, Keefe SM, et al. Incidence of bladder cancer in patients with type 2 diabetes treated with metformin or sulfonylureas. Diabetes Care. 2014;37:1910–7.
25. Liu Z, Ren L, Liu C, Xia T, Zha X, Wang S. Phenformin induces cell cycle change, apoptosis, and mesenchymal–epithelial transition and regulates the AMPK/mTOR/p70s6k and MAPK/ERK pathways in breast cancer cells. PLoS ONE. 2015;10:e0131207.
26. Pollak M. Potential applications for biguanides in oncology. J Clin Invest. 2013;123:3693–700.
27. Pryor R, Cabreiro F. Repurposing metformin: an old drug with new tricks in its binding pockets. Biochem J. 2015;471:307–22.
28. Dykens JA, Jamieson J, Marroquin L, Nadanaciva S, Billis PA, Will Y. Biguanide-induced mitochondrial dysfunction yields increased lactate production and cytotoxicity of aerobically-poised HepG2 cells and human hepatocytes in vitro. Toxicol Appl Pharmacol. 2008;233:203–10.
29. Vallo S, Michaelis M, Rothweiler F, Bartsch G, Gust KM, Limbart DM, et al. Drug-resistant urothelial cancer cell lines display diverse sensitivity profiles to potential second-line therapeutics. Transl Oncol. 2015;8:210–6.

First-generation *EGFR* tyrosine kinase inhibitor therapy in 106 patients with compound *EGFR*-mutated lung cancer: a single institution's clinical practice experience

Xiangyang Yu[1,2†], Xuewen Zhang[1,3†], Zichen Zhang[1,4†], Yongbin Lin[1,2], Yingsheng Wen[1,2], Yongqiang Chen[1,2], Weidong Wang[1,2] and Lanjun Zhang[1,2*] ⦿

Abstract

Background: The antitumour efficacy of tyrosine kinase inhibitors (TKIs) in lung cancer patients with compound epidermal growth factor receptor (*EGFR*) mutations has not been resolved. Our study summarizes a single institutional experience of first-generation TKI therapy for lung cancers with compound *EGFR* mutations.

Methods: A total of 106 consecutive patients with tumours bearing compound *EGFR* mutations were identified between January 2012 and May 2016; all patients received first-generation TKI therapy. Deletions in exon 19 and the *L858R* point mutation in exon 21 were considered common mutations; *T790M* was considered separately because of its association with TKIs resistances. Any other mutation was defined as a rare mutation. Patients were divided as follows: double common mutations (group A); common plus *T790M* mutations (group B); common plus rare mutations (group C); double rare mutations (group D); and rare plus *T790M* mutations (group E). A separate group of 115 consecutive patients with a single common mutation was created for comparative analysis (group F).

Results: The frequency of patients with compound *EGFR* was 2.9% (114/3925) and their response rate to first-generation TKIs was 50.9%, which was not significantly different from group F (67.0%, $P = 0.088$). The progression-free survival (PFS) of the 106 patients receiving TKI therapy was worse than that of group F (median, 9.1 vs. 13.0 months, respectively; $P < 0.001$). The PFS of the compound mutation group was shorter than that of the single common mutation group (median, 10.1 months in group A, $P = 0.240$; 9.1 months in group B, $P < 0.001$; 9.6 months in group C, $P = 0.010$; 6.5 months in group D, $P = 0.048$; 5.4 months in group E, $P = 0.017$). Patients with a co-occurring mutation in exon 20 (excluding T790M) exhibited significantly worse PFS than the patients with other compound mutations or with a single common mutation (median, 6.5 vs. 9.1 vs. 13.0 months, respectively, $P = 0.002$).

Conclusions: There was significant heterogeneity among the compound *EGFR* mutations and their response to first-generation TKIs. Individualized treatment in clinical practice should be considered for each case.

Keywords: *EGFR*, TKIs, Compound mutations

*Correspondence: zhanglj@sysucc.org.cn
†Xiangyang Yu, Xuewen Zhang and Zichen Zhang contributed equally to this work
² Department of Thoracic Surgery, Sun Yat-sen University Cancer Center, 651 Dongfeng Road East, Guangzhou 510060, Guangdong, China
Full list of author information is available at the end of the article

Introduction

Lung cancer continues to be the primary cause of cancer death both in China and worldwide. The 5-year survival rate for lung cancer has increased from 12% in the 1970s to 17.7% in 2016 [1], and these sufferers primarily include numerous patients with advanced lung cancer. Many advances have been made in the treatment of advanced lung cancer, especially with regard to targeted therapies, and these treatment strategies have resulted in considerable improvements in survival. Among them, the receptor tyrosine kinases (RTKs) super-family of cell surface receptors serve as mediators of cell signaling by extra-cellular growth factors. Members of the ErbB family of RTKs, such as ErbB1 (also known as *EGFR*), ErbB2, ErbB3 and ErbB4, have received much attention, given their strong association with malignant proliferation [2, 3].

Over the past decade, three small-molecule ErbB tyrosine kinases inhibitors (TKIs) have been shown to efficiently target tumour cell survival pathways in advanced non-small cell lung cancers (NSCLC) expressing the epidermal growth factor receptor (*EGFR*): gefitinib (approved by the US Food and Drug Administration in May 2003), erlotinib (approved by the US Food and Drug Administration in November 2004) and icotinib (approved by China's State Food and Drug Administration in June 2011). The use of these agents has resulted in higher overall response rates (ORRs, up to 60%–70%) and longer progression-free survival (PFS; 9–16 months) and overall survival (OS; exceeding 20 months) than current first-line platinum-based chemotherapies [1–5].

These patients with classical *EGFR* genetic mutations that are sensitive to TKIs involve in-frame deletions of exon 19 and L858R substitutions of exon 21 and occur in approximately 85%–90% of all *EGFR*-mutated patients [1, 4–6]. However, compound *EGFR* mutations with or without classical mutations have been detected within the same tumour tissues in some patients [7–14]. Previous studies reported that only 2%–15% of the population with *EGFR* mutations exhibits these rare compound mutations [7–14]. The characteristics of this rare population, the efficacy of *EGFR* TKIs, and the prognostic value of the compound mutations have not been clarified because of the very low rate of these mutations. Furthermore, the lack of adequate evidence-based medical research hinders treatment decisions when these co-existing double-site mutants are detected.

The present cohort analysis examined two major questions: first, we investigated the incidence of different compound *EGFR* mutation subtypes in a single institution; and second, we investigated this population's characteristics and the efficacy (ORRs and PFS) of first-generation small-molecule TKI treatment and prognosis compared with patients bearing the classical mutation alone.

Materials and methods

Patient selection

We retrospectively reviewed a molecular diagnostic database of lung cancer in the Sun Yat-sen University Cancer Center (SYSUCC) between January 2012 and May 2016. The database was screened for *EGFR*-mutated cases, and a cohort of consecutive cases with compound *EGFR* mutations was identified. The co-existence of two different *EGFR* mutation sites detected in a single tumour specimen was defined as a compound *EGFR* mutation. The hospital's ethics committee approved the research using this micro-database, and all subjects provided written informed consent.

Patients were eligible for enrolment if they had received daily oral *EGFR* TKIs, such as gefitinib (250 mg, qd), erlotinib (150 mg, qd) or icotinib (125 mg, tid), until disease progression or death; complete follow-up information was obtained from the medical record department. The co-existence of compound mutations with *T790M* must have been detected prior to initiation of targeted therapy.

Exclusion criteria included second primary neoplasms diagnosed before/after the lung cancer, intolerant levels of toxicity, loss to follow-up, and refusal of treatment.

Sequencing of EGFR mutations in exons 18–21

Details of the genetic sequencing and molecular analysis were described previously [6]. Briefly, tumour cell DNA was extracted from paraffin-embedded specimens that contained at least 50% tumour cells, including surgically resected tumour specimens, fine needle aspiration biopsies of lymph nodes or metastatic lesions, and tumour cells from pleural fluid, using a QIAamp DNA FFPE Tissue Kit (Qiagen, Hilden, Germany) in strict accordance with the manufacturer's recommendations. The tumour cell DNA was examined for *EGFR* mutation(s) in exons 18–21, including 36 TKI-responsive mutation sites and nine TKI-resistant mutation sites, using an amplification refractory mutation system polymerase chain reaction (ARMS-PCR) kit (GP Medical Technology Co. Ltd., Beijing, China) [6]. Mass ARRAY TYPER 4.0 software (Sequenom Inc., San Diego, CA, USA) was used to individually classify *EGFR*-positive mutation sites when the mutation frequency was higher than 1%.

Follow-up and end-point

A systemic baseline assessment, including chest and abdomen enhanced computed tomography (CT) scanning and brain enhanced magnetic resonance imaging examination, was routinely performed prior to *EGFR* TKI treatments for locally advanced, recurrent, or metastatic lung cancer. A follow-up assessment was generally performed every 3 months after the 1st day of TKI treatment until February 28, 2017, radiographic progression or death. Two board-certified radiologists independently evaluated the therapeutic effectiveness based on the Response Evaluation Criteria in Solid Tumours (RECIST) and classified the therapeutic effect into four levels: progressive disease (PD), stable disease (SD), partial response (PR), and complete response (CR). Patients exhibiting PD or SD were considered non-responders to targeted treatments, while patients with PR or CR were regarded as effective disease control by antitumour agents. Follow-up information was extracted from the patients' complete medical and radiological records.

The duration of PFS was calculated from the 1st day of *EGFR* TKI treatment to the last follow-up, the date of death or when disease progression was first observed. The duration of OS was also evaluated from the date of the 1st day of *EGFR* TKI treatment until the last follow-up or the date of death from any cause. Patients were censored at their last known progression-free or alive date.

Data analysis

Complete medical, pathological and radiological data and molecular diagnostics were analysed using the Statistical Package for the Social Sciences for Windows version 23.0 (SPSS Inc., Chicago, IL, USA). Categorical variables were compared between the *EGFR* mutant subgroups (i.e., single common mutation, double common mutations,

common plus *T790M* mutations, common plus rare mutations, rare plus rare mutations, and rare plus *T790M* mutations) using Chi square (χ^2) and Fisher's exact tests. The Kaplan–Meier method was used to construct the PFS and OS curves of each subgroup, and significant differences between survival curves were examined using the log-rank test. A two-sided *P* value less than 0.05 was used to confirm significant differences.

Results

Clinical and pathological features of the population with compound *EGFR* mutations

A total of 3925 NSCLC patients with *EGFR* mutations were identified using ARMS-PCR between January 2012 and December 2016 in SYSUCC. A total of 209 consecutive patients with compound *EGFR* mutations were identified among the 3925 NSCLC patients. However, 95 cases with the *19Del* or *L858R* mutations that acquired the *T790M* after TKI therapy and 8 cases that did not receive TKI therapy in our hospital were excluded. Only 106 patients (2.9%) with primary co-existing double *EGFR* mutations received first-generation TKI therapy and were entered into our analysis (Fig. 1).

Most of the 106 patients were non-geriatric (63/106, 59.4%; median age at initial diagnosis, 57 ± 10.7 years), non-smokers (69/106, 65.1%) and had advanced lung cancer (86/106, 81.1%) (Table 1). All initial pathological stage I -IIIA patients (20/106, 18.9%) received radical resection. No sex predilection (55 women and 51 men)

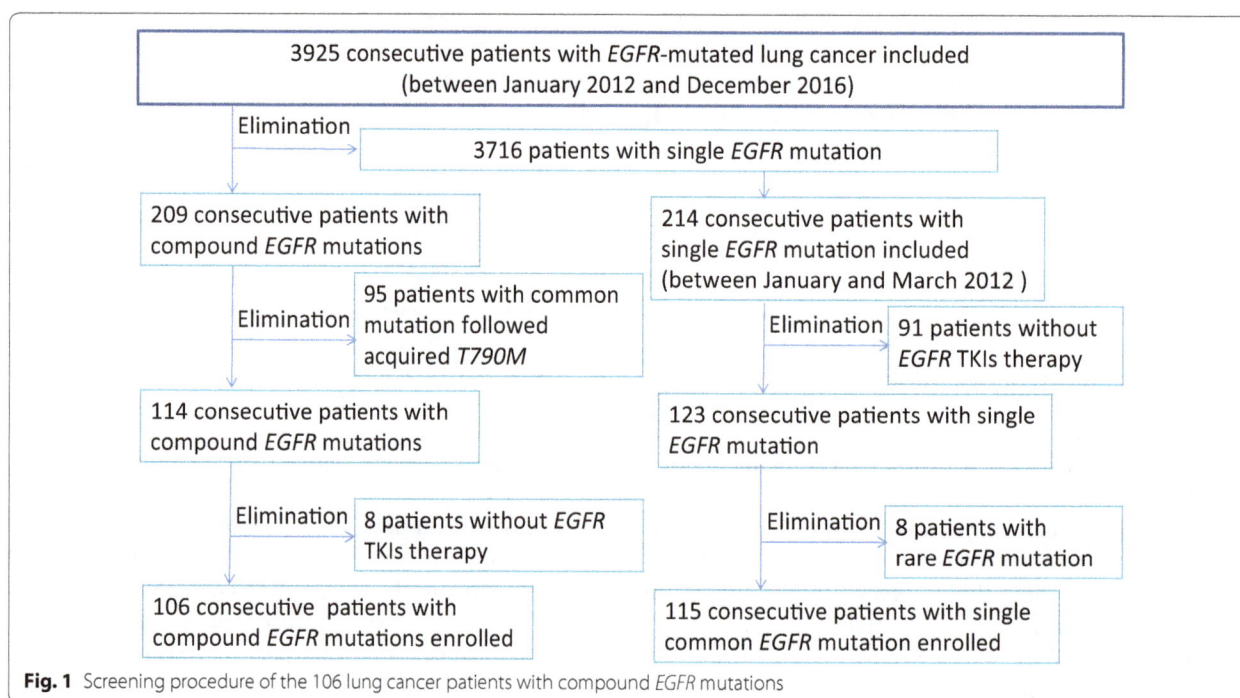

Fig. 1 Screening procedure of the 106 lung cancer patients with compound *EGFR* mutations

Table 1 Clinicopathological characteristics of lung cancer patients with compound *EGFR* mutations

Variable	Single common mutation (n=115)	Compound mutations (n=106)	$P^\dagger$	Double common mutations (n=5)	$P^\dagger$	Common + rare mutations (n=11)	$P^\dagger$	Rare + rare mutations (n=13)	$P^\dagger$	Rare + T790M mutations (n=8)	$P^\dagger$	Common + T790M mutations (n=69)	$P^\dagger$
Sex													
Female	56	55	0.635	1	0.368	6	0.711	6	0.862	4	0.943	38	0.402
Male	59	51		4		5		7		4		31	
Age (years)													
<60	57	63	0.141	2	0.675	5	0.794	8	0.413	7	0.063	41	0.195
≥60	58	43		3		6		5		1		28	
Smoking status													
Non-smoker	69	69	0.270	1	0.118	5	0.795	4	0.442	5	0.795	54	0.022
Smoker	34	24		3		3		4		3		11	
Unknown	12	13		1		0		5		0		4	
Tumour status													
Recurrence	36	20	0.034	1	0.592	3	0.782	3	0.753	0	0.103	13	0.064
Initial IIIb–IV	79	86		4		8		10		8		56	
ECOG PS													
0–1	107	96	0.501	4	0.327	9	0.212	13	0.326	6	0.071	64	0.941
2–4	8	10		1		2		0		2		5	
Pathology													
ADC	110	102	0.529	4	0.141	10	0.672	13	0.899	8	0.948	67	0.534
SCC	5	2		0		1		0		0		1	
LELC	0	1		1		0		0		0		0	
ASC	0	1		0		0		0		0		1	
Timing of TKI													
First line	52	55	0.720	2	0.914	5	0.835	6	0.803	3	0.805	39	0.460
Second line	55	46		3		6		7		5		25	
Third line	7	4		0		0		0		0		4	
Fourth line	1	1		0		0		0		0		1	
TKI selection													
Gefitinib	64	47	0.034	3	0.981	5	0.592	4	0.214	2	0.161	33	0.021
Erlotinib	26	41		1		4		4		4		28	
Icotinib	25	18		1		2		5		2		8	

Table 1 (continued)

Variable	Single common mutation (n=115)	Compound mutations (n=106)	$P^†$	Double common mutations (n=5)	$P^†$	Common+rare mutations (n=11)	$P^†$	Rare+rare mutations (n=13)	$P^†$	Rare+T790M mutations (n=8)	$P^†$	Common+T790M mutations (n=69)	$P^†$
Response to TKIs													
PD	10	14	0.088	1	0.148	2	0.652	2	0.328	4	0.012	5	0.293
SD	21	33		1		3		5		1		22	
PR	77	54		3		5		5		3		39	
CR	1	0		0		0		0		0		0	
NE	6	5		0		1		1		0		3	

ECOG PS Eastern Cooperative Oncology Group performance status, *ADC* adenocarcinoma, *SCC* squamous cell carcinoma, *LELC* lymphoepithelioma-like carcinoma, *ASC* adenosquamous carcinoma, *PD* progressive disease, *SD* stable disease, *PR* partial response, *CR* complete response, *NE* not evaluated, *TKI* tyrosine kinase inhibitor, *PFS* progression-free survival, *OS* overall survival

† All variables of different subgroups were compared with the single common mutation group; $P < 0.05$ was defined as significantly different

was present in our cohort. Notably, a compound *EGFR* mutation was detected in four non-adenocarcinoma patients, including two squamous cell carcinomas (SCC, *L858R+L858Q* and *L858R+T790M*), one lymphoepithelioma-like carcinoma (LELC, *19Del+L858R*) and one adenosquamous carcinoma (ASC, *19Del+T790M*). The first-generation *EGFR* TKIs were primarily administered as first (55/106, 51.9%) or second line (46/106, 43.4%) treatment.

A total of 115 consecutive patients with a single common mutation (*19Del* or *L858R*) who received first-generation *EGFR* TKI therapy between January and March 2012 were selected for comparative analysis (Fig. 1).

Distribution frequency of compound *EGFR* mutations

We divided the cohort with the compound *EGFR* mutations into five groups based on the categories of common and rare mutations sites reported in the literature: a double common mutation group (5/106, 4.7%), a common plus rare mutation group (11/106, 10.4%), a common plus *T790M* mutation group (69/106, 65.1%), a double rare mutation group (13/106, 12.3%), and a rare plus *T790M* mutation group (8/106, 7.5%) (Table 1) [3]. The most frequent mutation site was *T790M* (77/106, 72.6%), and the majority of patients harboured *19Del* (50/106, 47.2%) or *L858R* (40/106, 37.7%) as one of the compound mutations (Table 3). Notably, the most frequent compound mutation involved a common mutation co-existing with *T790M* (69/106, 65.1%), and these common mutations included *19Del* or *L858R* with *T790M*. The most frequent uncommon mutation was *L858Q* (13/106, 12.3%), followed by *S768I* (9/106, 8.5%), *G719X* (7/106, 6.6%), *G719S* (5/106, 4.7%), *D761Y* (2/106, 1.9%), *S720P* (1/106, 0.9%), *K757R* (1/106, 0.9%), *I744M* (1/106, 0.9%), *R776C* (1/106, 0.9%), *L833V* (1/106, 0.9%), *E709A* (1/106, 0.9%), and *V774M* (1/106, 0.9%).

PFS and patient response after TKI treatment

The median follow-up time in the compound *EGFR* mutation cohort was 29.4 months (range, 1.5–119.5 months), and the 1-, 2-, and 3-year PFS rates after *EGFR* TKI treatment were 32.7, 4.3, and 1.4%, respectively, which were all significantly lower than the population with a single common mutation (1-, 2-, and 3-year PFS rates were 54.1, 20.1, and 10.5%, respectively, $P < 0.001$) (Fig. 2a). Twenty-six tumour-related deaths occurred during follow-up, and the median OS was not reached for all patients with compound mutations. Univariate analysis of the total 221 patients who received first-generation TKI therapy revealed that compound mutations were significantly correlated with shorter duration of targeted therapy (HR: 1.883, 95% *CI*

1.404–2.526, $P < 0.001$), in addition to initial advanced status, non-adenocarcinoma, and more than second-line treatment (Table 2). Inclusion of these variables in the multivariate analysis revealed that these four factors were also independent significant PFS factors.

Among the five patients with double common *EGFR* mutations (*19Del* plus *L858R*), only one stage IV patient with brain metastases exhibited effective local control, i.e., SD in response to gefitinib, but progression of the primary pulmonary neoplasm was identified after 7.9 months. Three other patients with advanced lung cancer exhibited a PR to oral gefitinib or icotinib therapy, and their prolonged PFS times was longer than 10 months (10.1, 10.7 and 13.5 months, respectively) (Table 3). Notably, the patient with primary pulmonary LELC, whose tumour harboured a *19Del* plus *L858R* mutation, was diagnosed at stage IV because of osseous metastasis. However, no antitumour activity of erlotinib against this rare subtype of lung cancer was observed, i.e., there was PD. There were no significant differences in the response rates (RR, 25.0% vs. 67.0%, $P = 0.908$, using Chi square tests) or PFS (median, 10.1 months vs. 13.0 months, $P = 0.240$, using log-rank tests) compared with those of the group with a single common mutation.

The RR to TKI in the patients with common mutations (*19Del* or *L858R*) plus *T790M*, which was not a mutation acquired during oral *EGFR* TKI, was 56.5% (39/69); this rate was not significantly different than that of patients with a single *19Del* or *L858R* mutation ($P = 0.293$) (Table 1). These 69 patients exhibited a worse PFS than the 115 patients with a primary *T790M* (median, 9.1 months vs. 13.0 months, respectively; $P < 0.001$) (Fig. 2b). Approximately 33% of the patients (23/69) were enrolled in an AZD9291 international multicentre, single-arm phase 2 clinical trial after progression was detected using CT scanning during treatment with first-generation *EGFR* TKIs.

The compound *EGFR*-mutated patients with rare site involvement exhibited a lower RR (37.5% vs. 67.8%, $P = 0.023$) and a shorter median PFS than the single common mutation subgroup (median, 13.0 months vs. 6.5 months, respectively; $P < 0.001$) (Fig. 2c). However, there was no difference in PFS across the common plus rare mutations subgroup, double rare mutations subgroup, or the rare plus *T790M* mutations subgroup (median, 10.5 months vs. 6.5 months vs. 5.4 months, respectively; $P = 0.984$) (Table 1). The co-occurrence of mutations in exon 20 (excluding *T790M*) had a significant effect on PFS, which was worse than the other compound mutations and the single common mutation patients (median, 13.0 months vs. 9.1 months vs. 6.5 months, respectively; $P = 0.002$) (Fig. 2d).

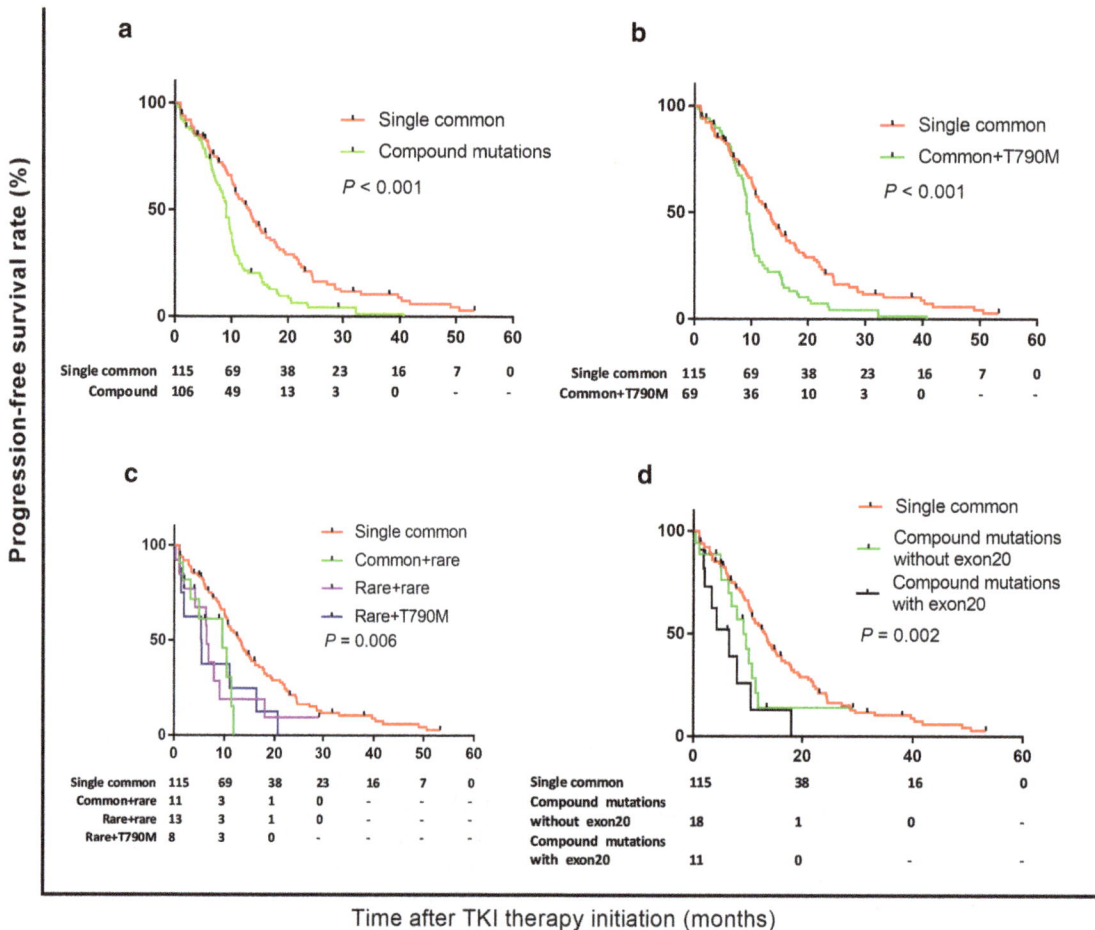

Fig. 2 Progression-free survival by mutation status: **a** a single common *EGFR* mutation vs. compound *EGFR* mutations (median PFS: 9.1 vs. 13.0 months, respectively; *P* < 0.001), **b** a single common *EGFR* mutation vs. common + *T790M* mutations (median: 9.1 months vs. 13.0 months, *P* < 0.001), **c** a single common *EGFR* mutation vs. common + rare mutations vs. rare + rare mutations vs. rare + *T790M* mutations (median: 13.0 months vs. 10.5 months vs. 6.5 months vs. 5.4 months, *P* = 0.006), and **d** a single *EGFR* mutation vs. compound mutations without exon 20 vs. compound mutations with exon 20 (median: 13.0 months vs. 9.1 months vs. 6.5 months, *P* = 0.002)

Discussion

Our single institution study identified 114 patients with compound *EGFR* mutations among 3925 patients with *EGFR* mutations (114/3925, 2.9%). The RR of this rare population to first-generation TKI therapy was 50.9%, which was lower than that of patients with a single common mutation, but the difference was not significant (*P* = 0.088). Patients with compound mutations exhibited a shorter duration of first-generation TKI therapy in multivariate analysis than patients with a single common mutation (HR, 1.981; 95% confidence interval (*CI*) 1.466–2.676; *P* < 0.001). Exclusion of patients with a co-occurrence of mutations in exon 20 (excluding *T790M*) revealed that the duration of targeted TKI therapy was even shorter for other types of compound mutations (*P* = 0.002).

The phenomenon of lung cancer cells harbouring multiple *EGFR* mutations is worth mentioning, and it reportedly has accompanied the clinical use of first-generation small-molecule TKIs since 2004 [7]. Most published studies on multiple mutations were case reports because the techniques for detecting *EGFR* mutations were used only to detect drug-sensitive mutations in exon 19 and 21, and some patients with compound mutations were likely undetected. Developments in mutational detection and analysis techniques, such as direct sequencing, multiplex PCR systems and next-generation sequencing, increased the number of reported cases with compound mutations between 2004 and 2017 (Table 4). The reported frequency of the rare population with compound mutations ranged from 2.6% to 15% [8–15], which was slightly higher than that observed in our cohort (2.9%).

Table 2 Univariate and multivariate analysis for progression-free survival to first-generation TKI therapy

	Univariate analysis		Multivariate analysis	
	HR (95% CI)	$P^{\dagger}$	HR (95% CI)	$P^{\dagger}$
Sex				
(Female/male)	1.061 (0.919–1.224)	0.420		
Age				
($<60/\geq 60$)	1.319 (0.987–1.763)	0.061		
Smoking status				
(Smoker/nonsmoker/unknown)	0.726 (0.518–1.018)	0.063		
Tumour status				
(Recurrence/initial IIIb–IV)	0.721 (0.560–0.926)	0.011	0.706 (0.548–0.909)	0.007
ECOG PS				
(0–1/2–4)	1.438 (0.872–2.372)	0.154		
Pathology				
(Non-adeno/adeno)	4.175 (2.113–8.250)	0.001	5.472 (2.623–11.417)	0.001
Timing of TKI				
($1/\geq 2$)	0.643 (0.480–0.862)	0.003	0.610 (0.452–0.823)	0.001
EGFR mutation status				
(Compound/single)	1.883 (1.404–2.526)	0.001	1.981 (1.466–2.676)	0.001
TKI selection				
(Gefitinib/erlotinib/icotinib)	0.978 (0.819–1.167)	0.806		

ECOG PS Eastern Cooperative Oncology Group performance status, *HR* hazard ratio, *CI* confidence interval

† All variables of different subgroups were compared with the single common mutation group; $P<0.05$ was defined as significantly different

19Del and *L858R* mutations are classical sensitizing mutations, and the strong response of these two mutations to TKIs has been demonstrated in many prospective studies [2–5, 9]. However, these two common mutations are frequently detected concomitant with other mutations in the compound *EGFR*-mutated population. A compound mutation co-existing with a *19Del* or *L858R* mutation was the most common combination in previous reports (203/278, 73.0%) (Table 4) and in our cohort (85/106, 80.2%) (Table 3). Xu et al. [16] reported that tumours with double common *EGFR* mutations (*19Del*+*L858R*, $n=18$) exhibited similar antitumour responses to small-molecule TKIs as tumours with single common mutations, and the median PFS and ORR rates were 9.53 months and 71.4% (10/14), respectively, which is consistent with our results (10.1 months and 60%, respectively) and those of Hata Akito (16.5 months and 86%, respectively) [11]. Some case reports also found that first-generation *EGFR* TKIs may be a desirable therapeutic strategy for patients with advanced lung cancer with synchronous *19Del* and *L858R* mutations [8, 9, 35].

In patients harbouring common plus rare mutation, the *L858R* mutation was more frequently observed than the *19Del* mutation. For example, approximately 10% and 17.3% of NSCLC patients harboured the L858R mutation concomitantly with rare mutations in the two cohorts reported by Wu et al. [17] and Kobayashi et al. [8],

respectively. Similarly, in our common plus rare mutation subgroup, *L858R*, was identified in the majority of the cases (9/11, 81.8%).

The response to TKIs in patients with common plus rare mutations and whether TKI therapy prolonged PFS remains controversial because of the relatively large heterogeneity. Keam [14] reported an RR of 68.8% and median PFS time of 8.1 months in 16 patients, which are similar to our observed RR (45.5%) and median PFS time (10.5 months) in 11 patients. Notably, this above finding was also reported previously [16, 18]. As a whole, this population may benefit from TKIs, but to lesser extent than the population harbouring a single common mutation. We found that the patients with *L858R*+*K757R* mutations (exon 21+exon 19) and *L858R*+*I744M* mutations (exon 21+exon 19) exhibited a partial response to gefitinib and obtained PFS of 9.0- and 9.6-month, respectively. Klughammer et al. [19] and Kempf et al. [20] reported that a single *I744M* mutation or a single *K757R* mutation in exon 19 may be TKI-sensitizing mutations, and these mutations were also observed to have PR to oral TKI therapy. Therefore, the above double or single mutation(s) patterns may be candidates for TKI therapy. Patients with exon 20 mutations are considered resistant to TKIs (discussed below), but our study included a patient with *L858R* plus the *R776H* mutation (exon

Table 3 Frequency, detailed combination patterns, progression-free survival, overall survival and response to first-generation TKIs of compound *EGFR* mutations

Subgroup of compound EGFR mutations	Frequency (n, %)	Mutated exons	Response (rate, %)	PFS (range, months)	OS (range, months)
Double common	5 (4.7)		25.0%	10.1±2.4	24.2±8.2
19Del+L858R	5	19 and 21	3PR, 1SD, 1PD	4.9–12	13.1–25.6
Common+rare	11 (10.4)		45.5%	10.5±3.9	Not reached
19Del+L861Q	2	19 and 21	1PR, 1SD	11.9–14.4	26.5–41.2
L858R+S720P	1	21 and 18	PD	2.1	2.1
L858R+K757R	1	21 and 19	PR	9.0	8.7
L858R+I744M	1	21 and 19	PR	17.6	41.2
L858R+S768I	3	21 and 20	1PR, 1PD, 1SD	1.8–6.2	4.0–12.5
L858R+R776H	1	21 and 20	PR	10.5	12.6
L858R+L858Q	1	21 and 21	NE	1	3
L858R+L833V	1	21 and 21	SD	5.0	15.9
Common+T790M	69 (65.1)		56.5%	10.3±0.6	Not reached
19Del+T790M	43	19 and 20	27PR, 12SD, 2 PD, 2NE	0.6–40.7	0.2–88.5
L858R+T790M	26	21 and 20	12PR, 10SD, 3PD, 1NE	0.9–24.1	1.2–56.6
Rare+rare	13 (12.3)		38.5%	6.5±1.3	Not reached
G719C+S768I	1	18 and 20	PR	6.5	13.2
G719S+S768I	2	18 and 20	1PR, 1SD	1–8.0	2.0–8.4
G719S+L858Q	1	18 and 21	SD	6.4	29.3
G719X+S768I	3	18 and 20	2PR, 1SD	2.0–18	2.0–44.0
G719X+L858Q	3	18 and 21	1SD, 1PD, 1NE	0.3–27.3	2.3–29.2
G719S+E709A	1	18 and 18	PR	4.1	4.1
G719S+L858Q	1	18 and 21	SD	6.4	29.3
S768I+V774M	1	20 and 20	PD	2.0	13.8
Rare+T790M	8 (7.5%)		37.5%	5.4±2.5	23.8±1.5
G719X+T790M	1	18 and 20	PR	11.1	55.6
D761Y+T790M	2	19 and 20	2PD	1.1–5.5	1.1–8.5
L858Q+T790M	5	21 and 20	2PR, 1SD, 2PD	1.4–20.6	18–88.3

TKI tyrosine kinase inhibitor, *PFS* progression-free survival, *OS* overall survival, *PR* partial response, *SD* stable disease, *CR* complete response, *PD* progressive disease, *NE* not evaluated

21 + exon 20) showing PR to TKIs for 10.5 months, which is also highly consistent with prior reports [8, 21]. Other patients with the *L858R* mutation associated with *S720P*, *S768I*, *L858Q* or *L833V* were classified in the insensitive to TKIs group, and most (5/6, 83.3%) exhibited PD or SD to TKI therapy. To the best of our knowledge, our study is the first to report the combinations of *L858R + S720P* mutations (exon 21 + exon 18) and *L858R + L833V* mutations (exon 21 + exon 21). No patient with *L833V + H835L* mutations (exon 21 + exon 21) was detected in our cohort; however, patients with this combination have been reported to have a good response to gefitinib [22, 23]. One case is especially notable. Leventakos et al. [24] demonstrated that patients with *L858R + S768I* mutations may be sensitive, or at least not resistant, to TKI therapy, which is in contrast to our results. Our patients with a

single *L861Q* mutation or compound mutations with *L861Q* exhibited a high RR (66%) and non-inferior PFS (median, 6 months) to TKI therapy. We also detected two cases with *19Del + L861Q* mutations, and a good response to TKIs (one PR and one SD) and prolonged PFS (11.4 and 11.9 months) were observed. However, the patient with *L858R + L861Q* exhibited PD after only 1 month of TKI therapy.

Notably, common mutations concomitant with an initial *T790M* mutation accounted for 65.1% of all compound mutations in our cohort, which was higher than in previous reports [13]. However, Su et al. [13] verified that pre-treatment of a co-existing *EGFR T790M* mutation was not a rare event (23/73, 31.5%), and the PFS was significantly shorter than that in patients without *T790M* (median, 6.7 months vs. 10.2 months, respectively; $P=0.035$) [13]. *T790M* status also affected PFS in our cohort compared with a single-sensitizing *EGFR*

Table 4 Literature review of patients harbouring compound *EGFR* mutations and PFS and response to first-generation TKIs between 2004 and 2017

Compound mutations	Double common (n, mPFS, response)	Common + rare (n, mPFS, response)	Rare + rare (n, mPFS, response)	Common + *T790M* (n, mPFS, response)	Rare + *T790M* (n, mPFS, response)
Kobayashi et al. [8]	None	3; 3 months[a]; 2 PR, 1 PD	4; 8 months; 4 PR	None	None
Zhang et al. [9]	3; 17.5 months; 1 CR, 1 PR, 1 NA	None	None	None	None
Hsieh et al. [10]	None	1; 1.9 months; 1 SR	6; 11.6 months; 4 PR, 2 PD	None	None
Hata et al. [11]	8; 12.7 months; 1 CR, 5 PR, 1 SD, 1 NA	8; 2.5 months; 2 PR, 1 SD, 2 PD, 3 NA	None	None	None
Keam et al. [14]	None	16; 8.1 months; 11 PR, 4 SD, 1 PD	3; 4.6 months; 1 PR, 1 PD, 1 NA	5; 8.0 months; 4 PR, 1 PD	None
Xu et al. [16]	14; 9.53 months; 10 PR, 3 SD, 1 PD	18; 9.8 months; 10 PR, 5 SD, 3 PD	None	9; 1.9 months; 2 PR, 3 SD, 4 PD	None
Wu et al. [17]	None	7; NA; 2 PR, 1 SD, 4 PD	3; NA; 2 PR, 1 PD	None	None
Chen et al. [18]	None	10; 8.9 months; 4 PR, 6 NA	None	3; 6.7 months; 1 PR, 1 SD, 1 NA	1; 6 months; SD
Wu et al. [21]	None	12; 13.5 months; 10 PR, 1 SD, 1 PD	7; 4.2 months; 2 PR, 4 SD, 1 PD	2; NA; 2 PR	None
Asahina et al. [26]	None	None	1; 1.1 months; PD	None	None
Zhang et al. [32]	2; 6.1 months; 2PR	7; NA; NA	11; NA; NA	8; 3.3 months; 1PR, 1SD, 6NA	3; NA; NA
Zhu et al. [33]	None	3; 5.3 months[a]; 2SD, 1PD	5; 3.5 months[a]; 2 PR, 2 SD, 1 NA	None	None
Wu et al. [34]	None	9; 8.6 months; 7 PR, 1 SD, 1 PD	4; 9.2 months; 2 PR, 1 PD, 1 SD	None	None
Yang et al. [35]	1; 2 months; 1 PD	None	None	None	None
Svaton et al. [36]	None	None	1; 8 months; 1 PR	None	None
Peng et al. [37]	2; 11.5 months; 1 PR, 1 SD	3; 10 months; 3 SD	None	1; 10 months; 1 SD	None
Baek et al. [38]	12; 7.4 months; 4 CR, 5 PR, 2 SD, 1 PD	None	11; 5.1 months; 5 CR, 4 PR, 2 SD	None	None
Peng et al. [39]	2; 11.5 months; 1 PR, 1 SD	4; 8 months; 4 SD	3; 3 months[a]; 1 CR, 1 SD	2; 9 months; 2 SD	None
Chung et al. [40]	None	1; 5 months[a]; PR	None	None	None
Yang et al. [41]	None	3; NA; 1 PR, 1 SD, 1 PD	2; NA; 2 SD	1; NA; PD	None
Ichihara et al. [42]	None	2; 2.4 months; 2 SD	None	1; 1.6 months; SD	None
Pugh et al. [43]	None	1; NA; PR	1; NA; PR	None	None
Kimura et al. [44]	None	1; 5 months; PR	None	None	None
Van Zandwijk et al. [45]	None	None	1; NA; PR	None	None
Jackman et al. [46]	None	1; 14.8 months[a]; SD	None	None	None
Pallis et al. [47]	None	3; NA; 1 PR, 1 SD, 1 PD	1; NA; PD	None	None
Han et al. [48]	None	1; 13.8 months; 1 SD	2; 3 months; 2 PR	None	None
Kosaka et al. [49]	None	2; 24.5 months; 2 PR	None	None	None
Choong et al. [50]	None	1; 8 months; PR	None	None	None
Oshita et al. [51]	None	2; 13.2 months; 2 PR	1; 12 months; SD	None	None
Tokumo et al. [52]	None	1; 2 months; PD	None	None	None
Chou et al. [53]	None	None	2; 4.1 months; 1 PD, 1 PD	None	None
Shih et al. [54]	None	2; NA; 2 PR	2; NA; 2 PR	None	None
Taron et al. [55]	None	1; 9.4 months; PR	None	None	None
Mitsudomi et al. [56]	None	1, NA,1 PD	None	None	None
Takano et al. [57]	None	2; 12.6 months; 2 PR	None	None	None
Pao et al. [58]	None	1; 13 months; 1 PR	None	None	None
Total, n	44	127	71	32	4
ORR, n (%)	31 (70.5%)	68 (53.5%)	34 (47.9%)	10 (31.2%)	NA
mPFS, range (months)	2–17.5	1.9–24.5	1.1–12	1.6–10	6

PFS progression-free survival, *TKI* tyrosine kinase inhibitor, *mPFS* median progression-free survival, *PR* partial response, *NA* not available, *SD* stable disease, *PD* progressive disease, *CR* complete response, *SR* serological response, *ORR* overall response rate

[a] mPFS not reached

mutation (9.1 months vs. 13.0 months, respectively; $P < 0.001$). We hypothesize that the scarcity of reports may be due to the bias of excluding patients with *T790M* [21]. Previous research on compound mutations may have overlooked the fact that—*T790M* may occur in patients before receiving *EGFR* TKI treatment [1, 21]. In addition, direct sequencing may be used to detect the classical sensitizing mutations in exons 19 and 21, which leads to a missed opportunity to discover patients with co-occurring *T790M*. The impact of *EGFR* TKIs in these patients with *19Del* or *L858R* plus *T790M* was not clarified because of the scarcity of patients and the varying durations of PFS in the published literature. However, approximately one-third and one-half of patients with concomitant initial *T790M* as one of the compound mutations in previous studies [13] and our cohort obtained more than 8 months of PFS with the aid of TKI therapy. Therefore, small molecule TKIs may be an optional therapeutic strategy to identify potential beneficiaries after explaining the bias of the therapy to patients in detail to ensure patient understanding and informed consent.

Patients who harbour a single exon 20 mutation in *EGFR* are reportedly insensitive to small-molecule TKIs [14, 19, 25–27]. However, whether patients with an *EGFR* exon 20 mutation accompanied by another mutation are candidates for TKI therapy remains unanswered. Marius Lund-Iversen and his colleagues reported seven exon 20-positive patients who received oral TKI, including five patients with single exon 20 mutation and two patients with double mutations. The five patients with single exon 20 mutation were found to have progressive disease at the first post-treatment follow-up, but the two patients with double mutations obtained 11 and 14 months of an ongoing response [28]. Chen et al. [18] also concluded that patients with compound mutations involving mutation in exon 20 benefited from TKIs more than single exon 20 mutations [18]. The duration of response to TKIs in compound *EGFR*-mutated patients with concomitant exon 20 mutation (excluding *T790M*) (6.5 months) was still shorter than compound mutated patients without exon 20 mutation (9.1 months) and patients with single common mutations (13.0 months), which is consistent with Keam et al. [14] (< 5 months). The analytical results of Kancha et al. [29] and Wu et al. [17] also support this finding. Together this suggests that first-generation *EGFR* TKIs may not be suitable for patients with an exon 20 mutation regardless of the presence of other mutations.

Overall, patients with double rare mutations or a rare mutation plus *T790M* exhibited a lower RR (38.5% and 37.5%, respectively) and worse PFS to TKI therapy (median, 6.5 and 5.4 months, respectively) in our cohort, which is consistent with a previous publication [14]. A patient with a single *L861Q* point mutation at exon 21 and a *G719X* point mutation at exon 18 may be classified into the TKI-sensitive mutation group [30]. However, patients with a *L861Q* or *G719X* mutation co-occurring with a rare mutation or *T790M* affected the effectiveness and sensitivity to TKI therapy in our clinical practice (RR, 28.6%; median PFS, 5.1 months). We found five patients with a rare mutation plus *T790M*, which is more than the overall number of reported cases. One patient with *G719X* + *T790M* mutations and one patient with *L858Q* + *T790M* mutations exhibited PR to TKI therapy and obtained more than 10 months PFS, which was similar to a case report from Chen et al. [18]. Balak et al. [31] found that the *D761Y* mutation in exon 19 was a novel secondary resistance mutation to *EGFR* TKIs [31]. Therefore, the two patients with two resistance mutations (*D761Y* + *T790M*) in our study exhibited disease progression very soon after initiating TKI therapy, which was not surprising.

The population in our study was a fairly large cohort to investigate the effectiveness of TKI therapy in patients with compound *EGFR*-mutated lung cancer. However, this study was a retrospective analysis, which may limit the reliability of the results. Potential selective bias may be unavoidable because of the low incidence of occurrence of these types of mutations. In addition, the RR and PFS of patients with compound *EGFR* mutations were compared only between patients who received *EGFR* TKI therapy without inclusion of patients who received chemotherapy. Our data were collected from a single institution, and patients from other areas of China should be examined. All reported cases between 2004 and 2017 were enrolled, but the literature from Asia still accounts for the majority of available data.

Conclusions

Although NSCLC patients with compound mutations exhibited a shorter RFS and lower RR in response to TKI therapy than those with a single common mutation, TKI therapy may still benefit patients with compound mutations. Therefore, after explaining the biases of TKI therapy to patients in detail to ensure their understanding and informed consent, a trial of first-generation small molecule TKIs may be an optional therapeutic strategy to identify potential beneficiaries.

Abbreviations
EGFR: epidermal growth factor receptor; TKIs: tyrosine kinase inhibitors; NSCLC: non-small cell lung cancer; PFS: progression-free survival; OS: overall survival; ADC: adenocarcinoma; SCC: squamous cell carcinoma; LELC: lymphoepithelioma-like carcinoma; ASC: adenosquamous carcinoma; PD: progressive disease; SD: stable disease; PR: partial response; CR: complete response; NE: not evaluated.

Authors' contributions
LJZ and YBL designed this study, participated in the interpretation of these results and reviewed the manuscript. XYY, YSW, WDW and YQC were responsible for data collection and assembly, data analysis and interpretation of the results. XWZ, ZCZ and XYY drafted this manuscript together. All authors read and approved the final manuscript.

Author details
[1] State Key Laboratory of Oncology in South China, Collaborative Innovation Center for Cancer Medicine, Guangzhou 510060, Guangdong, China. [2] Department of Thoracic Surgery, Sun Yat-sen University Cancer Center, 651 Dongfeng Road East, Guangzhou 510060, Guangdong, China. [3] Department of Medical Oncology, Sun Yat-sen University Cancer Center, Guangzhou 510060, Guangdong, China. [4] Department of Molecular Pathology, Sun Yat-sen University Cancer Center, Guangzhou 510060, Guangdong, China.

Acknowledgements
We express our gratitude for the support and suggestions in this study from the staff of the Department of Pathology, Sun Yat-sen University Cancer Center.

Competing interests
The authors declare that they have no competing interests.

Funding
The publishing and preparation of this manuscript were funded by the National Key Research and Development Plan (No. 2016YFC0905400), Ministry of Science and Technology of the People's Republic of China.

References
1. NCCN clinical practice guidelines in oncology (NCCN guidelines) non-small cell lung cancer, version 4; 2017.
2. Gaughan EM, Costa DB. Genotype-driven therapies for non-small cell lung cancer: focus on EGFR, KRAS and ALK gene abnormalities. Ther Adv Med Oncol. 2011;3(3):113–25.
3. Sharma SV, Bell DW, Settleman J, Haber DA. Epidermal growth factor receptor mutations in lung cancer. Nat Rev Cancer. 2007;7(3):169–81.
4. Mok TS, Wu YL, Thongprasert S, Yang CH, Chu DT, Saijo N, et al. Gefitinib or carboplatin-paclitaxel in pulmonary adenocarcinoma. N Engl J Med. 2009;361(10):947–57.
5. Zhou C, Wu YL, Chen G, Feng J, Liu XQ, Wang C, et al. Erlotinib versus chemotherapy as first-line treatment for patients with advanced EGFR mutation-positive non-small-cell lung cancer (OPTIMAL, CTONG-0802): a multicentre, open-label, randomised, phase 3 study. Lancet Oncol. 2011;12(8):735–42.
6. Wen YS, Cai L, Zhang XW, Zhu JF, Zhang ZC, Shao JY, et al. Concurrent oncogene mutation profile in chinese patients with stage Ib lung adeno-carcinoma. Medicine. 2014;93(29):e296.
7. Huang SF, Liu HP, Li LH, Ku YC, Fu YN, Tsai HY, et al. High frequency of epidermal growth factor receptor mutations with complex patterns in non-small cell lung cancers related to gefitinib responsiveness in Taiwan. Clin Cancer Res. 2004;10(24):8195–203.
8. Kobayashi S, Canepa HM, Bailey AS, Nakayama S, Yamaguchi N, Goldstein MA, et al. Compound EGFR mutations and response to EGFR tyrosine kinase inhibitors. J Thorac Oncol. 2013;8(1):45–51.
9. Zhang GC, Lin JY, Wang Z, Zhou Q, Xu CR, Zhu JQ, et al. Epidermal growth factor receptor double activating mutations involving both exons 19 and 21 exist in Chinese non-small cell lung cancer patients. Clin Oncol (R Coll Radiol). 2007;19(7):499–506.
10. Hsieh MH, Fang YF, Chang WC, Kuo HP, Lin SY, Liu HP, et al. Complex muta-tion patterns of epidermal growth factor receptor gene associated with variable responses to gefitinib treatment in patients with non-small cell lung cancer. Lung Cancer. 2006;53(3):311–22.
11. Hata A, Yoshioka H, Fujita S, Kunimasa K, Kaji R, Imai Y, et al. Complex mutations in the epidermal growth factor receptor gene in non-small cell lung cancer. J Thorac Oncol. 2010;5(10):1524–8.
12. Yokoyama T, Kondo M, Goto Y, Fukui T, Yoshioka H, Yokoi K, et al. EGFR point mutation in non-small cell lung cancer is occasionally accompa-nied by a second mutation or amplification. Cancer Sci. 2006;97(8):753–9.
13. Su KY, Chen HY, Li KC, Kuo ML, Yang JC, Chan WK, et al. Pretreatment epidermal growth factor receptor (EGFR) T790M mutation predicts shorter EGFR tyrosine kinase inhibitor response duration in patients with non-small-cell lung cancer. J Clin Oncol. 2012;30(4):433–40.
14. Keam B, Kim DW, Park JH, Lee JO, Kim TM, Lee SH, et al. Rare and complex mutations of epidermal growth factor receptor, and efficacy of tyrosine kinase inhibitor in patients with non-small cell lung cancer. Int J Clin Oncol. 2014;19(4):594–600.
15. Liu Y, Wu BQ, Zhong HH, Hui P, Fang WG. Screening for EGFR and KRAS mutations in non-small cell lung carcinomas using DNA extraction by hydrothermal pressure coupled with PCR-based direct sequencing. Int J Clin Exp Pathol. 2013;6(9):1880–9.
16. Xu J, Jin B, Chu T, Dong X, Yang H, Zhang Y, et al. EGFR tyrosine kinase inhibitor (TKI) in patients with advanced non-small cell lung cancer (NSCLC) harboring uncommon EGFR mutations: a real-world study in China. Lung Cancer. 2016;96:87–92.
17. Wu JY, Yu CJ, Chang YC, Yang CH, Shih JY, Yang PC. Effectiveness of tyros-ine kinase inhibitors on "uncommon" epidermal growth factor receptor mutations of unknown clinical significance in non-small cell lung cancer. Clin Cancer Res. 2011;17(11):3812–21.
18. Chen D, Song Z, Cheng G. Clinical efficacy of first-generation EGFR-TKIs in patients with advanced non-small-cell lung cancer harboring EGFR exon 20 mutations. Onco Targets Ther. 2016;9:4181–6.
19. Klughammer B, Brugger W, Cappuzzo F, Ciuleanu T, Mok T, Reck M, et al. Examining treatment outcomes with erlotinib in patients with advanced non-small cell lung cancer whose tumors harbor uncommon EGFR muta-tions. J Thorac Oncol. 2016;11(4):545–55.
20. Kempf E, Lacroix L, Soria JC. First reported case of unexpected response to an epidermal growth factor receptor tyrosine kinase inhibitor in the I744M uncommon EGFR mutation. Clin Lung Cancer. 2015;16(6):e259–61.
21. Wu SG, Chang YL, Hsu YC, Wu JY, Yang CH, Yu CJ, et al. Good response to gefitinib in lung adenocarcinoma of complex epidermal growth factor receptor (EGFR) mutations with the classical mutation pattern. Oncolo-gist. 2008;13(12):1276–84.
22. Frega S, Conte P, Fassan M, Polo V, Pasello G. A triple rare E709K and L833V/H835L EGFR mutation responsive to an irreversible Pan-HER inhibi-tor: a case report of lung adenocarcinoma treated with afatinib. J Thorac Oncol. 2016;11(5):e63–4.
23. Yang TY, Tsai CR, Chen KC, Hsu KH, Lee HM, Chang GC. Good response to gefitinib in a lung adenocarcinoma harboring a heterozygous complex mutation of L833V and H835L in epidermal growth factor receptor gene. J Clin Oncol. 2011;29(16):e468–9.
24. Leventakos K, Kipp BR, Rumilla KM, Winters JL, Yi ES, Mansfield AS. S768I mutation of EGFR in patients with lung cancer. J Thorac Oncol. 2016;11(10):1798–801.
25. Arcila ME, Nafa K, Chaft JE, Rekhtman N, Lau C, Reva BA, et al. EGFR exon 20 insertion mutations in lung adenocarcinomas: prevalence, molecular heterogeneity, and clinicopathologic characteristics. Mol Cancer Ther. 2013;12(2):220–9.
26. Asahina H, Yamazaki K, Kinoshita I, Yokouchi H, Dosaka-Akita H, Nishimura M. Non-responsiveness to gefitinib in a patient with lung adenocar-cinoma having rare EGFR mutations S768I and V769L. Lung Cancer. 2006;54(3):419–22.
27. Yasuda H, Kobayashi S, Costa DB. EGFR exon 20 insertion mutations in non-small-cell lung cancer: preclinical data and clinical implications. Lancet Oncol. 2012;13(1):e23–31.
28. Lund-Iversen M, Kleinberg L, Fjellbirkeland L, Helland Å, Brustugun OT. Clinicopathological characteristics of 11 NSCLC patients with EGFR-exon 20 mutations. J Thorac Oncol. 2012;7(9):1471–3.
29. Kancha RK, von Bubnoff N, Peschel C, Duyster J. Functional analysis of epidermal growth factor receptor (EGFR) mutations and potential impli-cations for EGFR targeted therapy. Clin Cancer Res. 2009;15(2):460–7.
30. Riely GJ, Politi KA, Miller VA, Pao W. Update on epidermal growth fac-tor receptor mutations in non-small cell lung cancer. Clin Cancer Res. 2006;12(24):7232–41.

31. Balak MN, Gong Y, Riely GJ, Somwar R, Li AR, Zakowski MF, et al. Novel D761Y and common secondary T790M mutations in epidermal growth factor receptor-mutant lung adenocarcinomas with acquired resistance to kinase inhibitors. Clin Cancer Res. 2006;12(21):6494–501.

32. Zhang Y, Wang Z, Hao X, Hu X, Wang H, Wang Y, et al. Clinical characteristics and response to tyrosine kinase inhibitors of patients with non-small cell lung cancer harboring uncommon epidermal growth factor receptor mutations. Chin J Cancer Res. 2017;29(1):18–24.

33. Zhu X, Bai Q, Lu Y, Qi P, Ding J, Wang J, et al. Response to tyrosine kinase inhibitors in lung adenocarcinoma with the rare epidermal growth factor receptor mutation S768I: a retrospective analysis and literature review. Target Oncol. 2017;12(1):81–8.

34. Wu JY, Shih JY. Effectiveness of tyrosine kinase inhibitors on uncommon E709X epidermal growth factor receptor mutations in non-small-cell lung cancer. Onco Targets Ther. 2016;9:6137–45.

35. Yang Y, Zhang B, Li R, Liu B, Wang L. EGFR-tyrosine kinase inhibitor treatment in a patient with advanced non-small cell lung cancer and concurrent exon 19 and 21 EGFR mutations: a case report and review of the literature. Oncol Lett. 2016;11(5):3546–50.

36. Svaton M, Pesek M, Chudacek Z, Vosmiková H. Current two EGFR mutations in lung adenocarcinoma—case report. Klin Onkol. 2015;28(2):134–7.

37. Peng L, Song Z, Jiao S. Comparison of uncommon EGFR exon 21 L858R compound mutations with single mutation. Onco Targets Ther. 2015;8:905–10.

38. Baek JH, Sun JM, Min YJ, Cho EK, Cho BC, Kim JH, et al. Efficacy of EGFR tyrosine kinase inhibitors in patients with EGFR-mutated non-small cell lung cancer except both exon 19 deletion and exon 21 L858R: a retrospective analysis in Korea. Lung Cancer. 2015;87(2):148–54.

39. Peng L, Song ZG, Jiao SC. Efficacy analysis of tyrosine kinase inhibitors on rare non-small cell lung cancer patients harboring complex EGFR mutations. Sci Rep. 2014;4:6104.

40. Chung KP, Shih JY, Yu CJ. Favorable response to gefitinib treatment of lung adenocarcinoma with coexisting germline and somatic epidermal growth factor receptor mutations. J Clin Oncol. 2010;28(34):e701–3.

41. Yang CH, Yu CJ, Shih JY, Chang YC, Hu FC, Tsai MC, et al. Specific EGFR mutations predict treatment outcome of stage IIIB/IV patients with chemotherapy-naive non-small-cell lung cancer receiving first-line gefitinib monotherapy. J Clin Oncol. 2008;26(16):2745–53.

42. Ichihara S, Toyooka S, Fujiwara Y, Hotta K, Shigematsu H, Tokumo M, et al. The impact of epidermal growth factor receptor gene status on gefitinib-treated Japanese patients with non-small-cell lung cancer. Int J Cancer. 2007;120(6):1239–47.

43. Pugh TJ, Bebb G, Barclay L, Sutcliffe M, Fee J, Salski C, et al. Correlations of EGFR mutations and increases in EGFR and HER2 copy number to gefitinib response in a retrospective analysis of lung cancer patients. BMC Cancer. 2007;7:128.

44. Kimura H, Suminoe M, Kasahara K, Sone T, Araya T, Tamori S, et al. Evaluation of epidermal growth factor receptor mutation status in serum DNA as a predictor of response to gefitinib (IRESSA). Br J Cancer. 2007;97(6):778–84.

45. van Zandwijk N, Mathy A, Boerrigter L, Ruijter H, Tielen I, et al. EGFR and KRAS mutations as criteria for treatment with tyrosine kinase inhibitors: retro- and prospective observations in non-small-cell lung cancer. Ann Oncol. 2007;18(1):99–103.

46. Jackman DM, Yeap BY, Lindeman NI, Fidias P, Rabin MS, Temel J, et al. Phase II clinical trial of chemotherapy-naive patients $\geq$ 70 years of age treated with erlotinib for advanced non-small-cell lung cancer. J Clin Oncol. 2007;25(7):760–6.

47. Pallis AG, Voutsina A, Kalikaki A, Souglakos J, Briasoulis E, Murray S, et al. 'Classical' but not 'other' mutations of EGFR kinase domain are associated with clinical outcome in gefitinib-treated patients with non-small cell lung cancer. Br J Cancer. 2007;97(11):1560–6.

48. Han SW, Kim TY, Jeon YK, Hwang PG, Im SA, Lee KH, et al. Optimization of patient selection for gefitinib in non-small cell lung cancer by combined analysis of epidermal growth factor receptor mutation, K-ras mutation, and Akt phosphorylation. Clin Cancer Res. 2006;12(8):2538–44.

49. Kosaka T, Yatabe Y, Endoh H, Yoshida K, Hida T, Tsuboi M, et al. Analysis of epidermal growth factor receptor gene mutation in patients with non-small cell lung cancer and acquired resistance to gefitinib. Clin Cancer Res. 2006;12(19):5764–9.

50. Choong NW, Dietrich S, Seiwert TY, Tretiakova MS, Nallasura V, Davies GC, et al. Gefitinib response of erlotinib-refractory lung cancer involving meninges–role of EGFR mutation. Nat Clin Pract Oncol. 2006;3(1):50–7 **(quiz 1 p. following 57)**.

51. Oshita F, Matsukuma S, Yoshihara M, Sakuma Y, Ohgane N, Kameda Y, et al. Novel heteroduplex method using small cytology specimens with a remarkably high success rate for analysing EGFR gene mutations with a significant correlation to gefitinib efficacy in non-small-cell lung cancer. Br J Cancer. 2006;95(8):1070–5.

52. Tokumo M, Toyooka S, Ichihara S, Ohashi K, Tsukuda K, Ichimura K, et al. Double mutation and gene copy number of EGFR in gefitinib refractory non-small-cell lung cancer. Lung Cancer. 2006;53(1):117–21.

53. Chou TY, Chiu CH, Li LH, Hsiao CY, Tzen CY, Chang KT, et al. Mutation in the tyrosine kinase domain of epidermal growth factor receptor is a predictive and prognostic factor for gefitinib treatment in patients with non-small cell lung cancer. Clin Cancer Res. 2005;11(10):3750–7.

54. Shih JY, Gow CH, Yu CJ, Yang CH, Chang YL, Tsai MF, et al. Epidermal growth factor receptor mutations in needle biopsy/aspiration samples predict response to gefitinib therapy and survival of patients with advanced nonsmall cell lung cancer. Int J Cancer. 2006;118(4):963–9.

55. Taron M, Ichinose Y, Rosell R, Mok T, Massuti B, Zamora L, et al. Activating mutations in the tyrosine kinase domain of the epidermal growth factor receptor are associated with improved survival in gefitinib-treated chemorefractory lung adenocarcinoma. Clin Cancer Res. 2005;11(16):5878–85.

56. Mitsudomi T, Kosaka T, Endoh H, Horio Y, Hida T, Mori S, et al. Mutations of the epidermal growth factor receptor gene predict prolonged survival after gefitinib treatment in patients with non–small-cell lung cancer with postoperative recurrence. J Clin Oncol. 2005;23(11):2513–20.

57. Takano T, Ohe Y, Sakamoto H, Tsuta K, Matsuno Y, Tateishi U, et al. Epidermal growth factor receptor gene mutations and increased copy numbers predict gefitinib sensitivity in patients with recurrent non-small-cell lung cancer. J Clin Oncol. 2005;23(28):6829–37.

58. Pao W, Miller V, Zakowski M, Doherty J, Politi K, Sarkaria I, et al. EGF receptor gene mutations are common in lung cancers from "never smokers" and are associated with sensitivity of tumors to gefitinib and erlotinib. Proc Natl Acad Sci USA. 2004;101(36):13306–11.

Age exerts a continuous effect in the outcomes of Asian breast cancer patients treated with breast-conserving therapy

Fuh Yong Wong[1*], Wei Ying Tham[1], Wen Long Nei[1], Cindy Lim[1] and Hui Miao[2]

Abstract

Background: Asians are diagnosed with breast cancer at a younger age than Caucasians are. We studied the effect of age on locoregional recurrence and the survival of Asian breast cancer patients treated with breast-conserving therapy.

Methods: Medical records of 2492 patients treated with breast-conserving therapy between 1989 and 2012 were reviewed. The Kaplan–Meier method was used to estimate locoregional recurrence, breast cancer-free survival, and breast cancer-specific survival rates. These rates were then compared using log-rank tests. Outcomes and age were modeled by Cox proportional hazards. Fractional polynomials were then used to test for non-linear relationships between age and outcomes.

Results: Patients ≤ 40 years old were more likely to have locoregional recurrence than were older patients (Hazard ratio [HR] = 2.32, $P < 0.001$). Locoregional recurrence rates decreased year-on-year by 4% for patients with luminal-type breast cancers, compared with 8% for those with triple-negative cancers. Similarly, breast cancer-free survival rates increased year-on-year by 4% versus 8% for luminal-type and triple-negative cancers, respectively. Breast cancer-specific survival rates increased with age by 5% year-on-year. Both breast cancer-free survival and breast cancer-specific survival rates in patients with luminal cancers exhibited a non-linear ("L-shaped") relationship—where decreasing age at presentation was associated with escalating risks of relapse and death. The influence of age on overall survival was confounded by competing non-cancer deaths in older women, resulting in a "U-shaped" relationship.

Conclusions: Young Asian breast cancer patients have a continuous year-on-year increase in rates of disease relapse and cancer deaths compared with older patients with no apparent threshold.

Keywords: Breast cancer, Breast-conserving therapy, Locoregional recurrence, Breast cancer-specific survival, Breast cancer-free survival, Younger age

Background

Breast cancer is relatively uncommon in young women. According to the Surveillance, Epidemiology, and End Results (SEER) program database, only 6.5% of breast tumors occur in women age < 40 years and only 0.6% in women age < 30 years [1].

Young age is, however, an important independent poor prognostic factor for breast cancer. Several studies have shown that young breast cancer patients have poorer local disease control, increased breast cancer mortality, and reduced overall survival compared with older premenopausal or postmenopausal patients [2–9]. However, the definition of "young age" has been arbitrary, with various age cut-offs ranging from 30 to 40 years.

Young women with breast cancer are faced with a choice between mastectomy and breast-conserving therapy (BCT). Women who chose BCT reported better body image, sexual functioning, and fewer disruptions to lifestyles compared with those who underwent mastectomy [10]. In some studies, age has been shown to be a

*Correspondence: wong.fuh.yong@singhealth.com.sg
[1] Division of Radiation Oncology, National Cancer Centre Singapore, 11 Hospital Drive, Singapore 169610, Singapore
Full list of author information is available at the end of the article

predictor for the choice of type of surgery [11]. Women who chose BCT were likely to be younger. Factors affecting women's choice of surgery included the risk of local recurrence and fears about losing a breast [12].

Several studies have shown that breast cancer presents earlier in Asian women than in their Western counterparts [13, 14]. In addition, patients in developing countries who are diagnosed with breast cancer are approximately one decade younger than those in developed countries [15]. The proportion of young patients (< 35 years) varies from approximately 10% in developed countries to up to 25% in developing Asian countries [13–15]. In developing countries, the majority of breast cancer patients continue to be diagnosed at a relatively late stage, and locally advanced cancers constitute over 50% of all patients [13–15]. The clinicopathology profile of the young Asian breast cancer patient differs from that of patients elsewhere in the world [16].

In addition, young women form a socioeconomically important segment, in both developing and developed societies. They are economically productive and often have young families and developing careers. For young women, the knowledge that their youth predisposes them to a worse prognosis affects them in two ways: it affects them in a profound manner psychosocially and sexually, and it undoubtedly influences their choices regarding child bearing and future plans, which may affect their choice of treatment and compliance with treatment [17, 18].

Due to the large proportion of young breast cancer patients in our Asian population, with their preference for breast-conserving, we conducted this study to better understand the effect of age on Asian breast cancer patients and their outcomes after BCT [19].

Patients and methods
Patients and data collection
Retrospective chart reviews of breast cancer patients treated with BCT at the National Cancer Centre Singapore between 1989 and 2012 were performed. All patients treated with curative intent are included. Patients who received mastectomy up front or completion mastectomy for positive margins are excluded. BCT refers to the wide local excision of the tumor with appropriate management of axillary nodes, followed by adjuvant whole breast radiotherapy and systemic treatment when indicated. Patients were staged according to the 7th edition of the American Joint Committee on Cancer (AJCC) system.

Follow-up and endpoints
Patients were followed up until death or until March 2013. Patients were seen at least twice a year in the first

5 years with digital breast examinations in the clinic. Mammograms and/or ultrasound of the breasts were scheduled annually in patients without symptoms. The endpoints studied were overall survival (OS), breast cancer-specific survival (BCSS), breast cancer-free interval (BCFI) and locoregional recurrence (LRR). Overall survival was defined as the time from diagnosis to death from any cause. BCSS was defined as the time from diagnosis to death from breast cancer-related events. BCFI referred to the time from surgery to the first breast cancer recurrence at any site. This included contralateral breast cancer and breast cancer-related deaths. LRR events comprised ipsilateral local, nodal, or locoregional recurrences. Concurrent local and distant recurrences were not considered local recurrences. Patients without events were censored at the time of their last follow-up.

Statistical analyses
Patients were divided into two age groups—using 40 years as the cut-off point. Associations between patient characteristics and age group were tested using the Pearson's Chi square test, the Fisher exact test, or the Wilcoxon rank sum test. The strength of association was estimated using the Cramer V test, the Kendall rank correlation coefficient, or the Spearman's rank correlation coefficient. The variables analyzed included (1) tumor size; (2) the number of nodes involved; (3) histological subtypes (approximated from immunohistochemical assessment of hormone receptor and HER-2 status); and (4) tumor grade. The Kaplan–Meier method was used to determine survival estimates. The log-rank test was used to test the differences in survival between the two groups of patients. In addition, a patient's age at diagnosis was analyzed as a continuous variable, using the Cox proportional hazards model. Fractional polynomials, with a maximum degree of 2, were used to test for nonlinear relationships with age. The closed-test algorithm was used for fractional polynomial model selection [20]. A 2-sided P value of less than 0.05 was considered statistically significant. All analyses were performed in Stata 11.2 (StataCorp, College Station, Texas, USA).

Relative survival analysis
A relative survival analysis was conducted to estimate the net survival and account for the variations in underlying background mortality of the different age groups. A 5-year relative survival ratio (RSR) was calculated as the ratio of observed 5-year cumulative survival of patients in the present study to the expected survival of the general population, matched by age and calendar year. The expected survival was derived from Singapore female population life tables, using the Ederer II method [21]. A generalized linear model for excess mortality was fitted,

according to the Hakulinen and Tenkanen method, to compare excess mortality by age and provide estimates of excess hazard ratios, relative excess risk (RER). This fitting was performed with patients older than 60 years of age as the reference group while adjusting for follow-up time and histological subtype [22]. The data were then analyzed using Stata (Version 12.1; StataCorp).

Results

Patient demographics and treatment received

The study included 2492 patients who had BCT, 447 (17.9%) of whom were 40 years or younger at the age of diagnosis (Table 1). The median age at diagnosis was 49 years (22–92 years). The median follow-up period was 4.14 years (range 0.03–24.83). With the exception of 5 patients, all patients completed adjuvant radiotherapy; 96.7% (2410) of patients had axillary clearance or sentinel lymph node biopsy. All patients with positive sentinel lymph nodes received axillary clearance.

The patients' clinicopathologic characteristics are summarized in Table 2. Older patients were more often diagnosed with stage I disease (56.9% vs. 45.9%, $P<0.001$), while younger patients had a significantly higher proportion of Grade 3 (47.0% vs. 35.6%, $P<0.001$) and estrogen receptor (ER)-negative tumors (28.2% vs. 23.3%, $P=0.020$). Younger patients were also more likely to have triple-negative breast cancers (15.2% vs. 9.9%, $P<0.001$) and lymphovascular invasion (22.6% vs. 18.4%; $P=0.012$) than were older patients. More younger than older patients received chemotherapy (62.0% vs. 45.7%, $P<0.001$).

Overall survival

The OS rates were similar for older and younger patients; the HR of OS for older patients was slightly higher but not significant statistically (HR $= 1.27$ $P=0.198$; Table 3, Fig. 1). However, when age was modeled as a continuous variable, we found that the relationship was significantly non-linear. A plot of the best fit fractional polynomial

Table 1 Age distribution for the 2492 Asian patients with breast cancer

Age at diagnosis (years)	Number	%
≤ 30	66	2.7
31–40	381	15.3
41–50	953	38.2
51–60	738	29.6
61–70	293	11.8
71–80	56	2.3
> 80	5	0.2

showed a U-shaped relationship between log relative hazard and age, indicating that the hazard of death first decreased and then increased with age, with the minimum at approximately 45 years (Fig. 2a). This trend may explain why age was not significant when modeled linearly or as 2 groups. The finding suggests that after age 45, there are increasingly larger competing background risks of death that exert a stronger influence on overall survival than on breast cancer deaths alone. When analyzed according to subtype, the luminal subtypes also showed a U-shaped relationship. HER2 and basal subtypes did not reach significance (Table 4).

Relative survival ratio

The 5-year relative survival ratio increased with age (Table 5). After adjusting for histological subtype and follow-up time, women younger than 45 years had the highest excess mortality (Relative Excess Risk 1.85, 95% CI 0.45–7.63), while the least excess mortality was observed for women aged between 51 and 60 years (RER 0.39, 95% CI 0.05–2.88). However, the differences were not significant in any age group.

Breast cancer-specific survival

Overall, 77 patients died from breast cancer-related events. Twenty-six of these patients were aged 40 or younger when diagnosed with breast cancer, while 51 were older than 40 years. Patients in the younger age group were more likely to die from a breast cancer- related event compared with those diagnosed later (HR $= 2.0$; 95% CI $= 1.23$–3.23; $P=0.004$). Five-year BCSS rates were 96.7% and 98.3% ($P=0.004$) for patients age ≤ 40 and > 40 years, respectively (Table 3).

When age was analyzed as a continuous variable, there was no evidence of a non-linear relationship between BCSS and age. The linear model was chosen by the model selection algorithm; it was estimated that the hazard of BCSS decreased linearly with increasing age by approximately 5% per year (95% CI $= 2\%$–8%; $P=0.001$). Therefore, the younger patient has a higher risk of dying from breast cancer compared to an otherwise similar but older patient; those patients at the youngest of age would have the highest risk of breast cancer death amongst all. Luminal breast cancers had a significant non-linear relationship with the hazard decreasing rapidly up until approximately age 50 at diagnosis and then more gradually thereafter. HER2 and triple-negative subtypes did not reach significance (Table 4, Fig. 2b).

Breast cancer-free interval

A total of 277 patients developed breast cancer-related events. Of these patients, 85 were 40 years or younger at diagnosis, while the remaining 192 were older than

Table 2 Characteristics of the 2492 Asian breast cancer patients treated with breast-conserving therapy (1989–2012)

Characteristic	Age ≤ 40 years (n = 447)	Age > 40 years (n = 2045)	P value	Strength of association
Age (years)				
Median (range)	36 (22–40)	51 (41–92)		
Race [n (%)]				
Chinese	342 (76.5)	1673 (81.8)		
Indian	21 (4.7)	94 (4.6)		
Malay	40 (8.9)	184 (9.0)		
Others	44 (9.8)	94 (4.6)	< 0.001	0.089
T category [n (%)]				
T0/T1/T1a/T1b/T1mic/Tx	85 (19.0)	542 (26.5)		
T1c	203 (45.4)	912 (44.6)		
T2–T4	159 (36.6)	591 (28.9)	0.001	− 0.060
N category [n (%)]				
N0	311 (69.6)	1525 (74.6)		
N1/N1mic	100 (22.4)	391 (19.1)		
N2/N3	36 (8.1)	129 (6.3)	0.086	− 0.030
TNM stage [n (%)]				
Stage 1	205 (45.9)	1163 (56.9)		
Stage 2A/2B	204 (45.6)	739 (36.1)		
Stage 3A/3C	34 (7.6)	130 (6.4)	< 0.001	− 0.064
Unknown	4 (0.9)	13 (0.6)		
Size (cm)				
Median (range)	1.8 (0–7.5)	1.6 (0–8)	0.001	
Unknown	31 (7)	72 (3.5)		
Grade [n (%)]				
Grade 1	61 (13.6)	440 (21.5)		
Grade 2	149 (33.3)	769 (37.6)		
Grade 3	210 (47.0)	727 (35.6)	< 0.001	− 0.086
Unknown	27 (6.0)	109 (5.3)		
Extensive intraductal component [n (%)]				
Not present	326 (72.9)	1567 (76.6)		
Present	74 (16.6)	372 (18.2)	0.751	0.007
Not mentioned/missing	47 (10.5)	106 (5.3)		
Margins (mm)				
0–5	215 (48.1)	982 (48.0)		
6–10	112 (25.1)	533 (26.1)		
> 10	87 (19.5)	442 (21.6)	0.744	0.012
Unknown	33 (7.4)	88 (4.3)		
Lymphovascular invasion [n (%)]				
No	304 (68.0)	1562 (76.4)		
Yes	101 (22.6)	376 (18.4)	0.012	− 0.052
Unknown	42 (9.4)	107 (0.2)		
No. of positive nodes				
Median (range)	0 (0–28)	0 (0–40)	0.024	− 0.045
Unknown	0 (0)	4 (0.2)		
ER[a] [n (%)]				
Negative	126 (28.2)	476 (23.3)		
Positive	284 (63.5)	1467 (71.7)	0.009	0.054
Equivocal	0 (0)	4 (0.2)		
Unknown	37 (8.3)	98 (4.8)		

Age exerts a continuous effect in the outcomes of Asian breast cancer patients treated...

73

Table 2 (continued)

Characteristic	Age ≤ 40 years (n = 447)	Age > 40 years (n = 2045)	P value	Strength of association
PR[a] [n (%)]				
Negative	141 (31.5)	605 (29.6)		
Positive	267 (59.7)	1332 (65.1)	0.190	0.027
Equivocal	0 (0)	4 (0.2)		
Unknown	39 (8.7)	104 (4.8)		
HER2[a] [n (%)]				
Negative	274 (61.3)	1365 (66.7)		
Positive	82 (18.3)	351 (17.2)	0.276	− 0.024
Equivocal	17 (3.8)	91 (4.4)		
Unknown	74 (16.6)	238 (11.6)		
Histologic subtype [n (%)]				
Luminal A/B	266 (59.5)	1421 (69.5)		
HER2 enriched	34 (7.6)	129 (6.3)		
Basal	68 (15.2)	202 (9.9)	< 0.001	0.087
Unknown	79 (17.7)	293 (14.3)		
Chemotherapy [n (%)]				
No	168 (37.6)	1106 (54.1)		
Yes	277 (62.0)	934 (45.7)	< 0.001	− 0.126
Unknown	2 (0.4)	5 (0.2)		
First event [n (%)]				
Locoregional recurrence	30 (6.7)	56 (2.7)		
Distant recurrence	38 (8.5)	91 (4.5)		
New contralateral breast cancer	17 (3.8)	43 (2.1)		
New non-breast or unknown cancers	5 (1.1)	40 (2.0)		
Death (any cause)	2 (0.5)	23 (1.1)		
Alive without disease	355 (79.4)	1792 (87.6)	< 0.001	0.125
Follow-up time (years)				
Median (range)	4.36 (0.18–24.83)	4.09 (0.03–22.14)	0.072	− 0.036

Patients were staged according to the 7th edition of the American Joint Committee on Cancer (AJCC) system

ER estrogen receptor, *PR* progesterone receptor

[a] Equivocal was excluded from the test of association

40 years. Patients 40 years or younger at diagnosis were more likely to have breast cancer recurrence compared with patients who were older at diagnosis (HR = 1.92; CI 1.49–2.50; P <0.001; Table 3).

When age was analyzed as a continuous variable, the relationship between BCFI and age was significantly non-linear. A plot of the best-fit fractional polynomial showed an L-shaped relationship between log relative hazard and age, indicating that an older age at diagnosis was associated with a lower hazard of breast cancer recurrence or death. Following an initial rapid decrease in the hazard with increasing age at presentation, the curve become more gradual at approximately 40 years of age, which suggests that beyond this point, the influence of age on breast cancer recurrence or death is diminished.

When we analyzed the histological subtypes, all three—Luminal A/B, HER2 enriched, and Basal subtypes—demonstrated increased risk in younger patients. A similar L-shaped relationship was found in luminal cancers, but non-linear relationships were not detected in HER2 and triple-negative subtypes. The hazard ratio for the basal subtype was 0.92, while the hazard ratio for the luminal subtype was 0.96. The decrease in the hazard each year related to the increase in age at diagnosis was larger for the basal subtype (8% decrease/year), than for the luminal subtype (4% decrease/year). The hazard decreased faster with age at diagnosis for the basal subtype than for the luminal subtype (Table 4 and Fig. 2c).

Local recurrence

Eighty-nine patients had local recurrences. Thirty-one of these patients were 40 years old or younger, while 58 of them were older than 40. The 5-year LRR rates were 5.2%

Table 3 Five-year survival/failure rates and hazard ratios by age group for the 2492 Asian breast cancer patients treated with breast-conserving therapy (1989–2012)

Clinical outcomes	No. of events/no. of patients	5-year rate [% (95% CI)]	Log-rank, P value	Hazard ratio (95% CI)	Cox model P value
Overall survival					
All patients	162/2492	95.7 (94.6–96.6)			
≤ 40 years at diagnosis	40/447	94.1 (90.6–96.4)		1.27 (0.88–1.82)	
> 40 years at diagnosis	122/2045	96.1 (94.9–97.0)	0.198	1.00	0.209
Breast cancer-specific survival					
All patients	77/2492	98.0 (97.1–98.6)			
≤ 40 years at diagnosis	26/447	96.7 (93.7–98.3)		2.00 (1.23–3.23)	
> 40 years at diagnosis	51/2045	98.3 (97.4–98.9)	0.004	1.00	0.007
Breast cancer-free interval					
All patients	277/2492	10.5 (9.0–12.1)			
≤ 40 years at diagnosis	85/447	15.3 (11.6–20.1)		1.92 (1.49–2.50)	
> 40 years at diagnosis	192/2045	9.4 (7.9–11.1)	< 0.001	1.00	< 0.001
Local recurrence					
All patients	89/2492	3.4 (2.6–4.4)			
≤ 40 years at diagnosis	31/447	5.2 (3.1–8.5)		2.33 (1.49–3.57)	
> 40 years at diagnosis	58/2045	3.0 (2.2–4.1)	< 0.001	1.00	< 0.001

Proportional hazards assumption was violated for overall survival

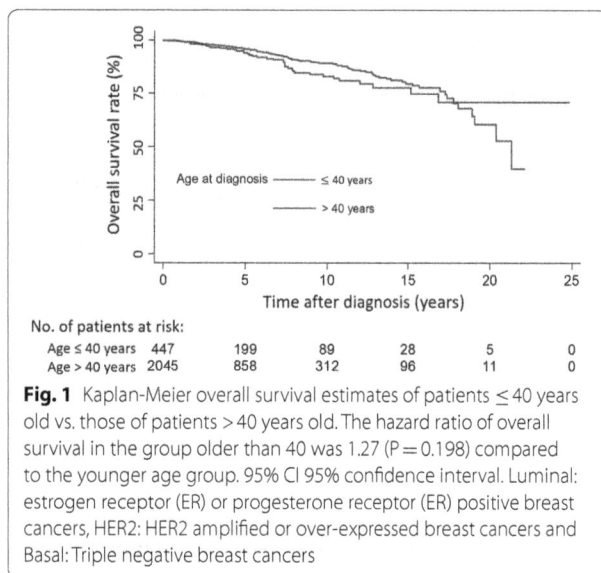

Fig. 1 Kaplan-Meier overall survival estimates of patients ≤ 40 years old vs. those of patients > 40 years old. The hazard ratio of overall survival in the group older than 40 was 1.27 (P = 0.198) compared to the younger age group. 95% CI 95% confidence interval. Luminal: estrogen receptor (ER) or progesterone receptor (ER) positive breast cancers, HER2: HER2 amplified or over-expressed breast cancers and Basal: Triple negative breast cancers

$P = 0.005$) in the triple-negative subtype. A multivariate analysis showed that age remained a significant factor in patients for local recurrence after controlling for histological subtype (Table 4, Fig. 2d).

Discussion

Our study shows that young Asian breast cancer patients treated with BCT have higher rates of local recurrence and breast cancer death than other patients. While previous investigations have examined the effect of age in a dichotomous fashion using arbitrary definitions of youth, our results showed no apparent threshold effect of age on breast cancer control or survival.

Outcomes of patients with breast cancer are influenced by the complex interactions between tumor biology, host biology and treatment received. Many aspects of tumor biology that influence treatment responses and outcomes have been clearly established, including (1) the stage of disease at presentation, (2) tumor grade, (3) the presence of hormone receptors, and (4) HER2 overexpression. Although many of these factors are associated with a patient's age and account for a significant portion of the variability in outcomes, age still remains a significant, independent prognostic factor [23].

The actual mechanism through which age influences outcomes is unknown. Recent studies have shown that breast cancer in young patients is replete with processes related to immature mammary epithelial cells (luminal progenitors, mammary stem, c-kit, and Receptor

and 3.0% ($P < 0.001$), respectively, for the ≤ 40 and > 40 age groups. Patients ≤ 40 years old were approximately twice as likely as their older counterparts to have a local disease recurrence (HR = 2.33, P < 0.001).

There was no evidence of non-linearity when age was analyzed as a continuous variable. The hazard of LRR decreased linearly with increasing age ($P = 0.001$), from a 4% decrease/year (95% CI = 1–7%, $P = 0.040$) in the luminal subtype to an 8% decrease/year (95% CI = 2–14%,

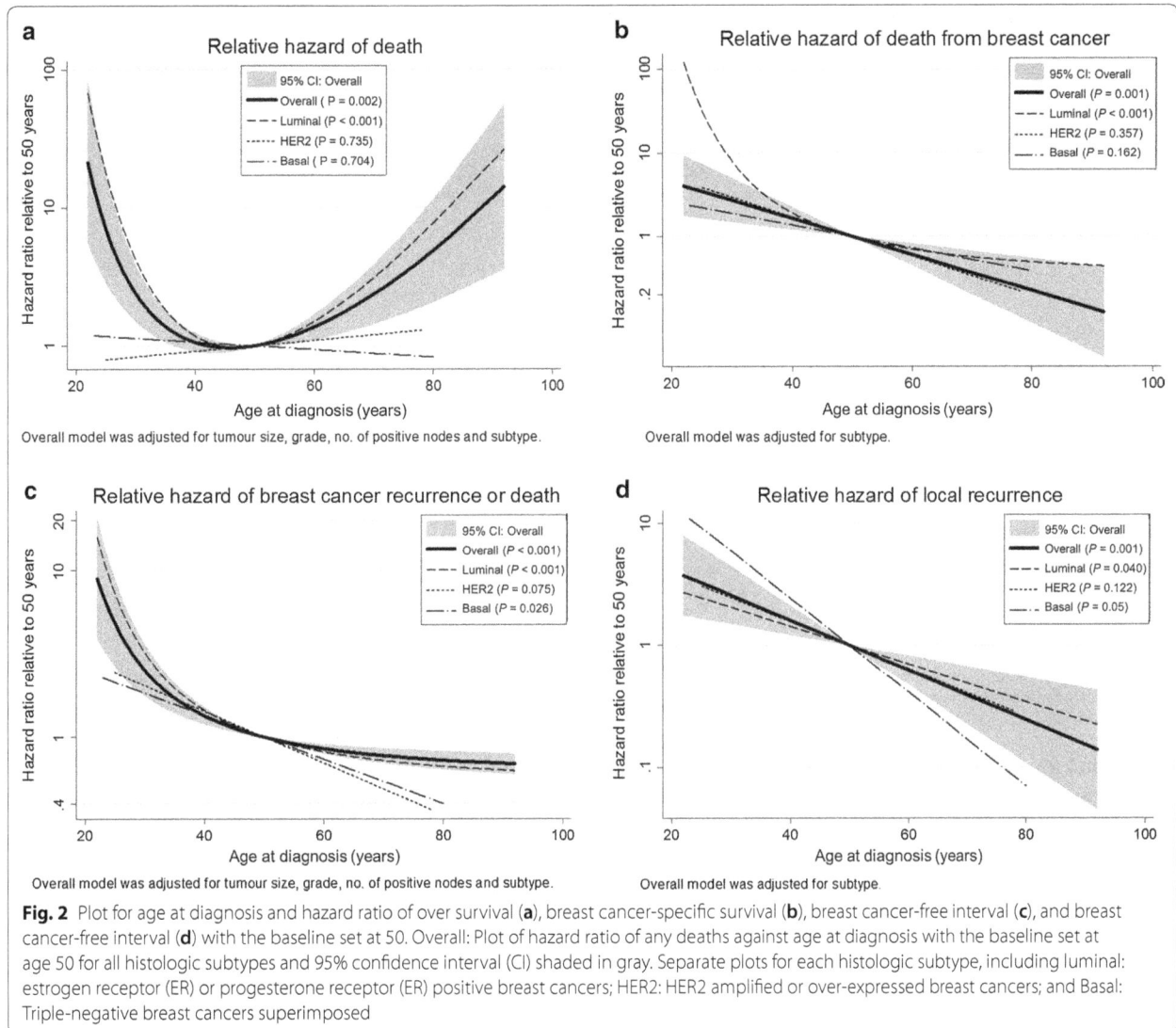

Fig. 2 Plot for age at diagnosis and hazard ratio of over survival (**a**), breast cancer-specific survival (**b**), breast cancer-free interval (**c**), and breast cancer-free interval (**d**) with the baseline set at 50. Overall: Plot of hazard ratio of any deaths against age at diagnosis with the baseline set at age 50 for all histologic subtypes and 95% confidence interval (CI) shaded in gray. Separate plots for each histologic subtype, including luminal: estrogen receptor (ER) or progesterone receptor (ER) positive breast cancers; HER2: HER2 amplified or over-expressed breast cancers; and Basal: Triple-negative breast cancers superimposed

activator of nuclear factor kappa-B ligand RANKL), growth factor signaling and mitogen activated protein kinase (MAPK), and phosphoinositide 3-kinase (PI3K)-related pathways [24–28]. Other studies that contradict the abovementioned reasoning postulate that age is no longer a significant prognostic factor, after correcting for clinicopathological and histopathological features such as grade, nodal status, ER status, and breast cancer subtypes [28, 29]. However, this argument only brings us back to the question of why younger women are more prone to aggressive subtypes of breast cancer in the first place and how the factors associated with younger patients, such as increased breast density and lower parity, contribute to these findings.

Although the same general trend for the age-outcome relationship is observed, it is clear that this interaction is complex and may well involve different mechanisms for each of the well-recognized breast cancer subtypes. The relationships of disease control and cancer death to age in luminal cancers are L-shaped, emphasizing the preponderance of risks in the youngest patients. This inflection point at 40–45 years of age may be indicative of a switch in factors driving disease initiation and progression. It has been similarly observed that luminal B cancers are particularly associated with poor outcomes in young breast cancer patients [30, 31]. However, the relationship between age and breast cancer events in HER2 enriched and triple-negative subtypes are more manifestly linear.

Our findings build on earlier studies carried out in dissimilar populations, indicating that women diagnosed with breast cancer at a younger age are more likely to have a poorer outcome. In patients younger than 40 years old, adjuvant radiotherapy following breast-conserving surgery reduced this risk by more than half [29, 30].

Table 4 Best fit multivariate models for the 2492 Asian breast cancer patients treated with breast-conserving therapy (1989–2012)

Clinicopathologic characteristics	Overall survival		Breast cancer-specific survival		Breast cancer-free interval		Time to local recurrence	
	Hazard ratio (95% CI)	P value	Hazard ratio (95% CI)	P value	Hazard ratio (95% CI)	P value	Hazard ratio (95% CI)	P value
No. of events/no. of patients	98/1988		54/2120		182/1988		64/2120	
Age at diagnosis	$25.21[(age/10)^{-2} - 0.04] + 0.06[(age/10)^2 - 25]^a$	<0.001	0.95 (0.92–0.98)	0.001	$13.14[(age/10)^{-2} - 0.04]^a$	<0.001	0.95 (0.93–0.98)	<0.001
Tumor size	1.21 (0.99–1.46)	0.064	Not included		1.15 (1.00–1.32)	0.050	Not included	
Grade		<0.001	Not included			<0.001	Not included	
1	1				1			
2	4.06 (1.59–10.38)				3.38 (1.78–6.41)			
3	4.94 (1.90–12.84)				4.08 (2.12–7.86)			
No. of positive nodes	1.05 (1.01–1.09)	0.031	Not included		1.06 (1.03–1.09)	0.001	Not included	
Histologic subtype		0.024		0.002		0.007		0.002
Luminal A/B	1		1		1		1	
HER2 enriched	1.02 (0.50–2.12)		0.80 (0.24–2.64)		1.39 (0.85–2.28)		3.42 (1.82–6.41)	
Basal	1.99 (1.22–3.25)		2.94 (1.64–5.28)		1.85 (1.27–2.69)		1.61 (0.82–3.15)	

[a] Where age was significantly non-linear, the fractional polynomial function was presented instead of the hazard ratio. Age was scaled by a factor of 10 and centered on 50 years in these models. Where the number of events was insufficient to include all the covariates in the model, only age and histologic subtype were included

Table 5 Relative survival ratio by age for the 2492 Asian breast cancer patients treated with breast-conserving therapy (1989–2012)

Age group	5-year cumulative survival rate (%)		5-year RSR [%(95% CI)]
	Observed	Expected	
≤ 40	94.3	99.7	94.6 (91.2–96.8)
41–50	96.7	99.2	97.4 (95.7–98.6)
51–60	96.9	98.1	98.8 (96.6–100.1)
> 60	92.3	93.0	99.2 (94.1–102.5)

RSR relative survival ratio

One study of 1703 patients from a single center showed that the relationship between recurrence hazard and age was continuous. Fitting with a log-linear function showed a 4% decrease in recurrence and a 2% decrease in cancer-specific death for every one-year increase in age, thus echoing our study findings [6].

A larger study carried out in Korea by Han et al. [7] showed that in patients younger than 35 years of age, there was an increasing risk of death with decreasing age; however, age did not affect patients between 35 and 50 years old. This finding is similar to our results for patients in the same age range. However, Han et al. [7] only included patients up to 50 years of age, whereas our study examined a wider age range. Our study examined records of patients older than 80 and showed that patients diagnosed at ages older than 50 faced increasing competing risks of death from non-breast cancer mortality; the evidence was a larger difference between breast cancer-specific survival and overall mortality in the older age group.

A relative survival analysis in our study population yielded results different from those reported in previous studies. Younger patients were found to have increased excess mortality compared with the older age groups, although this finding was not statistically significant in our study. The lack of statistical significance was possibly due to the smaller number of patients in the younger age group compared with that in the older age group, as well as the small number of events in the older age group.

Chia et al. [34] studied Singaporean breast cancer data and performed a population-based survival analysis. This study showed that younger patients have higher relative survival rates and lower excess risks of death compared with older patients. As demonstrated, this conclusion is opposite to that reached by our group. One possible explanation could be that the study by Chia et al. was conducted over an earlier period (1968–1992) that observed less effective systemic therapy for older patients. Older patients were often undertreated due to poorer health, reduced acceptance of treatment, or the denial of standard treatment arising from concerns of poorer tolerance to toxicity. In contrast, the increased use of systemic treatment, more effective chemotherapy, and better supportive care among older patients during our study period (1989–2012) enables older patients to enjoy the benefits of more effective treatment and improved outcomes. This finding reflects the relatively more indolent nature of their disease. A smaller, single-institution study by Foo et al. [35] showed that patients younger than 40 years did not have poorer overall survival, despite having tumors and a poorer prognostic profile. This result may be attributed to the more aggressive treatment the patients received. It is therefore likely that the differences in outcomes between age groups can be diminished with better treatment and better cancer subtyping.

These studies raise the issue of how we should define the relationship between age and the management of patients with breast cancer. Younger patients may need more aggressive treatment, while older patients may need less aggressive treatment. The current literature reveals conflicting results with regard to locoregional control in patients who have received BCT. Some studies have observed an increased risk of local recurrence with BCT, while others have not [32–36]. Nonetheless, there is no evidence that survival rates are inferior for younger patients who have received BCT relative to those for patients undergoing mastectomy [33]. Therefore, young age is not a contraindication to BCT.

Understanding the effect of age on breast cancer may allow us to better select patients for more appropriate therapy. Regan et al. studied SOFT and TEXT trials and found that the clinicopathologic characteristics that had the greatest contribution to the composite measure of recurrence risk relative to the complementary reference categories were young age (less than 35 years), four or more positive lymph nodes, and Grade 2–3 tumors. There was a gradual reduction in the hazard ratio from 2.2 to 1.2 for women 35 or younger to older than 50. It is now recommended that young women younger than 35 with hormone receptor positive breast cancer receive tamoxifen or exemestane plus ovarian suppression [37, 38].

At the other end of the spectrum, studies have shown that the survival of patients > 70 years old with estrogen-receptor (ER) positive tumors was not improved by the addition of adjuvant radiotherapy on top of lumpectomy and hormonal therapy; such an approach may therefore represent overtreatment in women of this age group [39, 40].

Mao et al. [41] showed that for women diagnosed at age 60 or younger, only the luminal A and basal molecular subtypes showed an overall survival benefit from radiotherapy. For women diagnosed at age 60 and older, there was no significant overall survival benefit of radiotherapy across all molecular subtypes.

Our study examined breast cancer outcomes with BCT in the Asian population. As the median age of diagnosis of breast cancer in Asians is 10 years younger than that in the Caucasian population, it is important for us to understand the effects of age on breast cancer. However, a drawback of our study was that the median follow-up period was only 4 years. A longer follow-up study in this population is being planned and would give us more information on the long-term outcome of BCT.

By intentionally limiting our study patients to only those with BCT, we may have inadvertently underestimated the effect of age, as long-term observational studies have shown improved overall outcomes with BCT compared with mastectomy. van Maaren et al. [42] carried out a population-based study on the Netherlands Cancer Registry and found that the 10-year overall survival for patients who received BCT was 21% higher than that for those who received mastectomy. The results were similar across all T and N stages. In particular, patients with T1N0 breast cancers had a 24% higher metastasis-free survival after BCT compared with that for patients undergoing mastectomy. In addition to our shorter follow-up, this observation may further explain the relatively high BCSS for patients in our study cohort, among whom more than half had Stage I cancer.

Our study population has a relatively small number of patients with HER2 or basal subtypes breast cancers. As such, the relationship between age and clinical outcomes cannot be determined accurately. To a large extent, our results have been affected by the large proportion of patients with luminal cancers. In the model construction, there might have been non-linear relationships that we missed, as we used significance testing (which is sensitive to sample size) to select models.

There were sufficient events to perform multivariate analysis for the relationship between age, overall survival and breast cancer-free interval. For other endpoints, these variables could not be adjusted for as the number of events was too small, particularly as size and number of positive nodes were modeled as continuous variables.

Conclusions

In conclusion, our study shows that young Asian breast cancer patients treated with BCT have higher local recurrence rates and rates of breast cancer death than do older patients. This effect is shown to be continuous, where every 1-year increase in age at presentation increases local control and decreases breast cancer death. The subtypes of breast cancers may display differing age-outcome relationships, reflecting differences in neoplastic mechanisms.

Abbreviations

BCT: breast-conserving therapy; HR: hazard ratio; ER: estrogen receptor; SEER: surveillance, epidemiology and end results; BCFS: breast-cancer-free-survival; LRR: locoregional recurrence; RSR: relative survival ratio; BCSS: breast cancer-specific survival; MAPK: mitogen activated protein kinase; RANKL: receptor activator of nuclear factor kappa-B ligand.

Authors' contributions

All authors participated in equal measure to the conception of the study, data collection, analysis and interpretation and drafting of the article. All authors read and approved the final manuscript.

Author details

[1] Division of Radiation Oncology, National Cancer Centre Singapore, 11 Hospital Drive, Singapore 169610, Singapore. [2] Saw Swee Hock School of Public Health, National University of Singapore, Singapore, Singapore.

Acknowledgements

We are grateful for the help given by our colleagues in the care of patients in this study and their contributions towards the study and preparation of this manuscript.

Competing interests

The authors declare that they have no competing interests.

Funding

This research received no specific grant from any funding agency in the public, commercial, or not-for-profit sectors.

References

1. Hankey BF, Miller B, Curtis R, Kosary C. Trends in breast cancer in younger women in contrast to older women. J Natl Cancer InstMonogr. 1994;16:7–14.
2. Han W, Kim SW, Park IA, Kang D, Kim SW, Youn YK, et al. Young age: an independent risk factor for disease-free survival in women with operable breast cancer. BMC Cancer. 2004;4:82.
3. Fowbie B, Schtulz DJ, Overmoyer B, Solin LJ, Fox K, Jardines L, et al. The influence of young age on outcome in early stage breast cancer. RadiatOncolBiolPhys. 1994;30:23–33.
4. Nixon AJ, Neuberg D, Hayes DF, Gelman R, Connolly JL, Schnitt S, et al. Relationship of patient age to pathologic features of the tumor and prognosis for patients with stage I or II breast cancer. J Clin Oncol Off J Am Soc Clin Oncol. 1994;12(5):888–94.
5. Wei X-Q, Li X, Xin X-J, Tong Z-S, Zhang S. Clinical features and survival analysis of very young (age < 35) breast cancer patients. APJCP. 2013;14(10):5949–52.
6. De la Rochefordiere A, Asselain B, Campana F, Scholl SM, Fenton J, Vilcoq JR, et al. Age as prognostic factor in premenopausal breast carcinoma. Lancet. 1993;341(8852):1039–43.
7. The Korean Breast Cancer Society, Han W, Kang SY. Relationship between age at diagnosis and outcome of premenopausal breast cancer: age less than 35 years is a reasonable cut-off for defining young age-onset breast cancer. Breast Cancer Res Treat. 2010;119(1):193–200.
8. Voogd AC, Nielsen M, Peterse JL, Blichert-Toft M, Bartelink H, Overgaard M, et al. Differences in risk factors for local and distant recurrence after breast-conserving therapy or mastectomy for stage I and II breast cancer: pooled results of two large European randomized trials. J Clin Oncol Off J Am Soc Clin Oncol. 2001;19(6):1688–97.
9. Bollet MA, Sigal-Zafrani B, Mazeau V, Savignoni A, de la Rochefordière A, Vincent-Salomon A, et al. Age remains the first prognostic factor for locoregional breast cancer recurrence in young (< 40 years) women treated with breast conserving surgery first. Radiother Oncol J Eur Soc Ther Radiol Oncol. 2007;82(3):272–80.
10. Engel J, Kerr J, Schlesinger-Raab A, Sauer H, Hölzel D. Quality of life following breast-conserving therapy or mastectomy: results of a 5-year prospective study. Breast J. 2004;10(3):223–31.
11. Morrow M, White J, Moughan J, Owen J, Pajack T, Sylvester J, et al. Factors predicting the use of breast-conserving therapy in stage I and II breast carcinoma. J Clin Oncol Off J Am Soc Clin Oncol. 2001;19(8):2254–62.
12. Molenaar S, Oort F, Sprangers M, Rutgers E, Luiten E, Mulder J, et al. Predictors of patients' choices for breast-conserving therapy or mastectomy: a prospective study. Br J Cancer. 2004;90(11):2123–30.
13. Pathy NB, Yip CH, Taib NA, Hartman M, Saxena N, Iau P, et al. Breast cancer in a multi-ethnic Asian setting: results from the Singapore-Malaysia hospital-based breast cancer registry. Breast Edinb Scotl. 2011;20(Suppl 2):S75–80.
14. The Hong Kong Breast Cancer Research Group, Kwong A, Mang OWK, Wong CHN, Chau WW, Law SCK. Breast cancer in Hong Kong, Southern China: the first population-based analysis of epidemiological characteristics, stage-specific, cancer-specific, and disease-free survival in breast cancer patients: 1997–2001. Ann Surg Oncol. 2011;18(11):3072–8.
15. Raina V, Bhutani M, Bedi R, Sharma A, Deo SV, Shukla NK, et al. Clinical features and prognostic factors of early breast cancer at a major cancer center in North India. Indian J Cancer. 2005;42(1):40–5.
16. Agarwal G, Pradeep PV, Aggarwal V, Yip C-H, Cheung PSY. Spectrum of breast cancer in Asian women. World J Surg. 2007;31(5):1031–40.
17. Arès I, Lebel S, Bielajew C. The impact of motherhood on perceived stress, illness intrusiveness and fear of cancer recurrence in young breast cancer survivors over time. Psychol Health. 2014;29(6):651–70.
18. Ruddy KJ, Greaney ML, Sprunck-Harrild K, Meyer ME, Emmons KM, Partridge AH. Young women with breast cancer: a focus group study of unmet needs. J Adolesc Young Adult Oncol. 2013;2(4):153–60.
19. Bhoo-Pathy N, Yip C-H, Hartman M, Uiterwaal CSPM, Devi BCR, Peeters PHM, et al. Breast cancer research in Asia: adopt or adapt Western knowledge? Eur J Cancer. 2013;49(3):703–9.
20. Royston P, Sauerbrei W. Multivariable model-building. Chichester: Wiley; 2008. http://doi.wiley.com/10.1002/9780470770771. Accessed 27 May 2015.
21. Ederer F, Axtell LM, Cutler SJ. The relative survival rate: a statistical methodology. Natl Cancer Inst Monogr. 1961;6:101–21.
22. Dickman PW, Sloggett A, Hills M, Hakulinen T. Regression models for relative survival. Stat Med. 2004;23(1):51–64.
23. Zhou P, Gautam S, Recht A. Factors affecting outcome for young women with early stage invasive breast cancer treated with breast-conserving therapy. Breast Cancer Res Treat. 2007;101(1):51–7.
24. Azim HA, Michiels S, Bedard PL, Singhal SK, Criscitiello C, Ignatiadis M, et al. Elucidating prognosis and biology of breast cancer arising in young women using gene expression profiling. Clin Cancer Res Off J Am Assoc Cancer Res. 2012;18(5):1341–51.
25. Van't Veer LJ, Dai H, van de Vijver MJ, He YD, Hart AAM, Mao M, et al. Gene expression profiling predicts clinical outcome of breast cancer. Nature. 2002;415(6871):530–6.
26. Eklund M, Esserman LJ. Screening: biology dictates the fate of young women with breast cancer. Nat Rev Clin Oncol. 2013;10(12):673–5.
27. Michailidou K, Hall P, Gonzalez-Neira A, Ghoussaini M, Dennis J, Milne RL, et al. Large-scale genotyping identifies 41 new loci associated with breast cancer risk. Nat Genet. 2013;45(4):353–61.
28. Anders CK, Hsu DS, Broadwater G, Acharya CR, Foekens JA, Zhang Y, et al. Young age at diagnosis correlates with worse prognosis and defines a subset of breast cancers with shared patterns of gene expression. J Clin Oncol. 2008;26(20):3324–30.
29. Anders CK, Fan C, Parker JS, Carey LA, Blackwell KL, Klauber-DeMore N, et al. Breast carcinomas arising at a young age: unique biology or a surrogate for aggressive intrinsic subtypes? J Clin Oncol. 2011;29:e18–20.
30. Cancello G, Maisonneuve P, Rotmensz N, Viale G, Mastropasqua MG, Pruneri G, et al. Prognosis and adjuvant treatment effects in selected breast cancer subtypes of very young women (< 35 years) with operable breast cancer. Ann Oncol. 2010;21:1974–81. https://doi.org/10.1093/annonc/mdq072.
31. Azim HA, Michiels S, Bedard PL, Singhal SK, Criscitiello C, Ignatiadis M, et al. Elucidating prognosis and biology of breast cancer arising in young women using gene expression profiling. Clin Cancer Res. 2012;18:1341–51. https://doi.org/10.1158/1078-0432.CCR-11-2599

32. Arriagada R, Lê MG, Guinebretière J-M, Dunant A, Rochard F, Tursz T. Late local recurrences in a randomised trial comparing conservative treatment with total mastectomy in early breast cancer patients. Ann Oncol Off J Eur Soc Med Oncol. 2003;14(11):1617–22.

33. Van der Leest M, Evers L, van der Sangen MJC, Poortmans PM, van de Poll-Franse LV, Vulto AJ, et al. The safety of breast-conserving therapy in patients with breast cancer aged < or = 40 years. Cancer. 2007;109(10):1957–64.

34. Chia KS, Du WB, Sankaranarayanan R, Sankila R, Wang H, Lee J, et al. Do younger female breast cancer patients have a poorer prognosis? Results from a population-based survival analysis. Int J Cancer J Int Cancer. 2004;108(5):761–5.

35. Foo CS, Su D, Chong CK, Chng HC, Tay KH, Low SC, et al. Breast cancer in young Asian women: study on survival. ANZ J Surg. 2005;75(7):566–72.

36. Cao JQ, Olson RA, Tyldesley SK. Comparison of recurrence and survival rates after breast-conserving therapy and mastectomy in young women with breast cancer. Curr Oncol. 2013;20(6):593.

37. Regan Meredith M, Francis Prudence A, Pagani Olivia, Fleming Gini F, Walley Barbara A, et al. Absolute benefit of adjuvant endocrine therapies for premenopausal women with hormone receptor-positive, human epidermal growth factor receptor 2–negative early breast cancer: TEXT and SOFT trials. J Clin Oncol. 2016;34(19):2221–31.

38. Gnant M, Harbeck N, Thomssen C. St. Gallen/Vienna 2017: a brief summary of the consensus discussion about escalation and de-escalation of primary breast cancer treatment. Breast Care. 2017;2017(12):102–7.

39. Hughes KS, Schnaper LA, Berry D, Cirrincione C, McCormick B, Shank B, et al. Lumpectomy plus tamoxifen with or without irradiation in women 70 years of age or older with early breast cancer. N Engl J Med. 2004;351(10):971–7.

40. Johnson K. Postop RT Study "Very Likely" to change breast cancer practice. 2013. http://www.medscape.com/viewarticle/817856. Accessed 16 Dec 2013.

41. Mao JH, Diest PJV, Perez-Losada J, Snijders AM. Revisiting the impact of age and molecular subtype on overall survival after radiotherapy in breast cancer patients. Sci Rep. 2017;7(1):12587.

42. van Maaren MC, de Munck L, de Bock GH, Jobsen JJ, van Dalen T, Linn SC, et al. 10 year survival after breast-conserving surgery plus radiotherapy compared with mastectomy in early breast cancer in the Netherlands: a population-based study. Lancet Oncol. 2016;17(8):1158–70.

7

Snail promotes metastasis of nasopharyngeal carcinoma partly by down-regulating TEL2

Yi Sang[1,2,3], Chun Cheng[3], Yi-Xin Zeng[1] and Tiebang Kang[1*]

Abstract

Background: Metastasis is the major cause of treatment failure in patients with nasopharyngeal carcinoma (NPC). We previously reported that TEL2, a negative regulator of SERPINE1, could inhibit NPC metastasis to lymph nodes.

Method: A series of in vivo and in vitro assays were performed to elucidate the regulation between Snail and TEL2. TEL2 expression was analyzed in three representative NPC cell lines expressing low levels of Snail (S26, 6-10B, HK1) and two cell lines expressing high levels of Snail (S18, 5-8F). Luciferase and chromatin immunoprecipitation assays were used to analyze the interaction between Snail and TEL2. The roles of the Snail/TEL2 pathway in cell migration and invasion of NPC cells were examined using transwell assays. Metastasis to the lungs was examined using nude mouse receiving NPC cells injection through the tail vein.

Results: Ectopic Snail expression down-regulated TEL2 at the mRNA and protein levels, whereas knockdown of Snail using short hairpin RNA up-regulated TEL2. Luciferase and chromatin immunoprecipitation assays indicated that Snail binds directly to the TEL2 promoter. Ectopic Snail expression enhanced migration and invasion of NPC cells, and such effects were mitigated by TEL2 overexpression. TEL2 overexpression also attenuated hypoxia-induced cell migration and invasion, and increased the number of metastatic pulmonary nodules. Snail overexpression reduced the number of metastatic pulmonary nodules.

Conclusions: TEL2 is a novel target of Snail and suppresses Snail-induced migration, invasion and metastasis in NPC.

Keywords: TEL2, Snail, Metastasis, Nasopharyngeal carcinoma

Background

Nasopharyngeal carcinoma (NPC) is highly prevalent in southern China and Southeast Asia [1–4]. In 2013, 42,100 new cases of NPC were diagnosed in China, with 21,320 NPC-related deaths [5]. Estimated rate of metastasis is 15%–30% despite of the exquisite sensitivity to radiation therapy [6, 7]. At the time of diagnosis, 74.5% of the patients have regional lymph node metastasis; 19.9% of the patients have distant metastasis, most often to the liver and lungs [2]. Distant metastasis is the major cause of treatment failure [8–10].

TEL2 (also referred to as ETV7) is a member of the ETS transcription factor family, and plays a key role in hematopoiesis [11, 12]. In a previous study, we identified an inverse relationship between TEL2 expression and metastasis potential in NPC cell lines [2]. We also showed EL2 inhibits NPC metastasis by binding to the promoter of SERPINE1 and down-regulating its expression [2].

Snail is a master regulator of epithelial-to-mesenchymal transition (EMT). High Snail expression is associated with high metastatic potential in colon cancer [13], liver cancer [14, 15], lung cancer [16], as well as NPC by our previous study [13]. Based on these findings, we speculate that TEL2 is a down-stream effector of Snail.

*Correspondence: kangtb@mail.sysu.edu.cn
[1] State Key Laboratory of Oncology in South China, Collaborative Innovation Center for Cancer Medicine, Sun Yat-sen University Cancer Center, No. 651 Dongfeng East Road, Guangzhou 510060, People's Republic of China
Full list of author information is available at the end of the article

The results of the current study indicated that Snail could down-regulate TEL2 via direct binding to promoter of the TEL2 gene. Consistent with such an action, Snail enhanced NPC cell migration invasion in cultured NPC cells and promoted metastasis to the lungs in nude mice carrying NPC xenograft.

Methods

Cell lines

The in vitro experiments were carried out in three representative NPC cell lines expressing low levels of Snail (S26, 6-10B, HK1) and two representative cell lines expressing high levels of Snail (S18, 5-8F) [2–4]. Cells were cultured in Dulbecco's modified Eagle's medium (DMEM; Invitrogen) supplemented with 10% fetal bovine serum (FBS; Gibco). All cell lines were authenticated using short-tandem repeat profiling within 6 months prior to the experiments. All five cell lines were obtained from Sun Yat-sen University Cancer Center (SYSUCC).

Plasmids

The full-length cDNAs of human TEL2 and Snail were cloned into pBABE-puro vector (Cell Biolabs, INC). An HA tag was inserted to the N-terminus of TEL2. The fusion protein Snail-T2A-TEL2, in which Snail and TEL2 were linked by a T2A linker, was also expressed using the pBABE-puro vector. Mutations were introduced using the Quick-Change Site-Directed Mutagenesis Kit (Stratagene), and verified with DNA sequencing.

Antibodies

Antibody against human TEL2 (Dilution, 1:1000) was obtained from Sigma (HPA029033). Antibodies against human Snail were obtained from R&D (AF3639) for chromatin immunoprecipitation (ChIP) assays and from Cell Signaling Technology (#3895) for Western blotting. Anti-E-cadherin antibody was obtained from BD Company. Antibodies against HA and Tubulin were obtained from Cell Signaling Technology. Antibody against human SERPINE1 was obtained from Santa Cruz (sc-5297).

RNA interference

Cell lines stably expressing short hairpin RNA (shRNA) targeting Snail transcripts or negative control scrambled shRNA were established using kits from Sigma. The sequences of the 2 human Snail shRNAs are: 5′-ATGCTC ATCTGGGACTCTGTC-3′ and 5′-TGCTCCACAAGC ACCAAGAGT-3′. Sequence of the short interfering RNA (siRNA) targeting human TEL2 is: 5′-GCCAGATGT GAAGCTCAAATTA-3′.

RNA extraction and qRT-PCR

These procedures were performed as described previously [3, 17, 18]. Briefly, total RNA was isolated using Trizol reagent (Invitrogen). First-strand cDNA was synthesized using the Revert Aid™ First Strand cDNA Synthesis Kit (MBI Fermentas). The primers were used to amplify target sequences (Additional file 1: Table S1).

Migration and invasion assays

For transwell migration assays, 1.5×10^4 cells (S18, 5-8F) or 3.5×10^4 cells (S26, 6-10B) in 200 µl of serum-free DMEM were added to cell culture inserts with an 8-µm microporous filter without extracellular matrix coating (Becton–Dickinson Labware). DMEM medium containing 10% FBS was added to the bottom chamber. After 24-h incubation, the cells in the lower surface of the filter were fixed, stained, and examined using a microscope. The numbers of migrated cells from triplicate filters were counted in three random optical fields (×100 magnification) and averaged.

Transwell invasion assays were carried out in the same way, except that the chamber inserts were precoated with Matrigel (Becton–Dickinson Labware).

Chromatin immunoprecipitation (ChIP) assay

The assay was conducted using a commercial ChIP kit from Active &Motif (cat#: 53040). Briefly, cells were seeded onto 15-cm plates and allowed to grow to 70%–80% confluence. Cells were fixed and collected, and the nuclear pellet was resuspended in ChIP Buffer, subjected to sonication and incubated overnight with 5-µg antibody, followed by incubation with protein G agarose beads for 3 h at 4 °C. DNA–protein complexes were eluted and de-cross-linked through a series of washes. Purified DNA was resuspended in TE buffer and analyzed with PCR using the following primers: E-cadherin-ChIP-F, 5′-ACTCCAGGCTAGAGGGTCACC-3′; E-cadherin-ChIP-R, 5′-CCGCAAGCTCACAGGTGC TTTGCAGTTCC-3′; TEL2-ChIP-E1-F, 5′-TGAATG TGCATTAGTTTATCAAGCC-3′; TEL2-ChIP-E1-R, 5′-CAATCTGCCTACCAGAAATTTATTC-3′; TEL2-ChIP-E2-F, 5′-CACAGTCACGGCTCACTGCAG-3′; TEL2-ChIP-E2-R, 5′-GAGTTGGACACCAGTCTGAAC AAC-3′; TEL2-ChIP-E3-F, 5′-GGAGCGCTCAAGACA GAAAGC-3′; TEL2-ChIP-E3-R, 5′-AAAATAGGTTTG GAAATCTAGGTGG-3′; TEL2-ChIP-E4-F, 5′-AGGCAG TAGAGTGGTTAACACAAAC-3′; TEL2-ChIP-E4-R, 5′-TTTATGGAGTTCTCTGTGGATCATG-3′; GAPDH-ChIP-F, 5′-TTCTTGCCTTGCTCTTGCTACTC-3′; and GAPDH-ChIP-R, 5′-AGCCTGCCTGGTGATAAT CTTTG-3′.

Luciferase assay

The assay was carried out as described previously [2, 4]. Briefly, cells were plated in 12-well plates at a density of 2×10^5 per well, and transfected with 0.8-µg promoter-luciferase plasmid. To normalize transfection efficiency, cells were co-transfected with 8-ng pRL-CMV encoding *Renilla* luciferase. After transfection for 48 h, luciferase activity was measured using the Dual-Luciferase Assay kit (Promega). Three independent experiments were performed, and means and standard deviations are presented.

Animal experiments

Experiments involving animal subjects and all protocols for animal studies were approved by the Research Animal Resource Center of Sun Yat-sen University, in full compliance with the guidelines of the Institutional Animal Care and Use Committee at Sun Yat-sen University Cancer Center. Male athymic mice aged 5–6 weeks were obtained from Shanghai Institutes for Biological Sciences (Shanghai, China). Human NPC cells were resuspended in 100-µl phosphate-buffered saline (PBS; Biological Industries) and injected into the lateral tail vein of mice (3×10^6 cells/animal). At 6 weeks after injection, mice were euthanized. Metastatic nodules were counted with the naked eyes.

Clinical samples

Experiments involving human tissue samples were approved by the Institutional Review Board of Sun Yat-sen University Cancer Center (YB2015-010). Written informed consent was obtained from all subjects prior to sample collection. Tissue blocks prepared from NPC tissues (10 cases) and lymph node metastases (4 cases) were stored for qRT-PCR.

Statistical analysis

Differences between two groups were assessed using Student's *t*-test. Differences among three or more groups were assessed using parametric ANOVA and the least significant difference (LSD) test. Statistical significance was set at $P < 0.05$ (2-sided).

Results

Snail down-regulates TEL2

In the present study, we found that levels of Snail mRNA were lower in primary NPC tissues than in metastatic NPC tissues in lymph nodes (Fig. 1a). Stably overexpressing Snail in S26 and 6-10B lines reduced the levels of TEL2 mRNA and protein, with E-cadherin serving as positive control (Fig. 1b–d). In contrast, knockdown of

Snail increased TEL2 expression in S18 and 5-8F lines (Fig. 1e, f).

Snail binds directly to the TEL2 promoter

In our efforts to investigate how Snail suppresses TEL2 expression in NPC, we analyzed the TEL2 promoter and identified four Snail binding motifs or E-box motifs. We generated several forms of the promoter and tested them in a luciferase reporter assay in order to identify which E-box motifs participate in Snail-mediated suppression of TEL2 (Fig. 2a). Mutation of E3 abolished the suppression of Snail-mediated (Fig. 2b, c). In the ChIP assay, Snail co-precipitated with E3, and this binding was greater in the cell lines S18, 5-8F and HK1 than in cell lines S26 and 6-10B (Fig. 2d, e). Snail did not bind to E1, E2 or E4 in S18 cells (Additional file 1: Figure S1). Throughout these experiments, Snail can bind the promoter of E-cadherin (Fig. 2f). Snail did not bind the promoter of the GAPDH gene (Fig. 2g).

Snail is involved in hypoxia-induced TEL2 down-regulation

We found that hypoxia increased migration and invasion of NPC cells in the transwell assay (Fig. 3a, b). As expected, 24-h hypoxia up-regulated Snail and down-regulated TEL2 at the mRNA and protein levels in S26 cells (Fig. 3c, d). This hypoxia-induced TEL2 down-regulation was attenuated by Snail knock-down (Fig. 3e, f).

A Snail/TEL2/SERPINE1 axis functions

To further determine the relationship among Snail, TEL2 and SERPINE1, we fused Snail and TEL2 using a T2A linker, commonly used for fusing multiple coding sequences [19] (Fig. 4a). The resulting fusion protein Snail-T2A-TEL2 (Sn/TE) was cleaved as expected into Snail and TEL2 in stably transfected 6-10B cells (Fig. 4b). SERPINE1 was dramatically overexpressed at the mRNA and protein levels in 6-10B cells stably expressing Snail, but not in cells expressing Sn/TE (Fig. 4c). Co-expression of the two proteins at the Sn/TE rescued the ability of TEL2 to down-regulate SERPINE1. The specificity of these results was confirmed with E-cadherin as negative control: 6-10B cells stably expressing either Snail or Sn/TE showed similar down-regulation of E-cadherin (Fig. 4d). Consistent with these results, we observed a negative correlation between Snail and TEL2 in NPC cells and tissues (Fig. 4e), and a positive correlation between Snail and SERPINE1 in NPC tissues (Fig. 4f).

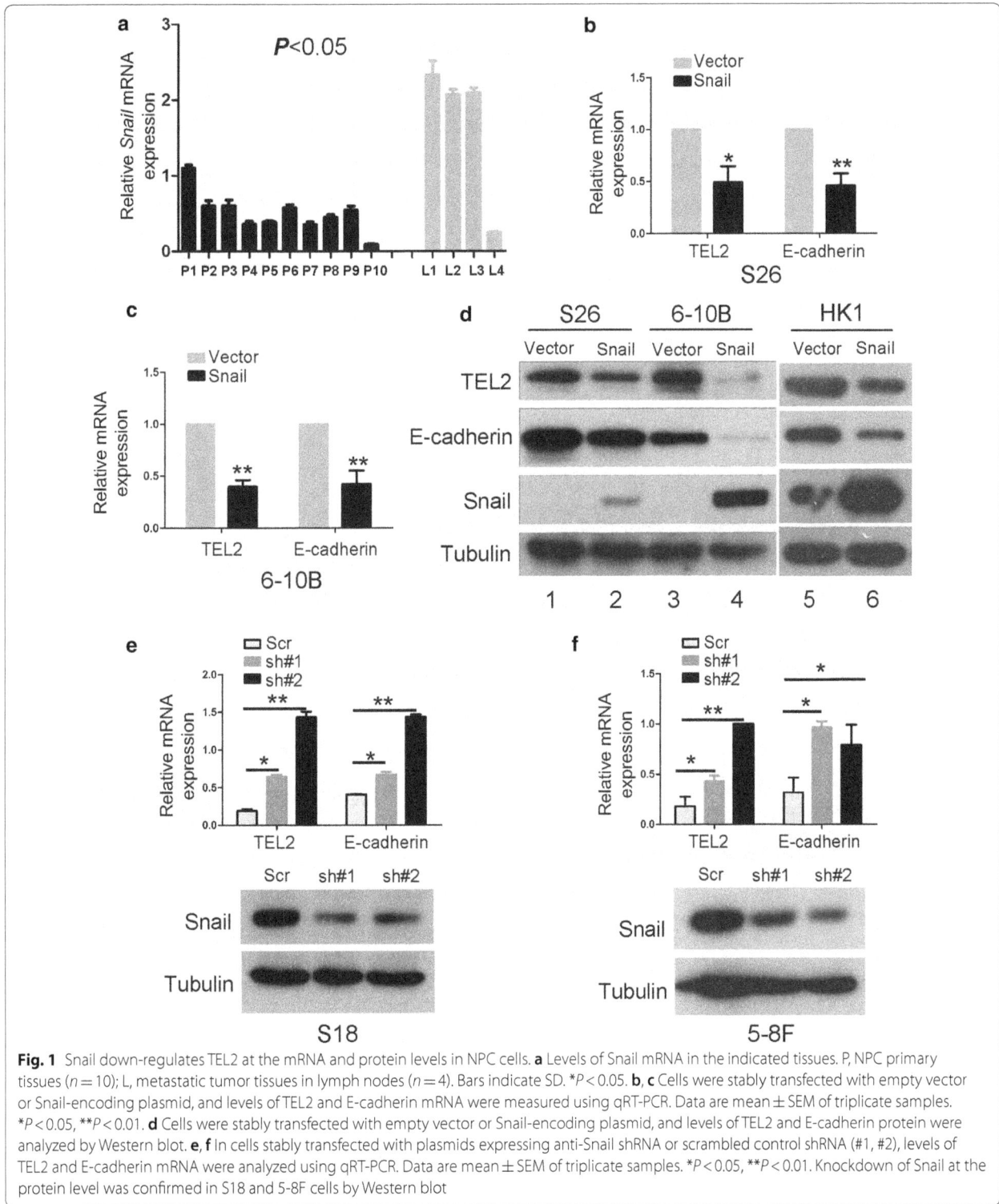

Fig. 1 Snail down-regulates TEL2 at the mRNA and protein levels in NPC cells. **a** Levels of Snail mRNA in the indicated tissues. P, NPC primary tissues ($n = 10$); L, metastatic tumor tissues in lymph nodes ($n = 4$). Bars indicate SD. $*P < 0.05$. **b, c** Cells were stably transfected with empty vector or Snail-encoding plasmid, and levels of TEL2 and E-cadherin mRNA were measured using qRT-PCR. Data are mean ± SEM of triplicate samples. $*P < 0.05$, $**P < 0.01$. **d** Cells were stably transfected with empty vector or Snail-encoding plasmid, and levels of TEL2 and E-cadherin protein were analyzed by Western blot. **e, f** In cells stably transfected with plasmids expressing anti-Snail shRNA or scrambled control shRNA (#1, #2), levels of TEL2 and E-cadherin mRNA were analyzed using qRT-PCR. Data are mean ± SEM of triplicate samples. $*P < 0.05$, $**P < 0.01$. Knockdown of Snail at the protein level was confirmed in S18 and 5-8F cells by Western blot

Snail promotes NPC cell migration and invasion by down-regulating TEL2

Ectopic expression of Snail increased the migratory and invasive abilities of NPC cells (Additional file 1: Figure S2). These effects were significantly reduced when TEL2 was overexpressed (Fig. 5a–d). Co-transfecting Snail-deficient cells with siRNA targeting TEL2 and shRNA targeting Snail partly rescued Snail-mediated cell

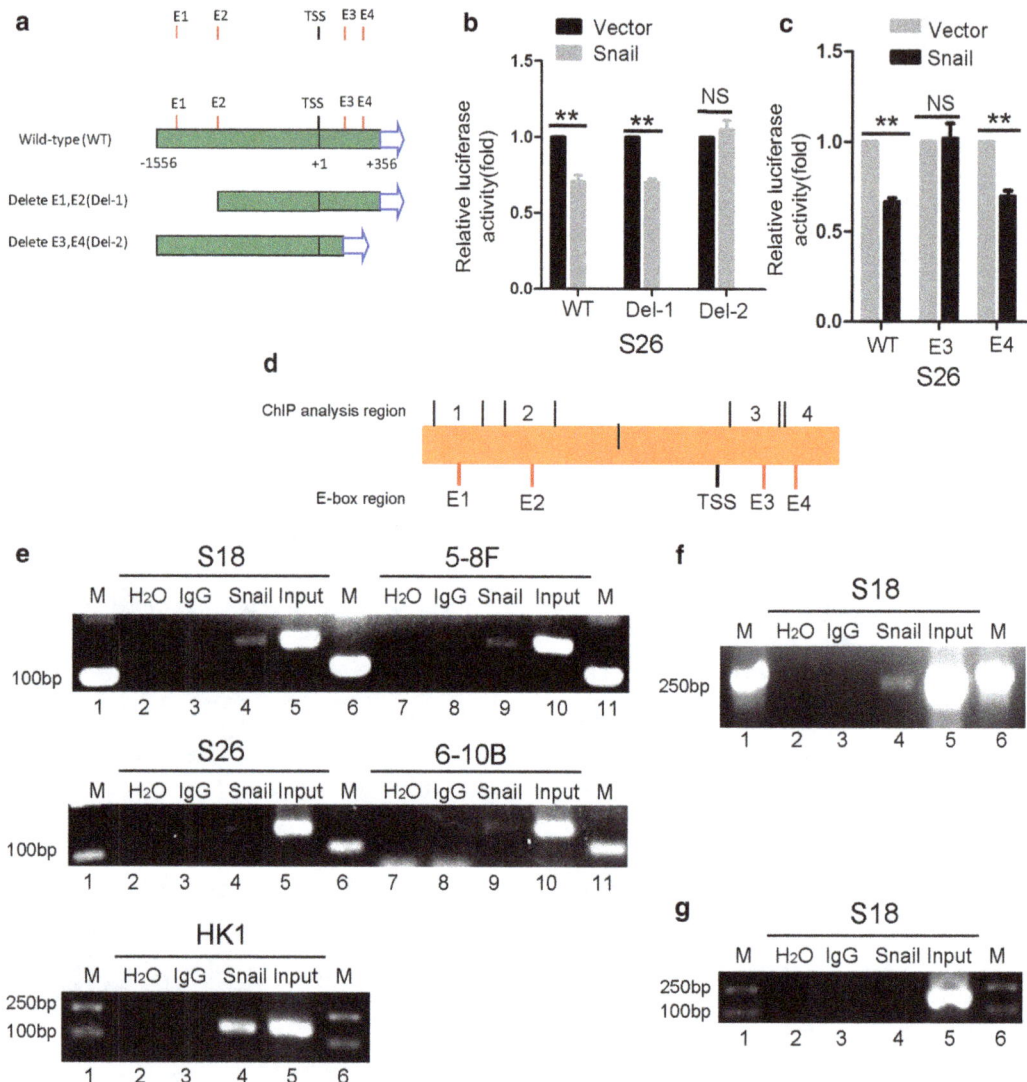

Fig. 2 Snail binds directly to the TEL2 promoter in NPC cells. **a** Schematic illustration of the wild-type TEL2 promoter and its mutants in luciferase reporter assays. **b, c** S26 cells stably transfected with empty vector or Snail-encoding plasmid were transfected with a luciferase reporter plasmid in which luciferase expression was driven by the wild-type or mutant TEL2 promoter. Luciferase activity was measured as described in Methods. Data are mean ± SEM of triplicate samples. *$P < 0.05$, **$P < 0.01$. **d** Schematic illustration of the location of primers for ChIP analysis. **e–g** Cells were analyzed in ChIP assays using anti-Snail antibody as described in "Methods"

invasiveness (Fig. 5e, f). TEL2 overexpression attenuated hypoxia-induced migration and invasion (Fig. 5g, h).

Snail promotes NPC metastasis by down-regulating TEL2

TEL2 overexpression was associated with significantly more metastatic pulmonary nodules, while Snail overexpression was associated with significantly fewer nodules (Fig. 6a–c). The mean number of metastatic nodules was higher in 6-10B cells stably expressing Snail than in cells stably expressing Sn/TE (Fig. 6a–c).

Discussion

The current study showed, for the first time, that TEL2 is a target of Snail in NPC. Snail is a key transcription factor that regulates cancer metastasis mainly by down-regulating E-cadherin, a key player during EMT and the reverse transition of mesenchymal-to-epithelial transition (MET). Our finding that TEL2 is a downstream target of Snail may explain why Snail overexpression up-regulates SERPINE1, as previously reported [20, 21]. Snail down-regulates TEL2, which in turn down-regulates SERPINE1. Results from the current study

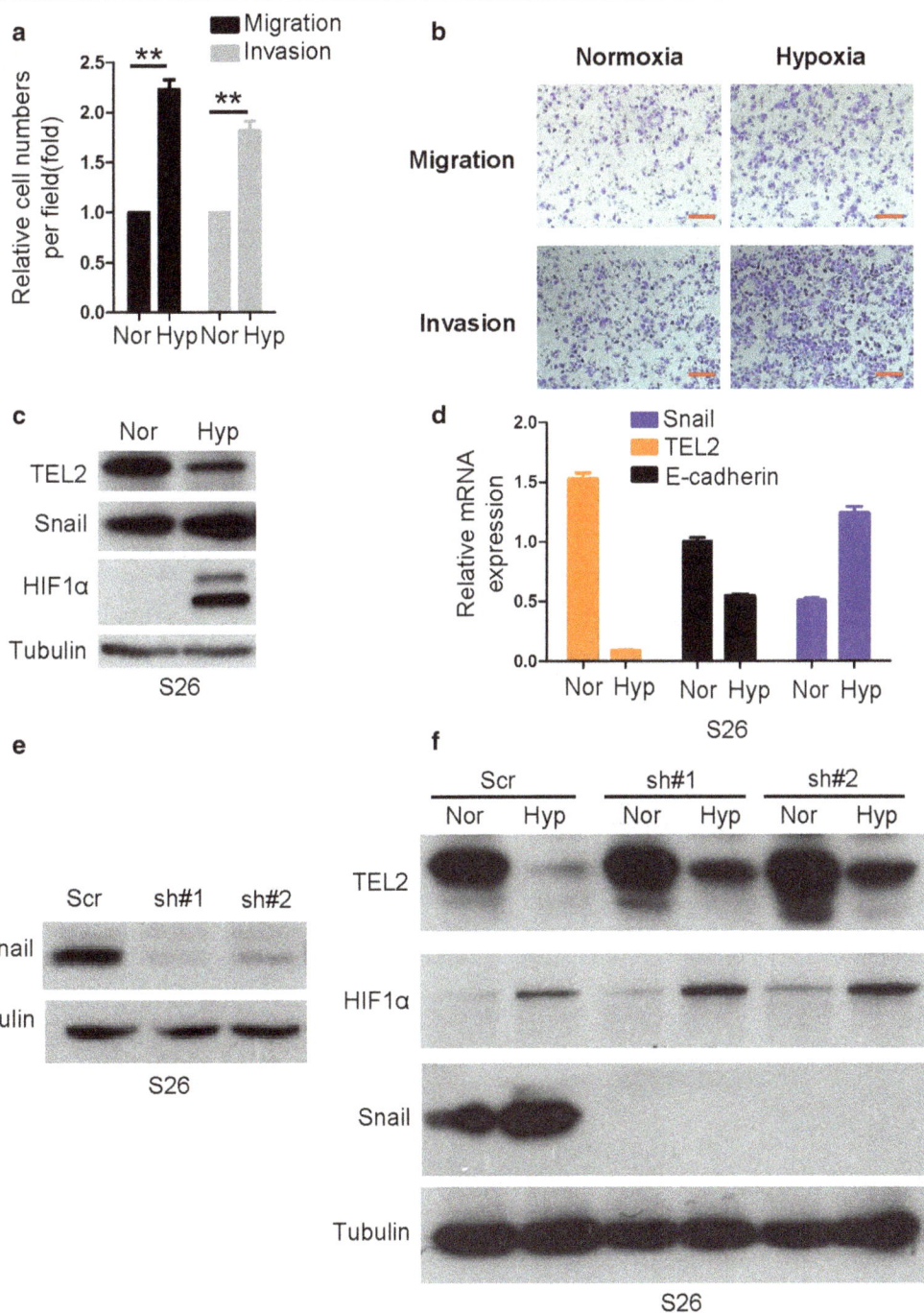

Fig. 3 Snail is involved in hypoxia-induced TEL2 down-regulation in NPC. **a** Migration and invasion activity was measured after 24 h in transwell assays under normoxia (Nor, 21% O_2) or hypoxia (Hyp, 1% O_2). Data are mean ± SEM. The number of cells passing through the membrane in each transwell was analyzed in triplicate and repeated three times with similar results. **P < 0.01. **b** Representative image of the assay in **a**. Red scale bar, 100 μm. **c** Levels of Snail, HIF1α and TEL2 proteins were analyzed by Western blot in S26 cells exposed for 24 h to normoxia (21% O_2) or hypoxia (1% O_2). **d** Levels of Snail, E-cadherin and TEL2 mRNA were measured by qRT-PCR in S26 cells treated as in (**c**). **e** Level of Snail protein in S26 cells was analyzed by Western blot after Snail knockdown. Tubulin was used as a loading control. **f** Levels of TEL2 and HIF1α proteins were measured in the indicated cells after treatment as in **c**. Tubulin was used as a loading control

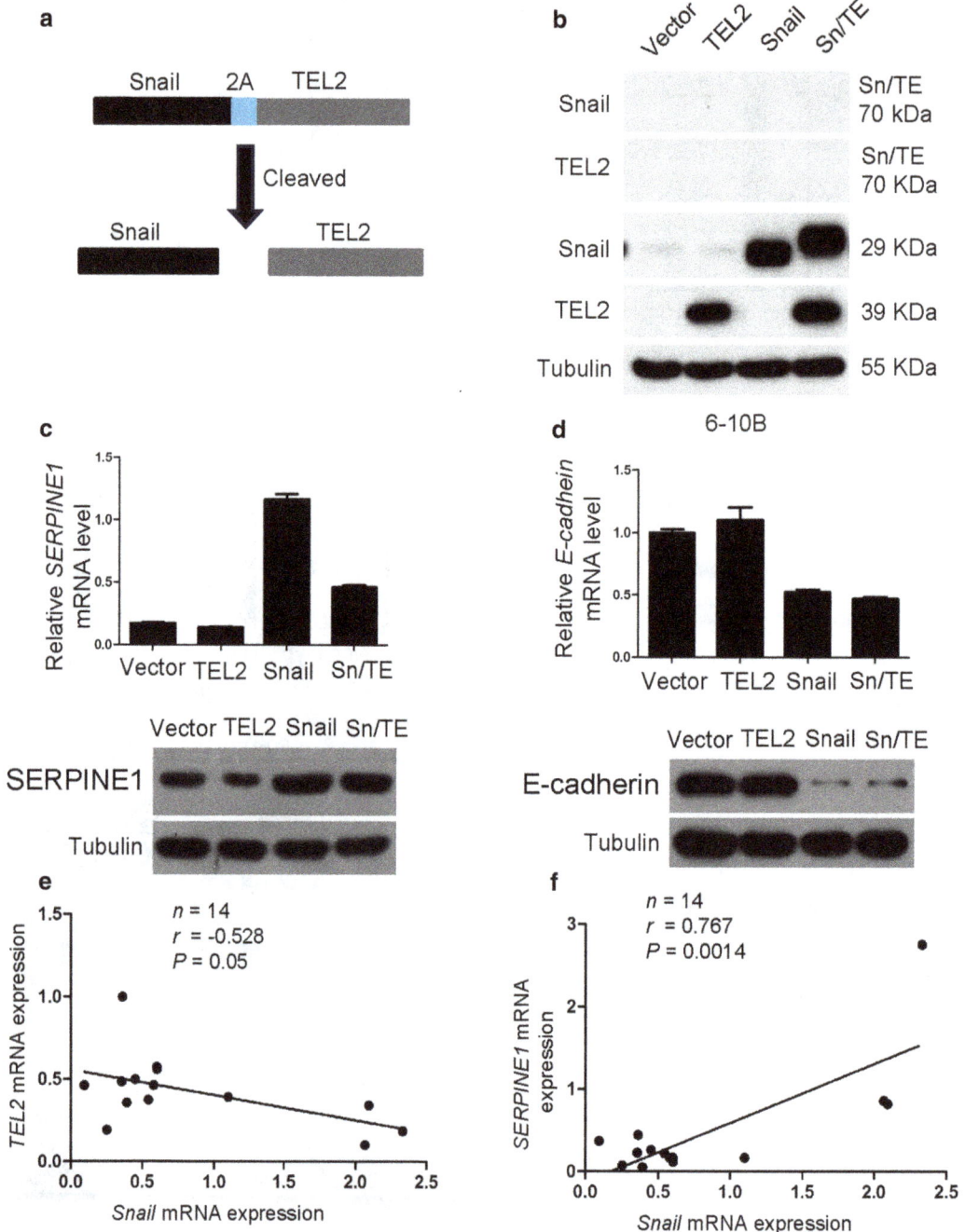

Fig. 4 The Snail/TEL2/SERPINE1 axis functions in NPC cells. **a** Schematic illustration for generating a fusion protein of Snail and TEL2 via a T2A linker. **b** Levels of Snail, TEL2 and Snail-TEL2 proteins were determined by Western blot in the indicated cells. Tubulin was used as a loading control. **c** Levels of SERPINE1 mRNA were measured by qRT-PCR and levels of SERPINE1 protein by Western blot. GAPDH served as a control. Data are mean ± SEM of triplicate samples. *$P < 0.05$, **$P < 0.01$, ***$P < 0.001$. **d** Levels of E-cadherin mRNA were measured by qRT-PCR and levels of E-cadherin protein by Western blot. GAPDH served as a control. Data are mean ± SEM of triplicate samples. *$P < 0.05$, **$P < 0.01$, ***$P < 0.001$. **e** In NPC tissues, a significant negative correlation was observed between Snail and TEL2 expression. **f** In NPS tissues, a significant positive correlation was observed between Snail and SERPINE1 expression

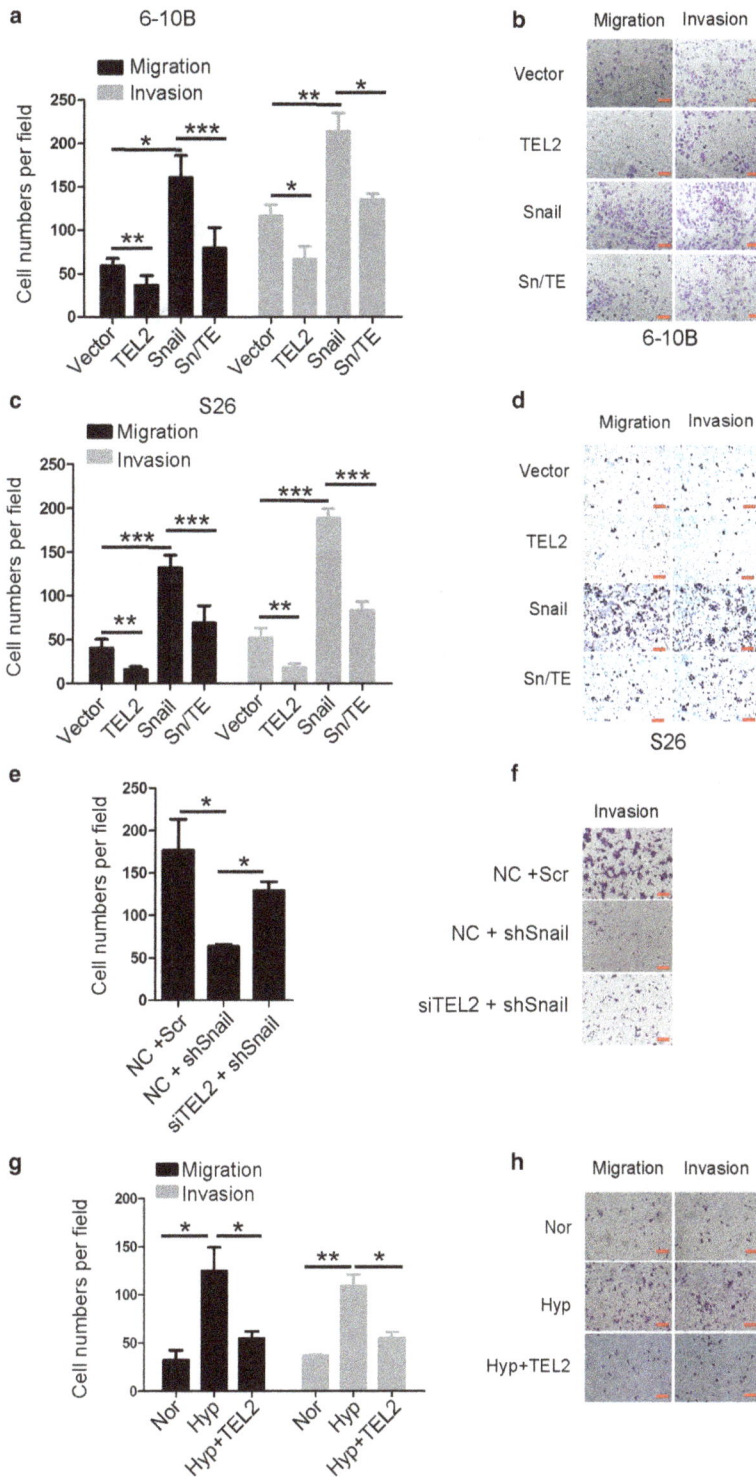

Fig. 5 Snail promotes NPC cell migration and invasion mostly by down-regulating TEL2. **a–f** Migration and invasion activity of indicated cells were measured at 24 h in transwell assays. The number of cells passing through the membrane in each well was analyzed in triplicate and repeated three times with similar results. Data are mean ± SEM. *$P < 0.05$, **$P < 0.01$, ***$P < 0.001$. **b, d, f** Representative images of transwell assays. Red scale bar, 100 μm. **e, f** The migration and invasion abilities of S26 cells with NC+scr, NC+shSnail or siTEL2+shSnail. The number of cells passing through the membrane in each well was analyzed in triplicate and repeated three times with similar results. Data are mean ± SEM. *$P < 0.05$, ** $P < 0.01$. **f** Representative image of the transwell assays described in **e**. Red scale bar, 100 μm. **g, h** TEL2 overexpression attenuated hypoxia-induced migration and invasion in S26 cells. **h** Representative image of the transwell assays described in **g**. Red scale bar, 100 μm

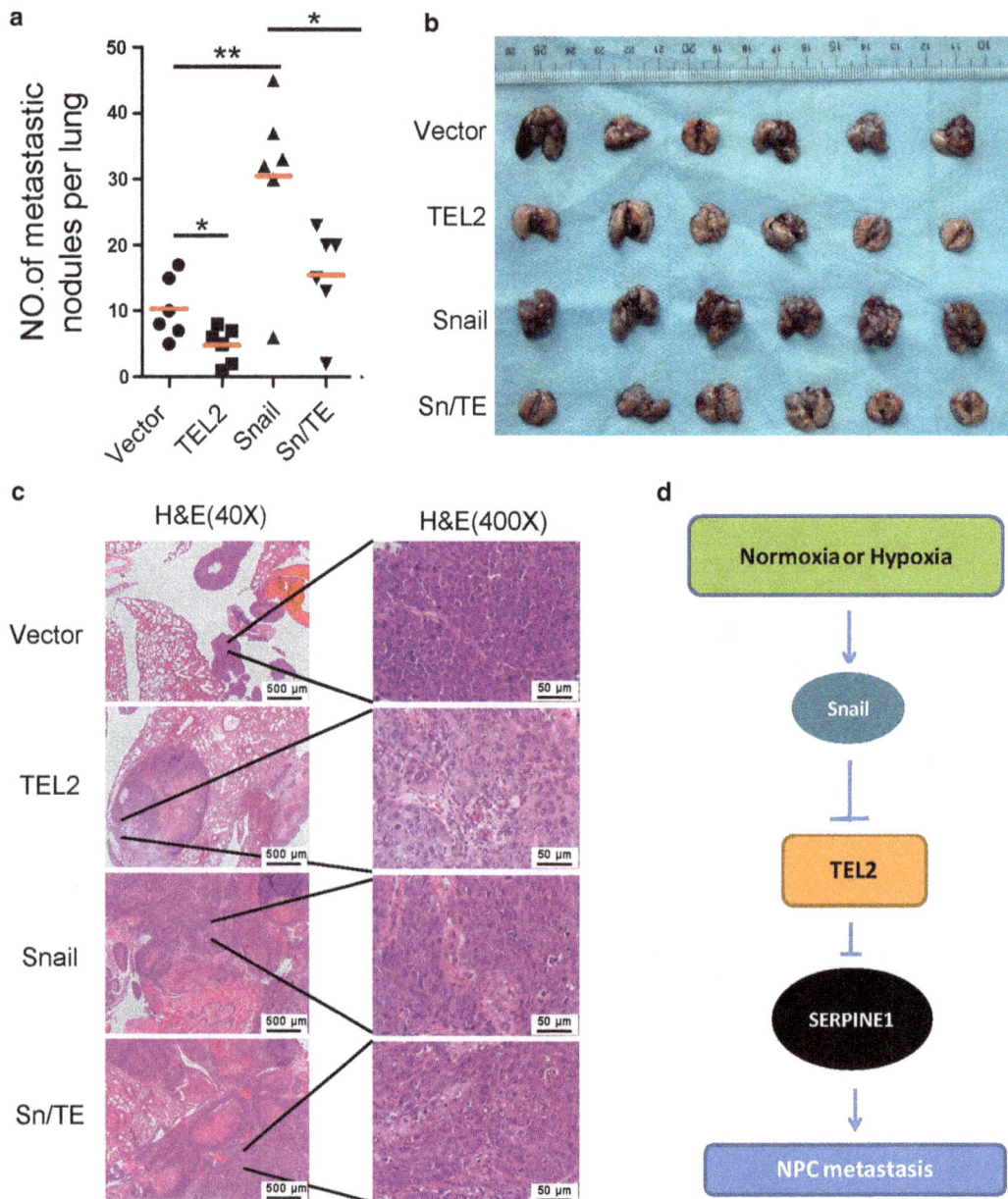

Fig. 6 Snail promotes NPC metastasis to lung mostly by down-regulating TEL2 in a nude mouse model. a–c Stably transfected cells were injected into the lateral tail vein of nude mice. a Quantitation of the number of metastases. Data are mean ± SEM ($n = 6$ per group). b Macroscopic appearance of metastatic lung tumors. c Tumor cross sections with hemotoxylin-eosin staining. Scale bars in (c): 500 μm (left), 50 μm (right). d Proposed model for the regulation and function of TEL2 in NPC metastasis. Snail down-regulates TEL2 during exposure to normoxia or hypoxia, up-regulating SERPINE1, which promotes NPC metastasis

suggest that the Snail/TEL2/SERPINE1 axis plays a key role in NPC metastasis.

Hypoxia is present in most NPC tumors, and could promote cancer metastasis [22, 23]. Consistent with a previous study reporting Snail induction by hypoxia [23], we showed increased Snail expression and decreased expression of TEL2 and E-cadherin upon hypoxia in cultured NPC cells. We speculate that the same processes occur in NPC tumors and mediate the ability of hypoxia to promote NPC metastasis.

Conclusions

Snail down-regulates TEL2 in NPC cells and tissues under both normoxic and hypoxic conditions, ultimately leading to up-regulation of SERPINE1, which promotes metastasis (Fig. 6d). This novel pathway may be valuable for designing new treatments for patients with NPC metastasis.

Authors' contributions

Conception and design: YS and TK. Development of methodology: YS and CC. Data acquisition: YS and CC. Data analysis and interpretation: YS and CC. Drafting and revision of the manuscript: YS and TK. Study supervision: TK. All authors read and approved the final manuscript.

Author details

[1] State Key Laboratory of Oncology in South China, Collaborative Innovation Center for Cancer Medicine, Sun Yat-sen University Cancer Center, No. 651 Dongfeng East Road, Guangzhou 510060, People's Republic of China.
[2] Department of Center Laboratory, The Eighth Affiliated Hospital of Sun Yat-Sen University, No. 3025 Shennan Middle Road, Shenzhen 518033, People's Republic of China. [3] Jiangxi Key Laboratory of Cancer Metastasis and Precision Treatment, The Third Affiliated Hospital of Nanchang University, No.128 Xianshan North Road, Nanchang 330008, People's Republic of China.

Acknowledgements

Not applicable.

Competing interests

The authors declare that they have no competing interests.

Funding

This work was supported by grants to YS from the National Science Foundation of China (81660449), the Jiangxi Provincial Natural Science Foundation of China (20161ACB21001, 20171BCD40026), and the Jiangxi Provincial Health and Family Planning Commission Foundation (20164005, 2015A077); as well as by a grant to TK from the Science and Technology Program of Guangzhou, China (201508020102).

References

1. Bei JX, Li Y, Jia WH, et al. A genome-wide association study of nasopharyngeal carcinoma identifies three new susceptibility loci. Nat Genet. 2010;42(7):599–603.
2. Sang Y, Chen MY, Luo D, et al. Tel2 suppresses metastasis by down-regulating serpine1 in nasopharyngeal carcinoma. Oncotarget. 2015;6(30):29240–53.
3. Sang Y, Wang L, Tang JJ, et al. Oncogenic roles of carbonic anhydrase ix in human nasopharyngeal carcinoma. Int J Clin Exp Pathol. 2014;7(6):2942–9.
4. Wang L, Sang Y, Tang J, et al. Down-regulation of prostate stem cell antigen (psca) by slug promotes metastasis in nasopharyngeal carcinoma. J Pathol. 2015;237(4):411–22.
5. Wei KR, Zheng RS, Zhang SW, et al. Nasopharyngeal carcinoma incidence and mortality in china, 2013. Chin J Cancer. 2017;36(1):90.
6. Sun X, Su S, Chen C, et al. Long-term outcomes of intensity-modulated radiotherapy for 868 patients with nasopharyngeal carcinoma: an analysis of survival and treatment toxicities. Radiother Oncol. 2014;110(3):398–403.
7. Tang XR, Li YQ, Liang SB, et al. Development and validation of a gene expression-based signature to predict distant metastasis in locoregionally advanced nasopharyngeal carcinoma: a retrospective, multicentre, cohort study. Lancet Oncol. 2018;19(3):382–93.
8. Jia WH, Huang QH, Liao J, et al. Trends in incidence and mortality of nasopharyngeal carcinoma over a 20–25 year period (1978/1983–2002) in Sihui and Cangwu counties in southern china. BMC Cancer. 2006;6:178.
9. Colaco RJ, Betts G, Donne A, et al. Nasopharyngeal carcinoma: a retrospective review of demographics, treatment and patient outcome in a single centre. Clin Oncol. 2013;25(3):171–7.
10. Wang MH, Sun R, Zhou XM, et al. Epithelial cell adhesion molecule overexpression regulates epithelial-mesenchymal transition, stemness and metastasis of nasopharyngeal carcinoma cells via the PTEN/AKT/mTOR pathway. Cell Death Dis. 2018;9(1):2.
11. Carella C, Potter M, Bonten J, et al. The ets factor tel2 is a hematopoietic oncoprotein. Blood. 2006;107(3):1124–32.
12. Gu X, Shin BH, Akbarali Y, et al. Tel-2 is a novel transcriptional repressor related to the ets factor tel/etv-6. J Biol Chem. 2001;276(12):9421–36.
13. Jagle S, Busch H, Freihen V, et al. Snail1-mediated downregulation of FOXA proteins facilitates the inactivation of transcriptional enhancer elements at key epithelial genes in colorectal cancer cells. PLoS Genet. 2017;13(11):e1007109.
14. Kuo TC, Chen CK, Hua KT, et al. Glutaminase 2 stabilizes dicer to repress snail and metastasis in hepatocellular carcinoma cells. Cancer Lett. 2016;383(2):282–94.
15. Qin Y, Zhao D, Zhou HG, et al. Apigenin inhibits nf-kappab and snail signaling, emt and metastasis in human hepatocellular carcinoma. Oncotarget. 2016;7(27):41421–31.
16. Zhang Y, Zhang X, Ye M, et al. Fbw7 loss promotes epithelial-to-mesenchymal transition in non-small cell lung cancer through the stabilization of snail protein. Cancer Lett. 2018;419:75–83.
17. Lv XB, Liu L, Cheng C, et al. Sun2 exerts tumor suppressor functions by suppressing the warburg effect in lung cancer. Sci Rep. 2015;5:17940.
18. Yin Y, Zhong J, Li SW, et al. Trim11, a direct target of mir-24-3p, promotes cell proliferation and inhibits apoptosis in colon cancer. Oncotarget. 2016;7(52):86755–65.
19. Shalem O, Sanjana NE, Hartenian E, et al. Genome-scale crispr-cas9 knockout screening in human cells. Science. 2014;343(6166):84–7.
20. Moreno-Bueno G, Cubillo E, Sarrio D, et al. Genetic profiling of epithelial cells expressing e-cadherin repressors reveals a distinct role for snail, slug, and e47 factors in epithelial-mesenchymal transition. Cancer Res. 2006;66(19):9543–56.
21. Fabre-Guillevin E, Malo M, Cartier-Michaud A, et al. Pai-1 and functional blockade of snai1 in breast cancer cell migration. Breast cancer research (BCR). 2008;10(6):R100.
22. Hong B, Lui VW, Hashiguchi M, et al. Targeting tumor hypoxia in nasopharyngeal carcinoma. Head Neck. 2013;35(1):133–45.
23. Lu X, Kang Y. Hypoxia and hypoxia-inducible factors: master regulators of metastasis. Clin Cancer Res. 2010;16(24):5928–35.

8

Overexpression of amplified in breast cancer 1 (*AIB1*) gene promotes lung adenocarcinoma aggressiveness in vitro and in vivo by upregulating C-X-C motif chemokine receptor 4

Liru He[1,2†], Haixia Deng[1†], Shiliang Liu[1,2], Jiewei Chen[1], Binkui Li[1], Chenyuan Wang[1], Xin Wang[1,3], Yiguo Jiang[4], Ningfang Ma[5], Mengzhong Liu[1,2*] and Dan Xie[1*]

Abstract

Background: We previously found that overexpression of the gene known as amplified in breast cancer 1 (*AIB1*) was associated with lymph node metastasis and poor prognosis in patients with lung adenocarcinoma. However, the role of AIB1 in that malignancy remains unknown. The present study aimed to investigate the function of AIB1 in the process of lung adenocarcinoma cell metastasis.

Methods: A series of in vivo and in vitro assays were performed to elucidate the function of AIB1, while real-time PCR and Western blotting were utilized to identify the potential downstream targets of AIB1 in the process of lung adenocarcinoma metastasis. Rescue experiments and in vitro assays were performed to investigate whether the invasiveness of AIB1-induced lung adenocarcinoma was mediated by C-X-C motif chemokine receptor 4 (CXCR4).

Results: The ectopic overexpression of AIB1 in lung adenocarcinoma cells substantially enhanced cell migration and invasive abilities in vitro and tumor metastasis in vivo, whereas the depletion of AIB1 expression substantially inhibited lung adenocarcinoma cell migration and invasion. CXCR4 was identified as a potential downstream target of AIB1 in lung adenocarcinoma. The knockdown of AIB1 greatly reduced CXCR4 gene expression at both the transcription and protein levels, whereas the knockdown of CXCR4 in cells with AIB1 ectopic overexpression diminished AIB1-induced migration and invasion in vitro and tumor metastasis in vivo. Furthermore, we found a significant positive association between the expression of AIB1 and CXCR4 in lung adenocarcinoma patients (183 cases), and the co-overexpression of AIB1 and CXCR4 predicted the poorest prognosis.

Conclusions: These findings suggest that AIB1 promotes the aggressiveness of lung adenocarcinoma in vitro and in vivo by upregulating CXCR4 and that it might be usable as a novel prognostic marker and/or therapeutic target for this disease.

Keywords: Lung adenocarcinoma, Amplified in breast cancer 1, C-X-C motif chemokine receptor 4, Metastasis, Prognosis

*Correspondence: liumzh@sysucc.org.cn; xiedan@sysucc.org.cn
†Liru He and Haixia Deng contributed equally to this work
[1] The State Key Laboratory of Oncology in South China, Collaborative Innovation Center for Cancer Medicine, Sun Yat-Sen University Cancer Center, No. 651, Dongfeng Road East, Guangzhou 510060, China
Full list of author information is available at the end of the article

Background

Lung cancer is responsible for the most cancer-related morbidity and mortality worldwide [1, 2], and lung adenocarcinoma is the major histologic subtype of lung cancer. Despite considerable therapeutic progress, the prognosis of patients with lung adenocarcinoma (LA) remains very poor [3], and metastasis is the main cause of cancer death [4]. It is known that the metastatic process of lung adenocarcinoma is due to multiple molecular abnormalities, such as the activation of numerous important oncogenes and/or inactivation of various tumor suppressor genes [5]. Therefore, a better understanding of the biological mechanisms underlying the metastasis of lung adenocarcinoma is crucial for the discovery of novel therapeutic targets and the consequent improvement of cancer treatment [6].

The amplified in breast cancer 1 (*AIB1*) gene was initially reported to be involved in a number of biological processes, including cell differentiation, proliferation, survival and migration in hormone-sensitive cancers [7, 8]. We recently reported that AIB1 was also overexpressed and closely correlated with advanced clinical stages and/or poor prognoses in a series of hormone-insensitive malignancies [9–14], including lung adenocarcinoma [13]. Our data suggest a potential selective advantage of AIB1 in promoting the lymph node metastasis of lung adenocarcinoma [13]. Very recently, Mo et al. [15] reported that AIB1 promotes colorectal cancer metastasis by enhancing Notch signaling. These data suggest that AIB1 may also be an important oncogene involved in tumor metastasis in hormone-insensitive cancers.

To date, only some signaling pathways, such as the matrix metalloproteinase (MMP) [16, 17], focal adhesion kinase (FAK) [18] and Notch signaling pathways [15], have been identified as molecular mechanisms by which AIB1 promotes cancer cell metastasis. C-X-C motif chemokine receptor 4 (CXCR4), which plays an important role in the cell proliferation and metastasis of lung adenocarcinoma, has also been demonstrated to be a transcriptional target of AIB1 involved in promoting cell proliferation in breast and bladder cancers [19, 20]. However, it is unknown whether CXCR4 is a functional downstream target in aggressive AIB1-mediated lung adenocarcinoma.

To elucidate the potential role of *AIB1* in the development of lung adenocarcinoma, we investigated the function and underlying molecular mechanisms by which *AIB1* mediates tumor cell metastasis in lung adenocarcinoma cell lines.

Methods
Patients and tissue specimens

Thirty pairs of lung adenocarcinoma and their adjacent normal tissue samples (10 localized, 10 regional and 10 metastatic cases) were obtained with informed consent under institutional review board-approved protocols between January 2012 and December 2012 from Sun Yat-sen University Cancer Center, Guangzhou, China. Tumors without regional lymph nodes or distant metastases, tumors with regional lymph node metastases but without distant metastases, and tumor with distant metastases were defined as localized, regional and metastatic cases, respectively. Paraffin-embedded pathological specimens from 183 lung adenocarcinoma patients treated between October 1994 and February 1998 were obtained from the archives of the Department of Pathology at the same institution. All the patients were treated with initial surgical resection with a curative or palliative intent. The cases were selected consecutively based on the availability of resection tissue and follow-up data. Tumor differentiation grades and pathological tumor-node-metastasis (TNM) status were assessed according to the criteria of the World Health Organization and the 8th edition of the TNM classification of the International Union Against Cancer (UICC, 2015). The medical ethics committee of the Cancer Center of Sun Yat-sen University approved this study.

Construction of tissue microarrays (TMAs)

TMAs were constructed according to the method described previously [21]. The tissues (183 lung adenocarcinomas and 30 normal lung tissues from the same patients) were sampled using a tissue arraying instrument (Beecher Instruments, Silver Spring, MD, USA).

Immunohistochemistry (IHC)

Endogenous peroxidase activity was blocked with 0.3% hydrogen peroxide for 15 min. Tissue slides were boiled in 10 mmol/L citrate buffer (pH 6.0) (Beyotime, Shanghai, China) in a pressure cooker for 10 min (AIB1) or microwave-treated for 10 min for antigen retrieval. The slides were incubated with anti-AIB1 [Clone 34, BD Transduction Laboratories, San Jose, CA, USA, diluted 1:50 in phosphate buffer saline (PBS)] and anti-CXCR4 (Clone 2074, Abcam, Cambridge, UK, diluted 1:1000 in PBS) overnight at 4 °C. Subsequently, the slides were sequentially incubated with biotinylated rabbit anti-mouse immunoglobulin (Dako, Carpinteria, CA, USA) at a concentration of 1:100 for 30 min at 37 °C and then reacted with a streptavidin-peroxidase (Dako) conjugate for 30 min at 37 °C and 3'-3' diaminobenzidine (Dako) as a chromogen substrate. The nucleus was counterstained using Meyer's hematoxylin (Sigma, St. Louis, MO, USA).

Since the positive nuclei staining of normal lung tissues ranged from 0% to 10% of the epithelium, normal expression and overexpression of AIB1 were identified when the nuclei of $\leq 10\%$ and $> 10\%$ of tumor cells were positively stained, respectively. To evaluate CXCR4 IHC staining, a previously validated semi-quantitative scoring criterion was used [22, 23]. A staining index (values 0–9) was calculated by multiplying a score reflecting the intensity of CXCR4-positive staining (negative $= 0$, weak $= 1$, moderate $= 2$, and strong $= 3$) and a score reflecting the proportion of immunopositive cells of interest ($< 10\% = 1$, 10% to 50% $= 2$, and $> 50\% = 3$).

Cell lines and culture conditions

Four lung adenocarcinoma cell lines (A549, H1975, H2073 and PC9) were cultured in RPMI1640 (Gibco, Grand Island, NY, USA) medium with 10% newborn calf serum. (Gibco, Grand Island, NY, USA) Another lung adenocarcinoma cell line, H1993, was maintained in Dulbecco's modified Eagle's medium supplemented with 10% fetal bovine serum (FBS) (Gibco). All 5 cell lines were obtained from the American Type Culture Collection (ATCC, Manassas, VA, USA).

Protein extraction and Western blotting

The protein was extracted from the lung adenocarcinoma cells using Radio-Immunoprecipitation Assay (RIPA) Lysis Buffer (Beyotime) at 4 °C. Protein concentrations were measured by the Bicinchoninic Acid Protein Assay (BioRad, Hercules, CA, USA). Equal amounts of whole-cell lysates were resolved by sodium dodecyl sulfate-polyacrylamide gel electrophoresis and transferred onto a polyvinylidene difluoride membrane (Millipore, Bedford, MA, USA) followed by incubation with primary mouse monoclonal antibodies against human AIB1 (1:1000 dilution), CXCR4 (1:500 dilution), tumor necrosis factor (ligand) superfamily member 10 (TNFSF10) (1:500 dilution), matrix metallopeptidase 11 (MMP11) (1:1000 dilution), matrix metallopeptidase 2 (MMP2) (1:500 dilution), and vascular endothelial growth factor A (VEGFA) (1:1000 dilution) (BD Transduction Laboratories) overnight at 4 °C. β-Actin was used as an internal control (1:1000 dilution, BD Transduction Laboratories). After washing, the polyvinylidene fluoride (PVDF) membranes were incubated with secondary antibody (goat anti-mouse, 1:10,000 dilution, Cell Signaling Technology, Danvers, MA, USA) for 2 hat room temperature. The immunoreactive proteins were detected with enhanced chemiluminescence detection reagents (Amersham Biosciences, Uppsala, Sweden) according to the manufacturer's instructions.

Knockdown of AIB1 and CXCR4 by lentiviral short hairpin RNA (shRNA)

We synthesized the sequences of AIB1 to construct lentiviral shRNA1 (5′-GGTCTTACCTGCAGTGGTGAA-3′) and shRNA2 (5′-AGACTCCTTAGGACC GCTT-3′), which have been previously found to efficiently knock down endogenous AIB1 expression in human cancer cells [14]. The shRNA sequence for CXCR4 is 5′-ACCGCG ATCAGTGTGAGTATATAAAGTTCTCTTATATAC TCACACTGATCGCTTTTTC-3′, which was also previously validated [24]. Virus packaging was performed by the transient transfection of 293FT cells with a transfer plasmid and three packaging plasmids: pMDLg/pRRE, pRSV-REV, and pCMV-VSVG, which were kindly provided by Professor Peng Xiang (Center for Stem Cell Biology and Tissue Engineering, Sun Yat-sen University). Seventy-two hours after transfection, the lentiviral particles were collected, filtered, and then concentrated. Subsequently, we infected the lung adenocarcinoma cell lines with the lentivirus in a 24-well plate. Four days after infection, the knockdown efficiency was examined by Western blotting.

Plasmid constructs and transfection

The construction of a plasmid expressing human AIB1 (pcDNA-AIB1) was conducted as described in our previous study [25]. In brief, full-length human AIB1 cDNA was amplified by PCR (primer: 5′-GTCATATGATGAGTG GATTAGGAGAAAAC -3′ (forward) and 5′- CGAGAT CTTCAGCAGTATTTCTGATCAGG-3′ (reverse), initial denaturation at 95 °C for 10 min and 35 cycles of 95 °C for 15 s, 55 °C for 30 s, and 72 °C for 5 min) and cloned into the NheI and EcoRI site pcDNA3.1 (+) expression vector (Invitrogen, Carlsbad, CA), then transfected into A549 cells using Lipofectamine 2000 (Invitrogen, Carlsbad, CA) according to the manufacturer's instructions. Cells transfected with empty vector were used as controls. Stable AIB1-expressing clones were selected by Geneticin (Rache Diagnostics, Indianapolis, IN) (500 μg/mL).

RNA interference (RNAi)

Short interfering RNAs (siRNAs) specifically directed against the CXCR4 gene (1: 5′-AUCACGUAAAGCUAGAAA -3′, 5′-GGGAUCAUUUCUAGCUUU-3′; 2: 5′-GCUGUU UAUGCAUAGAUA-3′, 5′-GAGAGAUUAUCUAUGCAU -3′) [26] and corresponding scrambled siRNAs (Ribo bio, Guangzhou, China) were transfected into A549 cells in six-well plates using Lipofectamine 2000 transfection reagent (Invitrogen) according to the manufacturer's instructions.

Migration and invasion assays

Cell migration was assessed by measuring the movement of cells into a scratch created by a 200 ml pipette tube.

(See figure on next page.)
Fig. 1 Amplified in breast cancer 1 (AIB1) expression in lung adenocarcinoma tissues. Immunohistochemical (IHC) staining of AIB1 in normal lung tissues (**a**) and the primary lesions of localized (n = 61, mean positive rate of AIB1 expression is 19.7%) (**b**), regional (n = 76, mean positive rate of AIB1 expression is 40.3%) (**c**), and metastatic (n = 30, mean positive rate of AIB1 expression is 70.5%) (**d**) lung adenocarcinoma tissues. **e** The box plots demonstrate the range of AIB1 expression within each group (non-tumor, localized tumor, regional tumor, and metastatic tumor). **f** Receiver operating characteristic (ROC) curve of AIB1 in lung adenocarcinomas with regional lymph node metastasis compared to non-regional metastatic lung adenocarcinomas. Blue line: ROC curve, green line: reference line. **g** ROC curve of AIB1 in metastatic lung adenocarcinomas compared to non-metastatic lung adenocarcinomas. Blue line: ROC curve, green line: reference line. **h** Overall survival curve according to AIB1 expression level for 167 lung adenocarcinoma patients

The degree of wound closure was observed after 24 h and photographed under a microscope. The fraction of cell coverage across the line was measured to determine the migration rate. Wound repair = [(Diameter of the wound before migration − Diameter of the wound after migration)/Diameter of the wound before migration] × 100%. Each independent experiment was repeated three times.

For invasion assays, cells (3×10^5) were added to a Matrigel invasion chamber (BD Biosciences, Becton Dickson Labware, Flanklin Lakes, New Jersey, USA) in the insert of a 24-well culture plate. Fetal bovine serum was added to the lower chamber as a chemoattractant. After 24 h, invasive cells located on the lower side of the chamber were fixed and stained with crystal violet, air dried, and photographed. The invasive cells were counted in five fields under an inverted microscope. Experiments were performed in triplicate with a minimum of 40 grids (400 magnification) per filter counted.

Real-time PCR

RNA was extracted from H1993 AIB1_shRNA2 and H1993_control_shRNA using Trizol (Invitrogen) and was cleaned using the RNeasy MinElute Cleanup Kit (Qiagen, Valencia, California, USA). The concentrations of the RNA samples were measured by NanoDrop 2000 (Thermo Fisher Scientific, Waltham Massachusetts, US). Subsequently, total RNA was reverse transcribed using Super- Script III reverse transcriptase (Invitrogen), and cDNA was amplified by PCR using 2×Super Array PCR Master Mix (SuperArray Bioscience, Frederick, Maryland, USA). Real-time PCR was then performed on each sample using the Human Tumor Metastasis RT2 Profiler-PCR array (SuperArray Bioscience) in an Opticon DNA Engine ABI PRISM7900 system (Applied Biosystems, Foster City, CA, USA), according to the manufacturer's instructions. Data were normalized to glyceraldehyde phosphate dehydrogenase (GAPDH) levels by the ΔΔCt method [27].

In vivo metastasis model

Animal experiments were carried out in accordance with the National Institutes of Health Guide for the Care and Use of Laboratory animals (NIH Publications No. 8023, revised 1978). Eight 4-week-old Balb/c nude mice, which were purchased from Shanghai Slac Laboratory Animal Co. Ltd. (Shanghai, China), were injected with A549-Vec, A549-AIB1, or A549-AIB1 + CXCR4 shRNA cells. Briefly, 2×10^5 cells (mixed with 100 µL PBS) were injected intravenously through the tail vein into each Balb/c nude mouse in a laminar flow cabinet. Six weeks after cell injection, the mice were killed by cervical dislocation. Their livers and lungs were harvested, fixed in 4% paraformaldehyde, and embedded in paraffin. Subsequently, serial 2-µm-thick sections of the whole lungs and livers were obtained and examined by hematoxylin and eosin (H&E) staining to identify the metastases. All the procedures were performed in accordance with the guidelines of the laboratory animal ethics committee of Sun Yat-sen University.

Statistical analysis

Statistical analysis was performed with SPSS software (SPSS Standard version 19.0, SPSS Inc. Chicago, IL). Receiver operating characteristic (ROC) curve analysis was applied to determine the cutoff scores of AIB1 expression for distinguishing localized, regional, and metastatic lung adenocarcinomas. The sensitivity, specificity, and areas under the ROC curves (AUC) were calculated. The association of AIB1 protein expression with clinicopathologic features and the correlations between molecular features were assessed by the Chi square test. Survival curves were assessed by the Kaplan–Meier method and compared by the log-rank test. Two-sided P values of less than 0.05 were considered to indicate statistical significance.

Results

IHC staining of AIB1 expression in the localized, regional, and metastatic stages of lung adenocarcinoma tissues

The mean positive rates of AIB1 expression in lung adenocarcinoma at the localized, regional, and metastatic stages of lung adenocarcinoma were about 20.0%, 40.0%, and 70.0% respectively, compared with 3.0% (range 0.0%–10.0%) for normal tissues ($P < 0.001$, Fig. 1a–e).

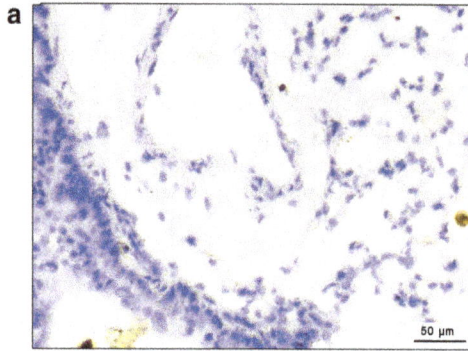
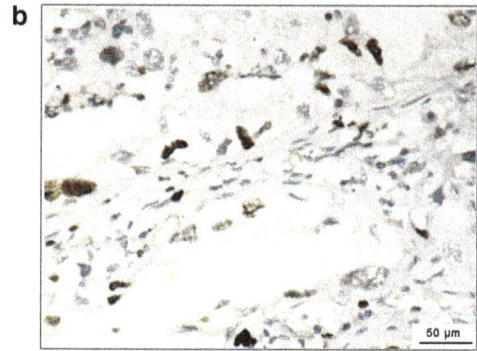
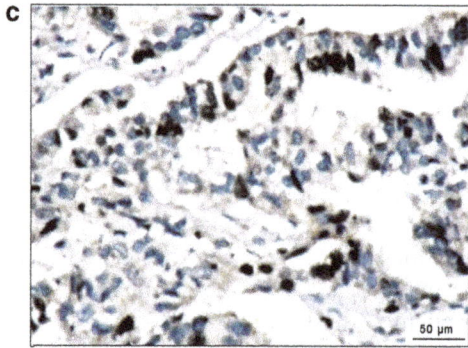
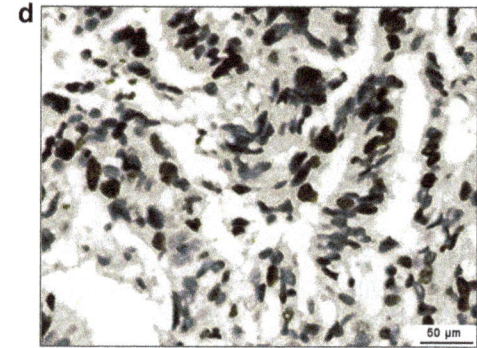
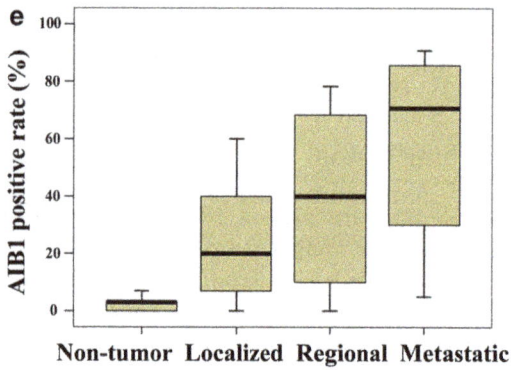
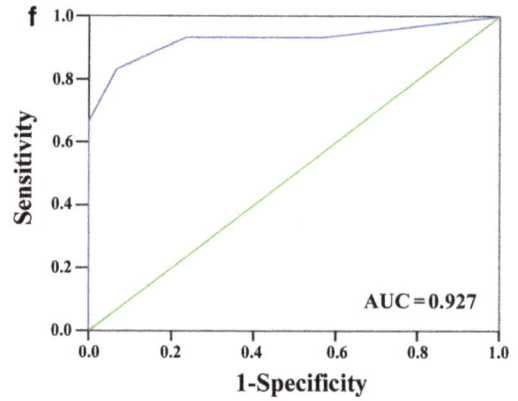
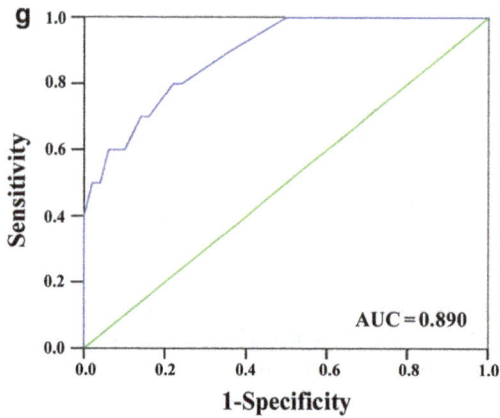
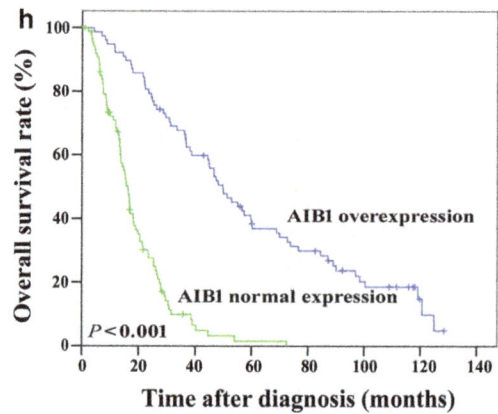

Table 1 Amplified in breast cancer 1 (AIB1) expression status and characteristics of the 167 lung adenocarcinoma patients

Characteristic	Total (cases)	AIB1 expression [cases (%)]		P
		Normal expression	Overexpression	
Age (years)				0.959
≤50[a]	81	38 (46.9)	43 (53.1)	
>50	86	40 (46.5)	46 (53.5)	
Gender				0.704
Male	118	54 (45.8)	64 (54.2)	
Female	49	24 (49.0)	25 (51.0)	
Tumor grade				0.110
G1	41	23 (56.1)	18 (43.9)	
G2	82	40 (48.8)	42 (51.2)	
G3	44	15 (34.1)	29 (65.9)	
T status				0.226
T1–2	88	45 (51.1)	43 (48.9)	
T3–4	79	33 (41.8)	46 (58.2)	
N status				0.015
N0	63	37 (58.7)	26 (41.3)	
N1–3	104	41 (39.4)	63 (60.6)	
M status				0.001
M0	137	72 (52.6)	65 (47.4)	
M1	30	6 (20.0)	24 (80.0)	
Stage				<0.001
I	32	24 (75.0)	8 (25.0)	
II	28	17 (60.7)	11 (39.3)	
III	77	31 (40.3)	46 (59.7)	
IV	30	6 (20.0)	24 (80.0)	

[a] Median age = 50 years old

The sensitivity, specificity, and area under the ROC curve (AUC) values of AIB1 expression levels for regional versus nonregional stages were 83.3%, 93.3%, and 0.927, respectively ($P < 0.001$, Fig. 1f), whereas the sensitivity, specificity, and AUC values of AIB1 expression levels for metastatic versus nonmetastatic stages were 80.0%, 78.0%, and 0.890, respectively ($P < 0.001$, Fig. 1g).

Association between the expression of AIB1 and lung adenocarcinoma patient clinicopathologic features and survival

We evaluated AIB1 expression in 167/183 (91.3%) of lung adenocarcinomas and 27/30 (90.0%) of normal lung tissues; lost samples, samples with too few tumor cells (<300 cells per case), and unrepresentative samples were not used in data compilation. Employing the previously described criterion (normal expression and overexpression of AIB1 were identified when at least 10% and more than 10%, respectively, of tumor cell nuclei were positively stained), overexpression of AIB1 was observed in 41.3%, 60.6%, 47.4%, and 80% of samples in the N0, N+, M0, and M1 stages of lung adenocarcinoma, respectively

(Table 1). Overexpression of AIB1 was correlated with an ascending clinical stage ($P < 0.001$, Table 1) and poor survival in lung adenocarcinoma patients ($P < 0.001$, Fig. 1h).

Silencing of AIB1 by RNA interference inhibits lung adenocarcinoma cell migration and invasion in vitro

Of the five lung adenocarcinoma cell lines analyzed, H1975, H1993, H2073, and PC9 cells showed relatively high levels of endogenous AIB1 protein expression, whereas A549 cells showed relatively low levels of AIB1 protein expression (Fig. 2a left).Two lung adenocarcinoma cell lines, H1975 and H1993, were then treated with two specific shRNAs against AIB1, and the shRNAs could efficiently knock down endogenous AIB1 in lung adenocarcinoma cells (Fig. 2a right). The knockdown of AIB1 caused an apparent suppression of cell migration in both H1975 and H1993 cell lines, as shown by using a wound-healing assay ($P < 0.01$, Fig. 2b). The ablation of endogenous AIB1 markedly reduced the invasive ability of both H1975 and H1993 cell lines in Matrigel invasion assays ($P < 0.05$, Fig. 2c).

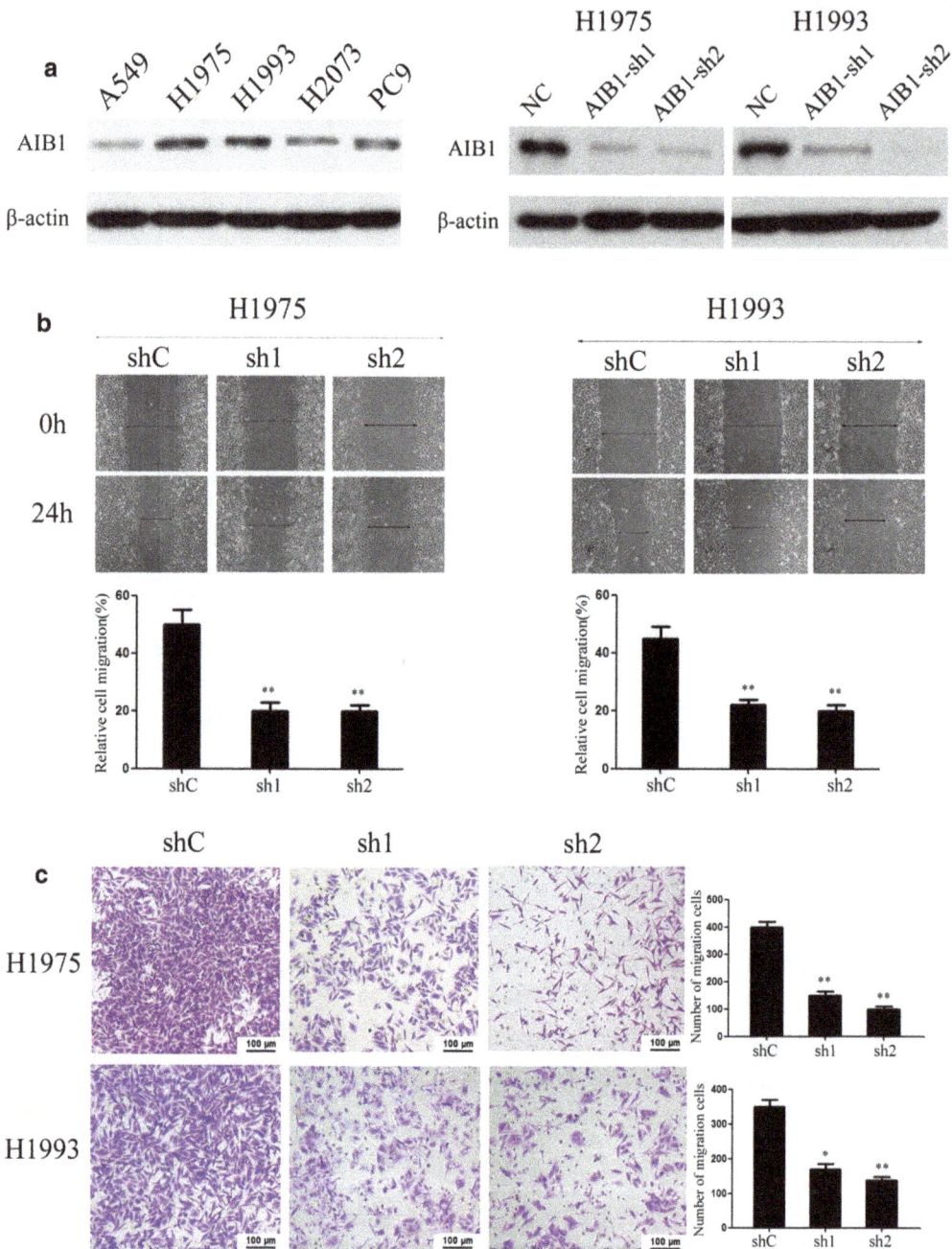

Fig. 2 Silencing of AIB1 by RNA interference inhibits lung adenocarcinoma cell migration and invasion in vitro. **a** Left: the levels of AIB1 expression in 5 lung adenocarcinoma cell lines by Western blotting analysis; right: Western blotting reveals that AIB1 was efficiently knocked down by the treatment with AIB1-shRNA1 and AIB1-shRNA2. **b** Wound-healing assays show that AIB1-silenced H1975 and H1993 cells had lower motility than control cells. **c** Cell invasion was evaluated using a Matrigel invasion chamber. Silencing of AIB1 decreased H1975 and H1993 cell invasive capacity. The numbers of invaded cells in the shAIB1 and control groups are shown in the right panel. Data are the mean ± standard error (SE) of three independent experiments; *P < 0.05, **P < 0.01 versus cells transfected with shC by Student's t test

Ectopic overexpression of AIB1 by plasmid transfection promotes lung adenocarcinoma cell migration and invasion in vitro

To determine whether the ectopic overexpression of AIB1 could enhance the migration and invasion capacity of lung adenocarcinoma cells, the A549-AIB1 cell line, which overexpressed AIB1, was constructed and used to perform wound-healing and invasion assays (Fig. 3a left) The wound-healing assay showed that the ectopic overexpression of AIB1 enhanced A549 cell migration at the

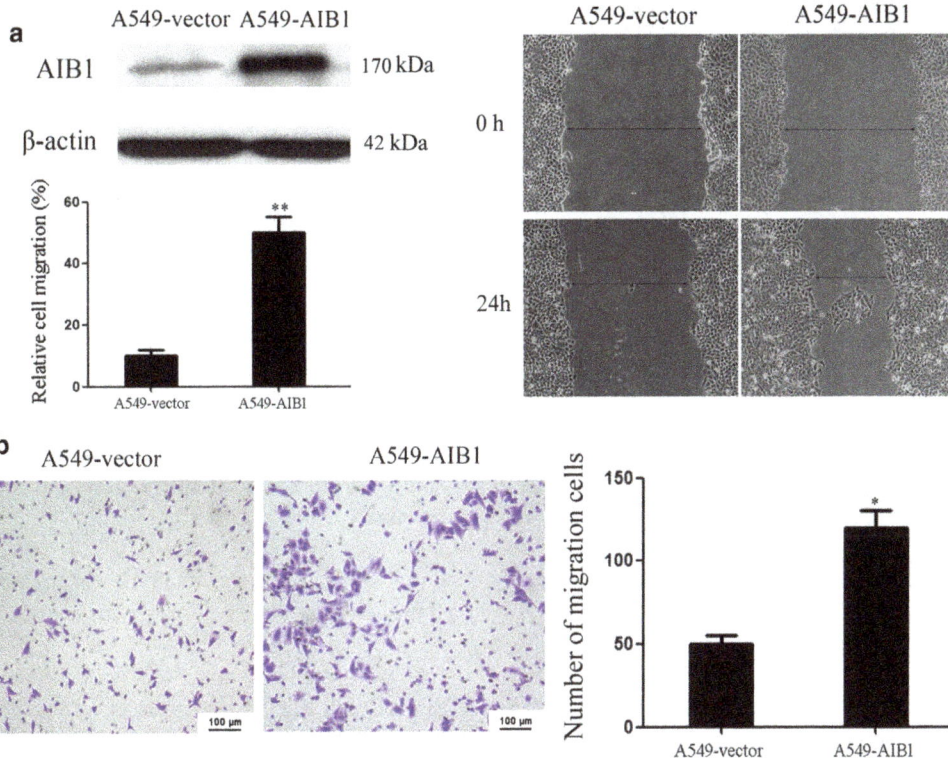

Fig. 3 Overexpression of AIB1 enhances lung adenocarcinoma A549 cell migration and invasion in vitro. **a** Left: Western blotting reveals that ectopic expression of AIB1 was substantially increased in A549-AIB1 cells compared with that in A549-vector cells (upper panel); right: representative results of wound-healing assays demonstrate that A549-AIB1 cells had higher motility than A549-vector cells. The numbers of migrating cells are shown in the left bottom panel. Data are the mean ± SE of three independent experiments; **$P < 0.001$ by Student's t test. **b** Ectopic overexpression of AIB1 enhanced A549 cell invasion in a Transwell assay. Data are the mean ± SE of three independent experiments; *$P < 0.05$ by Student's t test

Table 2 Differential expression of 5 metastasis-related genes in H1993-shAIB1 cells relative to expression in H1993-vector cells

Gene symbol	Gene name	Location	Fold change
CXCR4	Chemokine (C-X-C motif) receptor 4	2q21	− 22.49
TNFSF10	Tumor necrosis factor (ligand) superfamily, member 10	3q26	− 8.37
MMP11	Matrix metallopeptidase 11	22q11.23	− 4.63
MMP2	Matrix metallopeptidase 2	16q13-q21	− 4.31
VEGFA	Vascular endothelial growth factor A	6p12	− 3.85

edge of the exposed regions ($P < 0.01$, Fig. 3a right). The Matrigel invasion assay demonstrated that the invasive capacity of the A549-AIB1 cells was greater than that of the control A549-vector cells ($P < 0.05$, Fig. 3b).

AIB1 up-regulates CXCR4 expression in lung adenocarcinoma cells

To identify potential downstream targets regulated by AIB1 that were involved in lung adenocarcinoma cell invasion and/or metastasis, the mRNA expression profiles of shAIB1-transfected H1993 cells were compared with those of the control H1993 cells using a Human Tumor Metastasis RT2 Profiler TM PCR Array containing 84 cell metastasis-related genes. The results showed that a total of five downregulated genes (3.5-fold) were identified in shAIB1-transfected H1993 cells (Table 2, Additional file 1: Table S1). Subsequently, these five downstream targets (CXCR4, TNFSF10, MMP11, MMP2, and VEGFA) were selected and analyzed by Western blotting (Fig. 4a). Consistent with the mRNA

(See figure on next page.)
Fig. 4 The associations of AIB1 and C-X-C motif chemokine receptor 4 (CXCR4) expression in lung adenocarcinoma cells. **a** The five genes, CXCR4, tumor necrosis factor (ligand) superfamily member 10 (TNFSF10), matrix metallopeptidase 11 (MMP11), matrix metallopeptidase 2 (MMP2), and vascular endothelial growth factor A (VEGFA), showed more than a 3.5-fold mRNA differential expression in shAIB1-transfected H1993 cells compared with that in control H1993 cells, as shown by using a human tumor metastasis RT2 profiler PCR array. **b** Silencing of AIB1 by two shRNAs down-regulated CXCR4 expression in shAIB1 H1993 cells, as detected by Western blotting. **c** Upper left: treatment of 2 CXCR4-shRNAs in A549-AIB1 cells efficiently decreased the expression levels of CXCR4 as detected by Western blotting. Upper right and down: wound-healing assay showed that the enhanced migrative ability in A549-AIB1 cells was inhibited by silencing CXCR4. **d** Transwell assay demonstrated that the increased invasive capacity of A549-AIB1 cells was suppressed by CXCR4 silencing. Data are the mean ± SE of three independent experiments. **P < 0.01, *P < 0.05 versus cells transfected with A549-AIB1 by Student's t test. **e** Upper left: the level of CXCR4 decreased by silence of AIB1, and then increased after the treatment of CXCR4 as detected by Western blotting. Upper right and down: Wound-healing assay showed that the attenuated migrative ability in H1993-shAIB1 cells was enhanced by the overexpression of CXCR4. **f** Transwell assay demonstrated that the attenuated invasive capacity of H1993-shAIB1 cells was enhanced by the overexpression of CXCR4. Data are the mean ± SE of three independent experiments. **P < 0.01, *P < 0.05 versus cells transfected with AIB1-shNC by Student's t test

expression in the real-time PCR array, decreased protein expression of CXCR4 was shown by Western blotting in H1993 cells after AIB1 knockdown (Fig. 4b).

CXCR4 mediates the invasiveness of AIB1-induced lung adenocarcinoma

To determine whether CXCR4 is a functional downstream target involved in AIB1-induced lung adenocarcinoma cell aggressiveness, two RNAis were used to silence CXCR4 expression in AIB1-overexpressing A549 cells (Fig. 4c). We found that after the siCXCR4 treatment of A549-AIB1 cells, the AIB1-induced migration and invasive capacities of the A549 cells were dramatically inhibited ($P < 0.05$, Fig. 4c, d). In addition, we upregulated the expression of CXCR4 in H1993-shAIB1 cells and found that the attenuated migration and invasion cell abilities caused by AIB1 depletion were rescued by CXCR4 overexpression ($P < 0.05$, Fig. 4e, f).

Enforced expression of AIB1 enhances the metastasis potential of the lung adenocarcinoma cell line mediated by CXCR4 in vivo

To investigate whether AIB1 could affect the metastatic potential of lung adenocarcinoma cells in vivo and whether this effect could be mediated by CXCR4, we performed in vivo metastasis assays using a Balb/c nude mouse model. We did not detect any tumor nodules in the livers of all mice examined; however, metastatic tumor nodules were frequently found in the lungs of the mice (Fig. 5a). The expression levels of AIB1 and CXCR4, as detected by IHC, were simultaneously higher in the tumors of the A549-AIB1 group than in the tumors of the A549-vector group (Fig. 5b). The overexpression of AIB1 increased the number of lung metastases in mice injected with A549-AIB1 cells by approximately three-fold compared with the number in mice injected with A549 cells, whereas the depletion of CXCR4 dramatically decreased the number of AIB1-induced lung metastases ($P < 0.05$, Fig. 5b).

Expression of CXCR4 in lung adenocarcinoma tissues and its correlation with AIB1 expression and patient survival

The median staining index of CXCR4 in lung adenocarcinoma was 3; thus, the categories of high and low expression were defined as groups with a staining index above or below 3. In 156 of the 183 samples, AIB1 and CXCR4 IHC were detected successfully and simultaneously. The rate of high CXCR4 expression was significantly greater in carcinomas overexpressing AIB1 (58/83 cases, 69.9%) than in those cases with a normal expression of AIB1 (23/73 cases, 31.5%, $P < 0.001$, Table 3, Fig. 6a, b). Furthermore, high expression of CXCR4 was significantly associated with poorer survival in lung adenocarcinoma patients ($P < 0.001$, Fig. 6c). In addition, lung adenocarcinoma patients with high expression of both AIB1 and CXCR4 displayed the poorest survival, whereas patients with low expression of AIB1 and CXCR4 had the best survival ($P < 0.001$, Fig. 6d).

Discussion

In the present study, we report that the knockdown of AIB1 efficiently inhibits the migration and invasive abilities of lung adenocarcinoma in vitro, whereas the enforced overexpression of AIB1 substantially promotes lung adenocarcinoma migration and invasion in vitro and results in enhanced metastatic capacities in vivo. Importantly, we demonstrated that AIB1 enhances the migratory and metastasis abilities of lung adenocarcinoma cells by up-regulating the expression of chemokine receptor type 4 (CXCR4), an important downstream target. Furthermore, we showed that the simultaneous overexpression of AIB1 and CXCR4 predicts the poorest survival of LA patients.

Our previous study demonstrated the phenomenon of *AIB1* amplification in lung adenocarcinoma and showed that the overexpression of AIB1 was associated with pN status in M0 lung adenocarcinoma patients [13]. In the present study, we further found that the positive

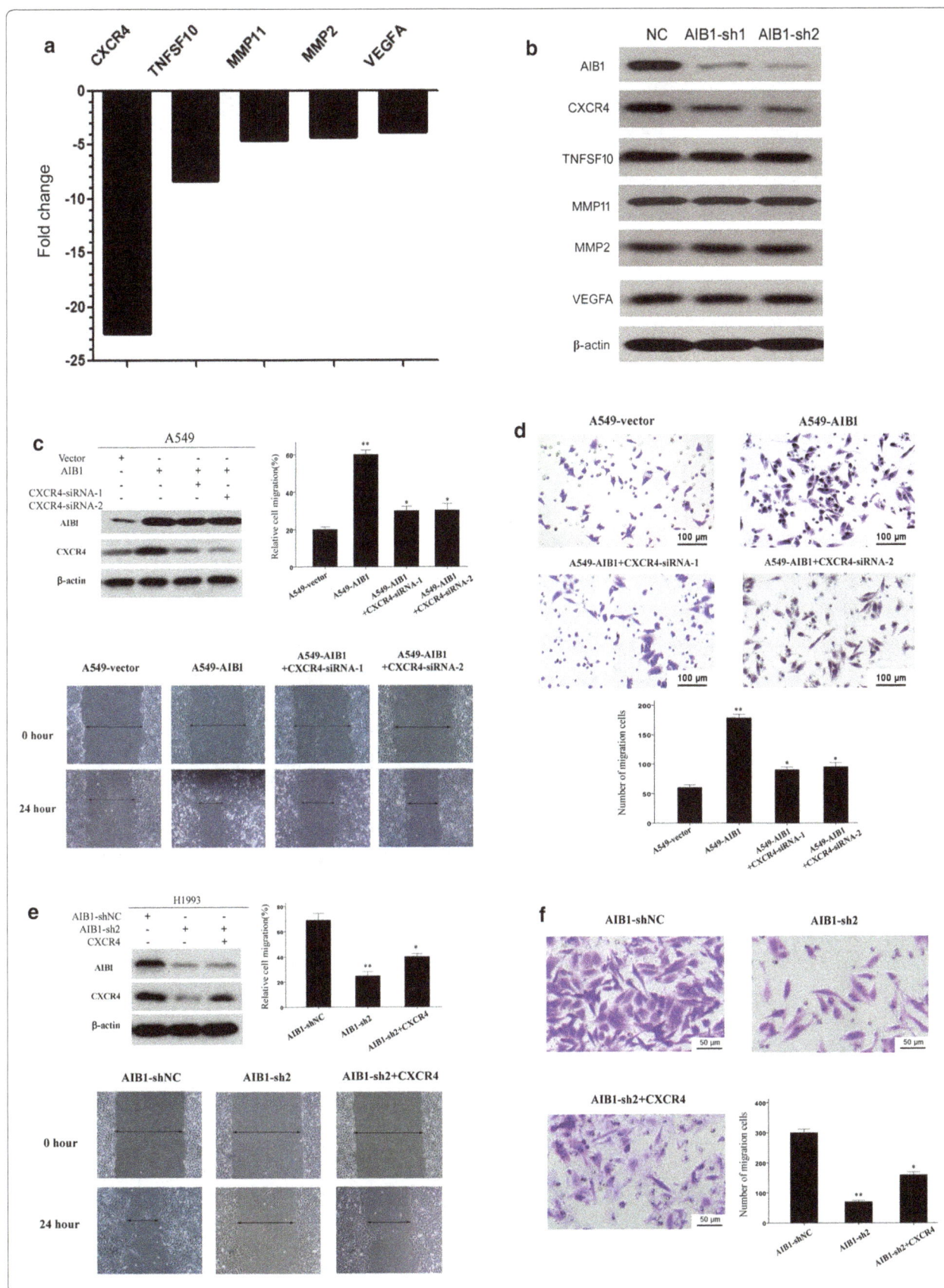

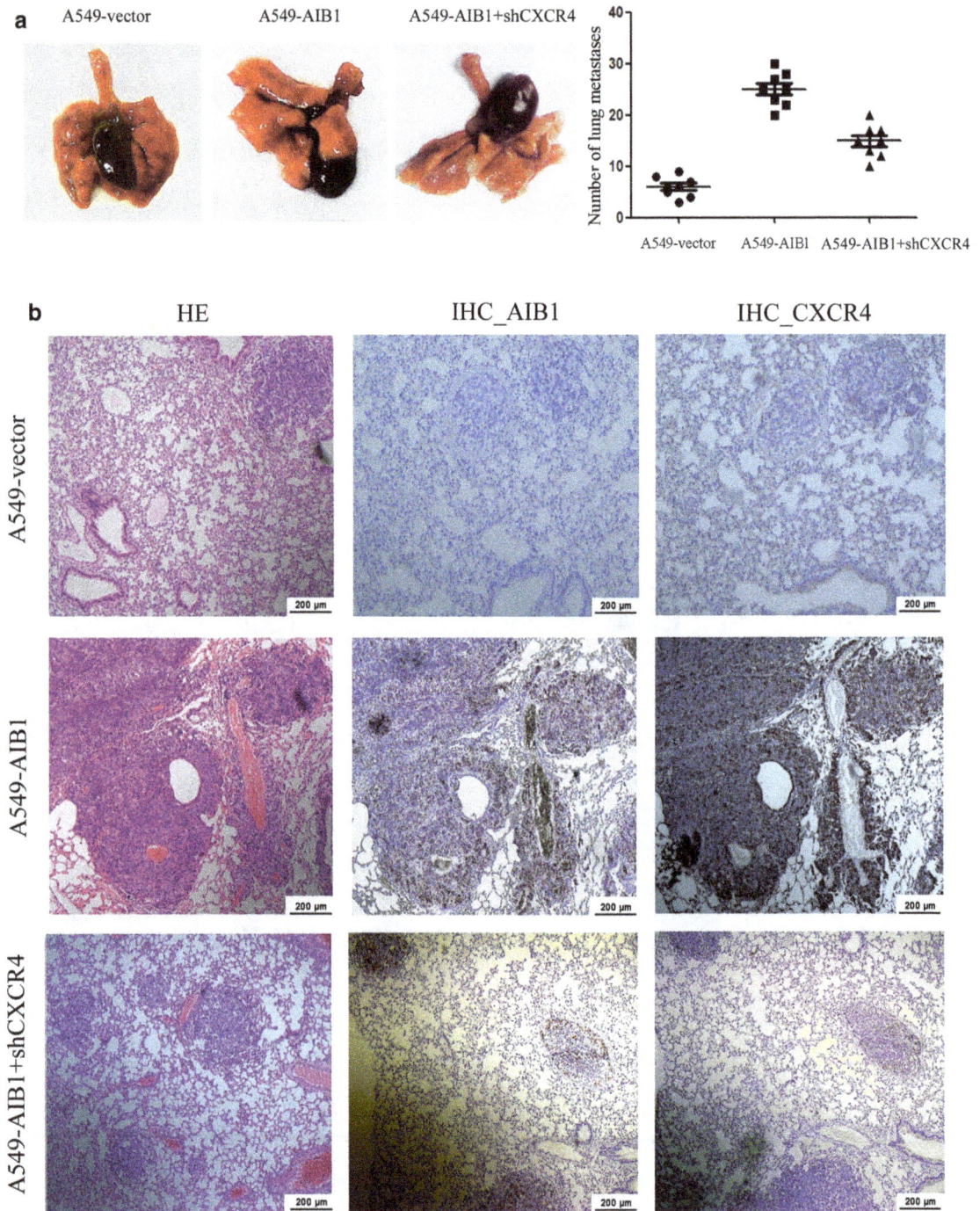

Fig. 5 Overexpression of AIB1 enhances lung adenocarcinoma A549 cell metastasis mediated by CXCR4 in vivo. **a** Left: representative lungs showing metastatic nodules originating from A549-vector, A549-AIB1, and A549-AIB1 + CXCR4-shRNA cells injected with Balb/c nude mice. Right: number of metastatic nodules formed in the lungs of mice 6 weeks after tail vein injection of A549-vector, A549-AIB1, and A549-AIB1 + CXCR4-shRNA cells (eight mice per group; *$P < 0.05$; independent Student's t test). **b** Representative hematoxylin and eosin (H&E) staining and IHC staining of AIB1 and CXCR4 in lung metastatic tumors originating from A549-vector, A549-AIB1, and A549-AIB1 + CXCR4-shRNA cells injected with Balb/c nude mice

Table 3 Associations of the expression status of AIB1 and CXCR4 in lung adenocarcinoma

CXCR4 expression	Cases	AIB1 expression [cases (%)]		P
		Normal	Over	
				<0.001
Low	75	50 (66.7)	25 (33.3)	
High	81	23 (28.4)	58 (71.6)	

expression rate of AIB1 increased from the localized to regional to metastatic stages of lung adenocarcinoma tissues. Similar results were observed in other human cancers, such as breast [16], prostate [17, 18], esophageal [28], pancreatic [29], and colon/rectum cancer [15], in which overexpression of AIB1 was reported to be associated with lymph node metastasis and/or distant organ

metastasis. In the present study, we demonstrated that AIB1 promotes lung adenocarcinoma migration in vitro and metastasis in vivo. These data support our emerging view that AIB1 is an important factor in promoting lung adenocarcinoma cell metastasis.

To the best of our knowledge, only two other studies have investigated the role of AIB1 in promoting cancer cell metastasis in vivo, one in breast cancer and the other in colorectal cancer, and only lung metastases were observed [15, 16]. Interestingly, in our mouse model, metastatic tumor nodules were also frequently found in lung tissues but not in liver tissues. It has been suggested that the expression of certain genes may lead to organ-specific metastasis in human cancers. For example, in colorectal cancer, the expression of transforming growth factor α (TGFα) often leads to liver-only metastasis [30], whereas in prostate cancer, the expression of platelet-derived growth factor receptor beta (PDGFR-β) often

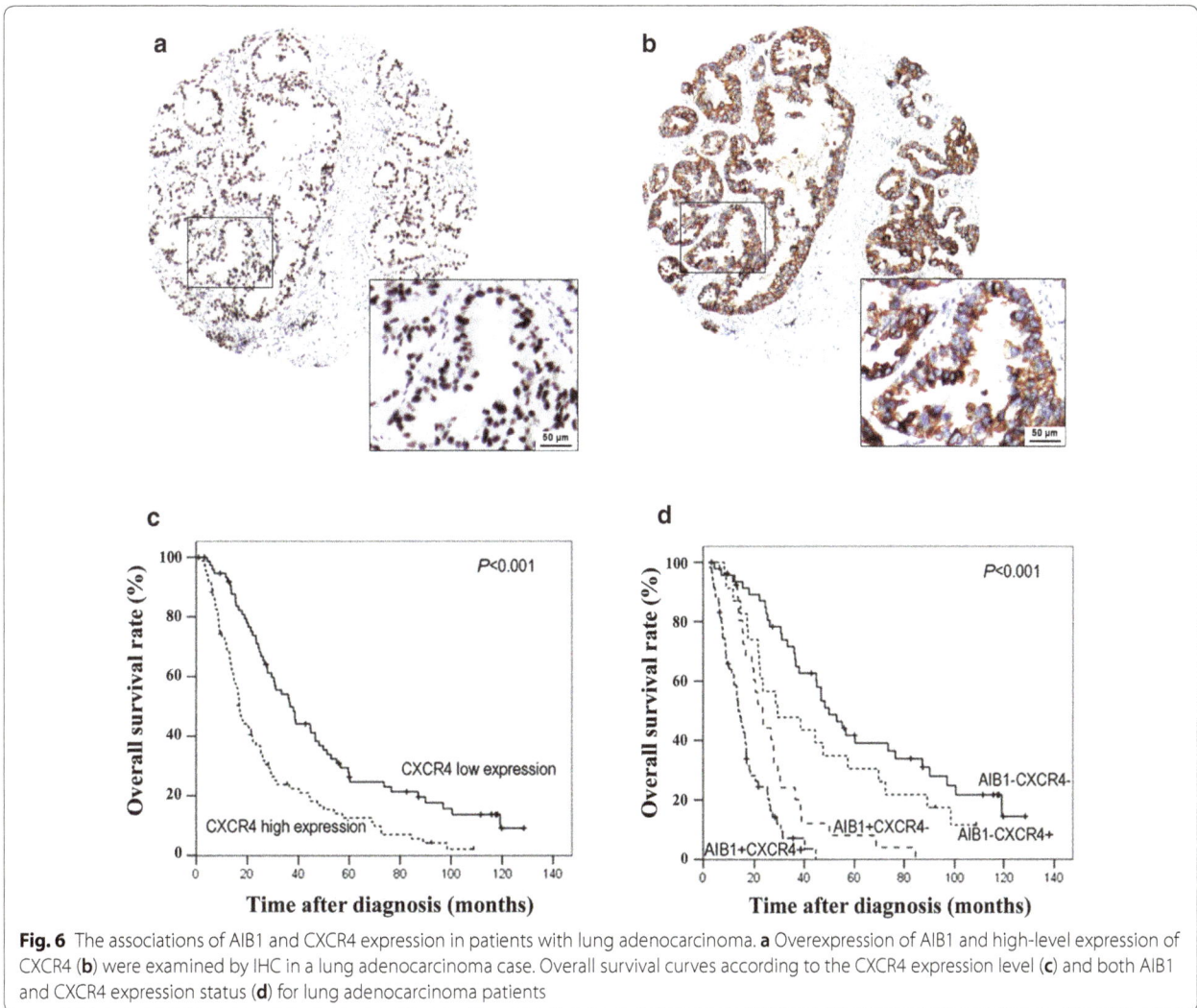

Fig. 6 The associations of AIB1 and CXCR4 expression in patients with lung adenocarcinoma. **a** Overexpression of AIB1 and high-level expression of CXCR4 (**b**) were examined by IHC in a lung adenocarcinoma case. Overall survival curves according to the CXCR4 expression level (**c**) and both AIB1 and CXCR4 expression status (**d**) for lung adenocarcinoma patients

leads to bone-only metastasis [31]. These data suggest that AIB1 may promote lung metastasis in certain human cancers.

To date, the molecular mechanisms by which AIB1 promotes cancer cell migration/metastasis are not yet fully understood. In 2008, Qin et al. [16] first reported that AIB1 can promote breast cancer cell metastasis through matrix metalloproteinases (MMPs). Later, Long et al. [18] and Yan et al. [17] reported that AIB1 can promote prostate and breast cancer cell metastasis through focal adhesion kinase (FAK). More recently, Mo et al. [15] revealed that AIB1 promotes colorectal cancer by the Notch signaling pathway. However, little is known about the mechanism by which AIB1 promotes lung adenocarcinoma cell metastasis. To investigate the downstream molecular events involving AIB1 and lung adenocarcinoma metastasis, we compared the mRNA expression profiles of shAIB1-transfected H1993 cells and H1993-vector cells using a human tumor metastasis real-time PCR array. Of the 84 genes, 5 genes (CXCR4, TNFSF10, MMP11, MMP2, and VEGFA) showed differential expression of 3.5-fold or more at the mRNA level. Subsequently, downregulated *CXCR4* was validated in protein levels by Western blot. Furthermore, a positive correlation between the overexpression of AIB1 and CXCR4 was observed in our cohort of lung adenocarcinoma tissues. These results collectively suggest that AIB1 may promote lung adenocarcinoma cell metastasis by regulating CXCR4.

In recent years, CXCR4, which belongs to the family of chemokines, has been reported to be overexpressed and to play an important role in the cell proliferation, migration, and metastasis of several cancers, including non-small cell lung cancer [32, 33]. Regarding lung adenocarcinoma histologic subtypes, it has been reported that the cytomembranous expression of CXCR4 in lung adenocarcinoma is associated with metastasis and patient survival [34]. More recently, Bertolini et al. [35] demonstrated that the subset of CD133+/CXCR4+ lung adenocarcinoma cells are highly tumorigenic and metastatic in vivo. To determine whether CXCR4 is functionally involved in AIB1-induced lung adenocarcinoma cell aggressiveness, we silenced CXCR4 by using siRNA in A549-AIB1 cells. The results clearly showed that the silencing of CXCR4 substantially prevented AIB1-induced A549 cell migration and invasion. These data, taken together, indicate that AIB1 might promote lung adenocarcinoma cell metastasis by regulating CXCR4.

With respect to the potential molecular mechanisms of how AIB1 regulates the expression of CXCR4, Cheng et al. [36] reported that SDF-1α/CXCL12 induced cell migration via SRC-mediated CXCR4-EGFR cross-talk in gastric cancer cells. It has also been demonstrated that SRC regulates breast cancer cell proliferation and invasion through the autocrine/paracrine activity of SDF-1α/CXCL12. Stromal derived factor-1 (SDF-1α), also termed CXCL12, is the main ligand for CXCR4 [20]. However, CXCL12 has not been found to be obviously downregulated in our real-time PCR array. CXCR4 is one of the most important molecule in promoting metastasis [37]. Further studies are needed to elucidate the detailed mechanisms by which AIB1 regulates CXCR4 expression in lung adenocarcinoma.

In conclusion, our results provide evidence that (1) AIB1 promotes lung adenocarcinoma aggressiveness in vitro and in vivo by upregulating the expression of an important downstream target, CXCR4, and (2) AIB1 and CXCR4 may potentially serve as novel prognostic markers and/or therapeutic targets for this disease.

Abbreviations
AIB1: the amplified in breast cancer 1; LA: lung adenocarcinoma; CXCR4: chemokine receptor 4; TMA: tissue microarrays; IHC: immunohistochemistry; SCID: severe combined immune-deficient; ROC: receiver operating characteristic; TNFSF10: tumor necrosis factor superfamily, member 10; VEGFA: vascular endothelial growth factor A; TGFα: transforming growth α; PDGFR-β: platelet-derived growth factor receptor-β; MMP: matrix metalloproteinases; FAK: focal adhesion kinase.

Authors' contributions
LRH participated in study design, collected the clinical data and drafted the manuscript. HXD, SLL, JWC, BKL, CYW and NFM contributed to the experimental work. YGJ and XW performed the statistical analysis. MZL and DX conceived of the study, participated in its design and revised the manuscript. All authors read and approved the final manuscript.

Author details
[1] The State Key Laboratory of Oncology in South China, Collaborative Innovation Center for Cancer Medicine, Sun Yat-Sen University Cancer Center, No. 651, Dongfeng Road East, Guangzhou 510060, China. [2] Department of Radiation Oncology, Sun Yat-Sen University Cancer Center, Guangzhou, China. [3] Department of Thoracic Oncology, Sun Yat-Sen University Cancer Center, Guangzhou, China. [4] The State Key Laboratory of Respiratory Disease, Guangzhou Medical University, Guangzhou, China. [5] Key Laboratory of Protein Modification and Degradation, School of Basic Medical Sciences, Affiliated Cancer Hospital & Institute of Guangzhou Medical University, Guangzhou, China.

Acknowledgements
We would like to thank LetPub (http://www.letpub.com) for providing linguistic assistance during the preparation of this manuscript.

Competing interests
The authors declare that they have no competing interests.

Funding
This work was supported by grants from National Key R&D Program of China (No. 2017YFC1309001), Nature Science Foundation of China (No. 81201842 and No. 81772483) and Open Project of State Key Laboratory of Respiratory Disease of China (No. SKLRD2016OP004 and No. 2007DA80154F1108).

References

1. Siegel RL, Miller KD, Jemal A. Cancer statistics, 2016. CA Cancer J Clin. 2016;66(1):7–30.
2. Dubey AK, Gupta U, Jain S. Epidemiology of lung cancer and approaches for its prediction: a systematic review and analysis. Chin J Cancer. 2016;35(1):71.
3. Liu YT, Hao XZ, Li JL, Hu XS, Wang Y, Wang ZP, et al. Survival of patients with advanced lung adenocarcinoma before and after approved use of gefitinib in China. Thorac Cancer. 2015;6(5):636–42.
4. Hung JJ, Jeng WJ, Wu YC, Chou TY, Hsu WH. Factors predicting organ-specific distant metastasis in patients with completely resected lung adenocarcinoma. Oncotarget. 2016;7(36):58261–73.
5. Tan Q, Cui J, Huang J, Ding Z, Lin H, Niu X, et al. Genomic alteration during metastasis of lung adenocarcinoma. Cell Physiol Biochem. 2016;38(2):469–86.
6. Fang B, Mehran RJ, Heymach JV, Swisher SG. Predictive biomarkers in precision medicine and drug development against lung cancer. Chin J Cancer. 2015;34(7):295–309.
7. Yan J, Tsai SY, Tsai MJ. SRC-3/AIB1: transcriptional coactivator in oncogenesis. Acta Pharmacol Sin. 2006;27(4):387–94.
8. Ma G, Ren Y, Wang K, He J. SRC-3 has a role in cancer other than as a nuclear receptor coactivator. Int J Biol Sci. 2011;7(5):664–72.
9. Xie D, Sham JS, Zeng WF, Lin HL, Bi J, Che LH, et al. Correlation of AIB1 overexpression with advanced clinical stage of human colorectal carcinoma. Hum Pathol. 2005;36:777–83.
10. Xu FP, Xie D, Wen JM, Wu HX, Liu YD, Bi J, et al. SRC-3/AIB1 protein and gene amplification levels in human esophageal squamous cell carcinomas. Cancer Lett. 2007;245:69–74.
11. Liu MZ, Xie D, Mai SJ, Tong ZT, Shao JY, Fu YS, et al. Overexpression of AIB1 in nasopharyngeal carcinomas correlates closely with advanced tumor stage. Am J Clin Pathol. 2008;129(5):728–34.
12. Luo JH, Xie D, Liu MZ, Chen W, Liu YD, Wu GQ, et al. Protein expression and amplification of AIB1 in human urothelial carcinoma of the bladder and overexpression of AIB1 is a new independent prognostic marker of patient survival. Int J Cancer. 2008;122:2554–61.
13. He LR, Zhao HY, Li BK, Zhang LJ, Liu MZ, Kung HF, et al. Overexpression of AIB1 negatively affects survival of surgically resected non-small-cell lung cancer patients. Ann Oncol. 2010;21(8):1675–81.
14. Tong ZT, Wei JH, Zhang JX, Liang CZ, Liao B, Lu J, et al. AIB1 predicts bladder cancer outcome and promotes bladder cancer cell proliferation through AKT and E2F1. Br J Cancer. 2013;108(7):1470–9.
15. Mo P, Zhou Q, Guan L, Wang Y, Wang W, Miao M, et al. Amplified in breast cancer 1 promotes colorectal cancer progression through enhancing notch signaling. Oncogene. 2015;34(30):3935–45.
16. Qin L, Liao L, Redmond A, Young L, Yuan Y, Chen H, et al. The AIB1 oncogene promotes breast cancer metastasis by activation of PEA3-mediated matrix metalloproteinase 2 (MMP2) and MMP9 expression. Mol Cell Biol. 2008;28(19):5937–50.
17. Yan J, Erdem H, Li R, Cai Y, Ayala G, Ittmann M, et al. Steroid receptor coactivator-3/AIB1 promotes cell migration and invasiveness through focal adhesion turnover and matrix metalloproteinase expression. Cancer Res. 2008;68(13):5460–8.
18. Long W, Yi P, Amazit L, LaMarca HL, Ashcroft F, Kumar R, et al. SRC-3Delta4 mediates the interaction of EGFR with FAK to promote cell migration. Mol Cell. 2010;37(3):321–32.
19. Zhang Y, Wang JH, Liu B, Qu PB. Steroid receptor coactivator-3 promotes bladder cancer through upregulation of CXCR4. Asian Pac J Cancer Prev. 2013;14(6):3847–50.
20. Kishimoto H, Wang Z, Bhat-Nakshatri P, Chang D, Clarke R, Nakshatri H. The p160 family coactivators regulate breast cancer cell proliferation and invasion through autocrine_paracrine activity of SDF-1alpha_CXCL12. Carcinogenesis. 2005;26(10):1706–15.
21. Kononen J, Bubendorf L, Kallioniemi A, Barlund M, Schraml P, Leighton S, et al. Tissue microarrays for high-throughput molecular profiling of tumor specimens. Nat Med. 1998;4(7):844–7.
22. Spano JP, Andre F, Morat L, Sabatier L, Besse B, Combadiere C, et al. Chemokine receptor CXCR4 and early-stage non-small cell lung cancer: pattern of expression and correlation with outcome. Ann Oncol. 2004;15(4):613–7.
23. Chen G, Wang Z, Liu XY, Liu FY. High-level CXCR4 expression correlates with brain-specific metastasis of non-small cell lung cancer. World J Surg. 2011;35(1):56–61.
24. André ND, Silva VA, Ariza CB, Watanabe MA, De Lucca FL. In vivo knock-down of CXCR4 using jetPEI/CXCR4 shRNA nanoparticles inhibits the pulmonary metastatic potential of B16-F10 melanoma cells. Mol Med Rep. 2015;12(6):8320–6.
25. Liu L, Dai Y, Chen J, Zeng T, Li Y, Chen L, et al. Maelstrom promotes hepatocellular carcinoma metastasis by inducing epithelial-mesenchymal transition by way of Akt/GSK-3beta/Snail signaling. Hepatology. 2014;59(2):531–43.
26. Jung MJ, Rho JK, Kim YM, Jung JE, Jin YB, Ko YG, et al. Upregulation of CXCR4 is functionally crucial for maintenance of stemness in drug-resistant non-small cell lung cancer cells. Oncogene. 2013;32(2):209–21.
27. Schmittgen TD, Livak KJ. Analyzing real-time PCR data by the comparative C(T) method. Nat Protoc. 2008;3:1101–8.
28. He LR, Liu MZ, Li BK, Rao HL, Deng HX, Guan XY, et al. Overexpression of AIB1 predicts resistance to chemoradiotherapy and poor prognosis in patients with primary esophageal squamous cell carcinoma. Cancer Sci. 2009;100(9):1591–6.
29. Guo S, Xu J, Xue R, Liu Y, Yu H. Overexpression of AIB1 correlates inversely with E-cadherin expression in pancreatic adenocarcinoma and may promote lymph node metastasis. Int J Clin Oncol. 2014;19(2):319–24.
30. Sasaki T, Nakamura T, Rebhun RB, Cheng H, Hale KS, Tsan RZ, et al. Modification of the primary tumor microenvironment by transforming growth factor alpha-epidermal growth factor receptor signaling promotes metastasis in an orthotopic colon cancer model. Am J Clin Pathol. 2008;173(1):205–16.
31. Uehara H, Kim SJ, Karashima T, Shepherd DL, Fan D, Tsan R, et al. Effects of blocking platelet-derived growth factor-receptor signaling in a mouse model of experimental prostate cancer bone metastases. J Natl Cancer Inst. 2003;95(6):458–70.
32. Burger JA, Kipps TJ. CXCR4: a key receptor in the crosstalk between tumor cells and their microenvironment. Blood. 2006;107(5):1761–7.
33. Liang JX, Gao W, Liang Y, Zhou XM. Chemokine receptor CXCR4 expression and lung cancer prognosis: a meta-analysis. Int J Clin Exp Med. 2015;8(4):5163–74.
34. Wagner PL, Hyjek E, Vazquez MF, Meherally D, Liu YF, Chadwick PA, et al. CXCL12 and CXCR4 in adenocarcinoma of the lung: association with metastasis and survival. J Thorac Cardiovasc Surg. 2009;137(3):615–21.
35. Bertolini G, D'Amico L, Moro M, Landoni E, Perego P, Miceli R, et al. Microenvironment-modulated metastatic CD133+/CXCR4+/EpCAM-lung cancer-initiating cells sustain tumor dissemination and correlate with poor prognosis. Cancer Res. 2015;75(17):3636–49.
36. Cheng Y, Qu J, Che X, Xu L, Song N, Ma Y, et al. CXCL12_SDF-1α induces migration via SRC-mediated CXCR4-EGFR cross-talk in gastric cancer cells. Oncol Lett. 2017;14(2):2103–10.
37. Mei Y, Yang JP, Qian CN. For robust big data analyses: a collection of 150 important pro-metastatic genes. Chin J Cancer. 2017;36(1):16.

9

Characterization of drug responses of mini patient-derived xenografts in mice for predicting cancer patient clinical therapeutic response

Feifei Zhang[1][†], Wenjie Wang[1][†], Yuan Long[1], Hui Liu[1], Jijun Cheng[1], Lin Guo[1], Rongyu Li[1], Chao Meng[1], Shan Yu[1], Qingchuan Zhao[2], Shun Lu[3], Lili Wang[4], Haitao Wang[4] and Danyi Wen[1][*]

Abstract

Background: Patient-derived organoids and xenografts (PDXs) have emerged as powerful models in functional diagnostics with high predictive power for anticancer drug response. However, limitations such as engraftment failure and time-consuming for establishing and expanding PDX models followed by testing drug efficacy, and inability to subject to systemic drug administration for ex vivo organoid culture hinder realistic and fast decision-making in selecting the right therapeutics in the clinic. The present study aimed to develop an advanced PDX model, namely MiniPDX, for rapidly testing drug efficacy to strengthen its value in personalized cancer treatment.

Methods: We developed a rapid in vivo drug sensitivity assay, OncoVee® MiniPDX, for screening clinically relevant regimens for cancer. In this model, patient-derived tumor cells were arrayed within hollow fiber capsules, implanted subcutaneously into mice and cultured for 7 days. The cellular activity morphology and pharmacokinetics were systematically evaluated. MiniPDX performance (sensitivity, specificity, positive and negative predictive values) was examined using PDX as the reference. Drug responses were examined by tumor cell growth inhibition rate and tumor growth inhibition rate in PDX models and MiniPDX assays respectively. The results from MiniPDX were also used to evaluate its predictive power for clinical outcomes.

Results: Morphological and histopathological features of tumor cells within the MiniPDX capsules matched those both in PDX models and in original tumors. Drug responses in the PDX tumor graft assays correlated well with those in the corresponding MiniPDX assays using 26 PDX models generated from patients, including 14 gastric cancer, 10 lung cancer and 2 pancreatic cancer. The positive predictive value of MiniPDX was 92%, and the negative predictive value was 81% with a sensitivity of 80% and a specificity of 93%. Through expanding to clinical tumor samples, MiniPDX assay showed potential of wide clinical application.

Conclusions: Fast in vivo MiniPDX assay based on capsule implantation was developed-to assess drug responses of both PDX tumor grafts and clinical cancer specimens. The high correlation between drug responses of paired MiniPDX and PDX tumor graft assay, as well as translational data suggest that MiniPDX assay is an advanced tool for personalized cancer treatment.

Keywords: Personalized cancer therapy, Cancer precision medicine, Patient-derived xenograft (PDX), MiniPDX, Drug response, In vivo

*Correspondence: danyi.wen@lidebiotech.com
†Feifei Zhang and Wenjie Wang contributed equally to this work
1 Shanghai LIDE Biotech Co., LTD, Shanghai 201203, P. R. China
Full list of author information is available at the end of the article

Background

Genomic profiling has been widely applied in precision cancer medicine for molecularly stratified oncologic treatment. However, limitations in functional tests compromise the effectiveness of these tests in predicting responses to targeted therapies, hampering precision cancer medicine development. Integrating next-generation sequencing with functional assays, such as patient-derived tumor organoids and patient-derived tumor xenografts (PDXs), in testing drug responses has significantly improved the predictive power of these assays [1–3]. Recently, several studies have established the patient-derived tumor organoid model in various cancers, including gastrointestinal, bladder and breast cancer, and have shown a high predictive value of this model in assessing patient clinical response to targeted therapy or chemotherapy [4–6].

PDXs, by directly implanting patient tumor fragments into immunodeficient mice, have become critical in preclinical drug assessment as they capture the heterogeneity, and the molecular and histopathologic signatures of the parent primary tumors better than cell lines or genetically engineered mouse models. In addition, the drug response profiles of PDXs well correlate with patient clinical responses [3, 7–16]. PDXs have been reported in many different solid tumor types and have been proven useful in predicting patient chemotherapeutic response and providing guidance for informed clinical decision-making [9, 11, 16–22]. To date, approximately 300 cases of 13 tumor types have been evaluated and the overall concordance between patient clinical response and therapeutic response in PDXs ranges from 70 to 100%. Although PDXs possess notable advantages, limitations prevent their widespread utilization in personalized medicine. An unduly long period of time, usually 4–8 months, is required for tumor xenograft engraftment [8, 21, 23], and additional time is required to generate sufficient tissues for testing therapeutic regimens in mice. In addition, the engraftment rate in mouse models is generally lower than 50% in many cancer types, which is even lower for breast cancer, prostate cancer, and renal cell carcinoma [9, 15, 22]. Thus, many patients with rapid progressing disease could not benefit from PDX studies, and there is an urgent need for a fast and reliable alternative method to assess drug sensitivity.

The hollow fiber assay is used at the USA National Cancer Institute (NCI) as a preliminary screening tool for novel anticancer drugs [24]. This assay has certain advantages, simultaneous evaluation of compounds against various cell lines, relatively short term, low cost, and good correlation with conventional tumor graft assay [25, 26]. However, the limitation of using cell lines and lack of good correlation to clinical activity has historically hampered the usage of this approach.

By taking advantage of the hollow fiber implant technology, we sought to develop a fast and accurate in vivo drug response assay, which we named mini-patient-derived xenograft (MiniPDX) assay, to effectively and faithfully predict patient clinical response to targeted therapy and chemotherapy. We analyzed the histopathological and immunohistochemical features of tumor cells in MiniPDX capsules and compared the therapeutic responses of tumor xenograft in the MiniPDX model and the PDX model. The results altogether demonstrate that the MiniPDX assay offers a rapid and effective alternative approach to the PDX model in assessing cancer therapeutic responses that mimics patient clinical therapeutic responses.

Materials and methods
Tumor tissue acquisition

Fresh surgical tumor specimens were acquired from patients with pathologically proven gastric cancer, lung cancer or pancreatic cancer at participating hospitals. The list of participating hospitals will be provided upon written request. Cancer pathology was confirmed by an experienced pathologist (SY). The study protocol was approved by the Institutional Ethics Committee of Shanghai LIDE. Tumor tissue acquisition was approved by the ethics committees of each participating hospital and agreed to by each patient via written informed consent and was carried out according to state and institutional regulations on experimental use of human tissues.

Animals

Six- to eight-week-old CB17-SCID or 5-week-old nu/nu mice (Charles River Co., Beijing, China) were housed at the AAALAC accredited animal facility at LIDE Biotech (Shanghai, China). CB17-SCID mice were used for PDX model recovery and nu/nu mice were used for drug efficacy tests. All study protocols were reviewed and approved by the Institutional Animal Care and Use Committee (IACUC) at LIDE Biotech, and conducted in accordance with established national and international regulations for laboratory animal protection.

Establishing the PDX model

Fresh surgically removed gastric cancer ($n=14$), lung cancer ($n=10$) and pancreatic cancer tissues ($n=2$) were used for establishing PDX models. Tumor cells were subcutaneously implanted into immune-deficient mice as previously described and stably propagated for three passages [8].

Establishing the MiniPDX model

We developed an in vivo drug sensitivity MiniPDX assay by using a modified microencapsulation and hollow fiber culture system (OncoVee MiniPDX®, LIDE Biotech) according to the manufacturer's instruction. Tumors ≥ 500 mm^3 in size with a necrotic area $< 30\%$ were used. Briefly, tumor tissues were washed with Hank's balanced salt solution (HBSS) to remove non-tumor tissues and necrotic tumor tissue in a biosafety cabinet. After the tumor tissues were morselized, they were digested with collagenase at 37 °C for 1–4 h. Cells were pelleted by centrifugation at 600g for 5 min followed by removal of blood cells and fibroblasts with magnetic beads. Cells were then washed with HBSS and filled into OncoVee® capsules. Capsules were implanted subcutaneously via a small skin incision with 3 capsules per mouse (5-week-old nu/nu mouse).

Histologic and immunofluorescence studies

Tumor tissues in the PDX assays and MiniPDX assays were fixed in buffered 10% formalin and routinely stained with hematoxylin and eosin (H&E) and examined by a certified pathologist.

For immunofluorescence studies, cellularized tumor cells (2×10^4 cells, 200 L) were cytospun onto a slide, fixed with 4% paraformaldehyde for 20 min, permeabilized with 0.3% Triton X-100 in PBS for 30 min, and then blocked with 5% normal goat serum for 1 h at room temperature. The cells were then divided into three fractions and incubated with primary mouse monoclonal antibodies at 4 °C overnight against the following proteins: pan-cytokeratin, indicating carcinoma components [27, 28] (1:200, AE1/AE3, sc-81714, Santa Cruz Biotechnology, Santa Cruz, CA, US), E-cadherin, generally found

in gastric adenocarcinomas [29] (1:50, HECD-1, ab1416, Abcam, Cambridge, UK), and MG7, a marker of gastric cancer [30] (1:300, NOTA-MG7) [30]. Subsequently, the cells were probed with secondary antibody donkey anti-mouse IgG H&L (Alexa Fluor® 488) (1:200, ab150105, Abcam). Finally, the cells were mounted with DAPI-containing mounting medium (S36973, Thermo Fisher, MA, US). Images were captured with a fluorescence microscope (Leica, Germany) with Leica Application Suite V4 software and edited with Photoshop (Adobe, US).

Pharmacokinetic assays

5-week-old nu/nu mice bearing MiniPDX capsules were administered orally with oxaliplatin (5 mg/kg) and approximately 200 μL blood was collected via a capillary in the retro-orbital plexus at different intervals post drug administration and directly mixed with 50 μL sodium citrate (3.8% solution). Blood samples were clarified by centrifugation and the supernatant was stored at -80 °C. In addition, MiniPDX capsules were retrieved at indicated time intervals, morselized, and suspended in 500 μL PBS. After clarification by centrifugation at 1580g for 5 min, the supernatant was collected and stored at -80 °C. The concentrations of oxaliplatin in the plasma and the MiniPDX capsules were analyzed by LC–MS/MS and pharmacokinetic parameters were calculated using the WinNonlin® 6.4 program.

MiniPDX drug sensitivity assays

Mice bearing MiniPDX capsules were treated with appropriate drugs or their combinations as detailed in Tables 1 and 2 for 7 days. Thereafter, the implanted capsules were removed and tumor cell proliferation was evaluated using the CellTiter Glo Luminescent Cell Viability Assay kit

Table 1 Drug preparations and treatment details

Drug	Supplier	Preparation[a]	PDX assay[b]	MiniPDX assay[b]
S-1	Hengrui	0.5% HPMC + 0.2% Tween 80	10 mg/kg, *po*, qd*5/w	10 mg/kg, *po*, qd*5
Docetaxel	DEMO	5% Tween 80 + 5% Ethanol + 90% Saline	20 mg/kg, *ip*, q4d	20 mg/kg, *ip*, q4d*2
Gemzar	Eli Lilly	Saline	60 mg/kg, *ip*, q4d	60 mg/kg, *ip*, q4d*2
Oxaliplatin	Hengrui	5% Glucose	5 mg/kg, *ip*, biw	5 mg/kg, *ip*, q4d*2
Irinotecan	DEMO	5% DMSO + 95% Saline	40 mg/kg, *ip*, q4d	50 mg/kg, *ip*, q4d*2
Cisplatin	Hansoh	Saline	5 mg/kg, *ip*, qw	5 mg/kg, *ip*, q4d*2
Epirubicin	Pfizer	Saline	5 mg/kg, *ip*, qw	5 mg/kg, *ip*, q4d*2
Capecitabine	Adamas	0.5% HPMC + 0.2% Tween 80	400 mg/kg, *po*, qd*14	400 mg/kg, *po*, qd*7
5-FU	Xudong-Haipu	Saline	25 mg/kg, *ip*, qd*5/w	25 mg/kg, *ip*, qd*5
Erlotinib	Topscience	0.5% HPMC + 0.2% Tween 80	50 mg/kg, po, qd	50 mg/kg, po, qd*7
Crizotinib	Aladdin	0.5% HPMC + 0.2% Tween 80	50 mg/kg, po, qd	50 mg/kg, po, qd*7
AZD9291	Topscience	0.5% HPMC + 0.2% Tween 80	5 mg/kg, po, qd	5 mg/kg, po, qd*7

po oral, *ip* intraperitoneal, *qd* once a day, *biw* twice a week, *qw* once a week, *q4d* once every 4 days

[a] Recipe of formulation

[b] Dose, dosing route, dosing frequency followed by, where indicated, dosing times and/or treatment duration

Table 2 Treatment details of combination regimens

Regimen	Drug 1	Drug 2	Drug 3
2	S-1 (6.9 mg/kg, *po*, qd*14)	Oxaliplatin (5 mg/kg, *ip*, qw)	NA
3	Capecitabine (400 mg/kg, *po*, qd*14)	Oxaliplatin (5 mg/kg, *ip*, qw)	NA
4	Capecitabine (400 mg/kg, *po*, qd*14)	Oxaliplatin (5 mg/kg, *ip*, qw)	Epirubicin (5 mg/kg, *ip*, qw)
5	Cisplatin (5 mg/kg, *ip*, qw)	5-FU (15 mg/kg, *ip*, qd*5)	Docetaxel (20 mg/kg, *ip*, qw)
7	Gemzar (60 mg/kg, *ip*, q4d)	Cisplatin (5 mg/kg, *ip*, qw)	NA
12	Oxaliplatin (5 mg/kg, *ip*, qw)	Irinotecan (40 mg/kg, *ip*, q4d)	NA

Drug combinations used to test efficacy in PDX models, including detailed treatment conditions in brackets (); Combination regimens have the same numbering as Table 3

NA not available, *po* per os, *ip* intraperitoneal, *qd* once a day, *biw* twice a week, *qw* once a week, *q4d* once every 4 days

(G7571, Promega, Madison, WI, US) as instructed by the manufacturer. Luminescence was measured in terms of relative luminance unit (RFU) using a spectrophotometer (SpectraMax M3, Molecular Devices, Sunnyvale, CA, US). Tumor cell growth inhibition (TCGI) (%) was calculated using the formula:

$$\text{TCGI (\%)} = \left(1 - \begin{array}{c}[\text{Mean RLU of the treatment group on day 7} - \text{Mean RLU on day 0)} \\ /(\text{Mean RLU of the vehicle group on day 7} - \text{Mean RLU on day 0}]\end{array}\right) \times 100\%$$

Each experiment was done in sextuplicate and mean values were reported. A positive drug response was considered present if TCGI was $\geq 45\%$ ($P < 0.05$), and a negative drug response was considered if TCGI was $< 45\%$ ($P < 0.05$).

Evaluation of therapeutic responses

The therapeutic response of primary tumors in PDX models to 12 clinically relevant regimens, including 9 chemotherapeutic drugs and 3 targeted drugs was examined (Table 3). Tumor volume was measured by a caliper twice a week and calculated as (length × width^2)/2, and tumors were harvested when they reached 500–700 mm^3 and were morselized and snap-frozen in liquid nitrogen. Morselized tumors were inoculated in the right flank of nu/nu mice and when they reached 100–300 mm^3, mice were randomized to receive vehicle or indicated regimens for 3 weeks as detailed in Tables 1 and 2. Antitumor efficacy was represented by tumor growth inhibition (TGI) (%) and calculated using the formula:

$$\text{TGI (\%)} = [1 - (V_{ti} - V_{t0})/(V_{ci} - V_{c0})] \times 100\%$$

where V_{t0} and V_{ti}; and V_{c0} and V_{ci} were the tumor volume at the first day of drug or vehicle treatment and the final tumor volume in the treatment group and the control group, respectively. The cutoff of TGI $\geq 45\%$ ($P < 0.05$)

was used to define positive response, and TGI $< 45\%$ ($P < 0.05$) was used to define negative response.

Statistical analysis

Statistical data and graphics were analyzed using GraphPad Prism 6. Statistical significances were assessed by Student's t test with $P < 0.05$ considered significant. The positive predictive value (PPV) was calculated using the formula:

$$\text{PPV} = \text{No. of true positives/No. of true positives} \\ + \text{No. of false positives} \times 100\%$$

and the negative predictive value (NPV) was calculated using the formula:

$$\text{NPV} = \text{No. of true negatives/No. of true negatives} \\ + \text{No. of false negatives} \times 100\%.$$

Results

The MiniPDX model could be used to assess therapeutic response of primary tumor cells

We developed a rapid in vivo drug sensitivity assay, the MiniPDX assay, for assessing therapeutic response of primary tumor cells. The integral process of MiniPDX assay included from sample preparation to drug response evaluation (Fig. 1). Our histologic and immunohistochemical study revealed that cells from the MiniPDX assay were morphologically and immunohistochemically similar to their original primary cancer cells (Fig. 2a, b–i), suggesting that tumor cells within the MiniPDX capsules closely mimic their parental primary tumor cells.

We further evaluated the dynamic changes of drug concentration of orally administered oxaliplatin in the MiniPDX capsules. We found that drug in MiniPDX capsules

Table 3 Drug efficacy in PDX models and OncoVee® MiniPDX capsules in mice

Model	Location	Pathology	Chemotherapeutic or targeted drug (Regimen)	TGI (%)	Response in PDX	TCGI(%)	Response in MiniPDX
GAYW5	Stomach	Poor/moderately differentiated AC, 80%	S-1 (1)	95 ± 6	+	94 ± 15	+
GAYW7	Stomach	Poorly differentiated AC, 90%	S-1 (1)	86 ± 10	+	92 ± 3	+
GAYL1	Stomach	Mucinous AC, 80%	S-1 (1)	37 ± 10	−	13 ± 29	−
GAYB7	Stomach	Poorly differentiated tubular AC, 70%	S-1 (1)	44 ± 16	−	14 ± 20	−
GAYP53	Stomach	Poor-moderately differentiated AC, 90%	S-1 (1)	35 ± 10	−	17 ± 13	−
GASIL2	Stomach	Moderately differentiated AC, 40%	S-1 + Oxaliplatin (2)	29 ± 20	−	40 ± 17	−
GABSI3	Stomach	Poorly differentiated AC, 80%	S-1 + Oxaliplatin (2)	37 ± 12	−	75 ± 4	+
GAYP93	Stomach	Moderately differentiated AC, 90%	S-1 + Oxaliplatin(2)	27 ± 20	−	29 ± 15	−
GAYP97	Stomach	Moderately differentiated AC, 90%	S-1 + Oxaliplatin (2)	7 ± 29	−	9 ± 10	−
GAJ07	Stomach	Poor-moderately differentiated AC, 50%	Capecitabine + Oxaliplatin (3)	80 ± 3	+	35 ± 13	−
GASI80	Stomach	Poorly differentiated AC, 80%	Capecitabine + Oxaliplatin (3)	112 ± 3	+	50 ± 11	+
GASI05	Stomach	Moderately differentiated AC, 40%	Epirubicin + Capecitabine + Oxaliplatin (4)	97 ± 16	+	45 ± 23	+
GASAB3	Stomach	Poorly differentiated AC, 90%	Cisplatin + 5-FU + Docetaxel (5)	43 ± 17	−	17 ± 14	−
GAYP16	Stomach	Poorly differentiated AC, 90%	Cisplatin + 5-FU + Docetaxel (5)	32 ± 16	−	−13 ± 39	−
GAYP53	Stomach	Poor-moderately differentiated AC, 90%	Cisplatin + 5-FU + Docetaxel (5)	125 ± 3	+	50 ± 7	+
LULI02	Lung	Poorly differentiated SCC, 98%	Docetaxel (6)	97 ± 12	+	51 ± 7	+
LULI03	Lung	Poorly differentiated AC, 98%	Docetaxel (6)	12 ± 23	−	15 ± 10	−
LULI20	Lung	Poorly differentiated AC, 98%	Docetaxel (6)	91 ± 14	+	86 ± 3	+
LULI21	Lung	Poorly differentiated SCC, 78%	Docetaxel (6)	42 ± 16	−	−61 ± 29	−
LULI27	Lung	Moderate-highly differentiated SCC, 80%	Docetaxel (6)	115 ± 3	+	32 ± 11	−
LULI55	Lung	Large cell carcinoma, 95%	Docetaxel (6)	109 ± 1	+	14 ± 4	−
CTYW012	Lung	Poor-moderately differentiated AC, 90%	Gemzar + Cisplatin (7)	116 ± 0	+	84 ± 7	+
LULI49	Lung	Poorly differentiated AC, 90%	Erlotinib (8)	40 ± 15	−	−16 ± 26	−
CTC15063	Lung	Poor-moderately differentiated AC, 95%	Erlotinib (8)	37 ± 19	−	21 ± 17	−
CTC15063	Lung	Poor-moderately differentiated AC, 95%	AZD9291 (9)	167 ± 5	+	61 ± 3	+
CTC16075	Lung	Poorly differentiated carcinoma, 90%	Crizotinib (10)	103 ± 2	+	102 ± 4	+
PAYY8	Pancreas	Poorly differentiated ductal AC, 90%	Gemzar (11)	27 ± 27	−	−14 ± 10	−
PAYY5	Pancreas	Poor-moderately differentiated ductal AC, 80%	Gemzar (11)	75 ± 9	+	56 ± 8	+
PAYY5	Pancreas	Poor-moderately differentiated ductal AC, 80%	Oxaliplatin + Irinotecan (12)	112 ± 2	+	54 ± 6	+

Model: Indicates a specific patient and patient-derived xenograft model

Pathology: Judged by licensed pathologist (SY); %, percentage of the diseased cells judged by pathology; *AC* adenocarcinoma, *SCC* squamous cell carcinoma

Regimen: Drug combinations used to test efficacy in specific PDX model and MiniPDX

Chemotherapeutic or targeted drug: Single or combination of drugs used in PDX assay and in MiniPDX

TGI: Tumor growth inhibition or TCGI: tumor cell growth inhibition. N = 6, results are mean ± SEM. Mean TGI or TCGI ≥ 45% is defined as positive therapeutic response (+)

turned out essentially the same as that in plasma (Fig. 3), indicating that the capsules do not limit in vivo distribution of oxaliplatin and the MiniPDX model could be used to assess systemically administered drugs.

The MiniPDX model and the PDX model exhibit largely consistent therapeutic responses

To further evaluate the consistency of therapeutic responses between MiniPDX assay and PDX model, we compared the therapeutic responses of 26 randomly selected primary tumors in the PDX model and the MiniPDX model (Table 3). If the therapeutic responses in PDX model and corresponding MiniPDX assay were both positive or negative, they would be defined as consistent therapeutic responses. Twelve (85.7%, 12/14) gastric cancer tissues showed consistent therapeutic responses to 15 drugs in the PDX model and the MiniPDX model. Five gastric cancer tissues had a TGI and TCGI ≥ 45% and eight gastric cancer tissues had a TGI and TCGI < 45% in both the PDX model and the MiniPDX model,

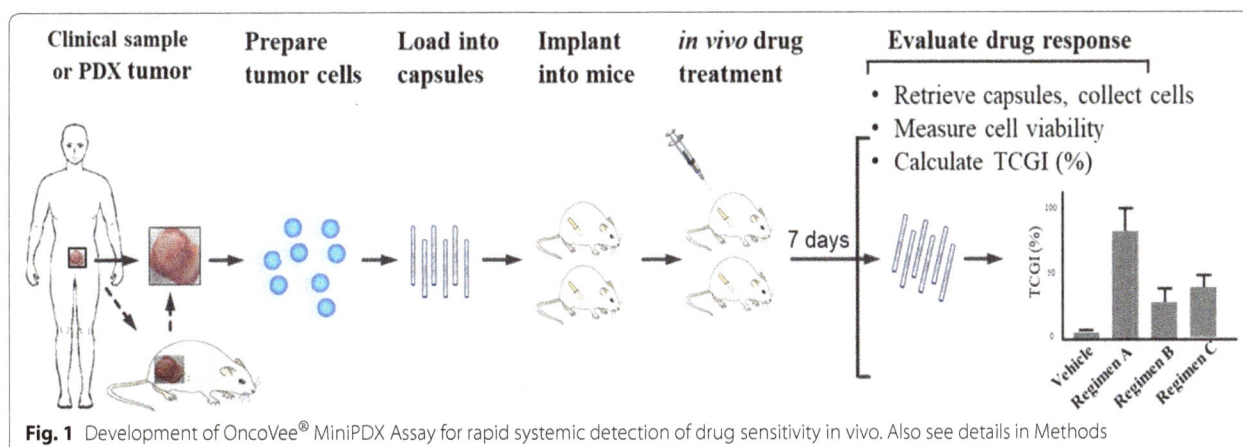

Fig. 1 Development of OncoVee® MiniPDX Assay for rapid systemic detection of drug sensitivity in vivo. Also see details in Methods

including one lung cancer tissue (GAYP53) with a TGI and TCGI ≥ 45% to cisplatin plus 5-FU and docetaxel, and a TGI and TCGI < 45% to S-1 in both the PDX model and the MiniPDX model. Similarly, 8 (80%, 8/10) lung cancer tissues showed consistent therapeutic responses in the PDX model and the MiniPDX model. Five lung cancer tissues had a TGI and TCGI ≥ 45% and 4 lung cancer tissues had a TGI and TCGI < 45% in both the PDX model and the MiniPDX model, including one lung cancer tissue (CTC15063) with a TGI and TCGI ≥ 45% to AZD9291 and a TGI and TCGI < 45% to erlotinib in the PDX model and the MiniPDX model. Two (100%, 2/2) pancreatic adenocarcinoma tissues were fully consistent in therapeutic responses in the MiniPDX model and the PDX model.

The MiniPDX model could predict clinical response of cancer patients

We further examined the therapeutic response of 4 gastric cancer tissues (GAYW5, GAYW7, GAYL1 and GAYB7) with known clinical responses to S-1. PDX assays showed that S-1 caused a significantly greater reduction in the tumor volume of GAYW5 and GAYW7 than vehicle control while no difference in tumor volume was seen in GAYL1 and GAYB7 between S-1 and control ($P < 0.05$) (Fig. 4a). The miniPDX assays further showed that S-1 significantly reduced the viabilities of GAYW5 and GAYW7 ($P < 0.001$) while no difference in the viabilities of GAYL1 and GAYB7 was seen (Fig. 4a). The results of the miniPDX assays are consistent with the findings of the PDX assays and the clinical response of the patients. The genomic sequencing data, therapeutic response from the PDX model and clinical response of lung cancer CTC15063 were previously published [31]. Consistently, CTC15063 showed greater sensitivity

to AZD9291 than erlotinib in terms of tumor volume reduction in the PDX assays but significantly lower viabilities in response to erlotinib in the PDX assays (Fig. 4b).

In addition, overall 29 pairwise efficacy tests were conducted on 26 PDX xenografts against 12 therapeutic regimens. Compared against the PDX assay, the MiniPDX assay had a PPV of 92%, a NPV of 81%, and a sensitivity of 80% and a specificity of 93%, suggesting that the MiniPDX assay is of high predictive power.

Application of MiniPDX assay in clinical settings

We also continuously looked into MiniPDX assay data using patients' tumor specimens. To date, 536 clinical samples comprising up to 40 malignancy types were obtained (Fig. 5). Four hundred twenty samples (79%) passed the quality control criterion and underwent MiniPDX tests. Quite interestingly, the MiniPDX assay yielded a 100% success rate achieved with these qualified samples.

Case report

Patient MDX245, a 48-year-old female, presented with bilateral multiple pulmonary metastases from low grade endometrial stromal sarcoma. She was initially treated with laparoscopic surgery and a regimen including lobaplatin, doxorubicin and ifosfamide. After only 2 cycles of chemotherapy, her disease progressed in the lungs and severe myelosuppression developed. Clinical investigation indicated that the patient could be a candidate for apatinib therapy. The MiniPDX tests with 4 different targeted drugs in 5 regimens showed that the lung metastasis responded to single agent apatinib and apatinib in combination with olapanib, but not to metformin, pazopanib or pazopanib combined with olapanib (Fig. 6a).

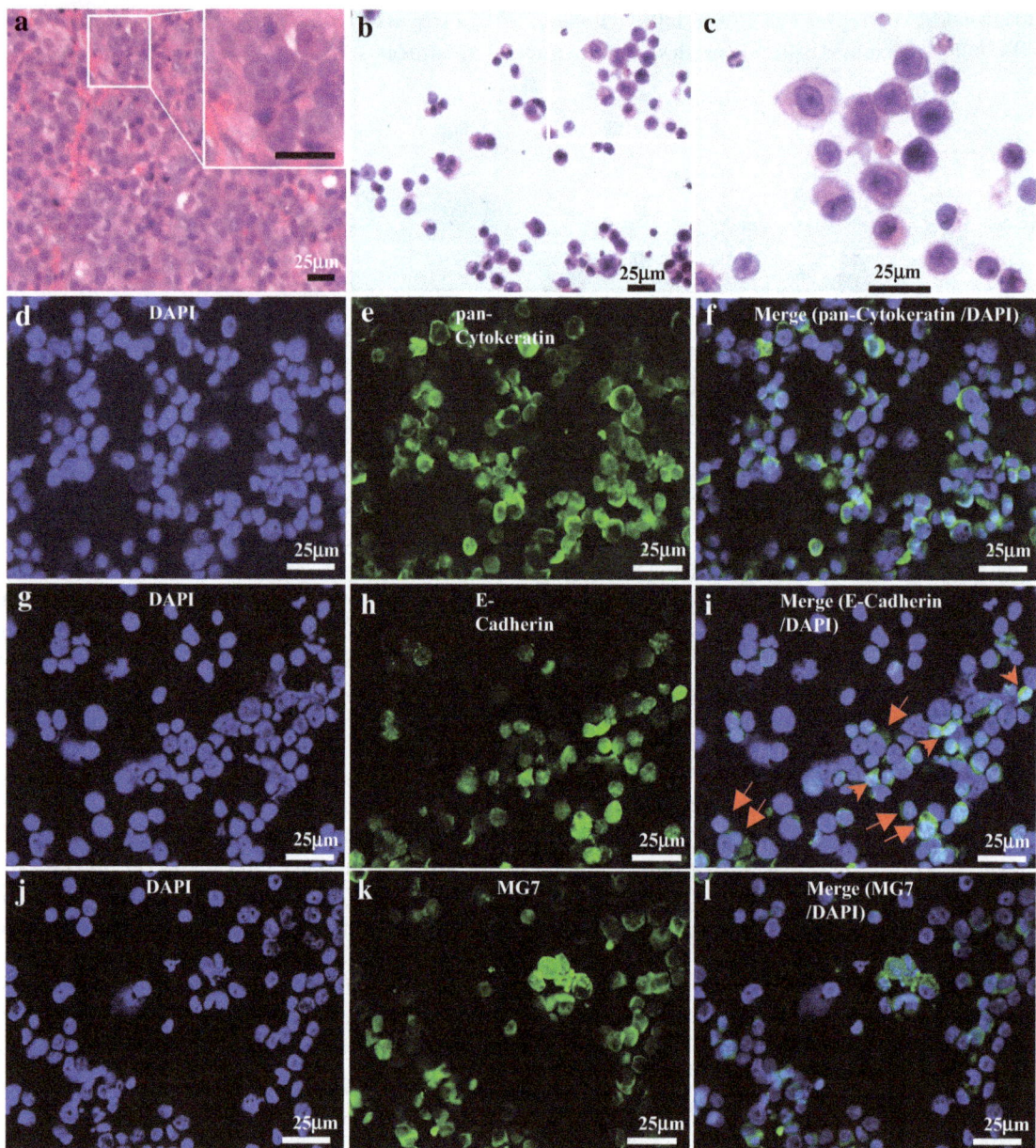

Fig. 2 Morphologic and immunohistochemical features of cells retrieved from the implanted capsules in MiniPDX-bearing mice. **a** Tissue section of a PDX xenograft tumor (GASI80) showing typical feature of poorly differentiated adenocarcinoma; inlet: High magnification view revealing tightly arranged poorly differentiated cells. **b, c** Cytospin of cells retrieved from the capsules implanted in MiniPDX-bearing mice, low- and high-power view, respectively (H&E stain), showing that the majority of the cells are associated with high nucleus to cytoplasm ratio, hyperchromatic nuclei, and scant cytoplasm. Immunofluorescent staining of pan-cytokeratin (**e**), E-cadherin (**h**) and MG7 (**i**); 4', 6-diamidino-2-phenylindole staining for individual panels (**d, g, j**). Merged images (**f, i, l**) show that the cells cultivated within the OncoVee® capsules expressed all of the three characteristic primary gastric cancer-related markers. Scale bars, 25 µm. The tumor cells cultivated in the MiniPDX capsules, which were derived from PDX tumor of gastric adenocarcinomas (PDX model GASI80, **a** H&E stain of tissue section), strongly expressed pan-cytokeratin (**e, f**) E-cadherin (**h, i**), and MG7 (**k, l**)

Indeed, 4 months post treatment, the patient achieved partial regression in her lung metastases that lasted for 8 months (Fig. 6b, c). The patient was currently being followed up.

Discussion

Experimental in vivo models that closely mimic the biology of cancer in patients are urgently needed to reliably predict optimal sensitivities to available regimens in personalized chemotherapy [9, 11, 16–22].

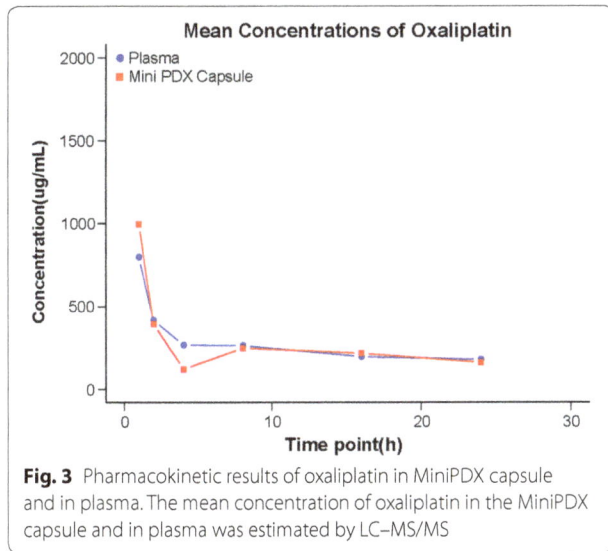

Fig. 3 Pharmacokinetic results of oxaliplatin in MiniPDX capsule and in plasma. The mean concentration of oxaliplatin in the MiniPDX capsule and in plasma was estimated by LC–MS/MS

Such models can yield drug test results within a short time frame to guide prompt cancer therapy [32–35]. The present study demonstrated that the MiniPDX sensitivity assay using fresh tumor samples is a rapid and effective alternative to the PDX model in capturing therapeutic responses of primary tumor tissues that mimic patient clinical therapeutic response and is of high predictive power with a sensitivity of 80% and a specificity of 93%.

The entire process of MiniPDX assay to test patient tumor response to chemotherapeutic or targeted drugs in immunodeficient mice can be completed within 7 days.

This is in contrast to duration of 4–8 months required for the PDX assay [8, 21, 23]. Recently, many patient-derived culture models such as patient-derived tumor organoid [4–6] and xenograft models have been utilized as rapid functional testing tools to predict therapeutic response. However, these ex vivo methods cannot mimic in vivo therapeutic response to systemically administered drugs in patients [36]. In addition, certain drugs can only be tested in vivo, not in vitro, as they undergo physiological metabolism before they become active. Thus, in vitro culturing assays such as patient derived tumor organoid cannot meet the need. In contrast, MiniPDX assays take the advantage of in vivo growth condition, which involves 3-dimentional growth (such as that in organoids), tumor microenvironment and tumor heterogeneity. Meanwhile, Mini-PDX-bearing mice received systemic drug administration as under clinical conditions. Thus, the MiniPDX assay is well positioned for wide clinical application in cancer precision medicine.

Streamlined conditions in MiniPDX assays allowed in vivo survival and growth of tumor cells, especially primary tumor cells of various cancer types, thus yielding a high success rate. According to our extensive MiniPDX studies, as long as quality control was met, a 100% success rate could be achieved using either PDX tumor grafts or surgically resected tumors, biopsy and thoracentesis specimens (Table 3 and Fig. 5a). The MiniPDX assay does not require prior PDX model establishment, which, a pre-requisite in in vivo PDX assay, often takes several months, and the model establishment rate is generally much lower than 50% [9, 15, 22].

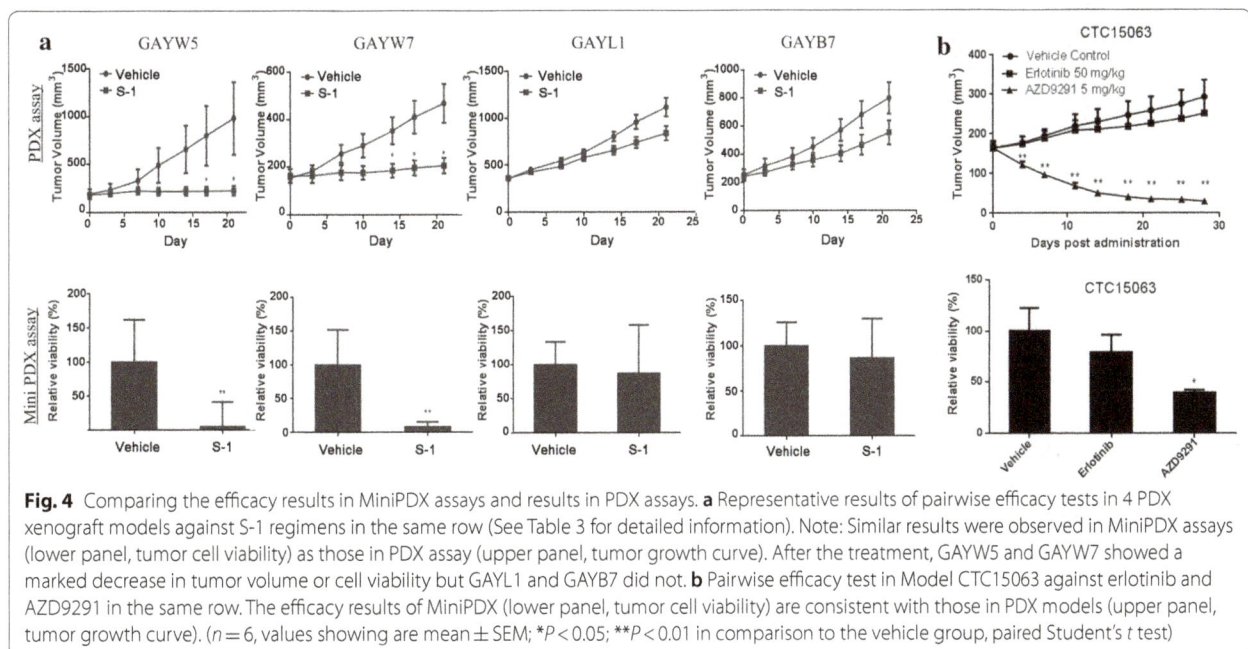

Fig. 4 Comparing the efficacy results in MiniPDX assays and results in PDX assays. **a** Representative results of pairwise efficacy tests in 4 PDX xenograft models against S-1 regimens in the same row (See Table 3 for detailed information). Note: Similar results were observed in MiniPDX assays (lower panel, tumor cell viability) as those in PDX assay (upper panel, tumor growth curve). After the treatment, GAYW5 and GAYW7 showed a marked decrease in tumor volume or cell viability but GAYL1 and GAYB7 did not. **b** Pairwise efficacy test in Model CTC15063 against erlotinib and AZD9291 in the same row. The efficacy results of MiniPDX (lower panel, tumor cell viability) are consistent with those in PDX models (upper panel, tumor growth curve). ($n=6$, values showing are mean ± SEM; *$P<0.05$; **$P<0.01$ in comparison to the vehicle group, paired Student's t test)

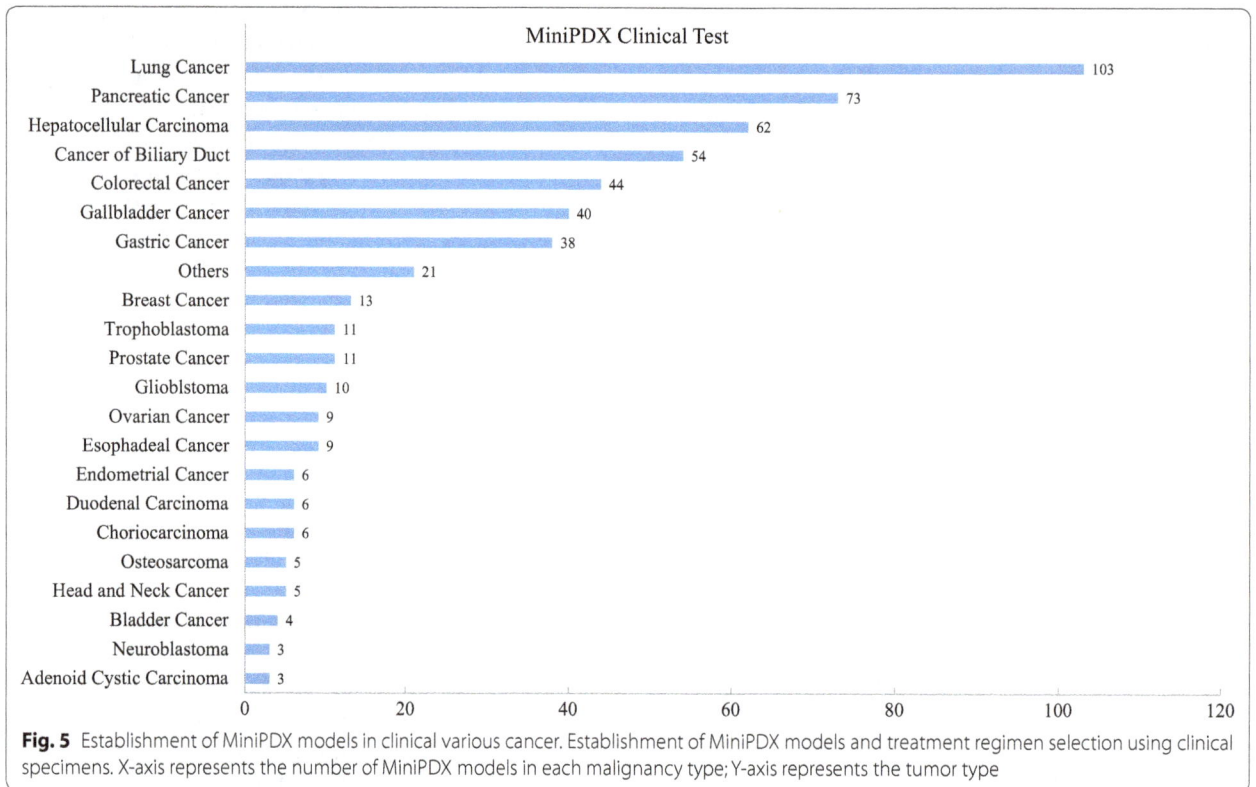

MiniPDX Clinical Test

Tumor type	Number
Lung Cancer	103
Pancreatic Cancer	73
Hepatocellular Carcinoma	62
Cancer of Biliary Duct	54
Colorectal Cancer	44
Gallbladder Cancer	40
Gastric Cancer	38
Others	21
Breast Cancer	13
Trophoblastoma	11
Prostate Cancer	11
Glioblstoma	10
Ovarian Cancer	9
Esophadeal Cancer	9
Endometrial Cancer	6
Duodenal Carcinoma	6
Choriocarcinoma	6
Osteosarcoma	5
Head and Neck Cancer	5
Bladder Cancer	4
Neuroblastoma	3
Adenoid Cystic Carcinoma	3

Fig. 5 Establishment of MiniPDX models in clinical various cancer. Establishment of MiniPDX models and treatment regimen selection using clinical specimens. X-axis represents the number of MiniPDX models in each malignancy type; Y-axis represents the tumor type

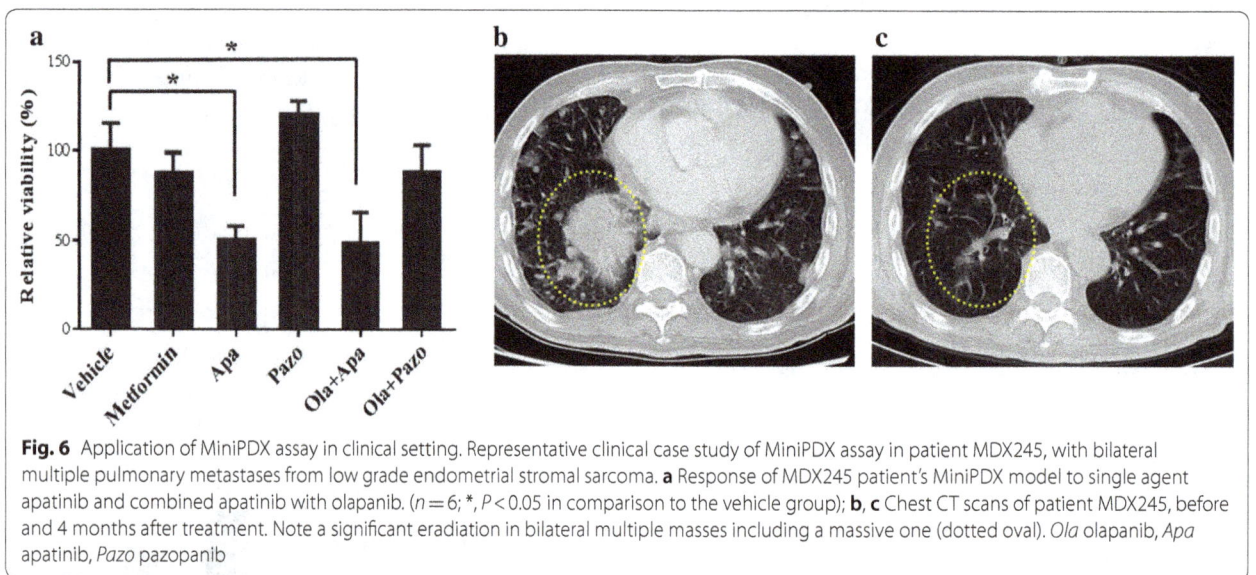

Fig. 6 Application of MiniPDX assay in clinical setting. Representative clinical case study of MiniPDX assay in patient MDX245, with bilateral multiple pulmonary metastases from low grade endometrial stromal sarcoma. **a** Response of MDX245 patient's MiniPDX model to single agent apatinib and combined apatinib with olapanib. ($n = 6$; *, $P < 0.05$ in comparison to the vehicle group); **b**, **c** Chest CT scans of patient MDX245, before and 4 months after treatment. Note a significant eradiation in bilateral multiple masses including a massive one (dotted oval). *Ola* olapanib, *Apa* apatinib, *Pazo* pazopanib

Tumor cells in the MiniPDX assays closely resemble parental primary tumors or original PDX tumors with regard to cancer type-specific morphologic and immunohistochemical features, as well as overall tumor heterogeneity (Fig. 2). During MiniPDX modeling tumor cells do not undergo any pressure selection like PDX tumor does during tumor engrafting in a host animal.

In the MiniPDX model, tumor cells were suspended in culture media and filled in implant capsules, which are made of hollow fiber membrane with a 500 kD pore size allowing molecules less than 500 kD to move in and out freely while keeping cells within the capsule. The surface of the implant membranes has been shown to be biocompatible in various animal models for periods exceeding 14 days [25, 26]. Recent studies using visualizing tools have demonstrated that tumor cells inside the fibers behave properly, including secreting cellular factors, communicating with the host mice and generating angiogenesis around cell-filled fibers. Furthermore, the fiber system delivers media to the cells in a manner akin to the delivery of blood through the capillary networks in vivo [37–39]. In addition, earlier studies of cell lines grown within the capsule, followed by implantation into a host animal, showed that human tumor cells are not subjected to host immunological attack [24]. In our streamlined conditions of MiniPDX assays, we observed that viability of untreated cells generally increased to 3 to 5 times after 7 days. Thus, MiniPDX assay holds high potential to evaluate various anticancer agents including antibody drugs. Collectively, tumor cells in MiniPDX are highly similar to original cancer cells with respect to phenotypic as well as molecular properties [27–30]. Clearly, the MiniPDX models used in this study are closely related to original malignancies, and assays based on such models for predicting drug responses would be highly relevant to the clinical situation.

For personalized chemotherapy, testing chemosensitivity for a few different chemotherapeutic regimens is desired for individual cancer patients. We have empirically determined that testing three drugs in Mini-PDX would require > 500 mm^3 tumor size and $\geq$ 70% tumor cell viability. The vast majority of cancer patients in which adjuvant chemotherapy is indicated according to the tumor-node-metastasis stage, have primary tumors of > 2 cm in diameter and thus providing sufficient tumor tissue for standard pathologic examination as well as for testing a variety of regimens in MiniPDX assays.

In summary, we developed, streamlined and validated a rapid systemic in vivo MiniPDX assay to predict clinical outcome. We systematically evaluated and compared the response rates of PDX assays and MiniPDX assays (Table 3) pair-wise in 26 PDX models of 3 types of cancers to 12 clinical relevant regimens, and we found a high correlation between drug responses of the two assays (Table 4). Although the sample tests were limited, our results indicated that the differential correlation response of the two assays could be present in different cancer types. We also confirmed this rapid testing method is feasible for various clinical samples to guide clinical treatment. Through a representative case of metastatic cancer patient, we demonstrated that clinical benefit was achieved using MiniPDX sensitivity results to guide clinical treatment.

Considering the current limited sample size and probable differential correlation response in different cancer types, several PI-initiated clinical trials for real world evidence (RWE) studies with FDA part 11 in compliance are registered and in progress for further evaluating the correlation between MiniPDX and clinical responses in a wide range of cancer types. The clinical effectiveness of proposed treatments, including determination of patient objective response rates, progression-free survival, and adverse effects, will be essential for expanding clinical usage of MiniPDX assays in personalized cancer precision treatment.

Table 4 Correlation response of MiniPDX _versus_ PDX assays in PDX models

	Response in PDX		
	R	NR	Total
Response in Mini-PDX			
R	12	1	13
NR	3	13	16
Total	15	14	29
Positive predictive value			92%
Negative predictive value			81%
Sensitivity			80%
Specificity			93%

R: responder; NR: non-responder

Conclusions

We developed a fast, systemic in vivo drug sensitivity assay, namely MiniPDX, in which patient primary tumor cells are capsulated and implanted in mouse to reliably and precisely test tumor responses to different antitumor drugs. MiniPDX method, as a complementary, if not an alternative, approach to PDX assay, is suitable for fast drug response assessment of primary cancer cells in order to select effective or to spare non-responding therapeutic regimens. MiniPDX holds promise to aid personalized therapy of cancer patients.

Abbreviations
PDX: patient-derived xenograft; MiniPDX: mini-patient-derived xenograft; TGI: tumor growth inhibition; TCGI: tumor cell growth inhibition; RLU: relative luminance unit; NCI: National Cancer Institute; RWE: real world evidence; IACUC: the Institutional Animal Care and Use Committees; H&E: hematoxylin and eosin; MEHFC: microencapsulation and hollow fiber culture; AC: adenocarcinoma; SCC: squamous cell carcinoma; LCC: large cell carcinoma; Ola: olapanib; Apa: apatinib; Pazo: pazopanib; po: oral; ip: intraperitoneal; qd: once a day; biw: twice a week; qw: once a week; q4d: once every 4 days.

Authors' contributions
Conceptualization, DW, FZ, YL, JC; Methodology and Validation, FZ, YL, HL; Investigation, JC, FZ, YL, LG; Clinical design, HW, QZ, SL, LW; Writing-and Editing, WW, JC, FZ, YL, HL, DW. All authors read and approved the final manuscript.

Author details
[1] Shanghai LIDE Biotech Co., LTD, Shanghai 201203, P. R. China. [2] Department of Surgery, Xijing Hospital, The Fourth Military Medical University, Xi'an 710032,

P. R. China. [3] Department of Oncology, Shanghai Chest Hospital Affiliated to Shanghai Jiao Tong University, Shanghai 200030, P. R. China. [4] The Second Hospital of Tianjin Medical University, Tianjin Key Laboratory of Urology, Tianjin 300211, P. R. China.

Acknowledgements
The authors thank Dr. Yurong Qu, Panpan Bao and Jie Liu for their technical assistance, and Dr. Xiaoqing Pan and Yang Yang for project co-ordination. We thank Professor Gang Zhao at Renji Hospital, School of Medicine, Shanghai Jiao Tong University for kindly support. We are also grateful to Professor Yongzhan Nie at the State Key Laboratory of Cancer Biology & Institute of Digestive Diseases, the Fourth Military Medical University, for helpful discussion and for providing MG7 antibody.

Competing interests
The authors declare that they have no competing interests.

Funding
Not applicable.

References
1. Letai A. Functional precision cancer medicine-moving beyond pure genomics. Nat Med. 2017;23(9):1028–35.
2. Pauli Chantal, Hopkins Benjamin D, Prandi Davide, Shaw Reid, Fedrizzi Tarcisio, Sboner Andrea, et al. Personalized in vitro and in vivo cancer models to guide precision medicine. Cancer Discov. 2017;7(5):1–16.
3. Friedman AA, Letai A, Fisher DE, Flaherty KT. Precision medicine for cancer with next-generation functional diagnostics. Nat Rev Cancer. 2015;15(12):747–56.
4. Vlachogiannis Georgios, Hedayat Somaieh, Vatsiou Alexandra, Jamin Yann, Fernandez-Mateos Javier, Khan Khurum, et al. Patient-derived organoids model treatment response of metastatic gastrointestinal cancers. Science. 2018;359:920–6.
5. Lee Suk Hyung, Wenhuo Hu, Matulay Justin T, Silva Mark V, Owczarek Tomasz B, Kim Kwanghee, et al. Tumor evolution and drug response in patient-derived organoid models of bladder cancer. Cell. 2018;173:515–28.
6. Sachs Norman, de Ligt Joep, Kopper Oded, Gogola Ewa, Bounova Gergana, Weeber Fleur, et al. A living biobank of breast cancer organoids captures disease heterogeneity. Cell. 2018;172:1–14.
7. Suggitt M, Bibby MC. 50 years of preclinical anticancer drug screening: empirical to target-driven approaches. Clin Cancer Res. 2005;11(3):971–81.
8. Rubio-Viqueira B, Jimeno A, Cusatis G, Zhang X, Iacobuzio-Donahue C, Karikari C, et al. An in vivo platform for translational drug development in pancreatic cancer. Clin Cancer Res. 2006;12(15):4652–61.
9. Zhang X, Claerhout S, Prat A, Dobrolecki LE, Petrovic I, Lai Q, et al. A renewable tissue resource of phenotypically stable, biologically and ethnically diverse, patient-derived human breast cancer xenograft models. Cancer Res. 2013;73:4885–97.
10. Bruna A, Rueda OM, Greenwood W, Batra AS, Callari M, Batra RN, et al. A biobank of breast cancer explants with preserved intra-tumor heterogeneity to screen anticancer compounds. Cell. 2016;167(1):260–74.
11. Bertotti A, Migliardi G, Galimi F, Sassi F, Torti D, Isella C, et al. A molecularly annotated platform of patient-derived xenografts ("xenopatients") identifies HER2 as an effective therapeutic target in cetuximab-resistant colorectal cancer. Cancer Discov. 2011;1:508–23.
12. Calles A, Rubio-Viqueira B, Hidalgo M. Primary human non-small cell lung and pancreatic tumorgraft models—utility and applications in drug discovery and tumor biology. Curr Protoc Pharmacol. 2013;Chapter 14:Unit 14.26.
13. Bihani T, Patel HK, Arlt H, Tao N, Jiang H, Brown JL, et al. Elacestrant (RAD1901), a selective estrogen receptor degrader (SERD), has antitumor activity in multiple ER+ breast cancer patient-derived xenograft models. Clin Cancer Res. 2017;23(16):4793–804.
14. Crystal AS, Shaw AT, Sequist LV, Friboulet L, Niederst MJ, Lockerman EL, et al. Patient-derived models of acquired resistance can identify effective drug combinations for cancer. Science. 2014;346:1480–6.
15. Lang H, Béraud C, Bethry A, Danilin S, Lindner V, Coquard C, et al. Establishment of a large panel of patient-derived preclinical models of human renal cell carcinoma. Oncotarget. 2016;7(37):59336–59.
16. Ricci F, Bizzaro F, Cesca M, Guffanti F, Ganzinelli M, Decio A, et al. Patient derived ovarian tumor xenografts recapitulate human clinicopathology and genetic alterations. Cancer Res. 2014;74:6980–90.
17. Marangoni E, Vincent-Salomon A, Auger N, Degeorges A, Assayag F, de Cremoux P, et al. A new model of patient tumor-derived breast cancer xenografts for preclinical assays. Clin Cancer Res. 2007;13:3989–98.
18. Topp MD, Hartley L, Cook M, Heong V, Boehm E, McShane L, et al. Molecular correlates of platinum response in human high-grade serous ovarian cancer patient-derived xenografts. Mol Oncol. 2014;8:656–68.
19. Huynh H, Ong R, Zopf D. Antitumor activity of the multikinase inhibitor regorafenib in patient-derived xenograft models of gastric cancer. J Exp Clin Cancer Res. 2015;34:132.
20. Nunes M, Vrignaud P, Vacher S, Richon S, Lievre A, Cacheux W, et al. Evaluating patient-derived colorectal cancer-xenografts as preclinical models by comparison with patient clinical data. Cancer Res. 2015;75:1560–6.
21. Hidalgo M, Bruckheimer E, Rajeshkumar NV, Garrido-Laguna I, De Oliveira E, Rubio-Viqueira B, et al. A pilot clinical study of treatment guided by personalized tumorgrafts in patients with advanced cancer. Mol Cancer Ther. 2011;10(8):1311–6.
22. Massimo M, Giulia B, Roberto C, Cristina B, Mattia B, Alessandra F, et al. Establishment of patient derived xenografts as functional testing of lung cancer aggressiveness. Sci Rep. 2017;7(1):6689.
23. Stebbing J, Paz K, Schwartz GK, Wexler LH, Maki R, Pollock RE, et al. Patient-derived xenografts for individualized care in advanced sarcoma. Cancer. 2014;120(13):2006–15.
24. Hollingshead MG, Alley MC, Camalier RF, et al. In vivo cultivation of tumor cells in hollow fibres. Life Sci. 1995;57:131–41.
25. Monga M, Sausville EA. Developmental therapeutics program at the NCI: molecular target and drug discovery process. Leukemia. 2002;16(4):520–6.
26. Lee KH, Rhee KH. Correlative effect between in vivo hollow fiber assay and xenografts assay in drug screening. Cancer Res Treat. 2005;37(3):196–200.
27. Hwang CS, Ahn S, Lee BE, Lee SJ, Kim A, Choi CI, et al. Risk of lymph node metastasis in mixed-type early gastric cancer determined by the extent of the poorly differentiated component. World J Gastroenterol. 2016;22(15):4020–6.
28. Carboni F, Levi Sandri GB, Valle M, Covello R, Garofalo A. Gastric sarcomatoid carcinoma. J Gastrointest Surg. 2013;17(11):2025–7.
29. Baniak N, Senger JL, Ahmed S, Kanthan SC, Kanthan R. Gastric biomarkers: a global review. World J Surg Oncol. 2016;14:212.
30. Xu B, Li X, Yin J, Liang C, Liu L, Qiu Z, et al. Evaluation of ^{68}Ga-labeled MG7 antibody: a targeted probe for PET/CT imaging of gastric cancer. Sci Rep. 2015;5:8626.
31. Yunhua Xu, Zhang Feifei, Pan Xiaoqing, Wang Guan, Zhu Lei, Zhang Jie, et al. Xenograft tumors derived from malignant pleural effusion of the patients with non-small-cell-lung cancer as models to explore drug resistance. Cancer Commun. 2018;38(1):19.
32. Biondi A, Lirosi MC, D'Ugo D, Fico V, Ricci R, Santullo F, et al. Neo-adjuvant chemo(radio)therapy in gastric cancer: current status and future perspectives. World J Gastrointest Oncol. 2015;7(12):389–400.
33. Chan BA, Jang RW, Wong RK, Swallow CJ, Darling GE, Elimova E. Improving outcomes in resectable gastric cancer: a review of current and future strategies. Oncology. 2016;30(7):635–45.
34. Nagasaka M, Gadgeel SM. Role of chemotherapy and targeted therapy in early-stage non-small cell lung cancer. Expert Rev Anticancer Ther. 2018;18(1):63–70.
35. Vreeland TJ, Katz MHG. Timing of pancreatic resection and patient outcomes: is there a difference? Surg Clin North Am. 2018;98(1):57–71.
36. Meijer TG, Naipal KA, Jager A, van Gent DC. Ex vivo tumor culture systems for functional drug testing and therapy response prediction. Future Sci OA. 2017;3(2):FSO190.
37. Suggitt M, Swaine DJ, Pettit GR, Bibby MC. Characterization of the hollow fiber assay for the determination of microtubule disruption in vivo. Clin Cancer Res. 2004;10:6677–85.

10

When fats commit crimes: fatty acid metabolism, cancer stemness and therapeutic resistance

Ching-Ying Kuo[1]* and David K. Ann[2,3]*

Abstract

The role of fatty acid metabolism, including both anabolic and catabolic reactions in cancer has gained increasing attention in recent years. Many studies have shown that aberrant expression of the genes involved in fatty acid synthesis or fatty acid oxidation correlate with malignant phenotypes including metastasis, therapeutic resistance and relapse. Such phenotypes are also strongly associated with the presence of a small percentage of unique cells among the total tumor cell population. This distinct group of cells may have the ability to self-renew and propagate or may be able to develop resistance to cancer therapies independent of genetic alterations. Therefore, these cells are referred to as cancer stem cells/tumor-initiating cells/drug-tolerant persisters, which are often refractory to cancer treatment and difficult to target. Moreover, interconversion between cancer cells and cancer stem cells/tumor-initiating cells/drug-tolerant persisters may occur and makes treatment even more challenging. This review highlights recent findings on the relationship between fatty acid metabolism, cancer stemness and therapeutic resistance and prompts discussion about the potential mechanisms by which fatty acid metabolism regulates the fate of cancer cells and therapeutic resistance.

Keywords: Fatty acid synthesis, Fatty acid oxidation, Fatty acid metabolism, Lipogenic phenotype, Cancer stem cells, Tumor-initiating cells, Cancer cell plasticity, Therapeutic resistance, Drug-tolerant persisters

Background

Fatty acid (FA) metabolism is composed of anabolic and catabolic processes that maintain energy homeostasis. FA synthesis, which converts various types of nutrients into metabolic intermediates, is essential for cellular processes such as maintaining cell membrane structure and function, storing energy and mediating signaling. Cells generate energy by breaking down FAs via FA oxidation (FAO), also known as β-oxidation [1, 2]. A loss of balance between FA synthesis and oxidation may result in inadequate FA levels, leading to lipid accumulation. Lipid accumulation has been observed in many types of cancer, including brain, breast, ovarian and colorectal cancers [3–5] and has recently drawn increased attention. This has motivated scientists to understand the molecular mechanisms by which FA metabolism participates in the pathophysiological processes of cancer.

Cancer stem cells (CSCs), also referred to as tumor-initiating cells (TICs), have been identified in many types of solid tumors and often result in tumor recurrence because of their self-renewal and tumorigenic properties. CSCs/TICs can be defined by in vitro tumorsphere formation assays and in vivo limiting dilution assays in conjunction with surface marker analyses [6, 7]. How CSCs originate remains under debate. Possible explanations are that: (1) adult stem cells acquire mutations to become malignant or (2) neoplastic, differentiated cells receive external stimuli and undergo reprogramming to a progenitor or stem-like state [8]. Recent findings on the interconversion of neoplastic

*Correspondence: cykuo27@ntu.edu.tw; dann@coh.org
[1] Department of Clinical Laboratory Sciences and Medical Biotechnology, College of Medicine, National Taiwan University, Taipei 10048, Taiwan, China
[2] Department of Diabetes Complications and Metabolism, Diabetes and Metabolism Research Institute, Beckman Research Institute, City of Hope, Duarte, CA 91010, USA
Full list of author information is available at the end of the article

epithelial cells to CSC-like cells within a mixed tumor population suggest that a dynamic reprogramming process may occur during the transition state [9–12]. This bidirectional conversion or so-called cancer cell plasticity may emerge as a challenge for cancer treatment [13, 14]. Therefore, delineating the mechanisms of cancer cell plasticity and identifying regulators of the process that can be manipulated to prevent the conversion of cancer cells to CSCs may reduce the incidence of cancer recurrence.

A similar idea applies to the development of therapeutic resistance. Cancer treatments typically kill most fast-growing tumor cells. However, a subpopulation of cells may become tolerant of the drug, enter a state of dormancy and later evolve mechanisms of resistance. The cells in this small population are called drug-tolerant persisters (DTPs) and are considered independent from cells that acquire mutations to develop resistance. The interconversion between the drug-sensitive state and the tolerant state is thought to be controlled by growth factor signaling or epigenetic regulation [15–18]. For example, DTPs arising from tyrosine kinase inhibitor-resistant lung cancer cells are regulated by insulin growth factor signaling and a lysine demethylase, KDM5A [18]. In addition, these DTPs express the stem cell marker CD133 and share some of the CSC properties. Therefore, when appropriate, CSCs/TICs/DTPs will be used hereafter to describe the small populations of cells possessing the abilities to confer drug resistance and to repopulate. Understanding the mechanisms by which cancer cells progress into CSCs/TICs/DTPs will offer opportunities to prevent therapeutic resistance.

The plasticity of cancer cells and the genetic-independent acquisition of therapeutic resistance may be tightly associated with metabolic reprogramming. Altered metabolism is one of the hallmarks of cancer and has also been observed in CSCs (reviews in [19–22]). Hirsch et al. have shown that metformin, a blood sugar-lowering drug specifically targets breast CSCs and sensitizes CSCs to doxorubicin [23]. Metformin not only activates AMP-activated kinase (AMPK), but also inhibits complex I of the mitochondrial respiratory chain [24], suggesting that CSCs may have distinct metabolic features that are targetable. A study reveals that the loss of fructose-1,6-biphosphatase (FBP1) in basal-like breast cancer inhibits oxidative phosphorylation (OXPHOS), increases glycolysis and CSC properties [25]. Moreover, mesenchymal glioma stem cells derived from clinical specimens demonstrate elevated glycolytic activity. In contrast, mitochondrial biogenesis and OXPHOS are also critical for maintaining CSC populations [26, 27]. These findings suggest that there is metabolic plasticity in the CSC population and that modulating the utilization of metabolic

pathways could influence the tumorigenic capacity of tumor cells.

While increasing evidence has revealed the role of altered energy metabolism during cancer progression, relatively fewer studies have focused on FA metabolism. In this review, we aim to evaluate recent studies and to summarize their findings on the role of FA metabolism in cancer malignant phenotypes, especially therapeutic resistance and stemness. We wish to stimulate discussion of the mechanisms by which cancer cells may acquire malignant properties via altered FA metabolism.

Fatty acid metabolism in cancer progression and therapeutic resistance

The lipogenic phenotype is one of the metabolic hallmarks of cancer. First observed in the 1950s, de novo FA synthesis is the major source of FAs for cancer cells [28]. Rapidly growing cancer cells require relatively large amounts of FAs to support processes such as membrane formation and signaling. Cytosolic acetyl-CoA is the building block for FAs, and can be generated from citrate or acetate. Citrate comes from either glycolysis followed by the tricarboxylic acid (TCA) cycle or from glutaminolysis followed by reductive carboxylation; it is then cleaved by ATP-citrate lyase (ACLY) to form cytosolic acetyl-CoA and oxaloacetate. Acetate obtained from either external or internal sources is ligated to CoA by acyl-CoA synthetase short-chain family member 2 (ACSS2) to form acetyl-CoA. Next, acetyl-CoA is carboxylated by acetyl-CoA carboxylase (ACC) to form malonyl-CoA. This is followed by a series of condensation processes catalyzed by fatty acid synthase (FASN) in the presence of nicotinamide adenine dinucleotide phosphate (NADPH) to primarily produce palmitate for subsequent FA elongation, desaturation and lipid synthesis [1, 29] (Fig. 1).

In tumors, many lipogenic enzymes are up-regulated and correlate with cancer progression (Fig. 1). Overexpression of *FASN* has been frequently reported in a wide variety of cancers, including breast, ovarian, endometrial and prostate cancers, and is associated with poor prognosis and resistance to chemotherapy [29–35]. For example, increased expression of *FASN* is associated with resistance to cisplatin in breast and ovarian cancers and the resistance can be reversed by blocking FASN with an inhibitor, C75 [30, 31]. FASN increases DNA repair activity by up-regulating poly(ADP-ribose) polymerase 1 resulting in resistance to genotoxic agents [35]. In cancer cells, expression of FASN is modulated by sterol regulatory element-binding protein 1c (SREBP1) and proto-oncogene *FBI-I* (Pokemon) via dysregulated mitogen activated protein kinase or phosphoinositide 3-kinase/AKT pathways under hormonal or nutritional regulation [1, 36]. FASN expression can

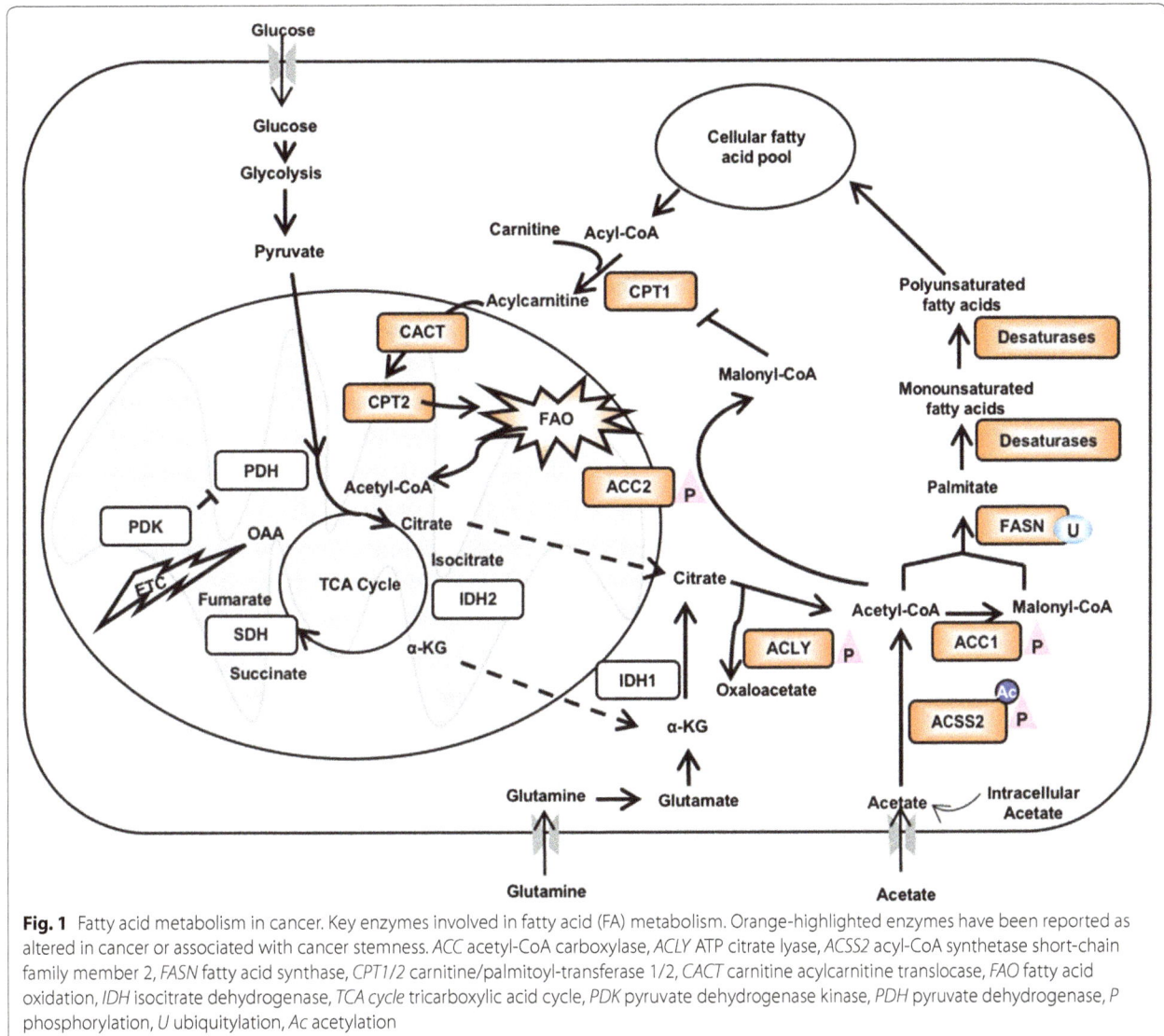

Fig. 1 Fatty acid metabolism in cancer. Key enzymes involved in fatty acid (FA) metabolism. Orange-highlighted enzymes have been reported as altered in cancer or associated with cancer stemness. *ACC* acetyl-CoA carboxylase, *ACLY* ATP citrate lyase, *ACSS2* acyl-CoA synthetase short-chain family member 2, *FASN* fatty acid synthase, *CPT1/2* carnitine/palmitoyl-transferase 1/2, *CACT* carnitine acylcarnitine translocase, *FAO* fatty acid oxidation, *IDH* isocitrate dehydrogenase, *TCA cycle* tricarboxylic acid cycle, *PDK* pyruvate dehydrogenase kinase, *PDH* pyruvate dehydrogenase, *P* phosphorylation, *U* ubiquitylation, *Ac* acetylation

also be regulated post-translationally. The deubiquit-inase USP2a is often up-regulated and stabilizes FASN in prostate cancer [37].

ACLY serves as a central hub for connecting glucose and glutamine metabolism with lipogenesis and initiating the first step of FA synthesis [38]. Elevated *ACLY* levels have been observed in gastric, breast, colorectal and ovarian cancers and are linked to malignant phenotypes and poorer prognosis [39–42]. In particular, overexpression of *ACLY* in colorectal cancer leads to resistance to SN38, an active metabolite of irinotecan [42]. Like *FASN*, the transcription of *ACLY* is also regulated by SREBP1 [43], and it can be regulated post-translationally. Phosphorylation at ACLY serine 454 by AKT is increased in lung cancer and is correlated with enhanced activity of ACLY [44]. ACLY can also

be phosphorylated by cAMP-dependent protein kinase and nucleoside diphosphate kinase [45, 46].

Overexpression of *ACC* has been found in breast, gastric and lung cancers [47–49]. Mammals express two isoforms of ACC, ACC1 and ACC2, which have distinct roles in regulating FA metabolism. ACC1 is present in the cytoplasm, where it converts acetyl-CoA to malonyl-CoA. ACC2 is localized to the mitochondrial membrane, where it prevents acyl-CoA from being imported into the mitochondria through carnitine/palmitoyl-transferase 1 (CPT1) for FAO and entering the TCA cycle to generate energy. Both ACC1 and ACC2 can be regulated transcriptionally and post-translationally by multiple physiological factors, including hormones and nutrients [50, 51]. mRNA expression of *ACC1* and *ACC2* is regulated by SREBP1, carbohydrate-responsive element-binding protein and liver X receptors [52, 53]. Additionally, ACC1 and ACC2 can be phosphorylated at serine 80 (serine 79 in mouse) and serine 222 (serine 212 in mouse), respectively, by tumor suppressor AMPK to inhibit their activities under ATP-depleted condition [50, 54–57]. The phosphorylation at serine 80 of ACC1 is associated with a metastatic phenotype in breast and lung cancers and is also responsible for resistance to cetuximab in head and neck cancer [58, 59].

There are 26 genes encoding acyl-CoA synthetase, which have distinct affinities for short-, medium-, long- or very long-chain FAs [60]. Overexpression of cyto-solic ACSS2, one of the three family members of short chain acyl-CoA synthetase, can lead to acetate addiction in breast, ovarian, lung and brain cancers when nutrients or oxygen are limited; this overexpression is correlated with cancer progression and worse progno-sis [61–63]. Mitochondrial ACSS1 is up-regulated in hepatocellular carcinoma and is associated with tumor growth and malignancy [64]. Although the regulation of ACSS expression remains poorly understood, it has been reported that ACSS genes are controlled by SREBP [65, 66].

In addition to the highly activated lipogenic pathway, FA catabolism is also important for maintaining cancer cell survival and contributing to chemotherapy resist-ance. The mitochondrial inner membrane is imperme-able to long-chain acyl-CoAs; thus, the CPT system is required for transporting long-chain acyl-CoAs into the mitochondria from the cytoplasm. Three components are involved in this transporting system: CPT1, the car-nitine acylcarnitine translocase (CACT) and CPT2 [67]. There are three currently known isoforms of CPT1 dis-tributed in different tissues: CPT1A, CPT1B and CPT1C [68]. Knockdown of CPT1A leads to down-regulation of mTOR signaling and increases of apoptosis, suggest-ing CPT1A promotes the growth of prostate cancer cells [69]. Moreover, CPT1A depletion can sensitize prostate cancer cells to anti-androgen treatment, enzalutamide [70]. It has also been reported that CPT1A is positively correlated with histone deacetylase activity to enhance the tumorigenesis of breast cancer [71]. The expres-sion of CPT1A can be regulated by nuclear receptors, PPARs and the PPARγ coactivator (PGC-1) [72]. PPARs have also been implicated as playing important roles in cancer progression [73]. CPT1A has also been shown to support the proliferation of leukemic cells and the knockdown or inhibition of CPT1A by a pharmacologi-cal inhibitor etomoxir (ETO) sensitizes leukemic cells to a chemotherapeutic drug, cytarabine [74]. In addition to CPT1A, AMPK regulates CPT1C expression to promote tumor growth upon metabolic stress in several types of cancer cells. Down-regulation of CPT1C enhances the

sensitivity to mTOR inhibitor, rapamycin in cancer cells [75]. Only a few studies have reported the dysregulated CPT1B expression in colorectal and bladder cancers [76, 77]. A recent study has revealed the relationship between STAT3-induced CPT1B expression and chemoresistance in breast cancer cells [78].

In comparison to CPT1, relatively less studies have pointed out the roles of CPT2 and CACT in cancer. Knockdown of CPT2 significantly impedes the growth of MYC-overexpressing triple-negative breast can-cer (TNBC) cells [79]. Another report also shows that depletion of CPT2 hinders TNBC growth via the down-regulation of the phosphorylated Src levels [80]. These data suggest an oncogenic role of CPT2 in TNBC. On the other hand, a meta-analysis has revealed that higher CPT2 expression is correlated with better outcome in colorectal cancer patients [81]. CACT has been found to be overexpressed in prostate cancer cells and down-regu-lated in bladder cancer [76, 82]. Therefore, the exact role of CACT in cancer progression and therapeutic resist-ance remains uncertain.

Fatty acid synthesis and cancer stemness
Similar to the expression patterns of lipogenic genes in cancer cells, several lipogenic genes are dysregulated in CSCs and are critical for CSC expansion and survival. However, how these genes are regulated in CSCs and why CSCs depend upon their lipogenic potential require fur-ther investigation. A recent study reported that glioma stem cells prefer to utilize glucose and acetate as carbon sources, compared with differentiated glioma cells [83]. In that study, FASN was concurrently expressed with glioma stem cell markers, including SOX2, CD133 and Nestin. In glioma stem cells, inhibition of FASN by the fatty acid synthesis inhibitor cerulenin decreases expres-sion of glioma stem cell markers and reduces the number of tumorspheres formed [83]. In pancreatic CSCs, FASN is up-regulated and the inhibition efficacy of cerulenin is greater on pancreatic CSCs than on pancreatic cancer cells [84]. In breast CSCs, down-regulation of FASN by metformin via the induction of miR-193b leads to inhi-bition of mammosphere formation [85]. The antioxidant-like plant polyphenol resveratrol also decreases FASN to promote apoptosis in breast CSCs [86]. Taken together, these studies suggest that FASN is involved in promoting CSC survival.

ACLY also plays an important role in CSCs. In an in vitro lung cancer cell model, knockdown of ACLY inhibits epithelial–mesenchymal transition (EMT), a phenomenon often linked to cancer stemness, and results in a decrease of tumorsphere formation [87]. Treating MCF7 breast cancer cells with soraphen A, a specific inhibitor of ACC, significantly reduces the population of CSCs, as defined by CSC marker ALDEFLUOR. The effects of this inhibition are even greater in MCF7 cells overexpressing the proto-oncogene human epidermal growth factor receptor 2 (HER2) [88].

Elevated levels of unsaturated FAs have been observed in ovarian CSCs and it was recently reported that desaturases control the fate of ovarian CSCs [89, 90]. In these studies, inhibition of desaturases by CAY10566 or SC-26196 diminishes cancer stemness by reducing stemness markers, including SCD1, ALDH1A1 and SOX2. Blockade of FA desaturation impairs NF-κB signaling, which also directly regulates the unsaturation of FAs.

FAO and cancer stemness

FAO is composed of a cyclical series of catabolic reactions and results in the shortening of fatty acids (two carbons per cycle). It is an essential source of reduced nicotinamide adenine dinucleotide (NADH), flavin adenine dinucleotide (FADH2), NADPH and ATP. NADH and FADH2 enter the electron transport chain to produce ATP, and NADPH protects cancer cells against metabolic stress and hypoxia [67]. As the key rate-limiting enzyme of FAO, CPT1 conjugates fatty acids with carnitine for translocation into the mitochondria; therefore, it controls FAO directly and thus facilitates cancer metabolic reprogramming. CPT1 also shares multiple connections with many other cellular signaling pathways often dysregulated in cancers, such as aerobic glycolysis, FAS, p53/AMPK axis, mutated RAS, mTOR and STAT3 [91, 92]. This evidence positions CPT1 as a multifunctional mediator in cancer pathogenesis and resistance to treatment.

In HER2-positive breast cancer cells, pharmacological inhibition of PPARγ by GW9662 results in a decrease in CSC number and down-regulated expression of CSC markers, presumably via increased production of reactive oxygen species (ROS) [93]. Whether the effects of PPARγ inhibition perturb the activity of FAO in HER2-positive breast CSCs remains unclear.

An interesting phenomenon has been observed in both leukemia and breast cancer. In leukemic cells, FAO is uncoupled from ATP synthesis and FA synthesis is enhanced to support FAO. Therefore, inhibiting FAO using ETO reduces the numbers of quiescent leukemic progenitors, which are able to initiate leukemia in the immune-deficient mice [74]. In breast cancer cells, prolonged treatment with the metabolic intermediate dimethyl α-ketoglutarate (DKG) leads to accumulation of succinate and fumarate, which induces hypoxia-inducible factor 1α (HIF-1α) to promote both glycolysis and OXPHOS to enable the plasticity of breast cancer cells. However, the increased OXPHOS is uncoupled from

ATP synthesis and can be dampened by ETO, so the detected oxygen consumption presumably comes from FAO. Moreover, inhibiting both glycolysis and FAO by dichloroacetate and ETO respectively can decrease DKG-induced tumorsphere formation and accumulation of FAs was observed in DKG-treated breast cancer cells, suggesting that increased FAs may be utilized to support FAO [94]. It is likely that FA synthesis and FAO feed-forward with one another. Additional possible sources of FAs may come from reductive carboxylation [95, 96] or extracellular lysophospholipids through macropinocytosis [97]. Indeed, altered lipid metabolism appears to play a role in TNBC: TNBC and non-TNBC patient tissues can be discriminated based on markers of lipid metabolism [98, 99].

NANOG, a transcription factor and known stem cell marker, was recently reported to promote mitochondrial FAO in CSCs and support liver oncogenesis and drug resistance [100]. In that report, inhibition of FAO by ETO limits the expansion of CSCs and sensitizes CSCs to sorafenib kinase inhibitor treatment. In this case, it is possible that NANOG-positive cells become CSCs/TICs/DTPs to exert resistance to sorafenib. How NANOG regulates FAO and how FAO promote resistance warrant further investigation.

More recently, breast adipocyte-derived leptin was shown to activate JAK/STAT3 signaling through the leptin receptor to up-regulate *CPT1B*, leading to enhanced FAO in breast CSCs [78]. FAO is critical for maintaining breast CSCs and is associated with chemoresistance. Blocking FAO with perhexiline, an FDA-approved drug for treatment of angina and heart failure [101], can sensitize chemoresistant breast cancer cells to the mitotic inhibitor paclitaxel.

Perspectives

CSCs/TICs, a minor population of cells capable of self-renewal and tumor initiation, are tightly associated with cancer relapse, metastasis and chemoresistance. The theory of CSC origin is currently based on two models: hierarchical and stochastic. The classic hierarchical model suggests that only a subset of cancer cells has the ability to self-renew and divide [8, 102]. On the other hand, accumulating evidence supports the stochastic model that every cancer cell has the potential to be reprogrammed into a CSC when the appropriate cues are present [9–12]. DTPs are a relatively new concept in cancer treatment resistance. This subpopulation is responsible for the development of drug resistance and shares similar properties with CSCs/TICs, but does not fully resemble them. The chromatin state is altered in DTPs [18], suggesting that the chromatin has undergone remodeling, leading to reprogramming. However, how cancer cells are reprogrammed and what the appropriate cues are remain largely unknown. Aberrant FA metabolism in cancer has also been correlated with malignant phenotypes, poor prognosis and chemoresistance. Dysregulation of FA metabolism not only accumulates FAs, but also generates extra metabolic intermediates, which may be utilized as signaling molecules for enhancing oncogenic signaling. In the previous sections, we summarized irregular FA metabolism in CSCs/TICs. However, the exact mechanism of FA metabolism in regulating CSCs/TICs/DTPs survival and expansion remains unclear. Understanding whether FAs serve as building blocks for CSCs/TICs/DTPs and/or whether the metabolic intermediates generated from FA metabolism are important signaling molecules for maintaining CSCs/TICs/DTPs or reprogramming cancer cells to CSCs/TICs/DTPs has implications for combating cancer therapeutic resistance.

How FA metabolism is regulated in CSCs also remains an outstanding question. Since FAs are not only important nutrients in human metabolism but also play a significant role in the composition of lipid bilayer membranes, it is likely that FA metabolism determines cell fate in a growing number of physiological and pathological conditions. The therapeutic manipulation of FAO holds great promise for the diagnosis and treatment of a wide range of human diseases in clinical settings. The master regulator of FA synthesis, SREBP1, regulates FASN expression to activate FA synthesis in cancer cells [1]. However, very little is known about the role of SREBP1 in CSCs/TICs/DTPs. SREBP1 binds to c-Myc to promote pluripotent gene expression in somatic cells [103], suggesting a potential role for SREBP1 in promoting cancer stemness. In breast cancer cells, leptin and transforming growth factor β (TGFβ) co-regulate AMPK-mediated ACC phosphorylation, implying that FAO is also affected by these signals [58]. Leptin signaling can also increase *CPT1B* expression via the JAK/STAT3 pathway to promote FAO [78]. Both leptin and TGFβ are secreted by adipose tissue [104–106], suggesting that FA metabolism in cancer cells may be regulated by the surrounding adipose tissue. Indeed, obesity has been associated with increased cancer risk and tumor progression [107, 108]. It is possible that adipose tissue in the tumor microenvironment secretes hormones and growth factors to reprogram FA metabolism in cancer cells and to drive cancer cell plasticity and promote cancer stemness.

Inhibition of FASN reduces numbers of CSCs [83, 85, 86], suggesting that FA synthesis is important for CSC maintenance, but how FAs facilitate CSC survival and expansion is unknown. Unsaturated FAs accumulate in ovarian CSCs and can activate NF-κB to regulate downstream stemness gene expression [89]. However, the detailed mechanism of how these unsaturated FAs

activate NF-κB remains unclear. The specific roles of various types of FAs in maintaining CSCs/TICs/DTPs are also unknown. Future studies could use lipidome analysis to identify the composition of FA species and their function in CSCs/TICs/DTPs. Further efforts focusing on the identification and quantification of many metabolites from FA metabolism in a biological sample as possible will serve as a translatable tool to provide personalized medicine for individuals.

We suggest that preclinical and clinical studies are needed to address several key mitochondrial FAO-related questions. The first question is why and how does FAO enable the survival of CSCs/TICs/DTPs. We posit that FAO could serve three purposes: first, as a means to reduce lipotoxicity from lipid intermediates [109]; second, to energetically and efficiently generate ATP (e.g. in long-lived cell types, such as memory T cells, that depend on FAO for survival [110]; and third, to contribute to the accumulation of acetyl-CoA in the cytoplasm for protein acetylation and FA synthesis. It is still not fully understood why CSCs/TICs/DTPs rely on FAO for survival. A possible explanation is that during the process of FAO, an increase of NADPH and ATP helps CSCs/TICs/DTPs to survive. Elevated ROS is detrimental to CSCs/TICs/DTPs [111, 112] and NADPH serves as an antioxidant to reduce ROS levels. Consistent with this, inhibition of FAO reduces NADPH and ATP, leading to an increase of ROS and cell death in glioma [113]. Another possibility is that increased FAO generates increased oxidized nicotinamide adenine dinucleotide (NAD^+), a cofactor for sirtuins (SIRTs). SIRT1–7 activity is regulated by the NAD^+/NADH ratio. This family of deacetylases plays an important role in regulating stemness, tumorigenesis and many other critical cellular processes [114]. Blocking FAO by ETO results in decreased NAD^+/NADH ratio and SIRT1 activity [115].

The next question is how does FA metabolism participate in the reprogramming process from cancer cells to CSCs/TICs/DTPs. Acetyl-CoA is a central metabolic intermediate at which multiple metabolic pathways converge. It is critical for initiating de novo FA synthesis and for incorporation into the TCA cycle to generate energy following FAO. Acetyl-CoA can also be an important source of histone or protein acetylation, which regulates a wide range of gene expression and protein functions. Acetyl-CoA homeostasis is controlled by several key enzymes. ACLY responsible for converting glucose-derived citrate into acetyl-CoA, which then affects histone acetylation to regulate gene expression [116]. ACC1 phosphorylation, which results in ACC1 inhibition, leads to accumulation of cytosolic acetyl-CoA. Accumulated acetyl-CoA causes total protein acetylation, including acetylation of the signal transducer Smad2; this enhances

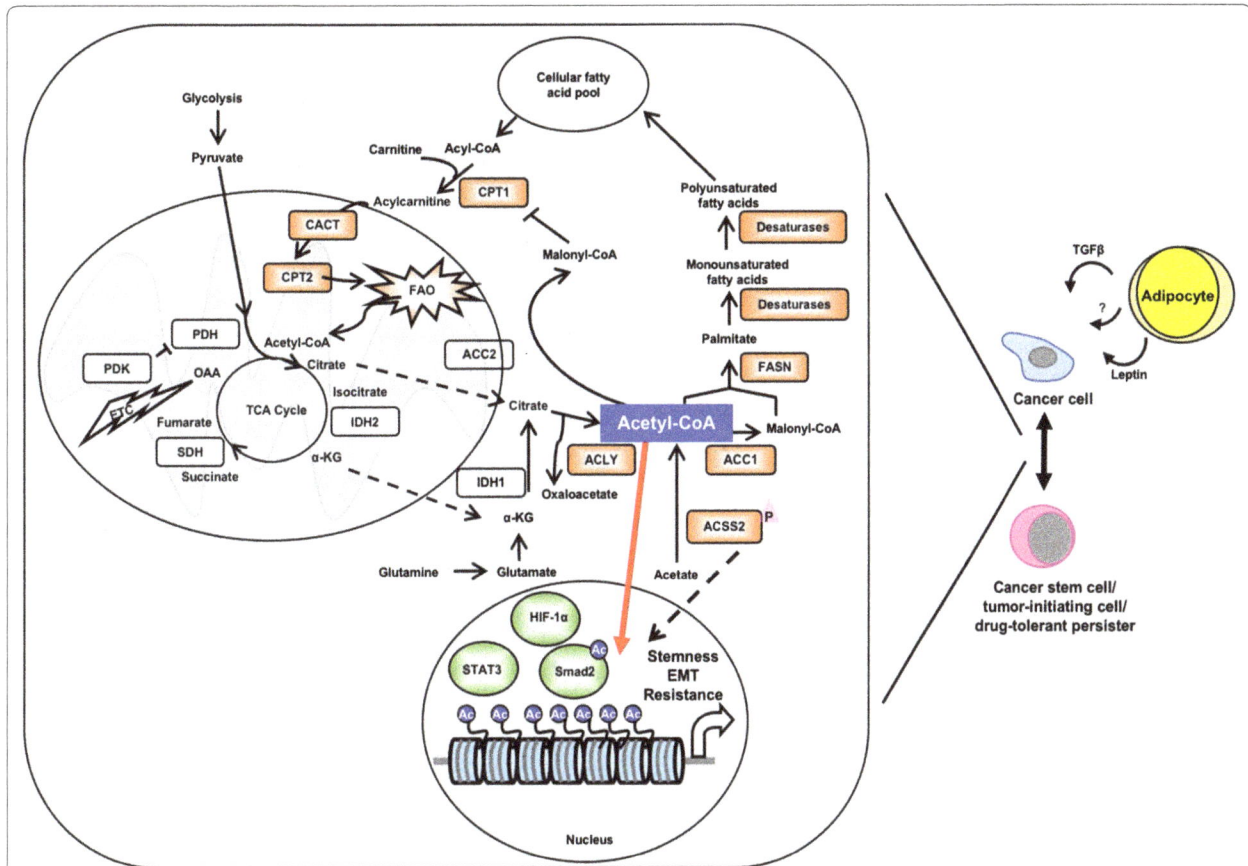

Fig. 2 Potential roles of fatty acid metabolism in regulating cancer cell plasticity. Cancer cells can be reprogrammed into a cancer stemness state or drug-tolerant state with appropriate cues. It has been shown that adipocytes in the tumor microenvironment secrete leptin, transforming growth factor β (TGFβ) or other hormones and growth factors that support conversion of cancer cells into more malignant cell types, including cancer stem cells/tumor-initiating cells or drug-tolerant persisters. Acetyl-CoA is a central hub for multiple metabolic pathways including FA synthesis and FAO. Therefore, acetyl-CoA might be a major carbon source for histone acetylation and regulating gene expression for reprogramming. ACSS2 is phosphorylated and transferred to nucleus for histone acetylation. Some transcription factors, including hypoxia inducible factor-1α (HIF-1α), signal transducer and activator of transcription 3 (STAT3) and SMAD family member 2 (Smad2), are also involved in the conversion and may drive cancer cell plasticity

Smad2 transcriptional activity and ultimately results in EMT and metastasis in breast cancer [58]. FAO-derived acetyl-CoA can acetylate mitochondrial proteins, but the function of this phenomenon remains unknown [117]. Moreover, acetylation of ACSS2 inhibits its activity; SIRT3 can reverse the acetylation and activate ACSS2 [118]. Cancer cells preferentially utilize acetate as their carbon source, not only for FA synthesis, but also for epigenetic regulation via modulation of histone acetylation and associated gene expression. ACSS2 plays an important role in converting acetate into acetyl-CoA. Therefore, it is also involved in acetate-mediated epigenetic regulation [119]. For example, ACSS2 is phosphorylated at serine 659 by AMPK under metabolic stress and translocated to nucleus to locally produce acetyl-CoA for histone acetylation at the promoter regions of genes involved in autophagosome and lysosome formation

[120]. That study provides strong evidence linking metabolism to epigenetic regulation of gene expression.

Another intriguing question is how are differentiated cancer cells reprogrammed into a stem-like or drug-tolerant state and what signals drive the process of reprogramming. Acetyl-CoA-mediated histone acetylation is controlled by glucose availability in embryonic stem (ES) cells and is responsible for maintaining the pluripotency of ES cells [121]. However, the gene expression profile associated with histone acetylation has not been revealed. Not only glucose, but also lipids, can be metabolized into acetyl-CoA, which then becomes a major carbon source for histone acetylation [122]. Moreover, the enhancement of both FAO and FA accumulation in breast cancer cells is linked to the acquisition of stem-like properties [94], implying that maximally functioning FA catabolism and anabolism may continuously provide acetyl-CoA for chromatin remodeling and reprogramming. Taken together, this suggests that lipid-derived acetyl-CoA is a major signaling metabolite that can reprogram cancer cells to acquire malignant phenotypes. Blockade of FAO with CPT inhibitors (e.g. ETO or perhexiline) or combination of FAO inhibitors with FASN inhibitors may hold hope for combating therapeutic resistance by eliminating CSCs/TICs/DTPs.

Lastly, both the lipogenic phenotype and cancer stemness can be induced by hypoxia [94, 123–126], suggesting that hypoxic signaling could be a converging pathway for both phenotypes. HIF-1α is the major regulator of hypoxic signaling, and a hypoxia- or pseudohypoxia-induced lipogenic phenotype can be HIF-1α-dependent [94, 126]. Moreover, HIF-1α induces expression of stemness factors, including Oct-4 and NANOG, and cancer cell plasticity observed in breast cancer is also dependent on HIF-1α [94, 125]. Therefore, HIF-1α may be an ideal target for shutting down both FA metabolism and stemness signaling in cancer cells, and ultimately preventing the conversion from cancer cells to CSCs/TICs/DTPs (Fig. 2).

Conclusions

FA metabolism has drawn increasing attention in recent years. Particularly, the association between FA synthesis and the resulting lipogenic phenotype with cancer progression has been well-documented. However, fewer studies have focused on the role of FAO in CSCs/TICs/DTPs. Here, we have summarized evidences showing the relationship among FA metabolism, cancer stemness and therapeutic resistance and also discussed potential issues that may warrant further investigations. In the future, with more detailed mechanistic findings, therapeutic targeting of FA metabolism may be used to eradicate CSCs/TICs/DTPs and combat cancer more effectively.

Abbreviations

ACC: acetyl-CoA carboxylase; ACLY: ATP-citrate lyase; ACSS2: acyl-CoA synthetase short-chain family member 2; AMPK: AMP-activated kinase; CACT : carnitine acylcarnitine translocase; CPT1: carnitine/palmitoyl-transferase 1; CSC: cancer stem cells; DKG: dimethyl α-ketoglutarate; DTP: drug-tolerant persisters; EMT: epithelial–mesenchymal transition; ES: embryonic stem; ETO: etomoxir; FA: fatty acid; FADH2: flavin adenine dinucleotide; FAO: fatty acid oxidation; FASN: fatty acid synthase; HER2: human epidermal growth factor receptor 2; HIF1α: hypoxia-inducible factor 1α; JAK: janus kinase; NAD$^+$: oxidized nicotinamide adenine dinucleotide; NADH: reduced nicotinamide adenine dinucleotide; NADPH: nicotinamide adenine dinucleotide phosphate; OXPHOS: oxidative phosphorylation; PPAR: peroxisome proliferator-activated receptors; ROS: reactive oxygen species; SIRT: sirtuin; SREBP1: sterol regulatory element-binding protein 1c; STAT3: signal transducer and activator of tran-

scription 3; TCA cycle: tricarboxylic acid cycle; TGF: transforming growth factor; TIC: tumor-initiating cells; TNBC: triple-negative breast cancer.

Authors' contributions

Both authors contributed substantially to the writing of this review. Both authors read and approved the final manuscript.

Author details

[1] Department of Clinical Laboratory Sciences and Medical Biotechnology, College of Medicine, National Taiwan University, Taipei 10048, Taiwan, China. [2] Department of Diabetes Complications and Metabolism, Diabetes and Metabolism Research Institute, Beckman Research Institute, City of Hope, Duarte, CA 91010, USA. [3] Irell and Manella Graduate School of Biological Sciences, City of Hope, Duarte, CA 91010, USA.

Acknowledgements

We thank the members of Dr. Ann's laboratory, Dr. Chun-Ting Cheng for critical discussions and support throughout this work and Dr. Sarah T. Wilkinson for editing.

Competing interests

The authors declare that they have no competing interests.

Funding

This work was supported in part by funds from the National Institutes of Health R01DE026304 and R01CA220693 (to D.K.A.) and Ministry of Science and Technology, R.O.C, Special Talents Award (to C.-Y. K).

References

1. Rohrig F, Schulze A. The multifaceted roles of fatty acid synthesis in cancer. Nat Rev Cancer. 2016;16(11):732–49. https://doi.org/10.1038/nrc.2016.89.
2. Beloribi-Djefaflia S, Vasseur S, Guillaumond F. Lipid metabolic reprogramming in cancer cells. Oncogenesis. 2016;5:e189. https://doi.org/10.1038/oncsis.2015.49.
3. Tirinato L, Pagliari F, Limongi T, Marini M, Falqui A, Seco J, et al. An overview of lipid droplets in cancer and cancer stem cells. Stem Cells Int. 2017;2017:17. https://doi.org/10.1155/2017/1656053.
4. Tirinato L, Liberale C, Di Franco S, Candeloro P, Benfante A, La Rocca R, et al. Lipid droplets: a new player in colorectal cancer stem cells unveiled by spectroscopic imaging. Stem Cells. 2015;33(1):35–44. https://doi.org/10.1002/stem.1837.
5. Koizume S, Miyagi Y. Lipid droplets: a key cellular organelle associated with cancer cell survival under normoxia and hypoxia. Int J Mol Sci. 2016;17(9):1430. https://doi.org/10.3390/ijms17091430.
6. Al-Hajj M, Wicha MS, Benito-Hernandez A, Morrison SJ, Clarke MF. Prospective identification of tumorigenic breast cancer cells. Proc Natl Acad Sci USA. 2003;100:3982–8. https://doi.org/10.1073/pnas.0530291100.
7. O'Brien CA, Kreso A, Jamieson CHM. Cancer stem cells and self-renewal. Clin Cancer Res. 2010;16(12):3113.
8. Lobo NA, Shimono Y, Qian D, Clarke MF. The biology of cancer stem cells. Annu Rev Cell Dev Biol. 2007;23(1):675–99. https://doi.org/10.1146/annurev.cellbio.22.010305.104154.
9. Chaffer CL, Brueckmann I, Scheel C, Kaestli AJ, Wiggins PA, Rodrigues LO, et al. Normal and neoplastic nonstem cells can spontaneously convert to a stem-like state. Proc Natl Acad Sci. 2011;108(19):7950–5. https://doi.org/10.1073/pnas.1102454108.
10. Chaffer Christine L, Marjanovic Nemanja D, Lee T, Bell G, Kleer Celina G, Reinhardt F, et al. Poised chromatin at the ZEB1 promoter enables

breast cancer cell plasticity and enhances tumorigenicity. Cell. 2013;154(1):61–74. https://doi.org/10.1016/j.cell.2013.06.005.

11. Gupta Piyush B, Fillmore Christine M, Jiang G, Shapira Sagi D, Tao K, Kuperwasser C, et al. Stochastic state transitions give rise to phenotypic equilibrium in populations of cancer cells. Cell. 2011;146(4):633–44. https://doi.org/10.1016/j.cell.2011.07.026.

12. Roesch A, Fukunaga-Kalabis M, Schmidt EC, Zabierowski SE, Brafford PA, Vultur A, et al. A temporarily distinct subpopulation of slow-cycling melanoma cells is required for continuous tumor growth. Cell. 2010;141(4):583–94.

13. Chen W, Dong J, Haiech J, Kilhoffer M-C, Zeniou M. Cancer stem cell quiescence and plasticity as major challenges in cancer therapy. Stem Cells Int. 2016;2016:1740936. https://doi.org/10.1155/2016/1740936.

14. Deheeger M, Lesniak MS, Ahmed AU. Cellular plasticity regulated cancer stem cell niche: a possible new mechanism of chemoresistance. Cancer Cell Microenviron. 2014;1(5):e295. https://doi.org/10.14800/ccm.295.

15. Borst P. Cancer drug pan-resistance: pumps, cancer stem cells, quiescence, epithelial to mesenchymal transition, blocked cell death pathways, persisters or what? Open Biol. 2012;2(5):120066. https://doi.org/10.1098/rsob.120066.

16. Dannenberg J-H, Berns A. Drugging drug resistance. Cell. 2010;141(1):18–20. https://doi.org/10.1016/j.cell.2010.03.020.

17. Ramirez M, Rajaram S, Steininger RJ, Osipchuk D, Roth MA, Morinishi LS et al. Diverse drug-resistance mechanisms can emerge from drug-tolerant cancer persister cells. Nat Commun. 2016;7:10690. https://doi.org/10.1038/ncomms10690 https://www.nature.com/articles/ncomms10690#supplementary-information.

18. Sharma SV, Lee DY, Li B, Quinlan MP, Takahashi F, Maheswaran S, et al. A chromatin-mediated reversible drug-tolerant state in cancer cell subpopulations. Cell. 2010;141(1):69–80. https://doi.org/10.1016/j.cell.2010.02.027.

19. Peiris-Pagès M, Martinez-Outschoorn UE, Pestell RG, Sotgia F, Lisanti MP. Cancer stem cell metabolism. Breast Cancer Res. 2016;18:55. https://doi.org/10.1186/s13058-016-0712-6.

20. Sancho P, Barneda D, Heeschen C. Hallmarks of cancer stem cell metabolism. Br J Cancer. 2016;114(12):1305–12. https://doi.org/10.1038/bjc.2016.152.

21. Vlashi E, Pajonk F. The metabolic state of cancer stem cells—a valid target for cancer therapy? Free Radic Biol Med. 2015;79:264–8. https://doi.org/10.1016/j.freeradbiomed.2014.10.732.

22. Dando I, Dalla Pozza E, Biondani G, Cordani M, Palmieri M, Donadelli M. The metabolic landscape of cancer stem cells. IUBMB Life. 2015;67(9):687–93. https://doi.org/10.1002/iub.1426.

23. Hirsch HA, Iliopoulos D, Tsichlis PN, Struhl K. Metformin selectively targets cancer stem cells, and acts together with chemotherapy to block tumor growth and prolong remission. Can Res. 2009;69(19):7507–11. https://doi.org/10.1158/0008-5472.CAN-09-2994.

24. Viollet B, Guigas B, Sanz Garcia N, Leclerc J, Foretz M, Andreelli F. Cellular and molecular mechanisms of metformin: an overview. Clin Sci. 2012;122(6):253–70. https://doi.org/10.1042/cs20110386.

25. Dong C, Yuan T, Wu Y, Wang Y, Fan Teresa WM, Miriyala S, et al. Loss of FBP1 by snail-mediated repression provides metabolic advantages in basal-like breast cancer. Cancer Cell. 2013;23(3):316–31. https://doi.org/10.1016/j.ccr.2013.01.022.

26. De Luca A, Fiorillo M, Peiris-Pagès M, Ozsvari B, Smith DL, Sanchez-Alvarez R, et al. Mitochondrial biogenesis is required for the anchorage-independent survival and propagation of stem-like cancer cells. Oncotarget. 2015;6(17):14777–95.

27. Pastò A, Bellio C, Pilotto G, Ciminale V, Silic-Benussi M, Guzzo G, et al. Cancer stem cells from epithelial ovarian cancer patients privilege oxidative phosphorylation, and resist glucose deprivation. Oncotarget. 2014;5(12):4305–19.

28. Medes G, Thomas A, Weinhouse S. Metabolism of neoplastic tissue. IV. A study of lipid synthesis in neoplastic tissue slices in vitro. Can Res. 1953;13(1):27.

29. Menendez JA, Lupu R. Fatty acid synthase and the lipogenic phenotype in cancer pathogenesis. Nat Rev Cancer. 2007;7(10):763–77.

30. Al-Bahlani S, Al-Lawati H, Al-Adawi M, Al-Abri N, Al-Dhahli B, Al-Adawi K. Fatty acid synthase regulates the chemosensitivity of breast cancer cells to cisplatin-induced apoptosis. Apoptosis. 2017;22(6):865–76. https://doi.org/10.1007/s10495-017-1366-2.

31. Bauerschlag DO, Maass N, Leonhardt P, Verburg FA, Pecks U, Zeppernick F, et al. Fatty acid synthase overexpression: target for therapy and reversal of chemoresistance in ovarian cancer. J Transl Med. 2015;13(1):146. https://doi.org/10.1186/s12967-015-0511-3.

32. Cai Y, Wang J, Zhang L, Wu D, Yu D, Tian X, et al. Expressions of fatty acid synthase and HER2 are correlated with poor prognosis of ovarian cancer. Med Oncol. 2015;32:391. https://doi.org/10.1007/s12032-014-0391-z.

33. Dehghan-Nayeri NGA, Goudarzi Pour K, Eshghi P. Over expression of the fatty acid synthase is a strong predictor of poor prognosis and contributes to glucocorticoid resistance in B-cell acute lymphoblastic leukemia. World Cancer Res J. 2016;3(3):e746.

34. Lupu R, Menendez JA. Targeting fatty acid synthase in breast and endometrial cancer: an alternative to selective estrogen receptor modulators? Endocrinology. 2006;147(9):4056–66. https://doi.org/10.1210/en.2006-0486.

35. Wu X, Dong Z, Wang CJ, Barlow LJ, Fako V, Serrano MA, et al. FASN regulates cellular response to genotoxic treatments by increasing PARP-1 expression and DNA repair activity via NF-κB and SP1. Proc Natl Acad Sci. 2016;113(45):E6965–73. https://doi.org/10.1073/pnas.1609934113.

36. Flavin R, Peluso S, Nguyen PL, Loda M. Fatty acid synthase as a potential therapeutic target in cancer. Future Oncol. 2010;6(4):551–62. https://doi.org/10.2217/fon.10.11.

37. Graner E, Tang D, Rossi S, Baron A, Migita T, Weinstein LJ, et al. The isopeptidase USP2a regulates the stability of fatty acid synthase in prostate cancer. Cancer Cell. 2004;5(3):253–61. https://doi.org/10.1016/S1535-6108(04)00055-8.

38. Zaidi N, Swinnen JV, Smans K. ATP-citrate lyase: a key player in cancer metabolism. Can Res. 2012;72(15):3709.

39. Qian X, Hu J, Zhao J, Chen H. ATP citrate lyase expression is associated with advanced stage and prognosis in gastric adenocarcinoma. Int J Clin Exp Med. 2015;8(5):7855–60.

40. Wang D, Yin L, Wei J, Yang Z, Jiang G. ATP citrate lyase is increased in human breast cancer, depletion of which promotes apoptosis. Tumor Biol. 2017;39(4):1010428317698338. https://doi.org/10.1177/1010428317698338.

41. Wang YU, Wang Y, Shen L, Pang Y, Qiao Z, Liu P. Prognostic and therapeutic implications of increased ATP citrate lyase expression in human epithelial ovarian cancer. Oncol Rep. 2012;27(4):1156–62. https://doi.org/10.3892/or.2012.1638.

42. Zhou Y, Bollu LR, Tozzi F, Ye X, Bhattacharya R, Gao G, et al. ATP citrate lyase mediates resistance of colorectal cancer cells to SN38. Mol Cancer Ther. 2013;12(12):2782–91. https://doi.org/10.1158/1535-7163.MCT-13-0098.

43. Sato R, Okamoto A, Inoue J, Miyamoto W, Sakai Y, Emoto N, et al. Transcriptional regulation of the ATP citrate-lyase gene by sterol regulatory element-binding proteins. J Biol Chem. 2000;275(17):12497–502. https://doi.org/10.1074/jbc.275.17.12497.

44. Migita T, Narita T, Nomura K, Miyagi E, Inazuka F, Matsuura M, et al. ATP citrate lyase: activation and therapeutic implications in non-small cell lung cancer. Can Res. 2008;68(20):8547.

45. Pierce MW, Palmer JL, Keutmann HT, Avruch J. ATP-citrate lyase. Structure of a tryptic peptide containing the phosphorylation site directed by glucagon and the cAMP-dependent protein kinase. J Biol Chem. 1981;256(17):8867–70.

46. Wagner PD, Vu N-D. Phosphorylation of ATP-citrate lyase by nucleoside diphosphate kinase. J Biol Chem. 1995;270(37):21758–64. https://doi.org/10.1074/jbc.270.37.21758.

47. Moncur JT, Park JP, Memoli VA, Mohandas TK, Kinlaw WB. The "Spot 14" gene resides on the telomeric end of the 11q13 amplicon and is expressed in lipogenic breast cancers: implications for control of tumor metabolism. Proc Natl Acad Sci USA. 1998;95(12):6989–94.

48. Svensson RU, Parker SJ, Eichner LJ, Kolar MJ, Wallace M, Brun SN et al. Inhibition of acetyl-CoA carboxylase suppresses fatty acid synthesis and tumor growth of non-small-cell lung cancer in preclinical models. Nat Med. 2016;22(10):1108–19. https://doi.org/10.1038/nm.4181 http://www.nature.com/nm/journal/v22/n10/abs/nm.4181.html#supplementary-information.

49. Fang W, Cui H, Yu D, Chen Y, Wang J, Yu G. Increased expression of phospho-acetyl-CoA carboxylase protein is an independent prognostic factor for human gastric cancer without lymph node metastasis. Med Oncol. 2014;31(7):15. https://doi.org/10.1007/s12032-014-0015-7.

50. Wakil SJ, Abu-Elheiga LA. Fatty acid metabolism: target for metabolic syndrome. J Lipid Res. 2009;50(Supplement):S138–43. https://doi.org/10.1194/jlr.R800079-JLR200.

51. Currie E, Schulze A, Zechner R, Walther TC, Farese RV. Cellular fatty acid metabolism and cancer. Cell Metab. 2013;18(2):153–61. https://doi.org/10.1016/j.cmet.2013.05.017.

52. Wang Y, Viscarra J, Kim S-J, Sul HS. Transcriptional regulation of hepatic lipogenesis. Nat Rev Mol Cell Biol. 2015;16:678. https://doi.org/10.1038/nrm4074.

53. Zhao LF, Iwasaki Y, Zhe W, Nishiyama M, Taguchi T, Tsugita M, et al. Hormonal regulation of acetyl-CoA carboxylase isoenzyme gene transcription. Endocr J. 2010;57(4):317–24. https://doi.org/10.1507/endocrj.K09E-298.

54. Hardie DG. AMPK: a key regulator of energy balance in the single cell and the whole organism. Int J Obes. 2008;32:S7. https://doi.org/10.1038/ijo.2008.116.

55. Cho YS, Lee JI, Shin D, Kim HT, Jung HY, Lee TG, et al. Molecular mechanism for the regulation of human ACC2 through phosphorylation by AMPK. Biochem Biophys Res Commun. 2010;391(1):187–92. https://doi.org/10.1016/j.bbrc.2009.11.029.

56. Munday MR, Campbell DG, Carling D, Hardie DG. Identification by amino acid sequencing of three major regulatory phosphorylation sites on rat acetyl-CoA carboxylase. Eur J Biochem. 1988;175(2):331–8. https://doi.org/10.1111/j.1432-1033.1988.tb14201.x.

57. Fullerton MD, Galic S, Marcinko K, Sikkema S, Pulinilkunnil T, Chen Z-P et al. Single phosphorylation sites in Acc1 and Acc2 regulate lipid homeostasis and the insulin-sensitizing effects of metformin. Nat Med. 2013;19:1649. https://doi.org/10.1038/nm.3372 https://www.nature.com/articles/nm.3372#supplementary-information.

58. Rios Garcia M, Steinbauer B, Srivastava K, Singhal M, Mattijssen F, Maida A, et al. Acetyl-CoA carboxylase 1-dependent protein acetylation controls breast cancer metastasis and recurrence. Cell Metab. 2017;26(6):842–55. https://doi.org/10.1016/j.cmet.2017.09.018.

59. Luo J, Hong Y, Lu Y, Qiu S, Chaganty BKR, Zhang L, et al. Acetyl-CoA carboxylase rewires cancer metabolism to allow cancer cells to survive inhibition of the Warburg effect by cetuximab. Cancer Lett. 2017;384:39–49. https://doi.org/10.1016/j.canlet.2016.09.020.

60. Watkins PA, Maiguel D, Jia Z, Pevsner J. Evidence for 26 distinct acyl-coenzyme A synthetase genes in the human genome. J Lipid Res. 2007;48(12):2736–50. https://doi.org/10.1194/jlr.M700378-JLR200.

61. Schug ZT, Peck B, Jones DT, Zhang Q, Grosskurth S, Alam IS, et al. Acetyl-CoA synthetase 2 promotes acetate utilization and maintains cancer cell growth under metabolic stress. Cancer Cell. 2015;27(1):57–71. https://doi.org/10.1016/j.ccell.2014.12.002.

62. Comerford SA, Huang Z, Du X, Wang Y, Cai L, Witkiewicz AK, et al. Acetate dependence of tumors. Cell. 2014;159(7):1591–602. https://doi.org/10.1016/j.cell.2014.11.020.

63. Mashimo T, Pichumani K, Vemireddy V, Hatanpaa KJ, Singh DK, Sirasanagandla S, et al. Acetate is a bioenergetic substrate for human glioblastoma and brain metastases. Cell. 2014;159(7):1603–14. https://doi.org/10.1016/j.cell.2014.11.025.

64. Björnson E, Mukhopadhyay B, Asplund A, Pristovsek N, Cinar R, Romeo S, et al. Stratification of hepatocellular carcinoma patients based on acetate utilization. Cell Rep. 2015;13(9):2014–26. https://doi.org/10.1016/j.celrep.2015.10.045.

65. Luong A, Hannah VC, Brown MS, Goldstein JL. Molecular characterization of human acetyl-CoA synthetase, an enzyme regulated by sterol regulatory element-binding proteins. J Biol Chem. 2000;275(34):26458–66. https://doi.org/10.1074/jbc.M004160200.

66. Sone H, Shimano H, Sakakura Y, Inoue N, Amemiya-Kudo M, Yahagi N, et al. Acetyl-coenzyme A synthetase is a lipogenic enzyme controlled by SREBP-1 and energy status. Am J Physiol Endocrinol Metab. 2002;282(1):E222.

67. Carracedo A, Cantley LC, Pandolfi PP. Cancer metabolism: fatty acid oxidation in the limelight. Nat Rev Cancer. 2013;13(4):227–32. https://doi.org/10.1038/nrc3483.

68. Schreurs M, Kuipers F, Van Der Leij FR. Regulatory enzymes of mitochondrial β-oxidation as targets for treatment of the metabolic syndrome. Obes Rev. 2010;11(5):380–8. https://doi.org/10.1111/j.1467-789X.2009.00642.x.

69. Schlaepfer IR, Rider L, Rodrigues LU, Gijón MA, Pac CT, Romero L, et al. Lipid catabolism via CPT1 as a therapeutic target for prostate cancer. Mol Cancer Ther. 2014;13(10):2361.

70. Flaig TW, Salzmann-Sullivan M, Su L-J, Zhang Z, Joshi M, Gijón MA, et al. Lipid catabolism inhibition sensitizes prostate cancer cells to antiandrogen blockade. Oncotarget. 2017;8(34):56051–65. https://doi.org/10.18632/oncotarget.17359.

71. Pucci S, Zonetti MJ, Fisco T, Polidoro C, Bocchinfuso G, Palleschi A, et al. Carnitine palmitoyl transferase-1A (CPT1A): a new tumor specific target in human breast cancer. Oncotarget. 2016;7(15):19982–96. https://doi.org/10.18632/oncotarget.6964.

72. Song S, Attia RR, Connaughton S, Niesen MI, Ness GC, Elam MB, et al. Peroxisome proliferator activated receptor α (PPARα) and PPAR gamma coactivator (PGC-1α) induce carnitine palmitoyltransferase IA (CPT-1A) via independent gene elements. Mol Cell Endocrinol. 2010;325(1–2):54–63. https://doi.org/10.1016/j.mce.2010.05.019.

73. Tachibana K, Yamasaki D, Ishimoto K, Doi T. The role of PPARs in cancer. PPAR Res. 2008;2008:102737. https://doi.org/10.1155/2008/102737.

74. Samudio I, Harmancey R, Fiegl M, Kantarjian H, Konopleva M, Korchin B, et al. Pharmacologic inhibition of fatty acid oxidation sensitizes human leukemia cells to apoptosis induction. J Clin Investig. 2010;120(1):142–56. https://doi.org/10.1172/JCI38942.

75. Zaugg K, Yao Y, Reilly PT, Kannan K, Kiarash R, Mason J, et al. Carnitine palmitoyltransferase 1C promotes cell survival and tumor growth under conditions of metabolic stress. Genes Dev. 2011;25(10):1041–51. https://doi.org/10.1101/gad.1987211.

76. Kim WT, Yun SJ, Yan C, Jeong P, Kim YH, Lee I-S, et al. Metabolic pathway signatures associated with urinary metabolite biomarkers differentiate bladder cancer patients from healthy controls. Yonsei Med J. 2016;57(4):865–71. https://doi.org/10.3349/ymj.2016.57.4.865.

77. Yeh C-S, Wang J-Y, Cheng T-L, Juan C-H, Wu C-H, Lin S-R. Fatty acid metabolism pathway play an important role in carcinogenesis of human colorectal cancers by microarray-bioinformatics analysis. Cancer Lett. 2006;233(2):297–308. https://doi.org/10.1016/j.canlet.2005.03.050.

78. Wang T, Fahrmann JF, Lee H, Li Y-J, Tripathi SC, Yue C, et al. JAK/STAT3-regulated fatty acid β-oxidation is critical for breast cancer stem cell self-renewal and chemoresistance. Cell Metab. 2018;27(1):136–50. https://doi.org/10.1016/j.cmet.2017.11.001.

79. Camarda R, Zhou Z, Kohnz RA, Balakrishnan S, Mahieu C, Anderton B, et al. Inhibition of fatty acid oxidation as a therapy for MYC-overexpressing triple-negative breast cancer. Nat Med. 2016;22(4):427–32. https://doi.org/10.1038/nm.4055.

80. Park JH, Vithayathil S, Kumar S, Sung P-L, Dobrolecki LE, Putluri V, et al. Fatty acid oxidation-driven src links mitochondrial energy reprogramming and regulation of oncogenic properties in triple negative breast cancer. Cell Rep. 2016;14(9):2154–65. https://doi.org/10.1016/j.celrep.2016.02.004.

81. Guo H, Zeng W, Feng L, Yu X, Li P, Zhang K, et al. Integrated transcriptomic analysis of distance-related field cancerization in rectal cancer patients. Oncotarget. 2017;8(37):61107–17. https://doi.org/10.18632/oncotarget.17864.

82. Valentino A, Calarco A, Di SA, Finicelli M, Crispi S, Calogero RA et al. Deregulation of microRNAs mediated control of carnitine cycle in prostate cancer: molecular basis and pathophysiological consequences. Oncogene. 2017;36:6030. https://doi.org/10.1038/onc.2017.216. https://www.nature.com/articles/onc2017216#supplementary-information.

83. Yasumoto Y, Miyazaki H, Vaidyan LK, Kagawa Y, Ebrahimi M, Yamamoto Y, et al. Inhibition of fatty acid synthase decreases expression of stemness markers in glioma stem cells. PLoS ONE. 2016;11(1):e0147717. https://doi.org/10.1371/journal.pone.0147717.

84. Brandi J, Dando I, Pozza ED, Biondani G, Jenkins R, Elliott V, et al. Proteomic analysis of pancreatic cancer stem cells: functional role of fatty acid synthesis and mevalonate pathways. J Proteomics. 2017;150(Supplement C):310–22. https://doi.org/10.1016/j.jprot.2016.10.002.

85. Wahdan-Alaswad RS, Cochrane DR, Spoelstra NS, Howe EN, Edgerton SM, Anderson SM, et al. Metformin-induced killing of triple-negative breast cancer cells is mediated by reduction in fatty acid synthase via

miRNA-193b. Horm Cancer. 2014;5(6):374–89. https://doi.org/10.1007/s12672-014-0188-8.

86. Pandey PR, Okuda H, Watabe M, Pai SK, Liu W, Kobayashi A, et al. Resveratrol suppresses growth of cancer stem-like cells by inhibiting fatty acid synthase. Breast Cancer Res Treat. 2011;130(2):387–98. https://doi.org/10.1007/s10549-010-1300-6.

87. Hanai Ji, Doro N, Seth P, Sukhatme VP. ATP citrate lyase knockdown impacts cancer stem cells in vitro. Cell Death Dis. 2013;4:e696. https://doi.org/10.1038/cddis.2013.215. https://www.nature.com/articles/cddis2013215#supplementary-information.

88. Corominas-Faja B, Cuyàs E, Gumuzio J, Bosch-Barrera J, Leis O, Martin ÁG, et al. Chemical inhibition of acetyl-CoA carboxylase suppresses self-renewal growth of cancer stem cells. Oncotarget. 2014;5(18):8306–16.

89. Li J, Condello S, Thomes-Pepin J, Ma X, Xia Y, Hurley TD, et al. Lipid desaturation is a metabolic marker and therapeutic target of ovarian cancer stem cells. Cell Stem Cell. 2017;20(3):303–14. https://doi.org/10.1016/j.stem.2016.11.004.

90. Parrales A, Ranjan A, Iwakuma T. Unsaturated fatty acids regulate stemness of ovarian cancer cells through NF-κB. Stem Cell Investig. 2017;4(6):49.

91. Qu Q, Zeng F, Liu X, Wang QJ, Deng F. Fatty acid oxidation and carnitine palmitoyltransferase I: emerging therapeutic targets in cancer. Cell Death Dis. 2016;7(5):e2226. https://doi.org/10.1038/cddis.2016.132.

92. Wang X, Yao J, Wang J, Zhang Q, Brady SW, Arun B, et al. Targeting aberrant p70S6K activation for estrogen receptor–negative breast cancer prevention. Cancer Prev Res. 2017;10(11):641–50. https://doi.org/10.1158/1940-6207.CAPR-17-0106.

93. Wang X, Sun Y, Wong J, Conklin DS. PPAR[gamma] maintains ERBB2-positive breast cancer stem cells. Oncogene. 2013;32(49):5512–21. https://doi.org/10.1038/onc.2013.217.

94. Kuo C-Y, Cheng C-T, Hou P, Lin Y-P, Ma H, Chung Y, et al. HIF-1-alpha links mitochondrial perturbation to the dynamic acquisition of breast cancer tumorigenicity. Oncotarget. 2016;7(23):34052–69. https://doi.org/10.18632/oncotarget.8570.

95. Jiang L, Shestov AA, Swain P, Yang C, Parker SJ, Wang QA et al. Reductive carboxylation supports redox homeostasis during anchorage-independent growth. Nature. 2016;532:255. https://doi.org/10.1038/nature17393. https://www.nature.com/articles/nature17393#supplementary-information.

96. Metallo CM, Gameiro PA, Bell EL, Mattaini KR, Yang J, Hiller K et al. Reductive glutamine metabolism by IDH1 mediates lipogenesis under hypoxia. Nature. 2011;481:380. https://doi.org/10.1038/nature10602. https://www.nature.com/articles/nature10602#supplementary-information.

97. Palm W, Park Y, Wright K, Pavlova NN, Tuveson DA, Thompson CB. The utilization of extracellular proteins as nutrients is suppressed by mTORC1. Cell. 2015;162(2):259–70. https://doi.org/10.1016/j.cell.2015.06.017.

98. Jung YY, Kim HM, Koo JS. Expression of lipid metabolism-related proteins in metastatic breast cancer. PLoS ONE. 2015;10(9):e0137204. https://doi.org/10.1371/journal.pone.0137204.

99. Kim S, Lee Y, Koo JS. Differential expression of lipid metabolism-related proteins in different breast cancer subtypes. PLoS ONE. 2015;10(3):e0119473. https://doi.org/10.1371/journal.pone.0119473.

100. Chen C-L, Uthaya Kumar D, Punj V, Xu J, Sher L, Tahara S, et al. NANOG metabolically reprograms tumor-initiating stem-like cells through tumorigenic changes in oxidative phosphorylation and fatty acid metabolism. Cell Metab. 2016;23(1):206–19. https://doi.org/10.1016/j.cmet.2015.12.004.

101. Yin X, Dwyer J, Langley SR, Mayr U, Xing Q, Drozdov I, et al. Effects of perhexiline-induced fuel switch on the cardiac proteome and metabolome. J Mol Cell Cardiol. 2013;55(Supplement C):27–30. https://doi.org/10.1016/j.yjmcc.2012.12.014.

102. Nguyen LV, Vanner R, Dirks P, Eaves CJ. Cancer stem cells: an evolving concept. Nat Rev Cancer. 2012;12:133. https://doi.org/10.1038/nrc3184.

103. Wu Y, Chen K, Liu X, Huang L, Zhao D, Li L, et al. Srebp-1 interacts with c-Myc to enhance somatic cell reprogramming. Stem Cells. 2016;34(1):83–92. https://doi.org/10.1002/stem.2209.

104. Cammisotto PG, Bukowiecki LJ. Mechanisms of leptin secretion from white adipocytes. Am J Physiol Cell Physiol. 2002;283(1):C244.

105. Choy L, Skillington J, Derynck R. Roles of autocrine TGF-β receptor and smad signaling in adipocyte differentiation. J Cell Biol. 2000;149(3):667.

106. Coelho M, Oliveira T, Fernandes R. Biochemistry of adipose tissue: an endocrine organ. Arch Med Sci. 2013;9(2):191–200. https://doi.org/10.5114/aoms.2013.33181.

107. De Pergola G, Silvestris F. Obesity as a major risk factor for cancer. J Obes. 2013;2013:291546. https://doi.org/10.1155/2013/291546.

108. Park J, Morley TS, Kim M, Clegg DJ, Scherer PE. Obesity and cancer—mechanisms underlying tumour progression and recurrence. Nat Rev Endocrinol. 2014;10(8):455–65. https://doi.org/10.1038/nrendo.2014.94.

109. Unger RH, Clark GO, Scherer PE, Orci L. Lipid homeostasis, lipotoxicity and the metabolic syndrome. Biochimica et Biophysica Acta Mol Cell Biol Lipids. 2010;1801(3):209–14. https://doi.org/10.1016/j.bbalip.2009.10.006.

110. Pearce EL, Walsh MC, Cejas PJ, Harms GM, Shen H, Wang L-S, et al. Enhancing CD8 T cell memory by modulating fatty acid metabolism. Nature. 2009;460(7251):103–7. https://doi.org/10.1038/nature08097.

111. Shi X, Zhang Y, Zheng J, Pan J. Reactive oxygen species in cancer stem cells. Antioxid Redox Signal. 2012;16(11):1215–28. https://doi.org/10.1089/ars.2012.4529.

112. Zhou D, Shao L, Spitz DR. Reactive oxygen species in normal and tumor stem cells. Adv Cancer Res. 2014;122:1–67. https://doi.org/10.1016/B978-0-12-420117-0.00001-3.

113. Pike LS, Smift AL, Croteau NJ, Ferrick DA, Wu M. Inhibition of fatty acid oxidation by etomoxir impairs NADPH production and increases reactive oxygen species resulting in ATP depletion and cell death in human glioblastoma cells. Biochimica et Biophysica Acta Bioenergetics. 2011;1807(6):726–34. https://doi.org/10.1016/j.bbabio.2010.10.022.

114. O'Callaghan C, Vassilopoulos A. Sirtuins at the crossroads of stemness, aging, and cancer. Aging Cell. 2017;16(6):1208–18. https://doi.org/10.1111/acel.12685.

115. Cantó C, Gerhart-Hines Z, Feige JN, Lagouge M, Noriega L, Milne JC et al. AMPK regulates energy expenditure by modulating NAD+ metabolism and SIRT1 activity. Nature. 2009;458:1056. https://doi.org/10.1038/nature07813. https://www.nature.com/articles/nature07813#supplementary-information.

116. Wellen KE, Hatzivassiliou G, Sachdeva UM, Bui TV, Cross JR, Thompson CB. ATP-citrate lyase links cellular metabolism to histone acetylation. Science. 2009;324(5930):1076.

117. Hirschey MD, Shimazu T, Goetzman E, Jing E, Schwer B, Lombard DB et al. SIRT3 regulates mitochondrial fatty-acid oxidation by reversible enzyme deacetylation. Nature. 2010;464:121. https://doi.org/10.1038/nature08778. https://www.nature.com/articles/nature08778#supplementary-information.

118. Schwer B, Bunkenborg J, Verdin RO, Andersen JS, Verdin E. Reversible lysine acetylation controls the activity of the mitochondrial enzyme acetyl-CoA synthetase 2. Proc Natl Acad Sci. 2006;103(27):10224–9. https://doi.org/10.1073/pnas.0603968103.

119. Gao X, Lin S-H, Ren F, Li J-T, Chen J-J, Yao C-B et al. Acetate functions as an epigenetic metabolite to promote lipid synthesis under hypoxia. Nat Commun. 2016;7:11960. https://doi.org/10.1038/ncomms11960. https://www.nature.com/articles/ncomms11960#supplementary-information.

120. Li X, Yu W, Qian X, Xia Y, Zheng Y, Lee J-H, et al. Nucleus-translocated ACSS2 promotes gene transcription for lysosomal biogenesis and autophagy. Mol Cell. 2017;66(5):684–97. https://doi.org/10.1016/j.molcel.2017.04.026.

121. Moussaieff A, Rouleau M, Kitsberg D, Cohen M, Levy G, Barasch D, et al. Glycolysis-mediated changes in acetyl-CoA and histone acetylation control the early differentiation of embryonic stem cells. Cell Metab. 2015;21(3):392–402. https://doi.org/10.1016/j.cmet.2015.02.002.

122. McDonnell E, Crown SB, Fox DB, Kitir B, Ilkayeva OR, Olsen CA, et al. Lipids reprogram metabolism to become a major carbon source for histone acetylation. Cell Rep. 2016;17(6):1463–72. https://doi.org/10.1016/j.celrep.2016.10.012.

123. Li Z, Rich JN. Hypoxia and hypoxia inducible factors in cancer stem cell maintenance. In: Simon MC, editor. Diverse effects of hypoxia on tumor progression. Berlin: Springer; 2010. p. 21–30.

124. Qin J, Liu Y, Lu Y, Liu M, Li M, Li J, et al. Hypoxia-inducible factor 1 alpha promotes cancer stem cells-like properties in human ovarian cancer cells by upregulating SIRT1 expression. Sci Rep. 2017;7(1):10592. https://doi.org/10.1038/s41598-017-09244-8.

125. Zhang C, Samanta D, Lu H, Bullen JW, Zhang H, Chen I, et al. Hypoxia induces the breast cancer stem cell phenotype by HIF-dependent and ALKBH5-mediated m6A-demethylation of NANOG mRNA. Proc Natl Acad Sci. 2016;113(14):E2047–56. https://doi.org/10.1073/pnas.1602883113.

126. Valli A, Rodriguez M, Moutsianas L, Fischer R, Fedele V, Huang H-L, et al. Hypoxia induces a lipogenic cancer cell phenotype via HIF1α-dependent and -independent pathways. Oncotarget.

11

Azithromycin enhances anticancer activity of TRAIL by inhibiting autophagy and up-regulating the protein levels of DR4/5 in colon cancer cells in vitro and in vivo

Xinran Qiao⦿, Xiaofei Wang, Yue Shang, Yi Li and Shu-zhen Chen*⦿

Abstract

Background: Azithromycin is a member of macrolide antibiotics, and has been reported to inhibit the proliferation of cancer cells. However, the underlying mechanisms are not been fully elucidated. Tumor necrosis factor-related apoptosis-inducing ligand (TRAIL) selectively targets tumor cells without damaging healthy cells. In the present study, we examined whether azithromycin is synergistic with TRAIL, and if so, the underlying mechanisms in colon cancers.

Methods: HCT-116, SW480, SW620 and DiFi cells were treated with azithromycin, purified TRAIL, or their combination. A sulforhoddamine B assay was used to examine cell survival. Apoptosis was examined using annexin V-FITC/PI staining, and autophagy was observed by acridine orange staining. Western blot analysis was used to detect protein expression levels. In mechanistic experiments, siRNAs were used to knockdown death receptors (DR4, DR5) and LC-3B. The anticancer effect of azithromycin and TRAIL was also examined in BALB/c nude mice carrying HCT-116 xenografts.

Results: Azithromycin decreased the proliferation of HCT-116 and SW480 cells in a dose-dependent manner. Combination of azithromycin and TRAIL inhibited tumor growth in a manner that could not be explained by additive effects. Azithromycin increased the expressions of DR4, DR5, p62 and LC-3B proteins and potentiated induction of apoptosis by TRAIL. Knockdown of DR4 and DR5 with siRNAs increased cell survival rate and decreased the expression of cleaved-PARP induced by the combination of azithromycin and TRAIL. LC-3B siRNA and CQ potentiated the anti-proliferation activity of TRAIL alone, and increased the expressions of DR4 and DR5.

Conclusion: The synergistic antitumor effect of azithromycin and TRAIL mainly relies on the up-regulations of DR4 and DR5, which in turn result from LC-3B-involved autophagy inhibition.

Keywords: Azithromycin, TRAIL, Apoptosis, Autophagy, Colon cancer

Background

Azithromycin is a macrolide antibiotic widely used to treat bacterial infection. Azithromycin accumulates and undergoes slow release in cells, especially in phagocytes, and thus has higher local concentration and longer half-life than older macrolides (i.e., erythromycin and clarithromycin) [1, 2]. Recent studies have indicated that azithromycin could produce potent anti-proliferation

---

*Correspondence: bjcsz@imb.pumc.edu.cn
Institute of Medicinal Biotechnology, Chinese Academy of Medical Sciences & Peking Union Medical College, Beijing 100050, P.R. China

effect by inducing apoptosis in HeLa cells and SGC-7901 cancer cells [3]. Clinical studies have suggested promising efficacy of azithromycin in combination with paclitaxel and cisplatin in stage III–IV NSCLC patients [4]. In addition, it has been reported that antibiotics could affect tumor growth by targeting mitochondria and eradicating cancer stem cells [5]. Macrolide antibiotics (e.g., azithromycin, clarithromycin and erythromycin) sensitize cancer cells to the apoptotic effect of bortezomib and EGFR-TKI by blocking autophagy flux, but the targets of azithromycin in the apoptosis pathway remain unknown [6, 7]. Preclinical and clinical data suggest that clarithromycin in combination with conventional chemo-therapeutic agents could produce robust antitumor activities [8, 9]. However, few studies have explored potential action of azithromycin.

Tumor necrosis factor-related apoptosis-inducing ligand (TRAIL) is a member of the tumor necrosis factor superfamily, and considered a promising tumor therapeutic agent since it selectively targets tumor cells without producing cytotoxicity in healthy cells. TRAIL interacts with, and causes the clustering of death receptors (DR) 4 and 5, and induces the assembly of DISC and the activation of a series of downstream caspase cascades [10]. This pathway is known as the extrinsic apoptosis pathway [10]. Interestingly, past studies have produced seemingly opposite effects: increasing the expression of DR4/5 is related to survival in colon cancer patients [11]. Primary human colon cancer cells and high-grade adenomas are sensitive to TRAIL and combinational chemotherapies (e.g., using chloroquine and shogaol with TRAIL) could inhibit the proliferation of colon cells more effectively [12–16].

In the present study, we examined whether azithromycin and TRAIL could produce synergistic effects in colon cancers. Potential action of autophagy inhibition and apoptosis in the interaction was also examined.

Materials and methods

Cells culture

A total of 4 human colon adenocarcinoma cell lines were used in the current study. SW480 and SW620 cells were obtained from the Cell Resource Center of the institute of Basic Medical Sciences (IBMS) of the Chinese Academy of Medical Sciences (CAMS) & Peking Union Medical College (PUMC) (Beijing, China), respectively, and cultured in Iscove's Modified Dulbecco's Medium and Eibovitz's L-15 Medium (ThermoFisher Scientific, Waltham, MA, USA). HCT-116 cells were kept in our laboratory in RPMI-1640 medium (ThermoFisher Scientific). DiFi cell line was a gift from Professor Wang Zhen at our institute and cultured in Dulbecco's Modified Eagle Medium: nutrient mixture F-12 (1:1) medium (ThermoFisher Scientific). For all cell lines, the culture medium was supplemented with 10% fetal bovine serum (Gibco, Carlsbad, California, USA), 100-U/mL penicillin and 100-μg/mL streptomycin (North China Pharmaceutical Inc, Beijing, China) at 37 °C in a 5% CO_2 incubator.

Reagents and antibodies

Azithromycin and N-acetylcysteine (NAC) were obtained from National Institutes for Food and Drug Control (Beijing, China). Azithromycin was dissolved in anhydrous ethanol; NAC was dissolved in distilled water. Anti-caspase-3, anti-Akt (pan), anti-p44/42 MAPK (Erk 1/2), anti-p38 MAPK, anti-PARP and p62 antibodies were purchased from Cell Signaling Technology (Danvers, MA, USA). Anti-LC3B antibody was purchased from Sigma (St. Louis, MO, USA). Azide-free anti-human CD261 (DR4) antibody was obtained from Diaclone (Besancon, France). Anti-DR5 antibody was obtained from ProSci (San Diego, California, USA). β-Actin (6G3) and GAPDH (1C4) monoclonal antibodies were purchased from AmeriBiopharma (Wilmington, Delaware, USA). Secondary antibodies included peroxidase-conjugated affiniPure goat anti-mouse IgG (H+L) and goat anti-rabbit IgG (H+L) (ZSGB-BIO, Beijing, China). Caspase inhibitor zVAD-fmk and RIP1 inhibitor necrostatin-1 were purchased from Selleck.cn (Houston, TX, USA). Chloroquine (CQ), acridine orange hemi (zinc chloride) salt (AO) and sulforhodamine B (SRB) were from Sigma.

Expression and purification of TRAIL protein

Recombinant TRAIL was constructed in this laboratory and expressed in P. pastoris. TRAIL expressing strains were inoculated in 100-mL BMGY medium (100 mmol/L potassium phosphate buffer, pH 6.0, 1% yeast extract, 2% peptone, 1% glycerol, 1.34% YNB, 0.00004% biotin) in a shaking incubator at 30 °C for 36 h. Yeast cells were precipitated and re-suspended in 100-mL BMMY with added 1.5% methanol every 24 h, at 26 °C for 72 h. Supernatant was collected by centrifugation at $7800 \times g$, 4 °C for 15 min. TRAIL protein was purified with Ni^{2+} affinity chromatography (His Trap HP, GE Healthcare, Pittsburgh, Pennsylvania, USA). Protein concentration was examined using a BCA method.

Cell survival assay

Cells were seeded in 96-well plates at 3×10^3 cells/well in 100-μL culture medium. Twenty-four hour later, cells were exposed to test drugs (azithromycin and TRAIL of varying concentrations, and combination) for 24, 48, or 72 h prior to survival assay using a sulforhodamine B (SRB) method [17]. Cell survival was calculated relative to the control group.

Western blot analysis

Cells were lysed with a lysis buffer (50 mmol/L Tris–HCl pH 8.0; 2% NP-40; 150 mmol/L NaCl; 0.2% SDS; 0.5% sodium deoxycholate) containing 1% protease inhibitor (Beyotime, Jiangsu, China) and 100-μmol/L phenylmethylsulfonyl fluoride (PMSF). The supernatant was collected after centrifugation at $13,000 \times g$ for 15 min at 4 °C, prior to Western blotting analyses, as described previously [18].

Apoptosis assay

Apoptosis was determined using an annexin V-FITC/PI apoptosis detection kit from DOJINDO (Shanghai, China). A schematic plot was used to display the results: the lower left quadrant represents live cells; the lower right and upper right quadrants represent early and late apoptotic cells, respectively; the upper left quadrant represents necrotic cells. Cell death refers to the sum of early and late apoptotic and necrotic cells.

Acridine orange (AO) staining

HCT-116 and SW480 cells were plated into 6-well plates and treated with drugs for 24 h. Later, cells were washed by PBS twice and stained with 700 µL/well AO (1 µg/mL) for 15 min at 37 °C in the dark. Then, the cells were washed by PBS twice. Watching the images under a fluorescence microscope through a 490 nm band-pass excitation filter and a 515 nm long-pass barrier filter. The green color represented the nucleus, while the red represented the acidic vesicles.

siRNA transfection

DR4 siRNA (sense: 5′-AACGAGATTCTGAGCAAC GCA-3′, anti-sense: 3′-TTGCTCTAAGACTCGTTG CGT-5′), DR5 siRNA (sense: 5′-AAGACCCTTGTG CTCGTTGTC-3′, anti-sense: 3′-TTCTGGGAACAC GAGCAACAG-5′), LC-3B siRNA (sense: 5′-GGTGTA TGAGAGTGAGAAA-3′, anti-sense: 3′-CCACATACT CTCACACTTT-5′) and negative siRNA were purchased from Ruibo Biotechnology (Guangzhou, China) and dissolved in RNase-free water as a 20 µmol/L stock. Negative siRNA was designed by Ruibo biotechnology and belonged to scrambled control. Cells were transfected with siRNAs using the Ruibo FECT™ CP transfection kit, plated in 96-well or 6-well plates and incubated at 37 °C for 24 h. siRNAs were diluted in transfection reagent and incubated for 15 min at room temperature to allow the formation of transfection complexes prior to addition to the cells (final concentration: 30 nmol/L). Experiments with test drugs started 24 h after the transfection. Efficiency of transfection was verified with Western blotting.

Colon cancer xenograft

All animal experiments were performed in accordance with relevant guidelines and regulations. Briefly, HCT-116 cells (1×10^7 cells in 200-µL PBS) were injected into the right armpits of 6-week-old female BALB/c nude mice (SPF Biotechnology Co., Ltd., Beijing, China). At 21 days after the inoculation, tumors were removed and cut into 2 m × 2 m × 2 m prisms, and transplanted into the right flanks of other mice through a trocar. Seven days later, mice were randomized to receive azithromycin (50 mg/kg/day, via oral administration, for 3 consecutive days in a week) or TRAIL (10 mg/kg, via the tail vein, once a week). Tumor volumes and body weights were monitored once every 2 days. The tumor volume was calculated by the following formula: $V = ab^2/2$ (a represents the length of the tumor and b represents the width). The animal experiment lasted for a total of 32 days. At the end of experiment, the tumors were removed and fixed with formalin to detect cell proliferation by immunohistochemistry.

Ki-67

Tissue sections (5 µm) were quenched with 3% H_2O_2 for 10 min at room temperature after dewaxing and antigen retrieval in hot citrate buffer. After blocking with 5% BSA for 30 min at 37 °C, tissue sections were incubated with a monoclonal anti-Ki-67 nuclear antigen antibody (ZSGB-BIO) at 4 °C overnight. Immunostaining was assessed in 3 randomly selected fields under a microscope with a 200 × objective lens and photographed. Images were analyzed using a microscope-matched analytical software (Leica QWin Standard).

Assessment of drug interaction

The mode of drug interaction was evaluated based on the coefficient of drug interaction (CDI), calculated as: $CDI = AB/(A \times B)$, where AB is the survival rate of the cells exposed to both agents and A or B is the survival rate of cells exposed to either agent alone. A CDI at < 1.0 indicates synergistic effect; a CDI at < 0.7 indicates strongly synergistic effect [17].

Statistical analysis

All experiments were repeated for at least three times. Data are expressed as the mean ± SD, and analyzed with Student's t test for independent samples. Statistical significance was set at $P < 0.05$.

Results

Azithromycin inhibited cell proliferation

In a pilot experiments with four colon cancer cell lines (SW620, DiFi, SW480 and HCT-116), only SW480 and HCT-116 cells were sensitive to azithromycin (Fig. 1a). Accordingly, subsequent experiments were conducted in SW480 and HCT-116 cells. Azithromycin inhibited cell proliferation in a dose- and time-dependent manner in both HCT-116 and SW480 cells (Fig. 1b). The half-inhibitory concentration (IC_{50}) upon 48-h treatment was 63.19 ± 24.60 and 140.85 ± 32.81 µmol/L in HCT-116 and SW480 cells, respectively. Western blot analysis failed to showed differences of Erk and p38 MAPK expression among the four cell lines (Fig. 1c). In contrast, DR4/5 and Akt proteins in DiFi cells were much lower than in other

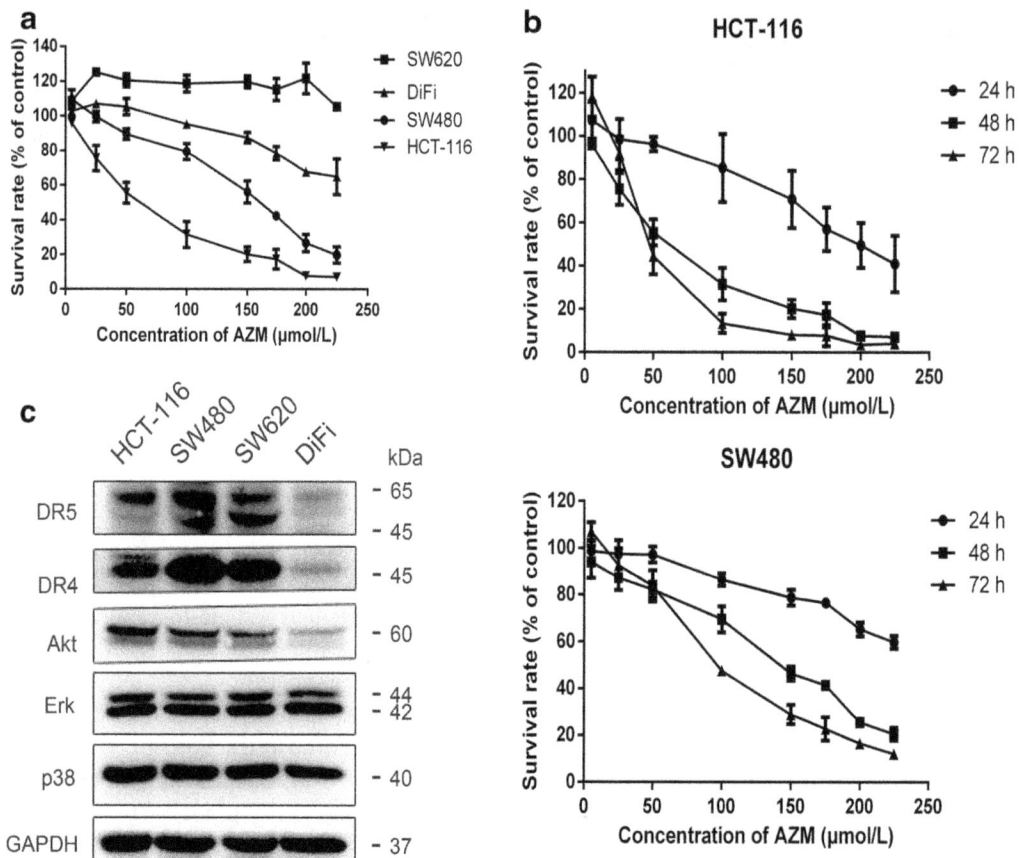

Fig. 1 Azithromycin inhibits cell proliferation of colon cancer cell lines. **a** The viability of SW620, DiFi, SW480 and HCT-116 cells after 48 h-of treatment with azithromycin at various concentrations was assessed with the SRB assay. **b** The proliferative activity of HCT-116 and SW480 cells after treatment with azithromycin (5–225 μmol/L) for 24–72 h was assessed by the SRB assay. The survival rate was calculated as a ratio to the control group (untreated cells). Values represent the mean ± SD of three independent samples. Each experiment was repeated three times. **c** DR4/5 expression, Akt and MAPK pathways of colon cancer cell lines. HCT-116, SW480, SW620 and DiFi cells not receiving any treatment were used as controls. AZM represents azithromycin

cell lines, suggesting that DR4/5, MAPK and Akt signal pathways may be not related to azithromycin sensitivity in our experimental system.

Azithromycin and TRAIL inhibit cell proliferation synergistically

The current study examined the potential interaction between azithromycin and TRAIL. Expression, purification and verification of TRAIL (using anti-His Tag and anti-TRAIL antibody) were illustrated in Fig. 2a. Although SW480 and HCT-116 cells were chose to subsequent experiments due to their sensitivity to azithromycin, we also needed to identify that if they were more sensitive to TRAIL than two other cells, so SRB assay was used to detect the anti-proliferation effects of TRAIL in four kinds of colon cancer cells and the results showed that TRAIL decreased the cell viability of SW480 and HCT-116 cells in a dose-dependent manner (Fig. 2b).

Next, we exposed these four kinds of cells to TRAIL alone, azithromycin alone, or the drug combination for 48 h. The results showed that there was no synergism between TRAIL alone, azithromycin in SW620 and DiFi cells (data not shown). However, the combination of azithromycin at 25–150 μmol/L with TRAIL (7.8125 and 16.625 nmol/L) was much more effective in reducing HCT-116 and SW480 cell proliferation than either single agent alone (Fig. 2c). The CDI was 0.5–1 in HCT-116 cells and 0.3–0.7 in SW480 cells.

Azithromycin enhanced TRAIL-induced cell death in HCT-116 and SW480 cells

Annexin V-FITC/PI staining was detected by flow cytometry analysis. Cell death rate in HCT-116 cells was $(12.73 \pm 1.76)\%$ in the control group, $(30.78 \pm 8.31)\%$ in the TRAIL group (15.625 nmol/L), $(15.73 \pm 5.07)\%$ in the azithromycin (50 μmol/L) group, $(33.08 \pm 7.9)\%$

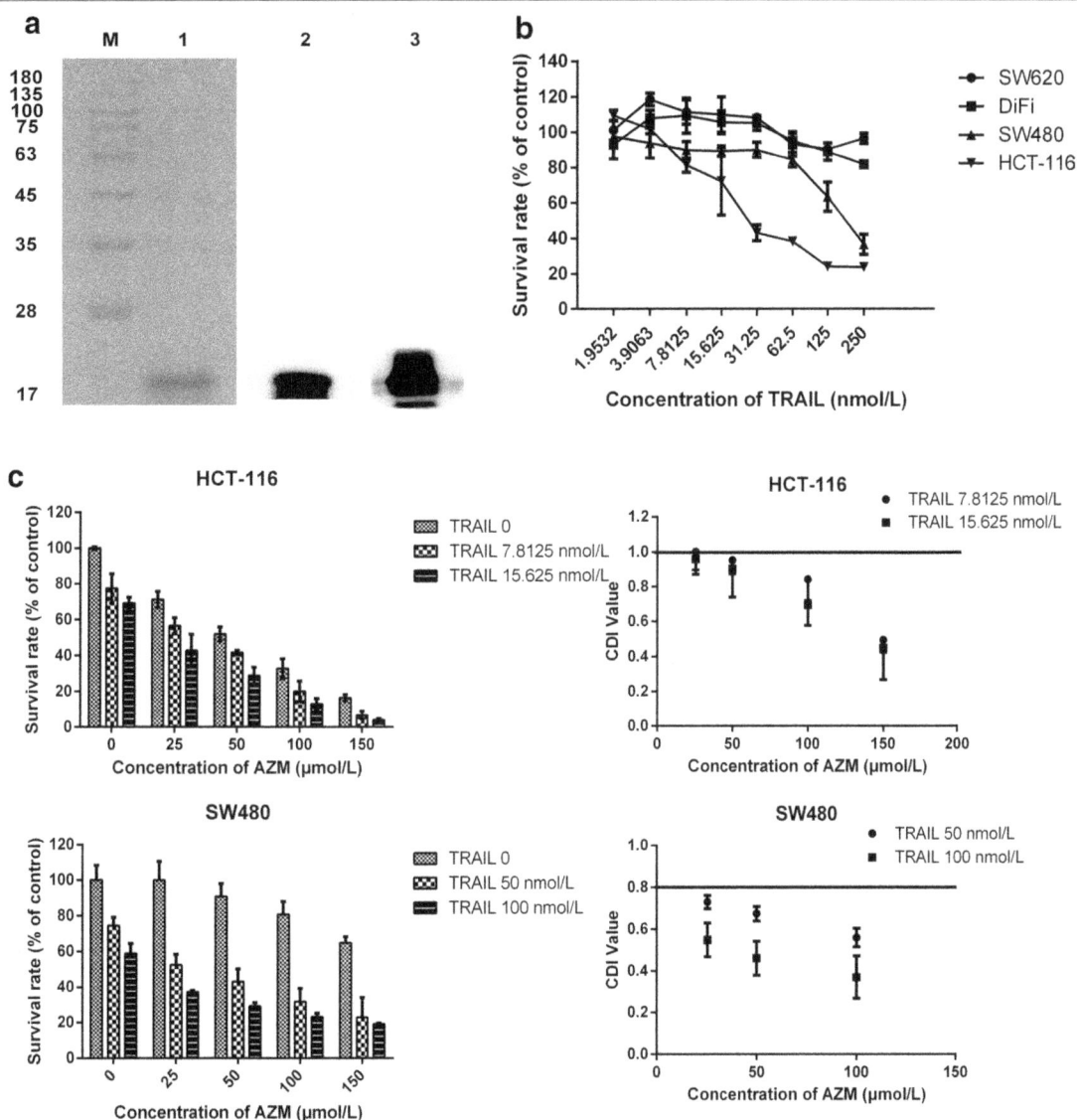

Fig. 2 The anti-survival effect of TRAIL alone and the combination of azithromycin and TRAIL in colon cancer cells. **a** The purification of TRAIL protein. M represents marker; 1 represents TRAIL protein; 2 represents Western blot by His-tag antibody; 3 represents Western blot by anti-TRAIL antibody. **b** The proliferation of four types of colon cancer cells (SW620, DiFi, SW480 and HCT-116) treated with various concentrations of TRAIL for 24 h, as detected by a SRB assay. **c** The synergistic inhibitory effect of azithromycin and TRAIL on the proliferation of SW480 and HCT-116 cells. HCT-116 cells were treated with azithromycin (25–150 μmol/L) and TRAIL (7.8125 and 15.625 nmol/L) for 48 h; SW480 cells were treated with TRAIL at 50 and 100 nmol/L. The survival rate was calculated as a ratio to the control group (untreated cells). CDI value < 1 represents a synergistic effect and CDI < 0.7 indicates a robust synergistic effect. Values represent the mean ± SD of three independent samples. Each experiment was repeated three times. AZM represents azithromycin

in the TRAIL + azithromycin (50 μmol/L) group, (24.06 ± 6.16)% in the azithromycin (100 μmol/L) group, and (66.88 ± 11.19)% in the TRAIL + azithromycin (100 μmol/L) group, respectively (Fig. 3a). At 100 μmol/L, azithromycin enhanced the antitumor activity of TRAIL more than at 50 μmol/L in HCT-116 cells. Cell death rate in SW480 cells was (13.49 ± 4.63)% in the control group, (56.17 ± 18.51)%

in the TRAIL (100 nmol/L) group, (14.20 ± 4.22)% in the azithromycin (50 μmol/L) group, (74.85 ± 7.53)% in the TRAIL + azithromycin (50 μmol/L) group, (21.24 ± 2.76)% in the AZM (100 μmol/L) group, and (89.37 ± 5.07)% in the TRAIL + azithromycin (100 μmol/L) group, respectively. At the concentrations used in the current study, azithromycin induced little cell apoptosis or necrosis, whereas combinations of

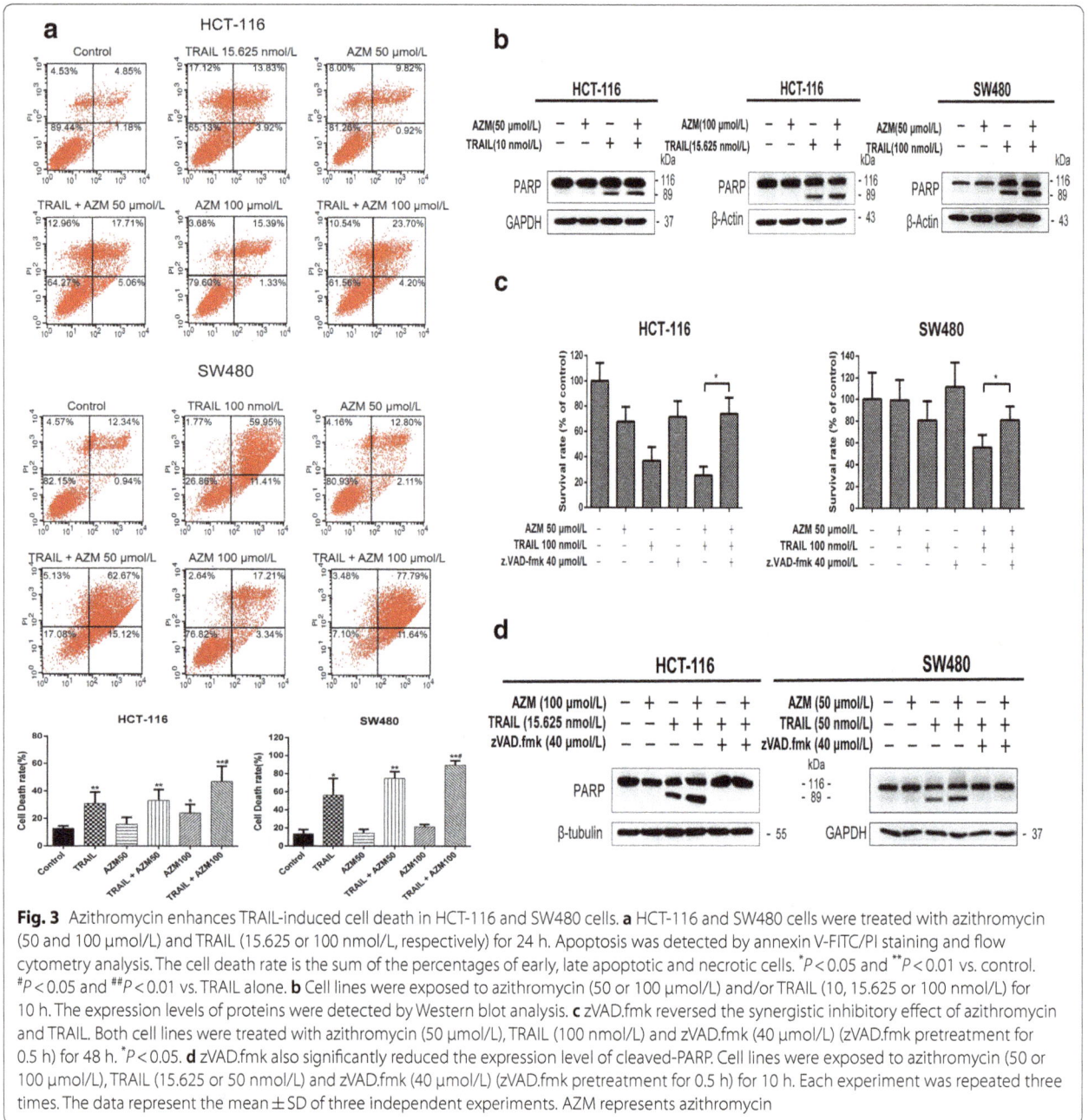

Fig. 3 Azithromycin enhances TRAIL-induced cell death in HCT-116 and SW480 cells. **a** HCT-116 and SW480 cells were treated with azithromycin (50 and 100 μmol/L) and TRAIL (15.625 or 100 nmol/L, respectively) for 24 h. Apoptosis was detected by annexin V-FITC/PI staining and flow cytometry analysis. The cell death rate is the sum of the percentages of early, late apoptotic and necrotic cells. *$P < 0.05$ and **$P < 0.01$ vs. control. #$P < 0.05$ and ##$P < 0.01$ vs. TRAIL alone. **b** Cell lines were exposed to azithromycin (50 or 100 μmol/L) and/or TRAIL (10, 15.625 or 100 nmol/L) for 10 h. The expression levels of proteins were detected by Western blot analysis. **c** zVAD.fmk reversed the synergistic inhibitory effect of azithromycin and TRAIL. Both cell lines were treated with azithromycin (50 μmol/L), TRAIL (100 nmol/L) and zVAD.fmk (40 μmol/L) (zVAD.fmk pretreatment for 0.5 h) for 48 h. *$P < 0.05$. **d** zVAD.fmk also significantly reduced the expression level of cleaved-PARP. Cell lines were exposed to azithromycin (50 or 100 μmol/L), TRAIL (15.625 or 50 nmol/L) and zVAD.fmk (40 μmol/L) (zVAD.fmk pretreatment for 0.5 h) for 10 h. Each experiment was repeated three times. The data represent the mean ± SD of three independent experiments. AZM represents azithromycin

azithromycin and TRAIL enhanced cell death in both HCT-116 and SW480 cell lines.

The expression of cleaved-PARP was increased in the combination treatment group relative to TRAIL or azithromycin alone (Fig. 3b), which was consistent with the results of flow cytometry analysis. SRB assay showed that zVAD.fmk, a broad-range caspase inhibitor, attenuated the synergistic inhibitory effect of azithromycin and TRAIL on cell proliferation (Fig. 3c).

In addition, zVAD.fmk significantly reduced the expression levels of cleaved-PARP (Fig. 3d).

Synergism between azithromycin and TRAIL in mouse xenograft

No death or significant body weight change was observed in any treatment group (Fig. 4a). Combined treatment with azithromycin and TRAIL significantly

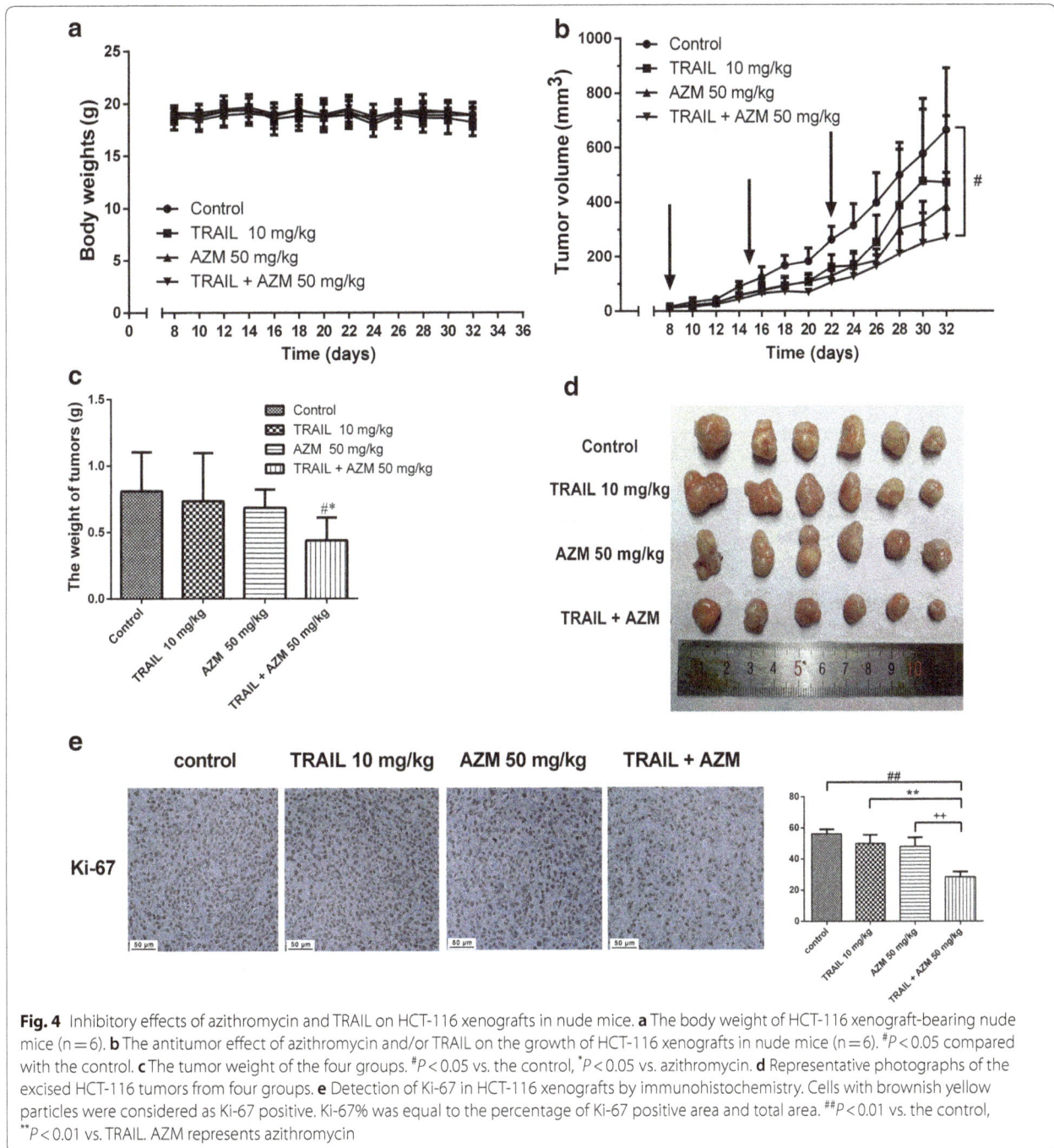

Fig. 4 Inhibitory effects of azithromycin and TRAIL on HCT-116 xenografts in nude mice. **a** The body weight of HCT-116 xenograft-bearing nude mice (n = 6). **b** The antitumor effect of azithromycin and/or TRAIL on the growth of HCT-116 xenografts in nude mice (n = 6). $^{#}P < 0.05$ compared with the control. **c** The tumor weight of the four groups. $^{#}P < 0.05$ vs. the control, $^{*}P < 0.05$ vs. azithromycin. **d** Representative photographs of the excised HCT-116 tumors from four groups. **e** Detection of Ki-67 in HCT-116 xenografts by immunohistochemistry. Cells with brownish yellow particles were considered as Ki-67 positive. Ki-67% was equal to the percentage of Ki-67 positive area and total area. $^{##}P < 0.01$ vs. the control, $^{**}P < 0.01$ vs. TRAIL. AZM represents azithromycin

inhibited the growth of HCT-116 xenografts (Fig. 4b, c for tumor volume and weight, respectively). The CDI was 0.87. The anti-tumor rate of the combined group was 45.88%. The synergistic effects were also apparent by inspecting the size and morphology of the xenografts (Fig. 4d). Ki-67 was significantly lower in the combination group than either azithromycin or TRAIL alone (Fig. 4e).

Azithromycin increased the expression of death receptors

Western blotting was used to examine the changes in DR4 and DR5 protein levels. Azithromycin at the concentration of 100 or 200 μmol/L increased the expression of DR4 and DR5 in 4–16 h in HCT-116 or SW480 cells, respectively (Fig. 5a). Doses of azithromycin at 50–150 or 150–250 μmol/L also elevated the levels of DR4 and DR5 in HCT-116 or SW480 cells, respectively (Fig. 5b).

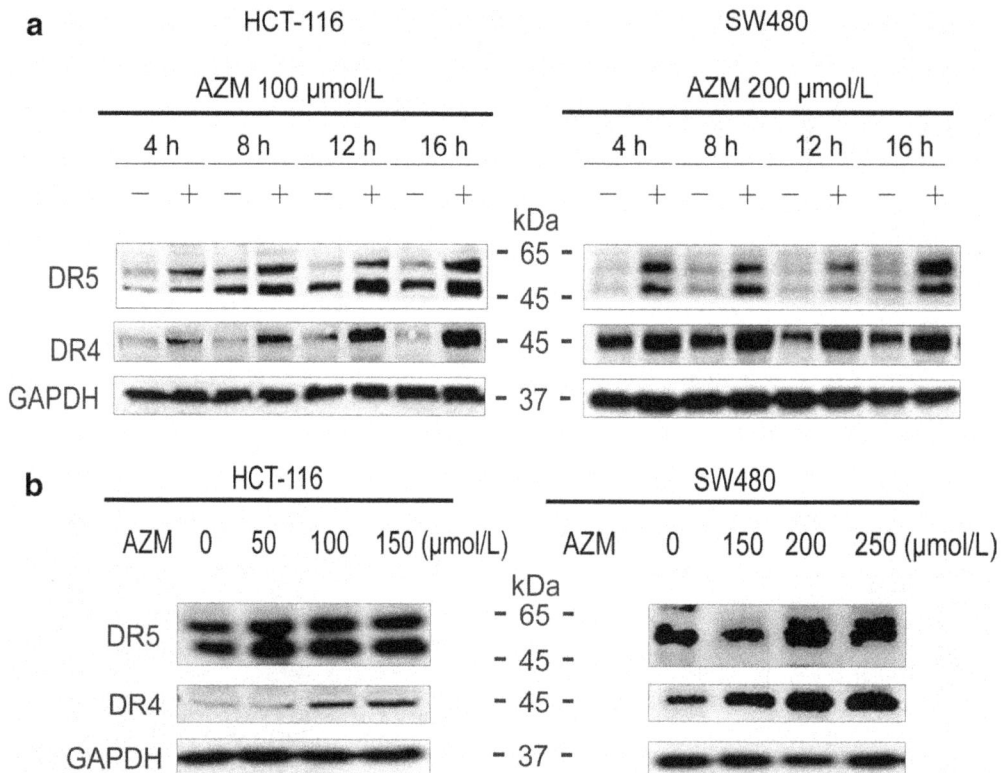

Fig. 5 Azithromycin increases the expression of the death receptor proteins. **a** HCT-116 and SW480 cells were treated with azithromycin for the indicated times. **b** Cells were treated with various concentrations of azithromycin for 10 h. The expression levels of proteins were determined using Western blot analysis. The data are shown as the mean ± SD of three independent samples. AZM represents azithromycin

Azithromycin blocked autophagy flux

In our experiments, HCT-116 and SW480 cells were treated with azithromycin (100 or 200 µmol/L) or various doses of azithromycin before determination of the expression levels of p62 and LC-3B using Western blot. Briefly, azithromycin increased p62 and LC-3B in both cell lines (Fig. 6a, b). Consistently, AO staining showed increased red fluorescence intensity in both cell lines after treatment with azithromycin for 24 h (Fig. 6c).

LC-3B-involved autophagy inhibition targeted death receptor 4 and 5 for increment to strengthen TRAIL activity

Knocking down of DR4 and DR5 with siRNAs increased survival rates and a decreased cleaved-PARP levels in the cells exposed to azithromycin (50 µmol/L) plus TRAIL (15.625 or 100 nmol/L) (Fig. 7a).

The RIPK1 allosteric inhibitor necrostatin-1 and ROS scavenger N-acetylcysteine did not affect the anti-proliferation activity of the combination of azithromycin and TRAIL (Additional file 1: Figure S1A, B), so we next examined whether LC-3B-involved autophagy inhibition is involved in the synergistic antitumor activity between azithromycin and TRAIL. LC-3B siRNA (30 nmol/L) or

CQ (20 µmol/L) potentiated the anti-proliferation activity of TRAIL (Fig. 7b). Also, LC-3B level elevated by azithromycin (50 µmol/L) did not change upon knocking down of DR4 or DR5 (Fig. 7c). In contrast, LC-3B siRNA (30 nmol/L) alone or combined with azithromycin (50 µmol/L) increased the expression of DR4 and DR5 (Fig. 7d). Similarly, CQ (20 and 30 µmol/L) elevated DR4 and DR5 levels in a dose-dependent manner (Fig. 7e).

Discussion

The current study showed that azithromycin could reduce the proliferation of SW480 and HCT-116 colon cancer cells. Varying sensitivity of different colon cancer cells to azithromycin could not be attributed to expression of DR4/5, MAPK and Akt signal pathways-related proteins. TRAIL decreased the viability of SW480 and HCT-116 cells. Most importantly, we showed synergistic inhibitory action between azithromycin and TRAIL on the proliferation in these two cell lines. Our results also suggested that azithromycin could enhance TRAIL-induced apoptosis via a caspase-dependent pathway in SW480 and HCT-116 cells. Experiments in nude mice

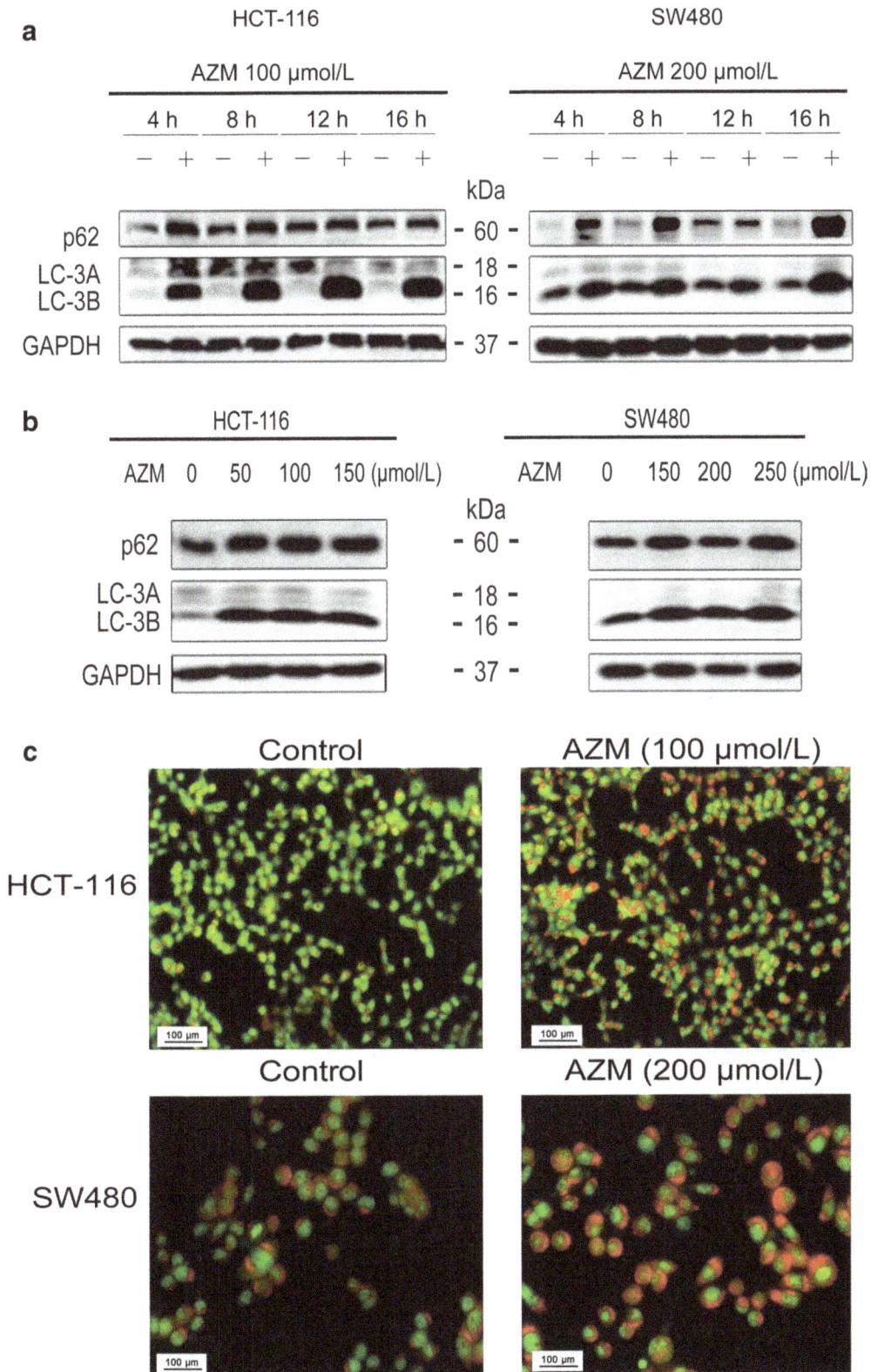

Fig. 6 Azithromycin blocks autophagy flux. **a, b** HCT-116 and SW480 cells were treated with azithromycin for the indicated times or treated with various concentrations of azithromycin for 10 h. The expression levels of proteins were determined using Western blot analysis. The data are shown as the mean ± SD of three independent experiments. **c** Acridine orange (AO) staining. The green signals represent the nuclei; red signals represent the acidic vesicles, including lysosomes and autophagolysosmes. AZM represents azithromycin

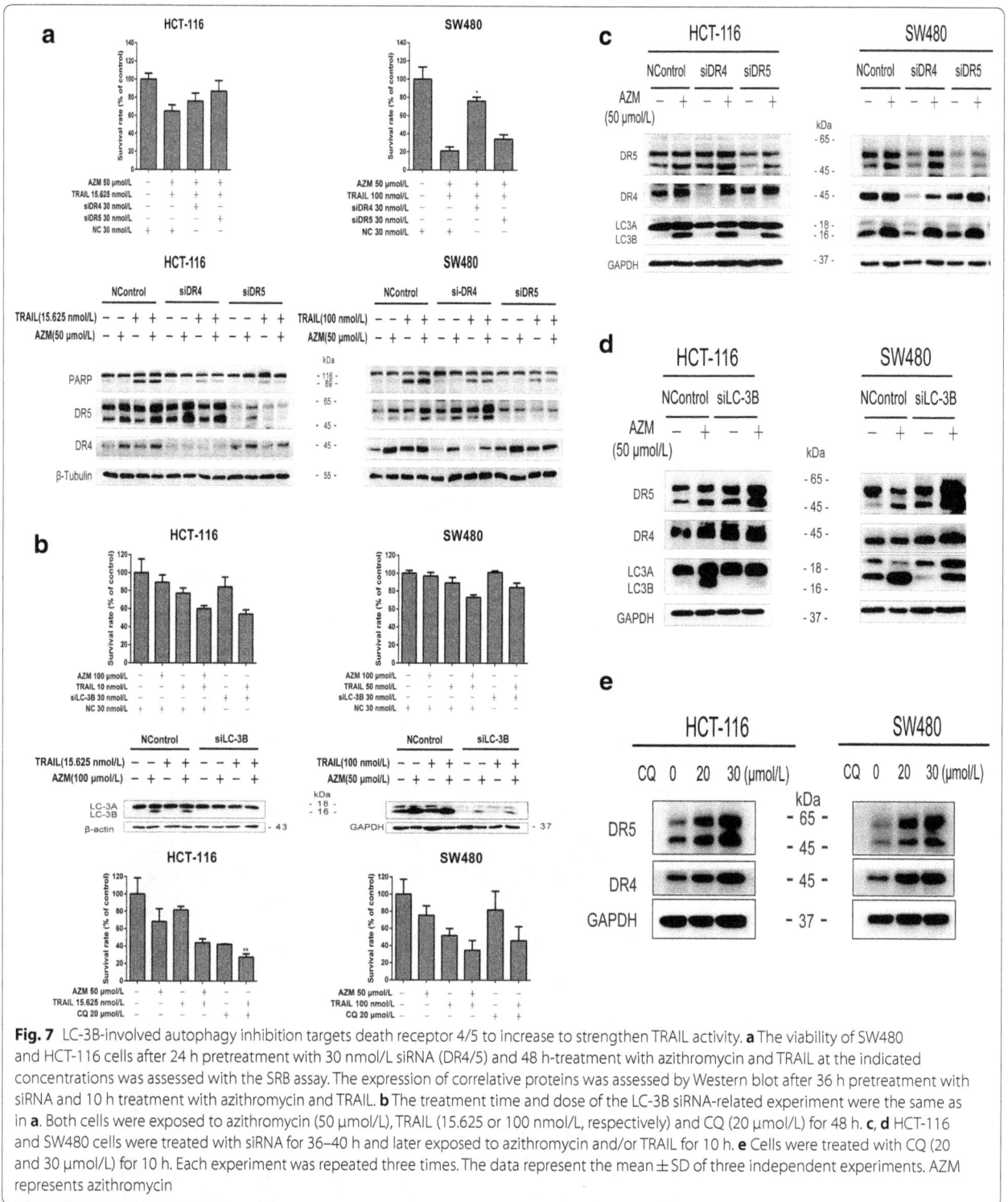

Fig. 7 LC-3B-involved autophagy inhibition targets death receptor 4/5 to increase to strengthen TRAIL activity. **a** The viability of SW480 and HCT-116 cells after 24 h pretreatment with 30 nmol/L siRNA (DR4/5) and 48 h-treatment with azithromycin and TRAIL at the indicated concentrations was assessed with the SRB assay. The expression of correlative proteins was assessed by Western blot after 36 h pretreatment with siRNA and 10 h treatment with azithromycin and TRAIL. **b** The treatment time and dose of the LC-3B siRNA-related experiment were the same as in **a**. Both cells were exposed to azithromycin (50 μmol/L), TRAIL (15.625 or 100 nmol/L, respectively) and CQ (20 μmol/L) for 48 h. **c, d** HCT-116 and SW480 cells were treated with siRNA for 36–40 h and later exposed to azithromycin and/or TRAIL for 10 h. **e** Cells were treated with CQ (20 and 30 μmol/L) for 10 h. Each experiment was repeated three times. The data represent the mean ± SD of three independent experiments. AZM represents azithromycin

carrying xenograft confirmed the synergistic action between azithromycin and TRAIL.

Azithromycin has been shown to induce apoptosis and necrosis in HeLa cells [4]. At 50 and 100 μmol/L, azithromycin alone did not induce cell apoptosis or necrosis in

the current study. Such a difference could reflect different sensitivity of the cells to azithromycin. Also, the concentration of azithromycin used in our system was lower than needed to induce apoptosis in the previous study. We found increased expression of death receptors DR4 and DR5 upon azithromycin treatment. TRAIL induces apoptosis via specific binding to DR4 and DR5. Moreover, several drugs (i.e., celecoxib, quinacrian, and bleomycin) sensitize certain types of cancer cells to apoptosis induced by TRAIL through increasing the protein levels of DR4 or DR5 [19–22]. We therefore suspect that the death receptor protein levels are implicated in the synergistic action between azithromycin and TRAIL.

Recent studies have shown that azithromycin is an autophagy inhibitor in myeloma and pancreatic cancer cells [6, 7], but whether azithromycin inhibits autophagy in colon cancer cells remains unknown. Autophagy is a lysosomal degradation process that involves two stages: the formation of autophagosomes (the early stage) and sequential fusion with lysosomes to form autolysosomes (the later stage) [23]. Autophagy could be inhibited by disrupting autophagosome formation, for example with 3-MA and ATG 5 siRNA, or by suppressing lysosomal activity, such as with chloroquine (CQ) and bafilomycin A1 [24]. The transformation of LC3 protein, from LC-3A in the cytoplasm to LC-3B that in turn binds the outer membranes, is essential to complete autophagosomes [10]. The p62 protein is a substrate of autophagy, and is widely used together with LC-3B to detect autophagy induction or inhibition. In our study, azithromycin increased the expression of LC-3B and p62 proteins, suggesting that azithromycin produces the anti-tumor effects by blocking autophagy flux.

Our results showed that azithromycin increased the expression of death receptors and blocked autophagy flux in colon cancer cells. The relationship between autophagy inhibition and death receptors-mediated cell death requires further investigation. Knockdown of DR4 and DR5 with siRNA increased survival rate of colon cancer cells and decreased cleaved-PARP. All together, these findings suggest that azithromycin treatment enhanced TRAIL-induced apoptosis via the up-regulation of DR4 and DR5 in colon cancer cells. A previous study showed that DR4 and DR5 co-localize with LC-3B on the surface of autophagosomes, which result in the decrease of the surface expression of DR4/5 and eventually induce TRAIL resistance in breast cancer cells [10]. Interestingly, in our experimental system, azithromycin and CQ simultaneously increased the expression of DR4, DR5 and LC-3B in colon cancer cells, despite of enhancing the anti-proliferation effects of TRAIL. In addition, the knockdown of DR4 or DR5 did not affect the expression of LC-3B. In contrast, the reduction in the LC-3B protein level increased the expression of DR4 and DR5 to some extent, and LC-3B siRNA also raised the anti-survival effect of TRAIL. Notably, not all autophagy inhibitors could increase the expression of DR4/5 protein. For instance, it has been reported that 3-MA decreased

DR4/5 proteins levels in colon cancer cells [25]. Thus we speculate that autophagy inhibition in early vs. late stages could lead to opposite results. Accordingly, azithromycin, CQ and LC-3B cooperate with TRAIL to produce antitumor effects via the induction of LC-3B-involved autophagy inhibition to up-regulate DR4/5 proteins.

In addition to apoptosis induction, TRAIL causes RIP1-dependent necroptosis [26–28]. By the RIPK1 allosteric inhibitor necrostatin-1 did not affect the anti-proliferation activity of the combination of azithromycin and TRAIL in our experimental system. Several previous studies have noted that the up-regulation of death receptors is associated with the activation of reactive oxygen species (ROS) [20, 29, 30]. The results obtained with the ROS scavenger N-acetylcysteine in the current study suggest that the ROS pathway is not involved in the mechanism of the synergistic antitumor effect between azithromycin and TRAIL.

There are some limitations in the current study. For example, in animal experiments, the standard deviation in tumor size was quite large. Also, participation of signaling pathways other than autophagy flux was not examined. Regardless of these limitations, the synergistic action between azithromycin and TRAIL is apparent. A schematic diagram of the working hypothesis is shown in Fig. 8.

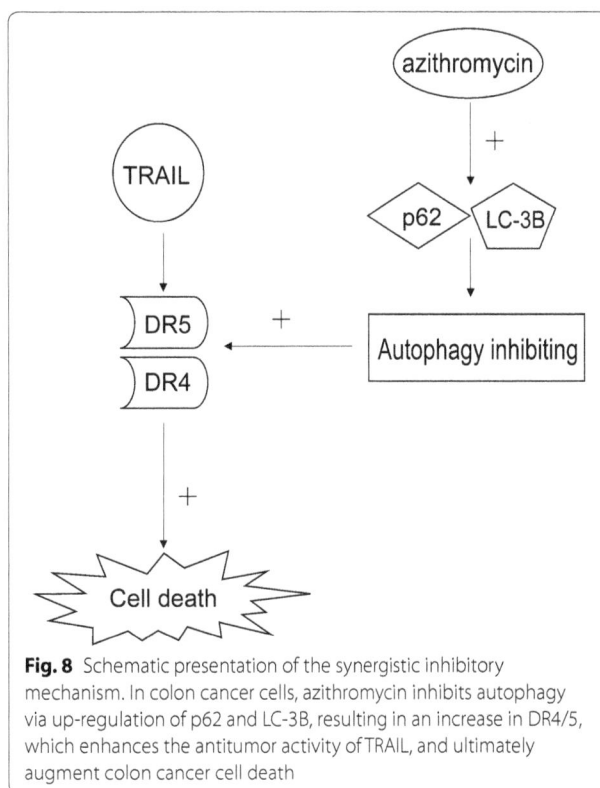

Fig. 8 Schematic presentation of the synergistic inhibitory mechanism. In colon cancer cells, azithromycin inhibits autophagy via up-regulation of p62 and LC-3B, resulting in an increase in DR4/5, which enhances the antitumor activity of TRAIL, and ultimately augment colon cancer cell death

Conclusions

Azithromycin could enhance the anticancer activity of TRAIL via LC-3B-involved autophagy inhibition to up-regulate DR4/5 in colon cancer cells both in vitro and in vivo. These results encourage further studies to explore using azithromycin in the treatment of colon cancer.

Additional file

Additional file 1: Figure S1. The ROS pathway and necroptosis are not involved in the combined antitumor effect of azithromycin and TRAIL. (A) NAC did not affect the synergistic inhibitory effect of azithromycin and TRAIL. The viability of HCT-116 and SW480 cells after 0.5 h-pretreatment with NAC (5 mmol/L) followed by a 48 h treatment with azithromycin (50 μmol/L) and TRAIL (15.625 or 100 nmol/L, respectively) was assessed using the SRB assay. (B) Necrostatin-1 did not affect the combined anti-tumor effect of azithromycin and TRAIL in the colon cells. Both cells were treated with azithromycin (100 μmol/L), TRAIL (100 nmol/L) and necrosta-tin-1 (25, 50, 75 and 100 μmol/L) for 48 h. Values represent the mean ± SD of three independent experiments. AZM represents azithromycin.

Abbreviations

3-MA: 3-methyl adenine; AO: acridine orange; CQ: chloroquine; DR4/5: death receptor 4/5; LC-3B: microtubule associated protein 1 light chain 3 beta; NAC: N-acetylcysteine; PARP: poly-ADP-ribose polymerase; RAPA: rapamycin; RIPK1: receptor interacting protein kinase 1; ROS: reactive oxygen species; SRB: sul-forhodamine B; TCA: trichloroacetic acid; TRAIL: tumor necrosis factor-related apoptosis-inducing ligand; zVAD.fmk: benzyloxycarbonyl-Val-Ala-Asp (OMe) fluoromethylketone.

Authors' contributions

SZC designed experiments and revised the manuscript. XRQ did all experiments and wrote the manuscript. XFW provided TRAIL for XRQ to do experiments. YS and YL help to do the animal experiments. For Figs 1, 2, 3, 4, 5, 6, 7, XRQ generated the data, constructed and assembled the figures. Figure 8 was conceptualized and generated by SZC. All authors read and approved the final manuscript.

Acknowledgements

We are grateful to Sun S-Y (Emory University, USA) for suggestion and editing of the manuscript.

Competing interests

The authors declare that they have no competing interests.

Funding

The manuscript was supported by grants from the National Natural Science Foundation of China (81373437 and 81621064) and CAMS Innovation Fund for Medical Sciences (CIFMS) (2016-I2M-02-002).

References

1. Eisenblatter M, Klaus C, Pletz MW, Orawa H, Hahn H, Wagner J, et al. Influence of azithromycin and clarithromycin on macrolide susceptibility of viridans streptococci from the oral cavity of healthy volunteers. Eur J Clin Microbiol Infect Dis. 2008;27(11):1087–92. https://doi.org/10.1007/s10096-008-0547-x.

2. Zheng S, Matzneller P, Zeitlinger M, Schmidt S. Development of a population pharmacokinetic model characterizing the tissue distribution of azithromycin in healthy subjects. Antimicrob Agents Chemother. 2014;58(11):6675–84. https://doi.org/10.1128/AAC.02904-14.

3. Zhou X, Zhang Y, Li Y, Hao X, Liu X, Wang Y. Azithromycin synergistically enhances anti-proliferative activity of vincristine in cervical and gastric cancer cells. Cancers. 2012;4(4):1318–32. https://doi.org/10.3390/cancers4041318.

4. Chu DJ, Yao DE, Zhuang YF, Hong Y, Zhu XC, Fang ZR, et al. Azithromycin enhances the favorable results of paclitaxel and cisplatin in patients with advanced non-small cell lung cancer. Genet Mol Res. 2014;13(2):2796–805. https://doi.org/10.4238/2014.April.14.8.

5. Lamb R, Ozsvari B, Lisanti CL, Tanowitz HB, Howell A, Martinezoutschoorn UE, et al. Antibiotics that target mitochondria effectively eradicate cancer stem cells, across multiple tumor types: treating cancer like an infectious disease. Oncotarget. 2015;6(7):4569–84. https://doi.org/10.18632/oncotarget.3174.

6. Moriya S, Che X-F, Komatsu S, Abe A, Kawaguchi T, Gotoh A, et al. Macrolide antibiotics block autophagy flux and sensitize to bort-ezomib via endoplasmic reticulum stress-mediated CHOP induction in myeloma cells. Int J Oncol. 2013;42(5):1541–50. https://doi.org/10.3892/ijo.2013.1870.

7. Mukai S, Moriya S, Hiramoto M, Kazama H, Kokuba H, Che X, et al. Macrolides sensitize EGFR-TKI-induced non-apoptotic cell death via blocking autophagy flux in pancreatic cancer cell lines. Int J Oncol. 2016;48(1):45. https://doi.org/10.3892/ijo.2015.3237.

8. Komatsu S, Miyazawa K, Moriya S, Takase A, Naito M, Inazu M, et al. Clarithromycin enhances bortezomib-induced cytotoxicity via endo-plasmic reticulum stress-mediated CHOP (GADD153) induction and autophagy in breast cancer cells. Int J Oncol. 2012;40(4):1029–39. https://doi.org/10.3892/ijo.2011.1317.

9. Van Nuffel AMT. Repurposing drugs in oncology (ReDO)—clarithromycin as an anti-cancer agent. ecancermedicalscience. 2015;9:513. https://doi.org/10.3332/ecancer.2015.513.

10. Di X, Zhang G, Zhang Y, Takeda K, Rosado LAR, Zhang B. Accumulation of autophagosomes in breast cancer cells induces TRAIL resistance through downregulation of surface expression of death receptors 4 and 5. Oncotarget. 2013;4(9):1349–64. https://doi.org/10.18632/oncotarget.1174.

11. Sung-Wook K, Ju-Hee L, Ji-Hong M, Nazim UMD, You-Jin L, Jae-Won S, et al. Niacin alleviates TRAIL-mediated colon cancer cell death via autophagy flux activation. Oncotarget. 2016;7(4):4356–68. https://doi.org/10.18632/oncotarget.5374.

12. Cousin FJ, Sandrine JL, Nathalie T, Catherine B, Elodie J, Le MMG, et al. The probiotic Propionibacterium freudenreichii as a new adjuvant for TRAIL-based therapy in colorectal cancer. Oncotarget. 2016;7(6):7161–78. https://doi.org/10.18632/oncotarget.6881.

13. Hwang JS, Lee HC, Oh SC, Lee DH, Kwon KH. Shogaol overcomes TRAIL resistance in colon cancer cells via inhibiting of survivin. Tumour Biol. 2015;36(11):8819–29. https://doi.org/10.1007/s13277-015-3629-2.

14. Kauntz H, Bousserouel S, Gossé F, Raul F. Silibinin triggers apoptotic signaling pathways and autophagic survival response in human colon adenocarcinoma cells and their derived metastatic cells. Apoptosis. 2011;16(10):1042–53. https://doi.org/10.1007/s10495-011-0631-z.

15. Park EJ, Min KJ, Choi KS, Kubatka P, Kruzliak P, Kim DE, et al. Chloroquine enhances TRAIL-mediated apoptosis through up-regulation of DR5 by stabilization of mRNA and protein in cancer cells. Sci Rep. 2016;6:22921. https://doi.org/10.1038/srep22921.

16. Zhang Z, Li Z, Wu X, Zhang CF, Calway T, He TC, et al. TRAIL pathway is associated with inhibition of colon cancer by protopanaxadiol. J Pharmacol Sci. 2015;127(1):83–91. https://doi.org/10.1016/j.jphs.2014.11.003.

17. Lv X, Liu F, Shang Y, Chen SZ. Honokiol exhibits enhanced antitumor effects with chloroquine by inducing cell death and inhibiting autophagy in human non-small cell lung cancer cells. Oncol Rep. 2015;34(3):1289–300. https://doi.org/10.3892/or.2015.4091.

18. Liu F, Shang Y, Chen SZ. Chloroquine potentiates the anti-cancer effect of lidamycin on non-small cell lung cancer cells in vitro. Acta Pharmacol Sin. 2014;35(5):645–52. https://doi.org/10.1038/aps.2014.3.

19. Chen S, Liu X, Yue P, Schonthal AH, Khuri FR, Sun SY. CCAAT/enhancer binding protein homologous protein-dependent death receptor 5 induction and ubiquitin/proteasome-mediated cellular FLICE-inhibitory

protein down-regulation contribute to enhancement of tumor necrosis factor-related apoptosis-inducing ligand-induced apoptosis by dimethyl-celecoxib in human non small-cell lung cancer cells. Mol Pharmacol. 2007;72(5):1269–79. https://doi.org/10.1124/mol.107.037465.

20. Das S, Tripathi N, Preet R, Siddharth S, Nayak A, Bharatam PV, et al. Quina-crine induces apoptosis in cancer cells by forming a functional bridge between TRAIL-DR5 complex and modulating the mitochondrial intrinsic cascade. Oncotarget. 2016;8(1):248–67. https://doi.org/10.18632/oncotarget.11335.

21. Liu X, Yue P, Zhou Z, Khuri FR, Sun SY. Death receptor regulation and celecoxib-induced apoptosis in human lung cancer cells. JNCI J Natl Cancer Inst. 2004;96(23):1769–80. https://doi.org/10.1093/jnci/djh322.

22. Timur M, Cort A, Ozdemir E, Sarikcioglu SB, Sanlioglu S, Sanlioglu AD, et al. Bleomycin induced sensitivity to TRAIL/Apo-2L-mediated apoptosis in human seminomatous testicular cancer cells is correlated with upregula-tion of death receptors. Anti-Cancer Agents Med Chem. 2015;15(1):99–106. https://doi.org/10.2174/1871520614666140829130047.

23. Lippai M, Szatmari Z. Autophagy-from molecular mechanisms to clinical relevance. Cell Biol Toxicol. 2017;33(2):145–68. https://doi.org/10.1007/s10565-016-9374-5.

24. Shi X, Chen Z, Tang S, Wu F, Xiong S, Dong C. Coxsackievirus B3 infection induces autophagic flux, and autophagosomes are critical for efficient viral replication. Adv Virol. 2016;161(8):2197–205. https://doi.org/10.1007/s00705-016-2896-6.

25. Chen L, Meng Y, Guo X, Sheng X, Tai G, Zhang F, et al. Gefitinib enhances human colon cancer cells to TRAIL-induced apoptosis of via autophagy-and JNK-mediated death receptors upregulation. Apoptosis. 2016;21(11):1291–301. https://doi.org/10.1007/s10495-016-1287-5.

26. Jouan-Lanhouet S, Arshad MI, Piquet-Pellorce C, Martin-Chouly C, Le Moigne-Muller G, Van Herreweghe F, et al. TRAIL induces necroptosis involving RIPK1/RIPK3-dependent PARP-1 activation. Cell Death Differ. 2012;19(12):2003–14. https://doi.org/10.1038/cdd.2012.90.

27. Karl I, Jossberger-Werner M, Schmidt N, Horn S, Goebeler M, Leverkus M, et al. TRAF2 inhibits TRAIL-and CD95L-induced apoptosis and necroptosis. Cell Death Dis. 2014;5(10):e1444. https://doi.org/10.1038/cddis.2014.404.

28. Liu XY, Lai F, Yan XG, Jiang CC, Guo ST, Wang CY, et al. RIP1 kinase is an oncogenic driver in melanoma. Can Res. 2015;75(8):1736–48. https://doi.org/10.1158/0008-5472.CAN-14-2199.

29. Jeong J-W, Lee WS, S-i Go, Nagappan A, Baek JY, Lee J-D, et al. Pachymic acid induces apoptosis of EJ bladder cancer cells by dr5 up-regulation, ROS generation, modulation of Bcl-2 and IAP family members. Phytother Res. 2015;29(10):1516–24. https://doi.org/10.1002/ptr.5402.

30. Liu YJ, Lin YC, Lee JC, Kuo SC, Ho CT, Huang LJ, et al. CCT327 enhances TRAIL-induced apoptosis through the induction of death receptors and downregulation of cell survival proteins in TRAIL-resistant human leukemia cells. Oncol Rep. 2014;32(3):1257–64. https://doi.org/10.3892/or.2014.3317.

12

Famitinib in combination with concurrent chemoradiotherapy in patients with locoregionally advanced nasopharyngeal carcinoma: a phase 1, open-label, dose-escalation Study

Qiuyan Chen[1,2†], Linquan Tang[1,2†], Na Liu[1], Feng Han[1,3], Ling Guo[1,2], Shanshan Guo[1,2], Jianwei Wang[1,3], Huai Liu[4], Yanfang Ye[5], Lu Zhang[6], Liting Liu[1,2], Pan Wang[1,2], Yingqin Li[1], Qingmei He[1], Xiaoqun Yang[1], Qingnan Tang[1,2], Yang Li[1,2], YuJing Liang[1,2], XueSong Sun[1,2], Chuanmiao Xie[1,7], Yunxian Mo[1,7], Ying Guo[1,8], Rui Sun[1,2], Haoyuan Mo[1,2], Kajia Cao[1,2], Xiang Guo[1,2], Musheng Zeng[1], Haiqiang Mai[1,2*] and Jun Ma[1,9*] (iD)

Abstract

Background: Famitinib is a tyrosine kinase inhibitor against multiple targets, including vascular endothelial growth factor receptor 2/3, platelet-derived growth factor receptor, and stem cell factor receptor (c-kit). Previous studies have demonstrated anti-tumour activities of famitinib against a wide variety of advanced-stage solid cancers. We aimed to determine the safety and efficacy of famitinib with concurrent chemoradiotherapy (CCRT) in patients with locoregionally advanced nasopharyngeal carcinoma (NPC). We also evaluated the feasibility of contrast-enhanced ultrasound (D-CEUS) as a predictor of early tumour response to famitinib and to correlate functional parameters with clinical efficacy.

Methods: The trial was conducted in subjects with stage III or IVa-b NPC using a 3 + 3 design of escalating famitinib doses. Briefly, subjects received 2 weeks of famitinib monotherapy followed by 7 weeks of famitinib plus CCRT. D-CEUS of the neck lymph nodes was performed at day 0, 8 and 15 after famitinib was administered before starting concurrent chemoradiotherapy. End points included safety, tolerability and anti-tumour activity.

Results: Twenty patients were enrolled (six each for 12.5, 16.5 and 20 mg and two for 25 mg). Two patients in the 25 mg cohort developed dose-limiting toxicities, including grade 4 thrombocytopenia and grade 3 hypertension. The most common grade 3/4 adverse events were leukopenia, neutropenia and radiation mucositis. D-CEUS tests showed that more than 60% of patients achieved a perfusion parameter response after 2 weeks taking famitinib alone, and the parameter response was associated with disease improvement. In the famitinib monotherapy stage, three patients (15%) showed partial responses. The complete response rate was 65% at the completion of treatment and 95% 3 months after the treatment ended. After a median follow-up of 44 months, the 3-year progression-free survival (PFS) and distant metastasis-free survival were 70% and 75%, respectively. Subjects with a decrease of perfusion

*Correspondence: maihq@sysucc.org.cn; majun@sysucc.org
†Qiuyan Chen and Linquan Tang contributed equally to this article
[1] State Key Laboratory of Oncology in South China, Collaborative Innovation Center for Cancer Medicine, Guangdong Key Laboratory of Nasopharyngeal Carcinoma Diagnosis and Therapy, Sun Yat-sen University Cancer Center, Guangzhou 510060, P. R. China
Full list of author information is available at the end of the article

parameter response, such as peak intensity decreased at least 30% after 1 week of famitinib treatment, had higher 3-year PFS (90.9% vs. 44.4%, 95% CI 73.7%–100% vs. 11.9%–76.9%, $P < 0.001$) than those with an increase or a reduction of less than 30%.

Conclusions: The recommended famitinib dose for phase II trial is 20 mg with CCRT for patients with local advanced NPC. D-CEUS is a reliable and early measure of efficacy for famitinib therapies. Further investigation is required to confirm the effects of famitinib plus chemoradiotherapy.

Keywords: Nasopharyngeal carcinoma, Famitinib, Concurrent chemoradiotherapy, Phase I, dynamic contrast-enhanced ultrasound

Background

Nasopharyngeal carcinoma (NPC) is highly endemic in Southern China and Southeast Asia, with a peak incidence of 50 cases per 100,000 [1]. Concurrent chemoradiotherapy (CCRT) with or without adjuvant chemotherapy is currently considered as the standard therapeutic regimen for locoregionally advanced NPC [2–6]. A previous study from this research group [7] demonstrated that induction chemotherapy with cisplatin, fluorouracil, and docetaxel in addition to CCRT significantly improved survival versus CCRT alone for advanced NPC patients. However, the role of induction chemotherapy remains debatable. Currently, experts agree that concurrent use of cisplatin with radiation improves progression-free survival (PFS) and overall survival (OS) [6, 8–11].

Intensity-modulated radiotherapy (IMRT) could target irregularly shaped tumour in a region surrounded by multiple critical organs, and has been increasingly used [12–15]. Irrespective of the availability of modern treatments, up to 30% of patients with locoregionally advanced NPC still die of distant metastasis [14].

Angiogenesis is essential for tumour growth and metastasis, and vascular endothelial growth factor (VEGF) is one of the most studied angiogenic factors. VEGF expression is associated with metastasis in NPC patients [16, 17]. Anti-VEGF antibody bevacizumab has direct antivascular effects with enhanced radiosensitivity [18]. A phase II study showed that the addition of bevacizumab to standard chemoradiation treatment in NPC patients is feasible and could delay the progression of subclinical distant disease [19].

Receptor tyrosine kinase (RTK) inhibitors with multiple targets are also promising for NPC treatment. Expression of the c-kit and platelet-derived growth factor receptor (PDGFR) has been detected in NPC tissues, cell lines and tumour xenografts [20–24]. In preclinical models, RTK inhibitors, such as sunitinib, demonstrated encouraging results in NPC [25, 26]. A phase II trial demonstrated significant responses in recurrent or metastatic NPC patients treated with sunitinib [27]. However, the trial was terminated due to haemorrhagic events occurred in 69% of the patients [27]. Therefore, new multi-target RTK

inhibitors with acceptable safety profiles are needed for NPC.

The sunitinib analogue famitinib is a novel and highly potent multi-target RTK inhibitor against VEGFR, C-Kit, and PDGFR, and has anti-tumour activity in a range of solid tumours [28–30]. The pharmacokinetic data showed that the mean half-lives and major metabolite of famitinib in healthy volunteers were shorter than those of sunitinib [28, 30, 31]. Furthermore, after administration for 28 days, the degrees of famitinib accumulation in vivo were significantly lower than sunitinib [28, 30, 31], indicating that famitinib may be a safer agent. Preclinical studies have demonstrated that both famitinib and sunitinib are synergistic with radiation [32, 33]. On the basis of promising preclinical data, we conducted this phase I study to evaluate the safety, tolerability and dose-limiting toxicities (DLTs) of famitinib with CCRT in NPC patients. The secondary objectives were to assess the anti-tumour activity of famitinib. Previous study has demonstrated that using contrast-enhanced ultrasound (D-CEUS) as a tool to predict early treatment response for metastatic renal cell carcinoma treated with sunitinib. We also evaluate whether D-CEUS could be used to predict famitinib response.

Patients and methods

Patients

This open-label, dose-escalation phase I study enrolled treatment-naïve patients with pathologically proven locoregionally advanced NPC who sought treatment between November 11, 2011 and September 23, 2013 at Sun Yat-sen University Cancer Center, Guangzhou, China. NPC was staged according to the 7th edition American Joint Committee on Cancer [AJCC] staging system. Patients with histologically confirmed undifferentiated NPC, WHO III and confirmed T3-4N1M0 or T1-4N2-3M0 locoregionally advanced NPC were eligible. Other inclusion and exclusion criteria are described in detail in Additional file 1: Methods.

The study protocol was approved by the Ethics Committee of Sun Yat-sen University Cancer Center (Approval No.: A2011-021-01). All patients provided written informed consent to the study. The study was registered at https://register.clinicaltrials.gov (NCT01462474).

Study design and procedures

This trial used a standard $3+3$ design to identify the maximum tolerated dose. Sequential dose-escalation cohorts of three to six patients were given oral famitinib at a starting dose of 12.5 mg/day, which was increased to 16.5, 20, and 25 mg/day. Famitinib alone was administered for 2 weeks prior to starting chemoradiotherapy, followed by 7 weeks of famitinib plus CCRT. Dose escalation was continued until DLTs or until the highest planned dose level without any DLT. If one out of three patients had a DLT, three additional patients were added at that dose. If two out of six patients had a DLT, the dose was declared to be above the maximum tolerated dose.

IMRT was conducted as previously reported [7]. Gross tumour volume included the primary tumour and the enlarged lymph nodes. The definition of planning target volumes (PTVs), high- (CTV-1) and low-risk clinical target volume (CTV-2) are detailed in Additional file 1: Methods.

Cisplatin was administered at 100 mg/m^2 on day 1, 22, and 43 of radiotherapy. Cisplatin dose reductions or delays were based on a predefined toxicity criterion, which is available in Additional file 1: Methods. Considering the maximum tolerated dose of famitinib was 25 mg for advanced solid malignancy [28], we chose an initial dose of 12.5 mg. If two out of three patients had a DLT at 12.5 mg, the concurrent cisplatin dose was reduced to 80 mg/m^2 for the remaining patients.

Assessments

Toxicities were assessed by the National Cancer Institute Common Terminology Criteria for Adverse Events (CTCAE, version 4.0). DLTs included grade 4 thrombocytopenia (or grade 3 with haemorrhage), grade 4 neutropenia ($< 1.0 \times 10^9$/L) lasting for more than 5 days (or grade 3 with fever at > 38.5 °C), grade 4 anaemia, and any other grade 3 non-hematologic toxicity. Tumour response [i.e., complete response (CR), partial response (PR), progressive disease (PD) and stable disease (SD)] was evaluated 2 weeks after taking famitinib, at completion of treatment and 12 weeks later according to

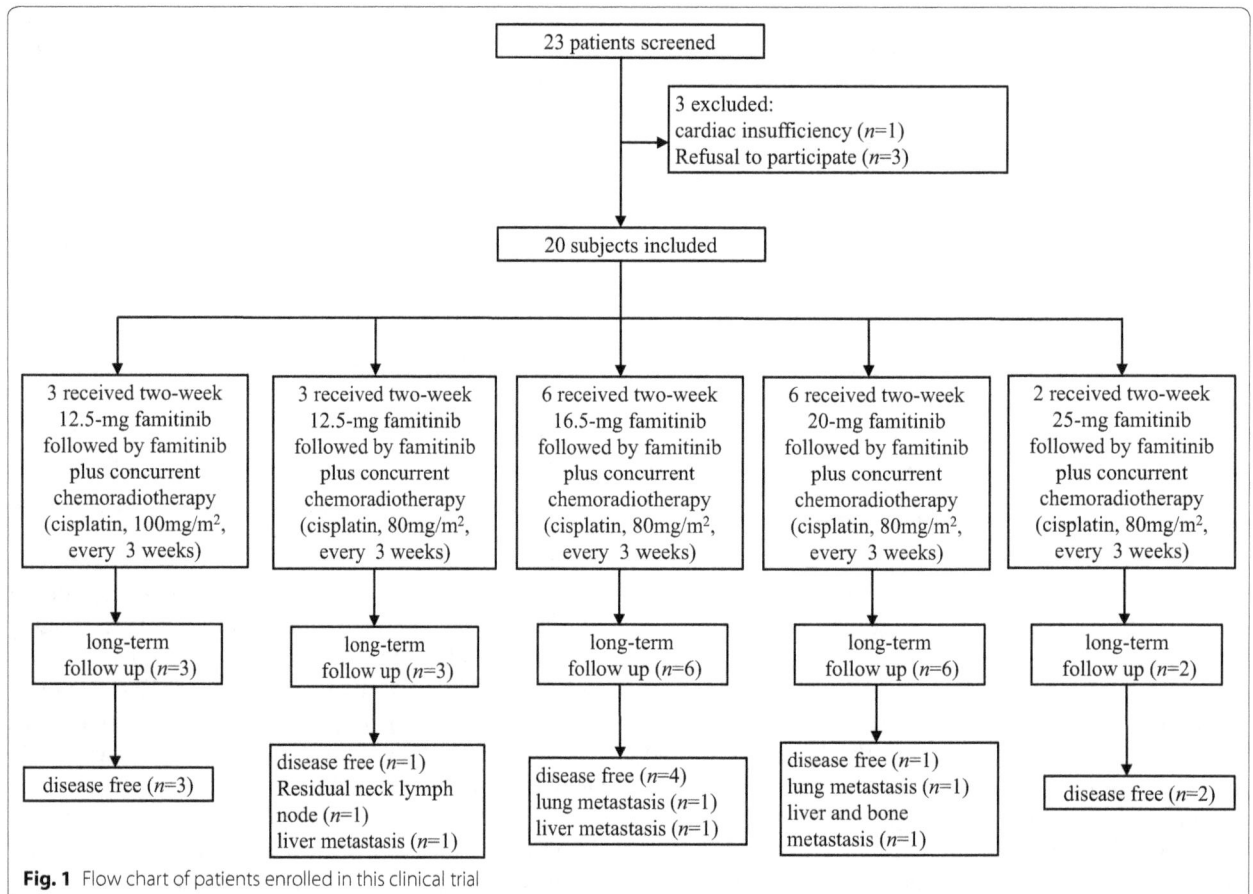

Fig. 1 Flow chart of patients enrolled in this clinical trial

Table 1 Demographic and baseline characteristics of patients with NPC who were treated with famitinib

Variables	Patients (n = 20)
Age, years	
Median (IQR)	43 (39–48)
Range	26–56
Male sex	18 (80%)
ECOG	
0	1 (5%)
1	19 (95%)
Histology, WHO type III	20 (100%)
Tumour stage	
T1	1 (5%)
T2	3 (15%)
T3	13 (65%)
T4	3 (15%)
Node stage	
N1	2 (10%)
N2	13 (65%)
N3	5 (25%)
Clinical stage	
III	12 (60%)
IVa	3 (15%)
IVb	5 (25%)
EBV DNA,	
≥ 4000 copy/ml	10 (50%)
VCA-IgA	
≥ 1:80	15 (75%)
EA-IgA	
≥ 1:10	13 (65%)
Smoking[a]	
Yes	9 (45%)
Family history of NPC	
Yes	3 (15%)

ECOG Eastern Cooperative Oncology Group, WHO World Health Organization, EBV DNA Epstein–Barr virus DNA, VCA viral capsid antigen, IgA immunoglobulin A, EA, early antigen, NPC nasopharyngeal carcinoma

[a] Defined as smoking ≥ 100 cigarettes/lifetime

Response Evaluation Criteria in Solid Tumours (RECIST version 1.1).

Contrast-enhanced ultrasound (D-CEUS)
Recent evidence has suggested that molecular anti-angiogenic agents often induce tumour necrosis or decrease tumour vascularity before a reduction in tumour volume [34–36]. Therefore, D-CEUS of the neck lymph nodes was performed at baseline (day 0), day 8 and 15 after famitinib was administered before starting CCRT. The ultrasonography protocol, enhancer agent Sono-Vue (Bracco, Milan, Italy), and quantitative analysis of

D-CEUS data are described in detail in Additional file 1: Methods [37, 38]. Six perfusion parameters sufficient to characterize both blood volume and blood flow were extracted from time-intensity curves: peak intensity (PI), area under the curve (AUC), time to PI (TP), mean transit time (MTT), slope of wash-in (PW) and wash-in perfusion index (WIPI). The above parameters are defined in Additional file 1: Methods. Intra-observer variability and inter-observer variability between two operators (FH and JWW) was calculated for the entire D-CEUS process (D-CEUS examination, ROI drawing and calculation of perfusion parameters) by evaluating 3 repeated examinations (SonoVue bolus injection repeated every 15 min) on 10 different patients.

Immunohistochemistry and quantitative PCR
Tissues were biopsied and routinely paraffin-embedded. VEGFR2, PDGFR2 and C-Kit expression was examined by immunohistochemistry as detailed in Additional file 1: Methods. Furthermore, blood samples were collected to determine plasma VEGF and PDGF and stem cell factor (SCF) levels at day 0 and 15 after famitinib therapy and 12 weeks after completing CCRT (Additional file 1: Methods). Plasma EBV DNA concentrations were routinely measured by quantitative PCR as we described previously [39, 40].

End points
The primary end points were safety of famitinib combined with CCRT. The secondary end point was tumour response. We also evaluated whether the functional parameters of D-CEUS could serve as effective predictors of early tumour response to famitinib and the correlation between the functional parameters and clinical efficacy. Follow-up assessments were performed every 3 months during the first 2 years, every 6 months during years 3–5, and then every year.

Statistical analysis
Non- normally distributed continuous variables were expressed as median (IQR) and normally distributed data were expressed as mean (SD). Categorical variables were presented as number and percentage (%). Progression-free survival (PFS) was calculated from the date of entry into the trial to the date of first failure (local and/or regional persistence/recurrence or distant metastasis) or death from any cause or the date of the last follow-up. Distant metastasis-free survival (DMFS) was calculated from the date of entry into the trial to the date of distant relapse or death from any cause or the date of the last follow-up. Survival analyses were performed by the Kaplan–Meier method, and log-rank test was used to compare two groups of patients with decreased D-CEUS

Table 2 Treatment-emergent adverse events occurring in NPC patients during the study in the safety analysis set

Adverse event	Famitinib alone					Famitinib with CCRT				
	Grade 1–2	Grade 3	Grade 4	Grade 5	Total	Grade 1–2	Grade 3	Grade 4	Grade 5	Total
Leukopenia	1 (5%)	0	0	0	1 (5%)	2 (10%)	17 (85%)	1 (5%)	0	20 (100%)
Neutropenia	1 (5%)	0	0	0	1 (5%)	9 (45%)	10 (50%)	1 (5%)	0	20 (100%)
Anaemia	2 (10%)	0	0	0	2 (10%)	16 (80%)	4 (20%)	0	0	20 (100%)
Radiation mucositis	0	0	0	0	0	16 (80%)	3 (15%)	1 (5%)	0	20 (100%)
Nausea and vomiting	0	0	0	0	0	16 (80%)	1 (5%)	0	0	17 (85%)
Radiation dermatitis	0	0	0	0	0	13 (65%)	0	0	0	13 (65%)
Weight loss	0	0	0	0	0	15 (75%)	0	0	0	15 (75%)
Proteinuria	1 (5%)	0	0	0	1 (5%)	15 (75%)	1 (5%)	0	0	16 (80%)
Thrombopenia	0	0	0	0	0	10 (50%)	3 (15%)	1 (5%)	0	14 (70%)
Hypertension	3 (15%)	0	0	0	3 (15%)	8 (40%)	1 (5%)	0	0	9 (45%)
Liver function impairment	3 (15%)	0	0	0	3 (15%)	10 (50%)	1 (5%)	0	0	11 (55%)
Hypertriglyceridemia	5 (25%)	0	0	0	5 (25%)	5 (25%)	0	0	0	5 (25%)
Hearing impairment	0	0	0	0	0	4 (20%)	0	0	0	4 (20%)
Renal impairment	0	0	0	0	0	4 (20%)	0	0	0	4 (20%)
Hematuria	2 (10%)	1 (5%)	0	0	3 (15%)	4 (20%)	1 (5%)	0	0	5 (25%)
Haemorrhage	0	0	0	0	0	2 (10%)	0	0	0	2 (10%)
Skin rash	2 (10%)	0	0	0	2 (10%)	1 (5%)	0	0	0	1 (5%)
Hypothyroidism	0	0	0	0	0	0	0	0	0	0
Hypercholesterolemia	1 (5%)	0	0	0	1 (5%)	0	0	0	0	0
Elevated total bilirubin	1 (5%)	0	0	0	1 (5%)	1 (5%)	0	0	0	1 (5%)
Elevated GGT	2 (10%)	0	0	0	2 (10%)	2 (10%)	0	0	0	2 (10%)

CCRT concurrent chemoradiotherapy, *GGT* gamma glutamyl transpeptidase, *NPC* nasopharyngeal carcinoma

functional parameters ($\geq 30\%$ vs. $< 30\%$). The percent coefficient of change (CV, calculated by dividing the SD by the mean and multiplying by 100) for the perfusion parameters was calculated to evaluate intra-observer variability, and the intra-class correlation coefficients for the six perfusion parameters were also estimated to evaluate inter-observer variability. All statistical analyses were performed using IBM SPSS version 20.0.

Results

Patient demographic and baseline characteristics

The study flowchart is shown in Fig. 1. Twenty-three patients were screened for eligibility. One patient was excluded due to cardiac insufficiency and two patients were not included because they refused to provide consent. Finally, 20 patients were enrolled in the study. The median age of the patients was 43 years (range 26–56 years) and 80% (18/20) of the patients were male. Patient demographic and baseline characteristics are shown in Table 1. Three patients received 2 weeks of famitinib (12.5 mg/day) followed by famitinib plus CCRT (cisplatin, 100 mg/m^2). Because two of the three patients receiving CCRT plus 12.5 mg cisplatin at the initial dose had a DLT, cisplatin was reduced to 80 mg/m^2

in the remaining patients. Finally, three, six, six and two patients were included in the 12.5, 16.5, 20 and 25 mg cohorts.

Co-primary end points

Neither radiotherapy interruptions nor deaths occurred during the study. Famitinib as a single agent was generally well tolerated. Except one patient with grade 3 adverse event (hematuria), all adverse events were grade 1 or 2 (Table 2).

More adverse events were observed with famitinib plus CCRT (Table 2). The majority of adverse events were grade 1 or 2. The five most frequent adverse events were leukopenia (100%), neutropenia (100%), anemia (100%), radiation mucositis (100%), and nausea and vomiting (85%). The five most frequent grade 3 or 4 adverse events were leukopenia (90%), neutropenia (55%), thrombopenia (20%), anaemia (20%) and radiation mucositis (20%). In addition, grade 1 or 2 hemorrhage occurred in 2 (10%) patients and no grade 3–4 haemorrhage was recorded. No grade 5 adverse event was reported. Two out of three patients receiving 12.5 mg cisplatin had DLTs; one patient suffered grade 4 neutropenia lasting more than 5 days, and the other patient suffered grade 3 neutropenia

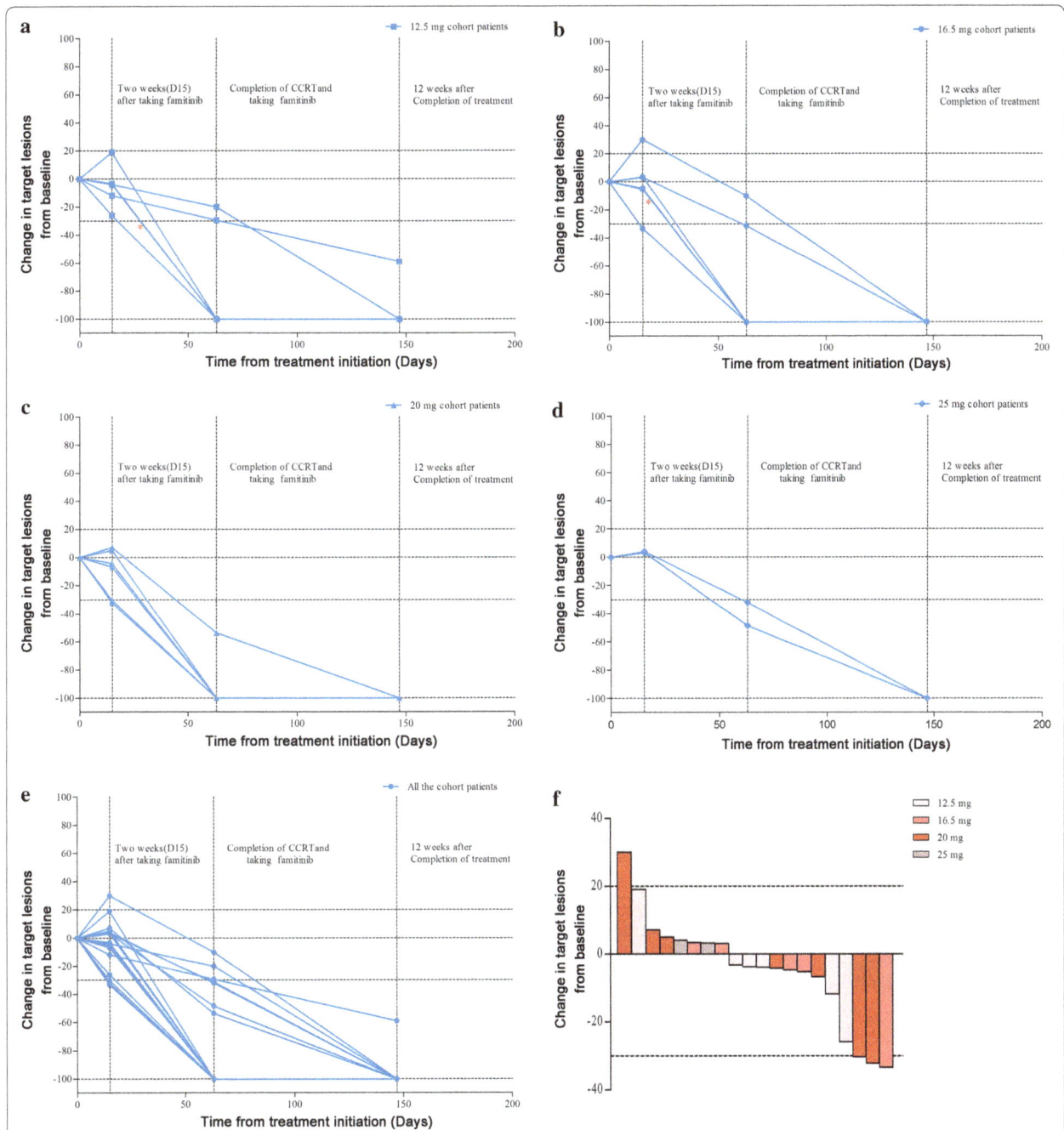

Fig. 2 Characteristics of neck lymph node regression in patients with nasopharyngeal carcinoma receiving famitinib and concurrent chemoradiotherapy. The response was measured as the largest percentage reduction in the sum of the longest diameters of target lesions for all assessable patients with a radiographic assessment (n = 20). Response kinetics in patients receiving famitinib **a** 12.5 or **b** 16.5 or **c** 20 or **d** 25 mg cohort and all the patients (**e**). Tumours were assessed 2 weeks after taking famitinib (D15), at the end of CCRT and 12 weeks after treatment according to the RECIST (version 1.0) guidelines; horizontal line at − 30% marks the threshold for defining objective response (partial tumour regression) according to RECIST, and a horizontal line at − 20% indicates the threshold for defining progressive disease. **f** Waterfall plot of best tumour response 2 weeks after taking famitinib (D15). *Indicated that two lines overlapped together

with fever. After cisplatin was reduced to 80 mg/m², in the remaining patients, one patient had grade 4 thrombocytopenia and one patient had grade 3 hypertension while receiving 25 mg cisplatin. Grade 3 hearing impairment occurred in one patient; no other grade 3 or 4 late adverse events were reported (Additional file 1: Table S1).

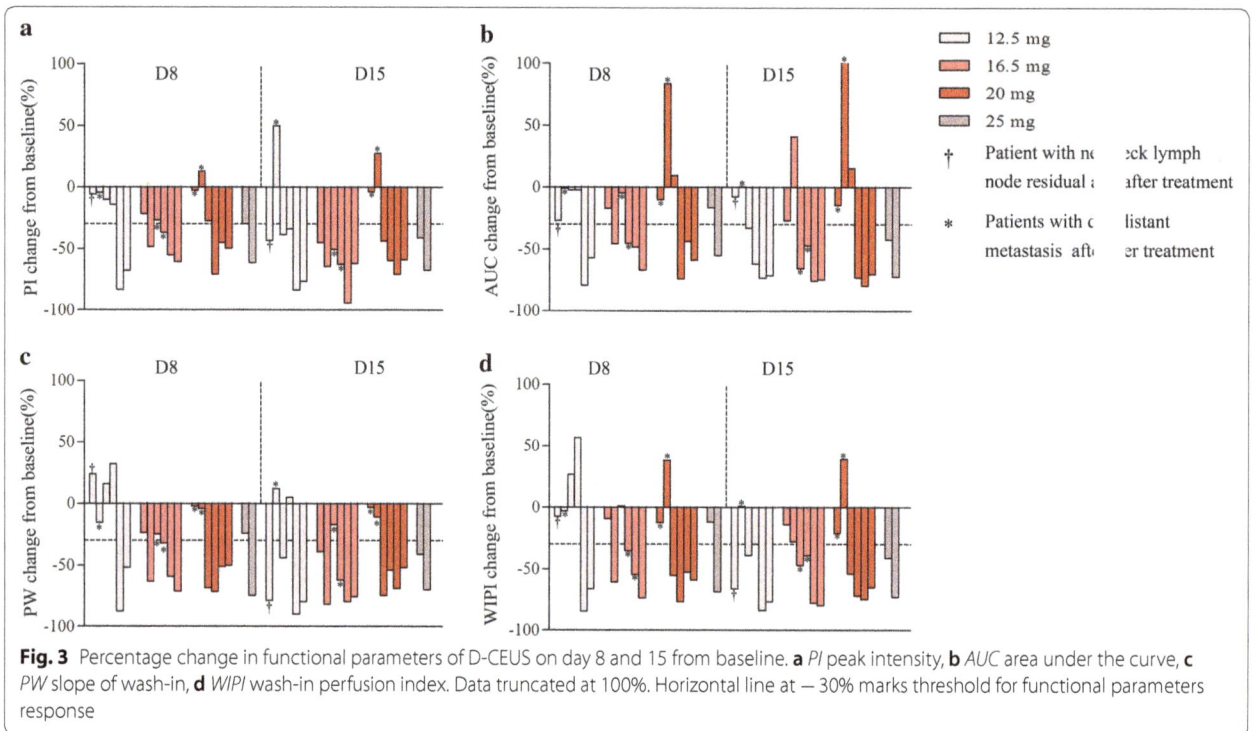

Fig. 3 Percentage change in functional parameters of D-CEUS on day 8 and 15 from baseline. **a** *PI* peak intensity, **b** *AUC* area under the curve, **c** *PW* slope of wash-in, **d** *WIPI* wash-in perfusion index. Data truncated at 100%. Horizontal line at − 30% marks threshold for functional parameters response

Fifteen (15/20, 75.0%) patients completed three cycles and 5 (25.0%) completed two cycles of cisplatin. The recommended phase II dose was defined as famitinib 20 mg/day with CCRT. Detailed treatments are presented in Additional file 1: Table S2.

Secondary end point

In famitinib monotherapy, 3 (15%) patients exhibited PR, 1 (5%) patient had PD, and 16 (80%) patients had SD (Fig. 2a–e). Overall, 12 (60%) patients demonstrated tumour shrinkage (from − 3.3% to− 33.3%, Fig. 2e, f).

Thirteen (65.0%) patients achieved CR and seven (35.0%) patients achieved PR at the completion of CCRT, and 19 (95%) patients achieved CR at 3 months after treatment (Fig. 2e). One patient, who had a residual neck lymph node that was evaluated 9 months after CCRT, subsequently underwent selective neck dissection. Five patients developed distant organ metastasis during 3 years of follow-up. After a median follow-up of 44 months, the 1-, 2-, and 3-year PFS was 85%, 70% and 70%, respectively. Additionally, the 1-, 2-, and 3-year DMFS was 90%, 75% and 75%, respectively (Additional file 1: Fig. S4). All five metastatic patients received palliative chemotherapy, and three patients were currently alive and two patients died.

Early Perfusion parameters response associated with clinical outcome

The mean CV was 4.05%, 6.63%, 3.64%, 24.40%, 6.44% and 6.33% for PI, AUC, TP, MTT, PW and WIPI, respectively. The intra-class correlation coefficients for the six perfusion parameters were between 0.95 and 0.99, indicating good agreement between observers.

Anti-angiogenic activity was noted across all four doses. At baseline, the frequency of VEGFR2-positive tumour cells was 50% or higher in 16 (80%) patients and that of C-kit-positive tumour cells was 50% or higher in 8 (40%) patients. PDGFR expression was not detected in NPC tissues (Additional file 1: Fig. S1). The plasma VEGF and PDGF levels decreased versus baseline after 2 weeks of single famitinib therapy and slightly increased after discontinuing famitinib 3 months later (Additional file 1: Fig. S2). Furthermore, 11 (55%), 10 (50%), 11 (55%), and 11 (55%) patients exhibited an at least 30% reduction in perfusion parameter response 1 week after taking famitinib for PI, AUC, PW, and WIPI, respectively. Seventeen (85%), 13 (65%), 17 (85%), and 11 (65%) patients exhibited response at 2 weeks, respectively (Fig. 3). There was no statistically significant difference in changes in the perfusion parameters at baseline, day 8 and 15 in terms of tumour response (PR vs SD/PD) after taking famitinib for 2 weeks (data not shown). However, tumour necrosis

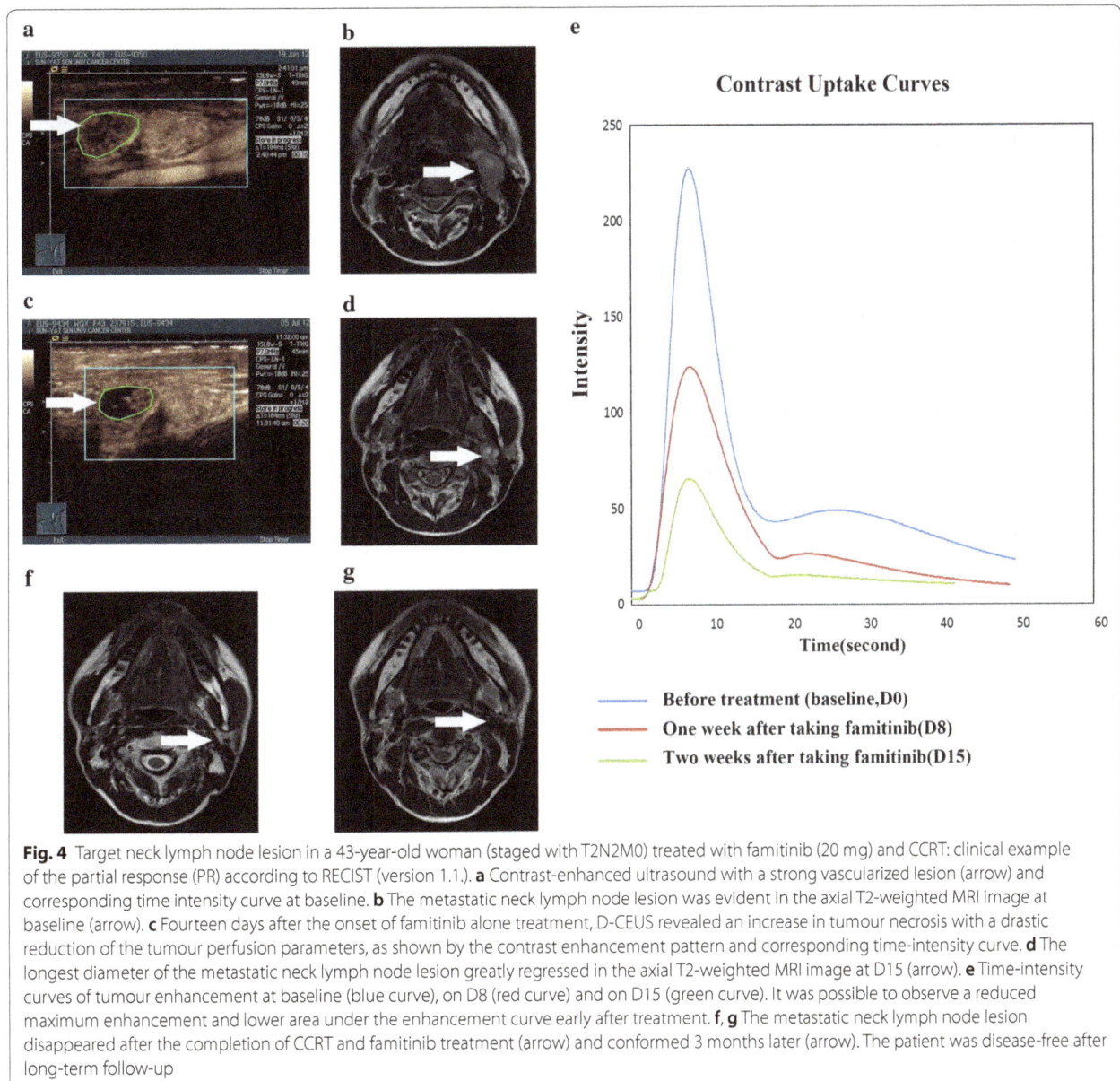

Fig. 4 Target neck lymph node lesion in a 43-year-old woman (staged with T2N2M0) treated with famitinib (20 mg) and CCRT: clinical example of the partial response (PR) according to RECIST (version 1.1.). **a** Contrast-enhanced ultrasound with a strong vascularized lesion (arrow) and corresponding time intensity curve at baseline. **b** The metastatic neck lymph node lesion was evident in the axial T2-weighted MRI image at baseline (arrow). **c** Fourteen days after the onset of famitinib alone treatment, D-CEUS revealed an increase in tumour necrosis with a drastic reduction of the tumour perfusion parameters, as shown by the contrast enhancement pattern and corresponding time-intensity curve. **d** The longest diameter of the metastatic neck lymph node lesion greatly regressed in the axial T2-weighted MRI image at D15 (arrow). **e** Time-intensity curves of tumour enhancement at baseline (blue curve), on D8 (red curve) and on D15 (green curve). It was possible to observe a reduced maximum enhancement and lower area under the enhancement curve early after treatment. **f, g** The metastatic neck lymph node lesion disappeared after the completion of CCRT and famitinib treatment (arrow) and conformed 3 months later (arrow). The patient was disease-free after long-term follow-up

of neck lymph nodes was observed on day 15 in several typical cases (Fig. 4).

The percentage changes in dynamic functional parameters stratified by progression are shown in Additional file 1: Table S3. The percentage changes in PI, AUC, PW and WIPI at day 0, 8 and 15 were significantly different between patients with and without progression. Furthermore, patients with a perfusion parameter response of less than 30% after taking famitinib for 1 week had a high risk of disease progression (Table 3 and Additional file 1: Fig. S4), suggesting that patients with disease progression had smaller percentage changes in perfusion parameters and were not sensitive to famitinib. Typical clinical

examples of the corresponding contrast uptake time-intensity curves for patients with progression at each time point after treatment are shown in Figs. 5 and 6.

Discussion

Findings from this phase I trial of 20 patients showed that the addition of famitinib to chemoradiation has an encouraging tolerability and anticancer profile for patients with NPC. Based on the assessment of safety and efficacy, we recommend famitinib 20 mg combined with chemoradiation (cisplatin 80 mg/m^2) for phase II testing. Haemorrhage is a well-known complication of sunitinib. However, we recorded no grade 3 or grade 4

Table 3 Correlation between D-CEUS parameters and PFS and DMFS

Parameter changes	< 30%	≥ 30%	P value
	3-year estimate (%, 95% CI)		
PFS (day 8)			
Peak intensity	90.9 (73.7–100)	44.4 (11.9–76.9)	0.021
Area under the curve	90.0 (71.4–100)	50.0 (31.0–81.0)	0.048
Slope of wash-in (coefficient)	90.9 (73.7–100)	44.4 (11.9–76.9)	0.021
Wash-in perfusion index	90.9 (73.7–100)	44.4 (11.9–76.9)	0.021
DMFS (day 8)			
Peak intensity	90.9 (73.7–100)	55.6 (23.1–88.1)	0.065
Area under the curve	90.0 (71.4–100)	60.0 (23.1–88.2)	0.119
Slope of wash-in (coefficient)	90.9 (73.7–100)	55.6 (23.1–88.1)	0.065
Wash-in perfusion index	90.9 (73.7–100)	55.6 (23.1–88.1)	0.065
PFS (day 15)			
Peak intensity	94.1 (82.9–100)	0.0	< 0.001
Area under the curve	92.3 (77.8–100)	42.9 (6.2–79.6)	0.038
Slope of wash-in (coefficient)	86.7 (69.5–100)	20.0 (0–55.1)	0.002
Wash-in perfusion index	80.0 (59.8–100)	40.0 (0–82.9)	0.072
DMFS (day 15)			
Peak intensity	88.2 (72.9–100)	0.0	< 0.001
Area under the curve	84.6 (65.0–100)	57.1 (20.4–93.8)	0.16
Slope of wash-in (coefficient)	93.3 (80.8–100)	20.0 (0–55.1)	< 0.001
Wash-in perfusion index	86.7 (69.5–100)	21.9 (0–82.9)	0.024

D-CEUS dynamic contrast enhanced ultrasound, *PFS* progression-free survival, *DMFS* Distant metastasis-free survival, *CI* confidence interval

haemorrhage when combining famitinib with chemoradiation in this trial. Although two of the first three patients exhibited DLTs when combining famitinib with cisplatin (100 mg/m^2), less toxicity was observed when cisplatin was reduced to 80 mg/m^2. Interestingly, we also found that D-CEUS could provide a reliable and early measure of efficacy for NPC patients treated with famitinib.

With the combination with famitinib, 75% of patients received three cycles of concurrent cisplatin, which showed slightly higher rates of compliance with cisplatin during radiation compared with those recorded in the Intergroup 0099 trial (63%) [41], Singapore trial (71%) [42], and Hong Kong NPC-9901 trial (52%) [9]. The 3-year PFS and DMFS were 70% and 75% for these local advanced NPC patients. At the single famitinib stage, most common famitinib-related toxicities were grade I–II, and fewer side effects were noted in this study in terms of leukopenia, neutropenia, thrombocytopenia, and hypertension compared with previously published incidence rates of advanced solid malignancy refractory to standard therapy [28, 29]. This is likely because the patients enrolled in this study had not received any previous treatment, and were in better general health. A meta-analysis of VEGFR tyrosine kinase inhibitors in 23 trials showed that the incidence of bleeding events was 16.7% [43]. Nevertheless, the incidence of haemorrhage in our

study was only 10%, which was much lower than the results of Hui et al., who reported high incidence rates of haemorrhage (64.3%) for recurrent or metastatic NPC patients [27]. The incidence of hypertension in this trial was 50%, which was similar to the incidence of hypertension (42.9%) for sunitinib administered to recurrent or metastatic NPC patients [27] and was significantly less than that for sunitinib (92%) in renal cell carcinoma [44]. The most common grade 3–4 adverse events were leukopenia (90%), neutropenia (55%), radiation mucositis (20%), and thrombopenia (20%). The rates of grade 3–4 toxicity of the bone marrow in this trial were higher than in other trials during CCRT in patients with NPC, which were recorded as 12.6%–32% [8, 9] for leukopenia and 13.2% [42] for neutropenia. We considered that famitinib plus CCRT increased the toxicities of the bone marrow, which, however, were tolerable. Grade 3–4 radiation mucositis was found in 20%, which compares favourably to the rates recorded in the Hong Kong NPC-9901 trial (62%) [9] and the Singapore trial (48.1%) [42] as well as with the addition of cetuximab or bevacizumab to standard chemoradiation (77%–87%) [19, 45].

D-CEUS tests found that more than 60% of patients achieved a perfusion parameter response after 2 weeks taking famitinib alone. Previous data have shown the potential of D-CEUS in monitoring the response of

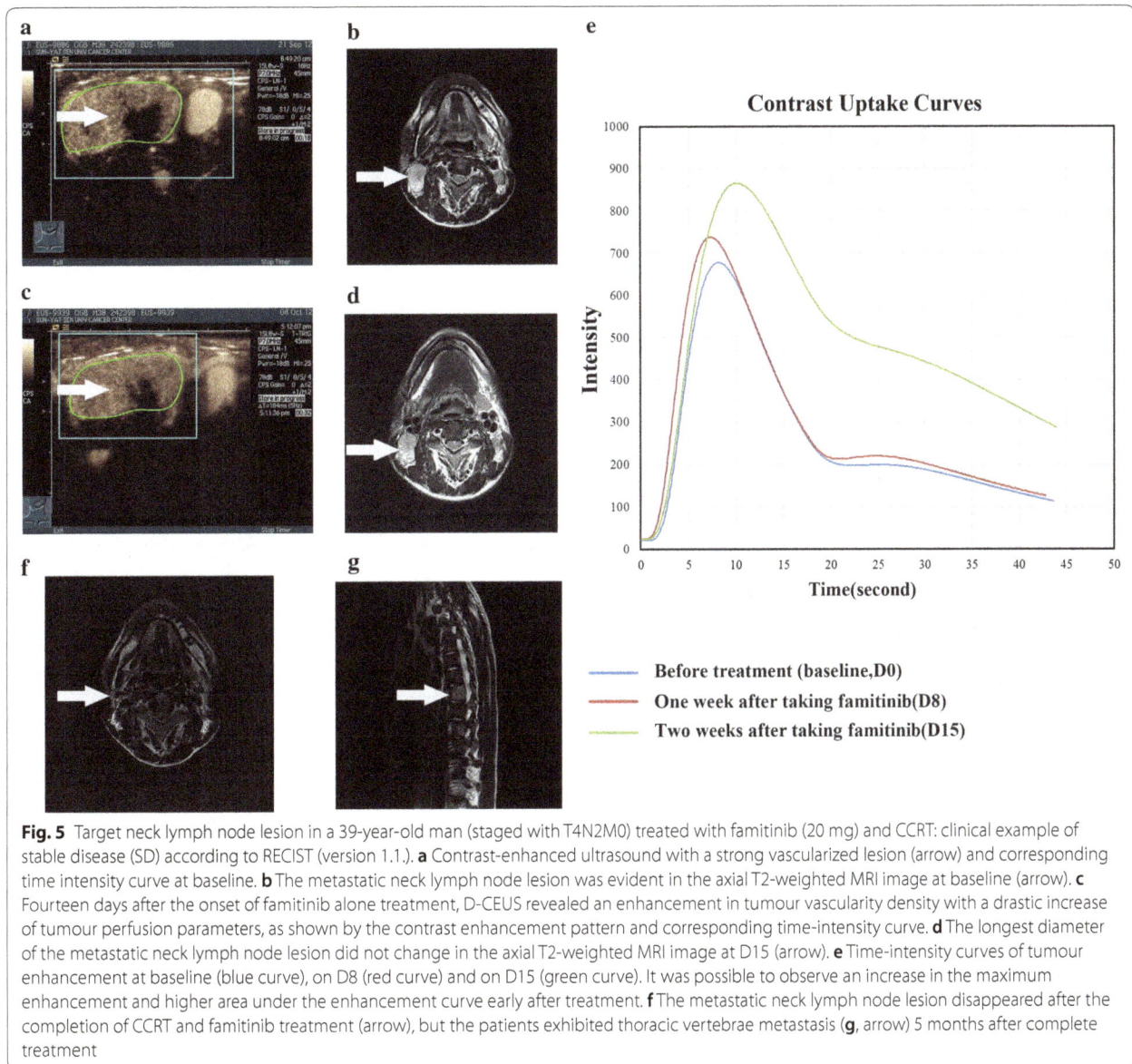

Fig. 5 Target neck lymph node lesion in a 39-year-old man (staged with T4N2M0) treated with famitinib (20 mg) and CCRT: clinical example of stable disease (SD) according to RECIST (version 1.1.). **a** Contrast-enhanced ultrasound with a strong vascularized lesion (arrow) and corresponding time intensity curve at baseline. **b** The metastatic neck lymph node lesion was evident in the axial T2-weighted MRI image at baseline (arrow). **c** Fourteen days after the onset of famitinib alone treatment, D-CEUS revealed an enhancement in tumour vascularity density with a drastic increase of tumour perfusion parameters, as shown by the contrast enhancement pattern and corresponding time-intensity curve. **d** The longest diameter of the metastatic neck lymph node lesion did not change in the axial T2-weighted MRI image at D15 (arrow). **e** Time-intensity curves of tumour enhancement at baseline (blue curve), on D8 (red curve) and on D15 (green curve). It was possible to observe an increase in the maximum enhancement and higher area under the enhancement curve early after treatment. **f** The metastatic neck lymph node lesion disappeared after the completion of CCRT and famitinib treatment (arrow), but the patients exhibited thoracic vertebrae metastasis (**g**, arrow) 5 months after complete treatment

anti-angiogenetic agents, and initial contrast uptake was a predictive factor of response to sorafenib and pazopanib in recurrent/metastatic NPC [46, 47]. To our knowledge, this is the first clinical trial to evaluate tumour response to famitinib combined with chemoradiation through D-CEUS for locally advanced NPC. In several patients, famitinib-treated tumours underwent central necrosis or decreases in tumour vascularity, as evidenced by D-CEUS measurements, indicating that famitinib is effective in decreasing tumour vascularity and inducing tumour necrosis before a reduction in tumour volume. In particular, among the parameters evaluated, PI, AUC, PW and WIPI showed an evident reduction early after the onset of famitinib treatment in

most of the patients who were free of disease long-term. Patients whose total blood volume described by functional parameters decreased at least 30% after 1 week of famitinib treatment had a higher PFS than those with an increase or a reduction of less than 30%. The same results were obtained when we considered DMFS. Once again, these findings suggest that D-CEUS could be a useful complement to standard anatomic imaging for monitoring early, even long-term, therapeutic effect of famitinib in patients with NPC.

Finally, we should emphasize several limitations of our study. First, this trial is a typical nonrandomized open-label phase I study, and efficacy was only a secondary endpoint. Since many patients were

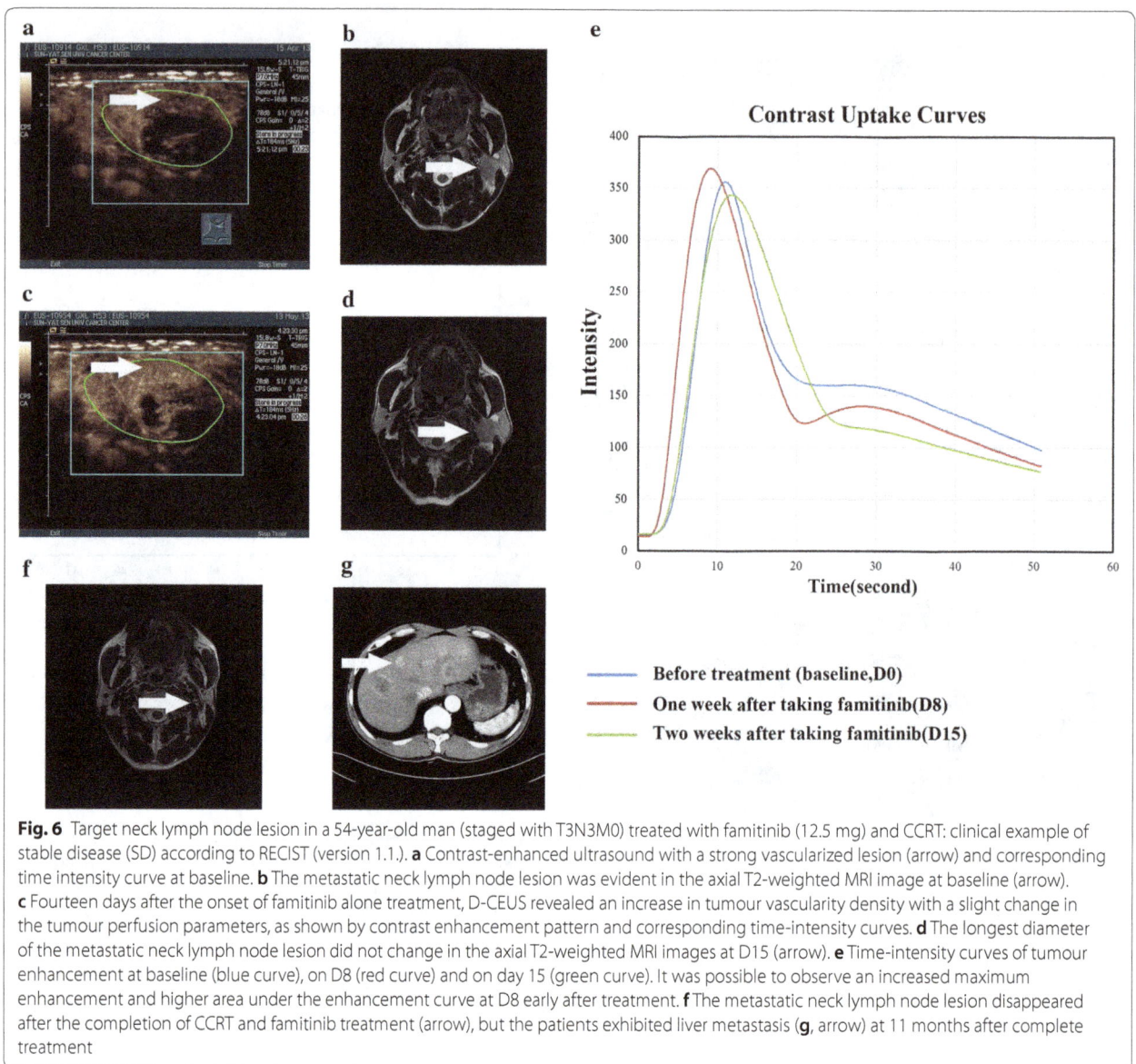

Fig. 6 Target neck lymph node lesion in a 54-year-old man (staged with T3N3M0) treated with famitinib (12.5 mg) and CCRT: clinical example of stable disease (SD) according to RECIST (version 1.1.). **a** Contrast-enhanced ultrasound with a strong vascularized lesion (arrow) and corresponding time intensity curve at baseline. **b** The metastatic neck lymph node lesion was evident in the axial T2-weighted MRI image at baseline (arrow). **c** Fourteen days after the onset of famitinib alone treatment, D-CEUS revealed an increase in tumour vascularity density with a slight change in the tumour perfusion parameters, as shown by contrast enhancement pattern and corresponding time-intensity curves. **d** The longest diameter of the metastatic neck lymph node lesion did not change in the axial T2-weighted MRI images at D15 (arrow). **e** Time-intensity curves of tumour enhancement at baseline (blue curve), on D8 (red curve) and on day 15 (green curve). It was possible to observe an increased maximum enhancement and higher area under the enhancement curve at D8 early after treatment. **f** The metastatic neck lymph node lesion disappeared after the completion of CCRT and famitinib treatment (arrow), but the patients exhibited liver metastasis (**g**, arrow) at 11 months after complete treatment

administered at considerably lower doses than the eventual MTD, all efficacy data should be interpreted with caution. Second, the small number of patients decreased the statistical power of our observations. We need phase II study to expand the sample size to further confirm our results. Indeed, variability in measurements is an issue within D-CEUS measurements, even if we found good agreement in a subset of patients. General predictions of the therapeutic effects by perfusion parameters of D-CEUS must be interpreted with caution. From another point of view, the residual cervical lymph nodes in the CCRT and IMRT era are very rare. The clinical applicability of D-CEUS in routine

NPC management may be limited. Future work should focus on the development of practical and widely accepted measurements for the calculation of necrosis and for the classification of tumour response based on D-CEUS findings.

Conclusions

Combined use of famitinib and CCRT (cisplatin, 80 mg/m^2) is well tolerated at 20 mg/day or lower in patients with NPC. The results also suggest that D-CEUS could be used to evaluate tumour vascularization and efficacy in patients with NPC treated with famitinib.

Additional file

Additional file 1: Table S1. Incidence of late toxicities in the combination group during follow up. Table S2. Actual delivered treatments for all enrolled patients. Table S3. Percentage changes from baseline of D-CEUS functional parameters stratified by progression after three years of follow up. Figure S1. Biomarker expression in NPC tumour tissue and normal nasopharyngeal epithelial cells. A VEGFR2; B PDGFR; C C-kit. VEGFR2, vascular endothelial growth factor receptor; PDGFR, platelet-derived growth factor receptor. Figure S2. Serum VEGF (A), PDGF (B) and SCF (C) concentration at baseline, two weeks after taking famitinib, and 12 weeks post-treatment (by ELISA), respectively. VEGF, vascular endothelial growth factor; PDGF, platelet-derived growth factor; SCF, stem cell factor. Figure S3. A and B show the results of longitudinal monitoring of the change in plasma EBV DNA concentrations of 14 patients in continuous remission and 6 patients who exhibited relapse, respectively. Figure S4. Progression-free survival (A) and distant metastasis-free survival (B) in patients with nasopharyngeal cancer treated with intensity-modulated radiotherapy, chemotherapy, and famitinib. Kaplan-Meier survival distributions according to the percentage variation in functional parameters (PI, AUC, PW, and PIWI) at day 8 for famitinib treatment alone. The curves show an association between an early decrease in functional parameters of PI, AUC, PW, and PIWI (after seven days of treatment, D8) and the disease progression. Patients were divided into two groups: those with a percentage decrease in PI (C), AUC (D), PW (E), and PIWI (F) greater than or equal to 30% (blue curve) and those with an increase or a percentage decrease lower than 30% (green curve). PI, peak intensity; AUC, area under the time-intensity curve; PW, slope coefficient of wash-in; WIPI, wash-in perfusion index.

Authors' contributions

JM and HM contributed to conception and design of the study and drafted the manuscript; QC and LT participated in data collection and literature research; NL, FH, LG, SG, JW, HL, YY, LZ, LL, PW, YL, QH, XY, QT, YL, YL, XS, CX, YM, YG, RS, HM, KC, XG and MZ contributed to data analysis and interpretation. All authors read and approved the final manuscript.

Author details

[1] State Key Laboratory of Oncology in South China, Collaborative Innovation Center for Cancer Medicine, Guangdong Key Laboratory of Nasopharyngeal Carcinoma Diagnosis and Therapy, Sun Yat-sen University Cancer Center, Guangzhou 510060, P. R. China. [2] Department of Nasopharyngeal Carcinoma, Sun Yat-sen University Cancer Center, Guangzhou 510060, P. R. China. [3] Department of Ultrasound, Sun Yat-sen University Cancer Center, Guangzhou 510060, P. R. China. [4] Department of Radiation Oncology, Key Laboratory of Translational Radiation Oncology, Hunan Cancer Hospital and The Affiliated Cancer Hospital of Xiangya School of Medicine, Central South University, Changsha 410013, P. R. China. [5] Department of Science and Education, Sun Yat-sen Memorial Hospital, Guangzhou 510120, P. R. China. [6] Department of Radiation Oncology, The First Affiliated Hospital of Guangzhou Medical University, Guangzhou 510120, P. R. China. [7] Department of Imaging, Sun Yat-sen University Cancer Center, Guangzhou 510060, P. R. China. [8] Department of Clinical Trial Center, Sun Yat-sen University Cancer Center, Guangzhou 510060, P. R. China. [9] Department of Radiation Oncology, Sun Yat-sen University Cancer Center, Guangzhou 510060, P. R. China.

Acknowledgements

Not applicable.

Competing interests

The authors declare that they have no competing interests.

Funding

The trial was supported by Jiangsu Hengrui Medicine Co., Ltd [The National Natural Science Foundation of China (Grant No. 81230056), The National Science & Technology Pillar Program during the Twelfth Five-year Plan Period (Grand No. 2014BAI09B10, The Natural Science Foundation of Guangdong Province (Grand Nos. S2013010012220, 2017A030312003), the Science and Technology Project of Guangzhou City, China (Grand No. 132000507), The Health & Medical Collaborative Innovation Project of Guangzhou City, China (Grand No. 201400000001), The Innovation Team Development Plan of the Ministry of Education (Grand No. IRT_17R110), the Program of Introducing Talents of Discipline to Universities (Grand No. B14035)].

References

1. Wei KR, Zheng RS, Zhang SW, Liang ZH, Li ZM, Chen WQ. Nasopharyngeal carcinoma incidence and mortality in China, 2013. Chin J Cancer. 2017;36(1):90. https://doi.org/10.1186/s40880-017-0257-9.
2. Langendijk JA, Leemans CR, Buter J, Berkhof J, Slotman BJ. The additional value of chemotherapy to radiotherapy in locally advanced nasopharyngeal carcinoma: a meta-analysis of the published literature. J Clin Oncol. 2004;22(22):4604–12.
3. Baujat B, Audry H, Bourhis J, Chan AT, Onat H, Chua DT, et al. Chemotherapy as an adjunct to radiotherapy in locally advanced nasopharyngeal carcinoma. Cochrane Database Syst Rev. 2006;4:CD004329.
4. Huncharek M, Kupelnick B. Combined chemoradiation versus radiation therapy alone in locally advanced nasopharyngeal carcinoma: results of a meta-analysis of 1,528 patients from six randomized trials. Am J Clin Oncol. 2002;25(3):219–23.
5. Chen L, Hu CS, Chen XZ, Hu GQ, Cheng ZB, Sun Y, et al. Concurrent chemoradiotherapy plus adjuvant chemotherapy versus concurrent chemoradiotherapy alone in patients with locoregionally advanced nasopharyngeal carcinoma: a phase 3 multicentre randomised controlled trial. Lancet Oncol. 2012;13(2):163–71.
6. Blanchard P, Lee A, Marguet S, Leclercq J, Ng WT, Ma J, et al. Chemotherapy and radiotherapy in nasopharyngeal carcinoma: an update of the MAC-NPC meta-analysis. Lancet Oncol. 2015;16(6):645–55.
7. Sun Y, Li WF, Chen NY, Zhang N, Hu GQ, Xie FY, et al. Induction chemotherapy plus concurrent chemoradiotherapy versus concurrent chemoradiotherapy alone in locoregionally advanced nasopharyngeal carcinoma: a phase 3, multicentre, randomised controlled trial. Lancet Oncol. 2016;17(11):1509–20.
8. Chan AT, Teo PM, Ngan RK, Leung TW, Lau WH, Zee B, et al. Concurrent chemotherapy-radiotherapy compared with radiotherapy alone in locoregionally advanced nasopharyngeal carcinoma: progression-free survival analysis of a phase III randomized trial. J Clin Oncol. 2002;20(8):2038–44.
9. Lee AW, Lau WH, Tung SY, Chua DT, Chappell R, Xu L, et al. Preliminary results of a randomized study on therapeutic gain by concurrent chemotherapy for regionally-advanced nasopharyngeal carcinoma: NPC-9901 Trial by the Hong Kong Nasopharyngeal Cancer Study Group. J Clin Oncol. 2005;23(28):6966–75.
10. Lin JC, Jan JS, Hsu CY, Liang WM, Jiang RS, Wang WY. Phase III study of concurrent chemoradiotherapy versus radiotherapy alone for advanced nasopharyngeal carcinoma: positive effect on overall and progression-free survival. J Clin Oncol. 2003;21(4):631–7.
11. Chen QY, Wen YF, Guo L, Liu H, Huang PY, Mo HY, et al. Concurrent chemoradiotherapy vs radiotherapy alone in stage II nasopharyngeal carcinoma: phase III randomized trial. J Natl Cancer Inst. 2011;103(23):1761–70.
12. Lee N, Harris J, Garden AS, Straube W, Glisson B, Xia P, et al. Intensity-modulated radiation therapy with or without chemotherapy for nasopharyngeal carcinoma: radiation therapy oncology group phase II trial 0225. J Clin Oncol. 2009;27(22):3684–90.
13. Lee N, Xia P, Quivey JM, Sultanem K, Poon I, Akazawa C, et al. Intensity-modulated radiotherapy in the treatment of nasopharyngeal carcinoma: an update of the UCSF experience. Int J Radiat Oncol Biol Phys. 2002;53(1):12–22.
14. Sun X, Su S, Chen C, Han F, Zhao C, Xiao W, et al. Long-term outcomes of intensity-modulated radiotherapy for 868 patients with nasopharyngeal carcinoma: an analysis of survival and treatment toxicities. Radiother Oncol. 2014;110(3):398–403.

15. Lee AW, Ng WT, Chan LL, Hung WM, Chan CC, Sze HC, et al. Evolution of treatment for nasopharyngeal cancer–success and setback in the intensity-modulated radiotherapy era. Radiother Oncol. 2014;110(3):377–84.
16. Hui EP, Chan AT, Pezzella F, Turley H, To KF, Poon TC, et al. Coexpression of hypoxia-inducible factors 1alpha and 2alpha, carbonic anhydrase IX, and vascular endothelial growth factor in nasopharyngeal carcinoma and relationship to survival. Clin Cancer Res. 2002;8(8):2595–604.
17. Wakisaka N, Wen QH, Yoshizaki T, Nishimura T, Furukawa M, Kawahara E, et al. Association of vascular endothelial growth factor expression with angiogenesis and lymph node metastasis in nasopharyngeal carcinoma. Laryngoscope. 1999;109(5):810–4.
18. Dings RP, Loren M, Heun H, McNiel E, Griffioen AW, Mayo KH, et al. Scheduling of radiation with angiogenesis inhibitors anginex and Avastin improves therapeutic outcome via vessel normalization. Clin Cancer Res. 2007;13(11):3395–402.
19. Lee NY, Zhang Q, Pfister DG, Kim J, Garden AS, Mechalakos J, et al. Addition of bevacizumab to standard chemoradiation for locoregionally advanced nasopharyngeal carcinoma (RTOG 0615): a phase 2 multi-institutional trial. Lancet Oncol. 2012;13(2):172–80.
20. Bar-Sela G, Kuten A, Ben-Eliezer S, Gov-Ari E, Ben-Izhak O. Expression of HER2 and C-KIT in nasopharyngeal carcinoma: implications for a new therapeutic approach. Mod Pathol. 2003;16(10):1035–40.
21. Huang PY, Hong MH, Zhang X, Mai HQ, Luo DH, Zhang L. C-KIT overexpression and mutation in nasopharyngeal carcinoma cell lines and reactivity of Imatinib on these cell lines. Chin J Cancer. 2010;29(2):131–5.
22. Sheu LF, Lee WC, Lee HS, Kao WY, Chen A. Co-expression of c-kit and stem cell factor in primary and metastatic nasopharyngeal carcinomas and nasopharyngeal epithelium. J Pathol. 2005;207(2):216–23.
23. Sheu LF, Young ZH, Lee WC, Chen YF, Kao WY, Chen A. STI571 sensitizes nasopharyngeal carcinoma cells to cisplatin: sustained activation of ERK with improved growth inhibition. Int J Oncol. 2007;30(2):403–11.
24. Jiang F, Hu W, Zhang B, Xu J, Shui Y, Zhou X, et al. Changes in c-Kit expression levels during the course of radiation therapy for nasopharyngeal carcinoma. Biomed Rep. 2016;5(4):437–42.
25. Qian CN, Min HQ, Lin HL, Feng GK, Ye YL, Wang LG, et al. Anti-tumor effect of angiogenesis inhibitor TNP-470 on the human nasopharyngeal carcinoma cell line NPC/HK1. Oncology. 1999;57(1):36–41.
26. Qian CN, Min HQ, Lin HL, Hong MH, Ye YL. Primary study in experimental antiangiogenic therapy of nasopharyngeal carcinoma with AGM-1470 (TNP-470). J Laryngol Otol. 1998;112(9):849–53.
27. Hui EP, Ma BB, King AD, Mo F, Chan SL, Kam MK, et al. Hemorrhagic complications in a phase II study of sunitinib in patients of nasopharyngeal carcinoma who has previously received high-dose radiation. Ann Oncol. 2011;22(6):1280–7.
28. Zhou A, Zhang W, Chang C, Chen X, Zhong D, Qin Q, et al. Phase I study of the safety, pharmacokinetics and antitumor activity of famitinib. Cancer Chemother Pharmacol. 2013;72(5):1043–53.
29. Zhang W, Zhou AP, Qin Q, Chang CX, Jiang HY, Ma JH, et al. Famitinib in metastatic renal cell carcinoma: a single center study. Chin Med J (Engl). 2013;126(22):4277–81.
30. Xie C, Zhou J, Guo Z, Diao X, Gao Z, Zhong D, et al. Metabolism and bioactivation of famitinib, a novel inhibitor of receptor tyrosine kinase, in cancer patients. Br J Pharmacol. 2013;168(7):1687–706.
31. Bello CL, Sherman L, Zhou J, Verkh L, Smeraglia J, Mount J, et al. Effect of food on the pharmacokinetics of sunitinib malate (SU11248), a multi-targeted receptor tyrosine kinase inhibitor: results from a phase I study in healthy subjects. Anticancer Drugs. 2006;17(3):353–8.
32. Mu X, Ma J, Zhang Z, Zhou H, Xu S, Qin Y, et al. Famitinib enhances nasopharyngeal cancer cell radiosensitivity by attenuating radiation-induced phosphorylation of platelet-derived growth factor receptor and c-kit and inhibiting microvessel formation. Int J Radiat Biol. 2015;91(9):771–6.
33. Schueneman AJ, Himmelfarb E, Geng L, Tan J, Donnelly E, Mendel D, et al. SU11248 maintenance therapy prevents regrowth after fractionated irradiation of murine tumour models. Cancer Res. 2003;63(14):4009–16.
34. Lassau N, Koscielny S, Albiges L, Chami L, Benatsou B, Chebil M, et al. Metastatic renal cell carcinoma treated with sunitinib: early evaluation of treatment response using dynamic contrast-enhanced ultrasonography. Clin Cancer Res. 2010;16(4):1216–25.
35. Lassau N, Lamuraglia M, Leclere J, Rouffiac V. Functional and early evaluation of treatments in oncology: interest of ultrasonographic contrast agents. J Radiol. 2004;85(5 Pt 2):704–12.
36. Zocco MA, Garcovich M, Lupascu A, Di Stasio E, Roccarina D, Annicchiarico BE, et al. Early prediction of response to sorafenib in patients with advanced hepatocellular carcinoma: the role of dynamic contrast enhanced ultrasound. J Hepatol. 2013;59(5):1014–21.
37. Zou RH, Lin QG, Huang W, Li XL, Cao Y, Zhang J, et al. Quantitative contrast-enhanced ultrasonic imaging reflects microvascularization in Hepatocellular Carcinoma and prognosis after resection. Ultrasound Med Biol. 2015;41(10):2621–30.
38. Zhou JH, Zheng W, Cao LH, Liu M, Luo RZ, Han F, et al. Contrast-enhanced ultrasonic parametric perfusion imaging in the evaluation of antiangiogenic treatment. Eur J Radiol. 2012;81(6):1360–5.
39. Tang LQ, Chen QY, Fan W, Liu H, Zhang L, Guo L, et al. Prospective study of tailoring whole-body dual-modality [18F]fluorodeoxyglucose positron emission tomography/computed tomography with plasma Epstein-Barr virus DNA for detecting distant metastasis in endemic nasopharyngeal carcinoma at initial staging. J Clin Oncol. 2013;31(23):2861–9.
40. Tang LQ, Li CF, Li J, Chen WH, Chen QY, Yuan LX, et al. Establishment and validation of prognostic nomograms for endemic Nasopharyngeal Carcinoma. J Natl Cancer Inst. 2016;108(1):djv291.
41. Al-Sarraf M, LeBlanc M, Giri PG, Fu KK, Cooper J, Vuong T, et al. Chemoradiotherapy versus radiotherapy in patients with advanced nasopharyngeal cancer: phase III randomized Intergroup study 0099. J Clin Oncol. 1998;16(4):1310–7.
42. Wee J, Tan EH, Tai BC, Wong HB, Leong SS, Tan T, et al. Randomized trial of radiotherapy versus concurrent chemoradiotherapy followed by adjuvant chemotherapy in patients with American Joint Committee on Cancer/International Union against cancer stage III and IV nasopharyngeal cancer of the endemic variety. J Clin Oncol. 2005;23(27):6730–8.
43. Je Y, Schutz FA, Choueiri TK. Risk of bleeding with vascular endothelial growth factor receptor tyrosine-kinase inhibitors sunitinib and sorafenib: a systematic review and meta-analysis of clinical trials. Lancet Oncol. 2009;10(10):967–74.
44. Feldman DR, Baum MS, Ginsberg MS, Hassoun H, Flombaum CD, Velasco S, et al. Phase I trial of bevacizumab plus escalated doses of sunitinib in patients with metastatic renal cell carcinoma. J Clin Oncol. 2009;27(9):1432–9.
45. Ma BB, Kam MK, Leung SF, Hui EP, King AD, Chan SL, et al. A phase II study of concurrent cetuximab-cisplatin and intensity-modulated radiotherapy in locoregionally advanced nasopharyngeal carcinoma. Ann Oncol. 2012;23(5):1287–92.
46. Xue C, Huang Y, Huang PY, Yu QT, Pan JJ, Liu LZ, et al. Phase II study of sorafenib in combination with cisplatin and 5-fluorouracil to treat recurrent or metastatic nasopharyngeal carcinoma. Ann Oncol. 2013;24(4):1055–61.
47. Lim WT, Ng QS, Ivy P, Leong SS, Singh O, Chowbay B, et al. A Phase II study of pazopanib in Asian patients with recurrent/metastatic nasopharyngeal carcinoma. Clin Cancer Res. 2011;17(16):5481–9.

13

Guided chemotherapy based on patient-derived mini-xenograft models improves survival of gallbladder carcinoma patients

Ming Zhan[1†], Rui-meng Yang[1†], Hui Wang[1], Min He[1], Wei Chen[1], Sun-wang Xu[1], Lin-hua Yang[1], Qiang Liu[2], Man-mei Long[3] and Jian Wang[1*]

Abstract

Background: Gallbladder carcinoma is highly aggressive and resistant to chemotherapy, with no consistent strategy to guide first line chemotherapy. However, patient-derived xenograft (PDX) model has been increasingly used as an effective model for in preclinical study of chemosensitivity.

Methods: Mini-PDX model was established using freshly resected primary lesions from 12 patients with gallbladder to examine the sensitivity with five of the most commonly used chemotherapeutic agents, namely gemcitabine, oxaliplatin, 5-fluorouracil, nanoparticle albumin-bound (nab)-paclitaxel, and irinotecan. The results were used to guide the selection of chemotherapeutic agents for adjunctive treatment after the surgery. Kaplan–Meier method was used to compare overall survival (OS) and disease free survival (DFS) with 45 patients who received conventional chemotherapy with gemcitabine and oxaliplatin.

Results: Cell viability assays based on mini-PDX model revealed significant heterogeneities in drug responsiveness. Kaplan–Meier analysis showed that patients in the PDX-guided chemotherapy group had significantly longer median OS (18.6 months; 95% CI 15.9–21.3 months) than patients in the conventional chemotherapy group (13.9 months; 95% CI 11.7–16.2 months) ($P = 0.030$; HR 3.18; 95% CI 1.47–6.91). Patients in the PDX-guided chemotherapy group also had significantly longer median DFS (17.6 months; 95% CI 14.5–20.6 months) than patients in the conventional chemotherapy group (12.0 months; 95% CI 9.7–14.4 months) ($P = 0.014$; HR 3.37; 95% CI 1.67–6.79).

Conclusion: The use of mini-PDX model to guide selection of chemotherapeutic regimens could improve the outcome in patients with gallbladder carcinoma.

Keywords: Gallbladder cancer, Mini-PDX, Chemosensitivity, Overall survival, Personalized therapy

*Correspondence: dr_wangjianrenji@163.com
†Ming Zhan and Rui-meng Yang contributed equally to this work
[1] Department of Biliary-Pancreatic Surgery, Renji Hospital, School of Medicine, Shanghai Jiao Tong University, 160 Pujian Road, Shanghai 200127, P. R. China
Full list of author information is available at the end of the article

Introduction

Gallbladder carcinoma, the most common biliary tract malignancy, is characterized by its aggressive growth and high lethality [1]. The disease generally carries a dismal prognosis due to its advanced stage at initial diagnosis and its recalcitrance to treatment [2, 3]. Despite advances in therapeutic strategies against gallbladder neoplastic disorders, surgical resection in combination with neo-adjuvant or adjuvant therapies still remains the optimal treatment modality [4]. Unfortunately, only a small proportion of gallbladder carcinoma patients are eligible for surgical intervention. Despite the controversial role of adjuvant therapy, a multimodal therapeutic approach may benefit patients at high risk for recurrence, such as for those with lymph node metastasis or positive resection margins [5].

Recently, several new cytotoxic agents have been proven effective for advanced biliary tract cancer, with a reduction in the rate of morbidity and mortality [6]. A number of clinical trials are underway to examine the effectivity of adjuvant chemotherapy with gemcitabine, capecitabine, or S-1 in combination with platinum. Two phase III trials have shown that the combination of gemcitabine with cisplatin or oxaliplatin is superior to single-agent chemotherapy in improving the overall survival (OS) of biliary tract cancer patients and is now used as the standard palliative regimen [7]. Several phase II studies have also investigated the efficacy of targeted agents against EGFR, VEGF, HER2, and MEK [8].

Irinotecan is a camptothecin derivative that exerts antitumor activities against a variety of tumor types by targeting topoisomerase I, consequently leading to the formation of DNA double-strand breaks and inhibition of DNA synthesis. A retrospective study in patients with advanced biliary tract cancer suggested that the combination therapy of irinotecan with gemcitabine and fluorouracil confers promising survival benefits with manageable toxicities [9]. In addition, a phase II trial of gemcitabine in combination with irinotecan indicated comparable efficacy with historic control [10]. However, given the rarity of these tumors, evidence is still largely based on retrospective studies, surveillance, epidemiological, and end results database inquiries, single or multi-institutional prospective studies, and meta-analysis of studies on adjuvant therapy [11]. Therefore, systematic prospective investigations are urgently needed.

Continued efforts in gene expression profiling and genomic sequencing have uncovered the underlying complexity and molecular heterogeneity of gallbladder carcinoma, shedding light on the daunting challenges of therapeutic interventions [12]. The highly intrinsic heterogeneity of gallbladder carcinoma and varied responses to chemotherapeutic drugs mandate a personalized approach to gallbladder carcinoma treatment [13]. Recently, there have been increasing interests in the development and characterization of patient-derived xenograft (PDX) tumor models for cancer research [14]. PDX models retain the principal histologic and genetic characteristics of donor tumors and remain stable throughout passages. These models have been shown to be predictive of clinical outcomes and are used for preclinical drug evaluation, biomarker identification, biological studies, and personalized medicine strategies [15–17]. Thus, PDX models are useful in recapitulating the complexity and heterogeneity of gallbladder carcinoma. However, there are limitations for direct application of traditional PDX models on gallbladder carcinoma patients. It typically takes 4–8 months for an established PDX model to be ready for assessing drug sensitivity, which is unduly long for initiation of drug-sensitivity guided treatment of gallbladder carcinoma patients. Mini-PDX model offers an effective alternative as it only takes about 7 days for the model to complete drug sensitivity test and could thus provide guidance for prompt personalized selection of individual drugs for each patient.

In the present study, we first established a mini-PDX model using fresh primary tumor cells from 12 surgically resected gallbladder carcinomas. Responses to five of the most commonly used chemotherapeutic agents including gemcitabine, oxaliplatin, 5-fluorouracil, nanoparticle albumin-bound (nab)-paclitaxel, and irinotecan were examined. We treated 12 gallbladder carcinoma patients with the top two efficient agents as obtained from the results of drug sensitivity tests. Patient outcomes then were compared with 45 gallbladder carcinoma patients who were conventionally treated with gemcitabine and oxaliplatin. Our results demonstrated that drug sensitivity-guided chemotherapy yielded significantly better outcomes as revealed by increased OS and disease free survival rate (DFS) than conventional chemotherapy. Analysis of the clinicopathologic features of gallbladder carcinoma patients further revealed that gemcitabine sensitivity was associated with nerve invasion while irinotecan sensitivity was associated with tumor size, lymph node metastasis and TNM stage. Lastly, we also found strong association between responses to drug sensitivity-guided therapy and the expression of several important chemoresistance-related proteins (e.g., p53 and P-gp).

Materials and methods

Tissue specimen acquisition

Fresh tissue specimens were obtained from 57 treatment naïve gallbladder carcinoma patients who underwent surgery at the Department of Biliary-Pancreatic Surgery of Renji Hospital, School of Medicine, Shanghai Jiao

Tong University between September 2014 and September 2016. Gallbladder carcinoma was staged according to the TNM classification (AJCC 7th edition).

Follow-up

Follow-ups were conducted once every month during the first year post surgery and once every 3 months thereafter. Phone calls were made to patients and their relatives according to the follow-up guidelines of the National Comprehensive Cancer Network of China. OS was calculated from the date of surgery until the date of the final follow-up visit or death and DFS was calculated from the date of surgery until the final follow-up visit or tumor recurrence. The final follow-up visit was September 2017.

Mini-PDX models and drug sensitivity assays

Mini-PDX models were established using freshly removed gallbladder carcinoma tissues from 12 patients. Drug sensitivity was examined using the OncoVee™-Mini PDX assay (LIDE Biotech, Shanghai, China). Briefly, gallbladder carcinoma samples were washed with Hank's balanced salt solution (HBSS) to remove non-tumor tissues and necrotic tumor tissues. After morselization, the tumor tissues were digested with collagenase at 37 °C for 1–2 h. Cells were collected followed by removal of blood cells and fibroblasts. Then, gallbladder carcinoma cell suspension was transferred to the HBSS washed capsules.

Four-weeks-old BALB/c nude mice (SLARC Inc., Shanghai, China), weighing 15–20 g each, were used for subcutaneous implantation. A small skin incision was made and the capsule was embedded in the subcutaneous tissue. Generally, each mouse received 3 capsules. Drugs (gemcitabine, 60 mg/kg, IP, Q4D × 2; oxaliplatin, 5 mg/kg, IP, Q4D × 2; 5-fluorouracil, 25 mg/kg, IP, QD × 5; nab-paclitaxel, 20 mg/kg, IV, QD × 5; irinotecan, 50 mg/kg, IP, Q4D × 2) were administered for 7 days respectively. Normal saline was used as the control. Anti-tumor activity was evaluated based on the relative fluorescence units (RFU) using the CellTiter-Glo® Luminescent Cell Viability Assay (Promega, Madison, WI, USA). Proliferation rate was calculated using the equation:

$$\text{Proliferation rate} = \left(\text{RFU}^{D7} - \text{RFU}^{D0}\right)_{\text{drug}} \Big/ \left(\text{RFU}^{D7} - \text{RFU}^{D0}\right)_{\text{placebo}}$$

The study flowchart is shown in Fig. 1a. All procedures were performed under specific pathogen free conditions and carried out in accordance with the guidelines for the Care and Use of Laboratory Animals of the National Institutes of Health.

Immunohistochemistry

Formalin-fixed, paraffin-embedded tissues were immunohistochemically stained as described previously [18]. Primary antibodies against the following proteins were used: p53 (1:200, ab1101, Abcam, Cambridge, UK), Ki-67 (1:600, ab15580, Abcam), P-gp (1:800, 13978, CST, MA, USA), MRP1 (1:200, 72202, CST), Bcl2 (1:400, 15071, CST), TS (1:100, ab58287, Abcam), GST-π (1:200, ab58287, Abcam), and Bcl-2 (1:400, 12286, CST). Immunohistochemical staining was semi-quantitatively scored by rating staining intensity of a protein of interest (I: negative, 0; weak, 1; moderate, 2; intense, 3) and the percentage of positively stained cells (P: 0%–5%, scored 0; 6%–35%, scored 1; 36%–70%, scored 2; and >70%, scored 3) to obtain a final score (Q), which was defined as the product of I × P. Two senior pathologists evaluated the tissues independently in a blinded manner.

Statistical analysis

Data are presented as mean ± standard deviation (SD). Normally distributed continuous variables were analyzed using unpaired Student's t-test. For multiple comparisons, the Tukey–Kramer honestly significant difference test was applied following ANOVA. Kaplan–Meier method and log-rank test were used to analyze OS and DFS. Data were censored for patients who were lost to follow-up. Pearson χ^2 test was used to analyze the correlation between clinicopathological variables and drug sensitivity. SPSS 17.0 software (SPSS Inc., Chicago, IL, USA) was used for all statistical analyses. For all analysis, $P < 0.05$ was considered statistically significant.

Ethical approval

The present study was approved by the Ethical Committee of Renji Hospital, School of Medicine, Shanghai Jiao Tong University. Written informed consents were provided by all participants before enrollment. All procedures were performed in accordance with the Ethical Standards of Institutional/National Research Committees and the 1964 Helsinki Declaration, its later amendments, or similar ethical standards.

Results
The mini-PDX model yields drug sensitivity patterns of gallbladder carcinoma patients

Cell viability assays showed that the mean proliferation rate of gallbladder carcinoma cells treated with gemcitabine, oxaliplatin, 5-fluorouracil, nab-paclitaxel, or irinotecan was 46.1%, 69.8%, 69.7%, 59.9%, and 43.0%, respectively (Fig. 1b). Drug sensitivity varied substantially, with the highest relative proliferation rate at

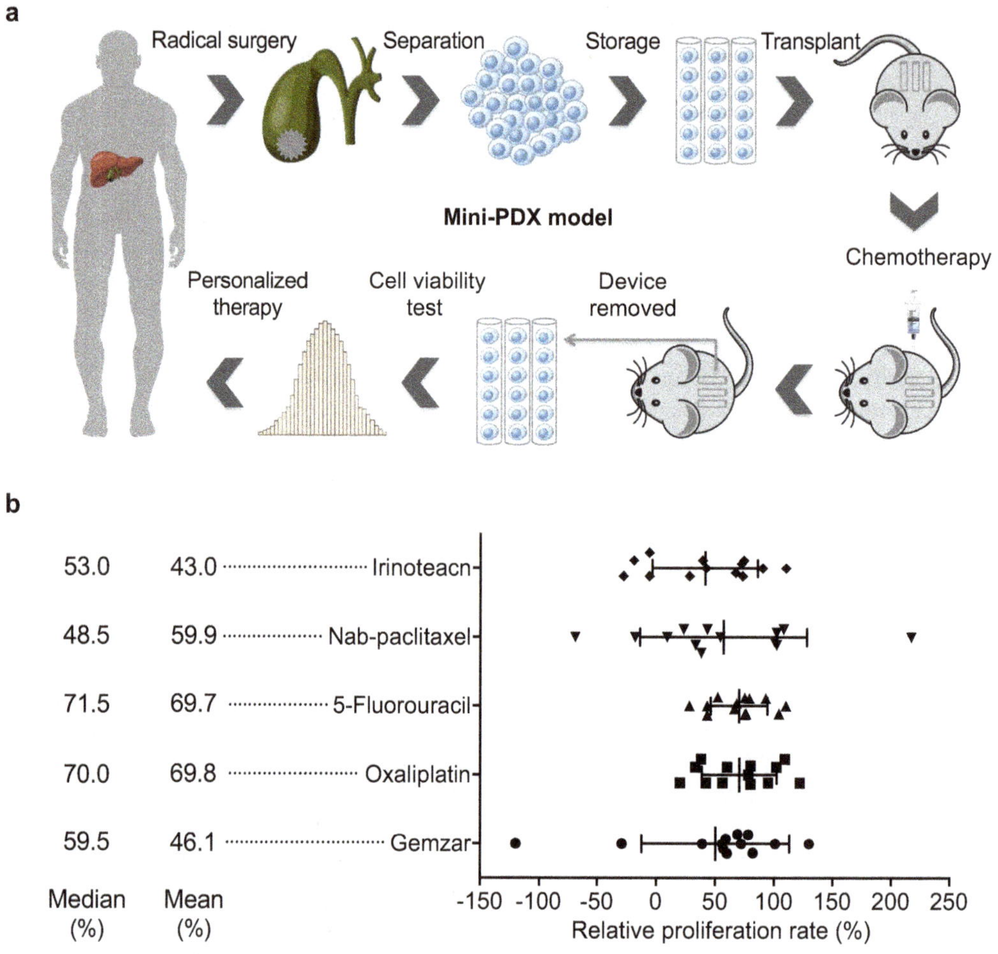

Groups	Chemotherapy programs											
Mini-PDX	NO.1	NO.2	NO.3	NO.4	NO.5	NO.6	NO.7	NO.8	NO.9	NO.10	NO.11	NO.12
	1+3	3+5	1+2	2+5	1+5	2+3	3+5	2+4	2+5	1+5	2+4	1+2
Conventional	4+5											

1: Irinoteacn; 2: Nab-paclitaxel; 3: 5-Fluorouracil; 4: Oxaliplatin; 5: Gemzar

Fig. 1 An overview of the generation of the mini-PDX model. **a** Gallbladder carcinoma cells from gallbladder carcinoma patients under surgical resection were transferred to the HBSS washed capsules and then subcutaneously implanted in BALB/c nude mice. Drugs or placebo (saline) were injected via the tail veins or intraperitoneally. Finally, the capsules were taken out and the anti-tumor activity was evaluated by detecting cell viabilities via CTG assays. Based on the anti-tumor activity data of the mini-PDX models, the optimal chemotherapy regimens were selected for different gallbladder carcinoma patients. **b** Scatter plot shows the results of the relative proliferation rate of the five drugs tested on the mini-PDX model among the 12 gallbladder carcinoma patients. **c** Detailed results reveal the two most effective agents chosen for treating the patients in the mini-PDX group and the conventional chemotherapy group

110% and the lowest at 28% of irinotecan implying the requirement of individualized therapy (Fig. 1b). The agents used in the investigated patients are shown in Fig. 1c.

Mini-PDX-guided chemotherapy is superior to conventional chemotherapy in prolonging survival of gallbladder carcinoma patients

The cohort included 24 males and 33 females with a mean age 66.6 ± 9.5 years. Patients in the PDX-guided chemotherapy group included 5 male (41.7%) and 7 female patients (58.3%) with a median age of 67 years (range 56–87 years). The PDX-guided chemotherapy group and the conventional chemotherapy group had comparable demographic and baseline characteristics (Table 1). Kaplan–Meier analysis showed that

patients in the PDX-guided chemotherapy group had significantly longer median OS (18.6 months; 95% CI 15.9–21.3 months) than patients in the conventional chemotherapy group (13.9 months; 95% CI 11.7–16.2 months) (P = 0.030; HR 3.18; 95% CI 1.47–6.91) (Fig. 2a). Patients in PDX-guided chemotherapy group

Table 1 Patient demographic and baseline characteristics

Characteristic	All	Conventional chemotherapy	PDX-guided chemotherapy	OR (95% CI)	P^a
No.	57	45	12		
Female gender, n (%)	33 (57.89)	26 (57.78)	7 (58.33)	1.02 (0.28–3.72)	0.972
Age, years, n (%)					
<65	23 (40.35)	18 (40)	5 (41.67)	1.07 (0.29–3.91)	0.917
Gallstone, n (%)					
Yes	44 (77.19)	36 (80)	8 (66.67)	0.5 (0.12–2.04)	0.555
CA19-9, U/mL, n (%)					
<37	16 (28.07)	13 (28.89)	3 (25)	0.82 (0.19–3.52)	0.924
Tumor size, cm, n (%)					
<4	37 (64.91)	31 (68.89)	6 (50)	0.45 (0.12–1.65)	0.223
Tumor differentiation, n (%)					
Well and moderate	31 (54.39)	23 (51.11)	8 (66.67)	1.91 (0.5–7.27)	0.525
Nerve invasion, n (%)					
Yes	21 (36.84)	15 (33.33)	6 (50)	0.5 (0.14–1.82)	0.288
Lymph node metastasis, n (%)					
Yes	21 (36.84)	14 (31.11)	7 (58.33)	0.4 (0.1–1.66)	0.375
^{b}TNM stage, n (%)					
IIIA	36 (63.16)	31 (68.89)	5 (41.67)	0.32 (0.09–1.2)	0.082
IIIB and IV	21 (36.84)	14 (31.11)	7 (58.33)		

PDX patient-derived xenograft

^{a} Chi square test

^{b} Tumor stage was defined according to the American Joint Committee on Cancer (AJCC) TNM staging system (AJCC 7th edition)

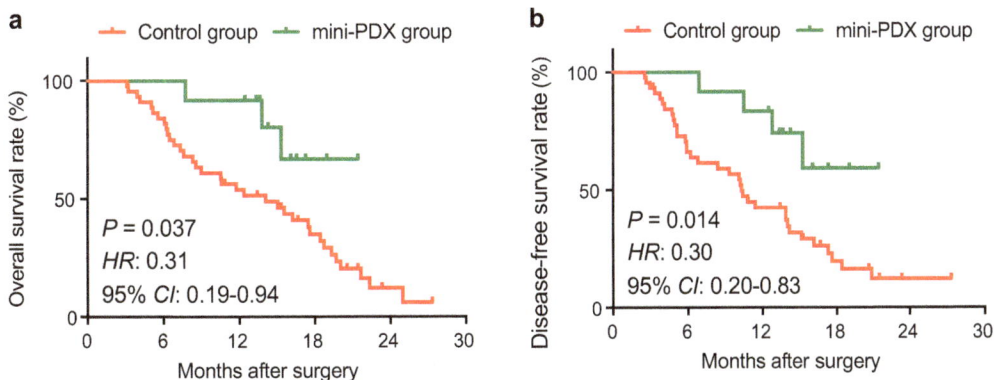

Fig. 2 Comparison of the prognosis of gallbladder carcinoma patients between the conventional chemotherapy group and the mini-PDX-guided chemotherapy group. The 12 gallbladder carcinoma patients who received agents based on the mini-PDX results had higher overall survival (**a**) and disease-free survival rates (**b**) than the 45 gallbladder carcinoma patients treated with conventional chemotherapeutic drugs. **b** The two curves were compared using log-rank test

also had significantly longer median DFS (17.6 months; 95% CI 14.5–20.6 months) than patients in the conventional chemotherapy group (12.0 months; 95% CI 9.7–14.4 months) ($P = 0.014$; HR 3.37; 95% CI 1.67–6.79) (Fig. 2b).

Correlation between drug sensitivity and clinicopathological variables and biomarkers

Our correlation analysis revealed that gemcitabine sensitivity was correlated with nerve invasion, while irinotecan efficacy was correlated with tumor size, lymph node metastasis and TNM stage (Table 2). In our mini-PDX models, irinotecan exhibited significantly greater cytotoxic effects on gallbladder carcinoma cells with high p53 or Ki-67 expression versus those with low p53 or Ki-67 expression (Fig. 3a, b). Furthermore, nab-paclitaxel demonstrated significantly greater anti-tumor effects on gallbladder carcinoma cells with low P-gp expression versus those with high P-gp expression (Fig. 3c). Oxaliplatin demonstrated significantly greater inhibitory effects on gallbladder carcinoma cells with high MRP1, Bcl-2 or GST-π expression; in contrast, 5-fluorouracil exhibited significantly greater inhibitory effects on gallbladder carcinoma cells with low Bcl-2 or TS expression (Fig. 3d–g).

Discussion

Cancer drug development has been hampered by a lack of preclinical models that could reliably predict the efficacy of novel compounds in cancer patients. PDX models have gained more popularity in the past several years over conventional models in predicting postoperative chemosensitivity of various tumors [19]. Here, we present the first piece of preclinical and clinical evidence for the utility of optimized mini-PDX model in guiding adjuvant chemotherapy of gallbladder cancer patients. Moreover, when prospectively comparing the efficacy of PDX-guided chemotherapy versus conventional chemotherapy, we found that PDX-guided chemotherapy significantly improved the survival outcome of gallbladder carcinoma patients. Additionally, the correlations between some clinicopathological features, biomarkers and drug efficacy were also analyzed. Our present study showed that the mini-PDX models well-recapitulated the tumor behaviors of gallbladder carcinoma patients and could provide important guidance for oncologists in making informed decision on individualized chemotherapy.

Most translational cancer studies require effective preclinical models [20–23]. Human cancer models for drug screening started in the 1970s with the help of conventional cell lines. Although convenient and easy to use,

Table 2 Association analysis between clinicopathologic characteristics and chemosensitivity

Proliferation rate (%)	Gemcitabine	P	Oxaliplatin	P	5-Fluorouracil	P	Nab-paclitaxel	P	Irinotecan	P
Tumor size, cm										
<4	65.3±11.5	0.316	72.2±27.9	0.814	66.5±30.0	0.684	84.8±28.5	0.257	71.0±26.4	*0.049*
≥4	26.8±88.6		67.3±40.2		72.8±21.7		35.0±97.4		15.0±51.9	
Tumor differentiation										
Well and moderate	38.5±78.2	0.699	55.0±28.7	0.127	61.7±24.6	0.292	35.3±67.5	0.264	31.7±46.8	0.449
Poor	53.7±51.2		84.5±32.6		77.7±25.2		84.5±76.1		54.3±52.7	
Nerve invasion										
No	10.3±72.1	*0.044*	74.8±26.8	0.618	71.2±30.2	0.848	82.7±94.2	0.303	37.2±56.5	0.700
Yes	81.8±24.8		64.7±40.4		68.2±21.9		37.2±40.9		48.8±44.8	
Lymph node metastasis										
No	30.2±85.7	0.491	55.4±34.3	0.219	69.8±34.1	0.989	21.4±66.3	0.128	7.4±38.5	*0.024*
Yes	57.4±46.3		80.0±30.5		69.6±19.7		87.4±69.1		68.4±40.0	
TNM stage										
I–IIIA	18.3±94.0	0.305	61.0±36.9	0.543	64.0±36.4	0.606	13.3±73.6	0.122	−7.5±22.2	*0.004*
IIIB–IV	60.0±43.5		74.1±32.7		72.5±20.0		83.3±65.1		68.3±37.0	

P values were calculated by unpaired t-test (2-sided)

(See figure on next page.)

Fig. 3 Correlation between drug sensitivity and various biomarkers. The relationship between the efficacy of the five drugs (gemcitabine, oxaliplatin, 5-fluorouracil, nab-paclitaxel, and irinotecan) and p53 (**a**), Ki-67 (**b**), P-gp (**c**), MRP1 (**d**), Bcl-2 (**e**), TS (**f**), GST (**g**) as well as TOP II (**h**) expressions in gallbladder carcinoma patients. Error bar, SD, *$P < 0.05$; **$P < 0.01$; ***$P < 0.001$; Student's t test (two-tailed)

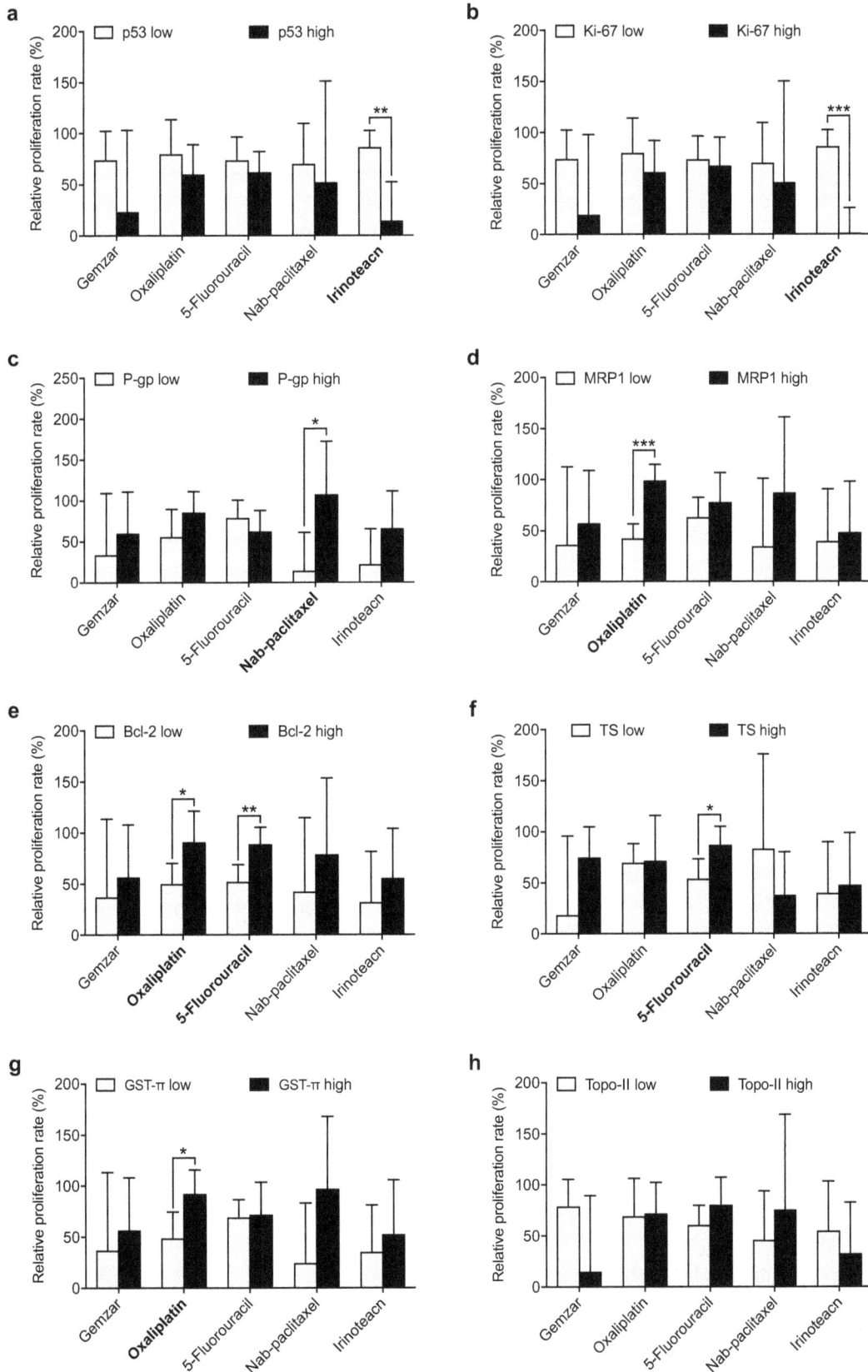

these cell lines-based studies lack the predictive value of specific cancer types for clinical application. The pre-clinical PDX models has circumvent the limitations of conventional cell line-based models and are now more commonly used. These models can provide drug sensitivities that mimic the clinical response of cancer patients to cytotoxic agents [24]. Also, since PDX models correlate well with the pathologic characteristics and genetic features of the tumors of individual patients, they are becoming the preferred preclinical tool to improve the drug development process [24]. However, the long time in establishing PDX models restrains their usage in more aggressive cancers like gallbladder carcinoma; not to mention that several transplantation cycles are needed for tumor xenograft formation in PDX models and which might alter the properties of the originally transplanted tumor. Reports have demonstrated that the finally formed tumor xenograft is subsequently a more aggressive phenotype and behaves more like metastatic tumor [25]. Most gallbladder carcinoma patients are diagnosed at advanced stages, and thus require prompt initiation of anti-tumor therapy. In this perspective, mini-PDX model is the more suitable alternative.

Currently, gemcitabine, oxaliplatin, 5-fluorouracil, nab-paclitaxel, and irinotecan are the five most potentially effective agents for gallbladder carcinoma patients [26]. Single or combination chemotherapies of these drugs have shown improved median survival rates of gallbladder carcinoma patients. However, further clinical application of these drugs are often impeded by the uncommon nature of gallbladder carcinoma and efficacy data are mostly based on studies from other biliary tract tumors like intrahepatic or extrahepatic cholangiocarcinoma, which are now considered to be different from gallbladder carcinoma [12, 27]. In this study, an improved prognosis was observed when the effectiveness of five chemotherapeutic drugs were separately tested using mini-PDX models, after which the two most effective drugs identified were prospectively prescribed to gallbladder carcinoma patients. This personalized treatment provides a scientific rationale for clinical therapy and avoids the side effects from clinical experience-guided medication. Aside from cytotoxic chemotherapeutic agents, several targeted agents against EGFR, VEGF or MEK have also been reported to be useful in treating gallbladder cancer. Therefore, our mini-PDX model could be suitable for preclinical testing of the effectiveness of these drugs in the coming future.

Aside from providing reliable references for the choice of drugs clinically, the mini-PDX models, when combined with other technical methods, could also accelerate the understanding of the underlying mechanisms of oncogenesis, tumor progression and chemoresistance. In this present study, we have found that gemcitabine sensitivity was correlated with nerve invasion, and irinotecan efficacy was associated with tumor size, lymph node metastasis and TNM stage. Future studies with a larger sample set are required to confirm these relationships and help elucidate the underlying mechanisms. P53, Ki-67, P-gp, MRP1, Bcl-2, TS, GST-π and Topo-II are important in modulating chemosensitivity [28, 29]. The reactivity to irinotecan in our mini-PDX model was found to correlate with p53 and Ki-67 expression in gallbladder carcinoma patients. Oxaliplatin sensitivity was associated with MRP1 and Bcl-2 expression. These findings demonstrate that the mini-PDX model is effective in predicting chemosensitivity of gallbladder carcinoma patients and lends support to the future application of this method in clinical practice. In addition, based on our obtained results, chemo resistant and chemosensitive PDX tumor models could be developed to study the molecular mechanisms of chemoresistance in gallbladder carcinoma, which would be conducive in finding potential therapeutic targets and predictive markers of chemosensitivity for gallbladder cancer patients. Hence, mini-PDX models has potential prospect of being extended in the treatment of other types of malignant tumors.

Conclusions

Our results show that the mini-PDX model is an effective tool in guiding the choice of chemotherapeutic regimens for gallbladder carcinoma patients and that PDX-guided chemotherapy can significantly improve the survival of gallbladder carcinoma patients compared to conventional chemotherapy. However, further confirmations from studies with larger sample size are needed.

Abbreviations
PDX: patient-derived xenograft; OS: overall survival; DFS: disease free survival rate; HBSS: Hank's balanced salt solution; RFU: relative fluorescence units; SD: standard deviation.

Authors' contributions
JW was responsible for coordination of the project and contributed to the study design. The writing team consisted of JW, MZ, and RMY. MZ, RMY, MH, and WC performed most of in vitro and in vivo experiments. MH, LHY, and HW took part in the collection of clinical samples and features. QL and MML performed IHC data analysis. All authors read and approved the final manuscript.

Author details
[1] Department of Biliary-Pancreatic Surgery, Renji Hospital, School of Medicine, Shanghai Jiao Tong University, 160 Pujian Road, Shanghai 200127, P. R. China. [2] Department of Pathology, Renji Hospital, School of Medicine, Shanghai Jiao Tong University, Shanghai 200127, P. R. China. [3] Department of Pathology, Shanghai Ninth People's Hospital, School of Medicine, Shanghai Jiao Tong University, Shanghai 200011, P. R. China.

Acknowledgements
We appreciate Dr. Wen Danyi (LIDE Biotech Inc.) for providing technical support on mini-PDX models.

Competing interests
The authors declare that they have no competing interests.

Funding
This work was supported by the Foundation of Shanghai Shen Kang Hospital Development Center (Nos. 16CR2002A and 16CR3028A), National Science Foundation of China (Nos. 81472240 and 81773184), and Shanghai Outstanding Academic Leaders Plan (2016, JW).

References

1. de Groen PC, Gores GJ, LaRusso NF, Gunderson LL, Nagorney DM. Biliary tract cancers. N Engl J Med. 1999;341(18):1368–78. https://doi.org/10.1056/NEJM199910283411807.

2. Lazcano-Ponce EC, Miquel JF, Munoz N, Herrero R, Ferrecio C, Wistuba II, et al. Epidemiology and molecular pathology of gallbladder cancer. CA Cancer J Clin. 2001;51(6):349–64.

3. Miller KD, Siegel RL, Lin CC, Mariotto AB, Kramer JL, Rowland JH, et al. Cancer treatment and survivorship statistics, 2016. CA Cancer J Clin. 2016;66(4):271–89. https://doi.org/10.3322/caac.21349.

4. Hueman MT, Vollmer CM Jr, Pawlik TM. Evolving treatment strategies for gallbladder cancer. Ann Surg Oncol. 2009;16(8):2101–15. https://doi.org/10.1245/s10434-009-0538-x.

5. Chan E, Berlin J. Biliary tract cancers: understudied and poorly understood. J Clin Oncol. 2015;33(16):1845–8. https://doi.org/10.1200/JCO.2014.59.7591.

6. Huang Y, Li X, Zhao Y. Progression of targeted therapy in advanced cholangiocarcinoma. Chin J Cancer Res. 2015;27(2):122–7. https://doi.org/10.3978/j.issn.1000-9604.2015.04.01.

7. Lee J, Park SH, Chang HM, Kim JS, Choi HJ, Lee MA, et al. Gemcitabine and oxaliplatin with or without erlotinib in advanced biliary-tract cancer: a multicentre, open-label, randomised, phase 3 study. Lancet Oncol. 2012;13(2):181–8. https://doi.org/10.1016/S1470-2045(11)70301-1.

8. Jensen LH. Biliary-tract cancer: improving therapy by adding molecularly targeted agents. Lancet Oncol. 2012;13(2):118–9. https://doi.org/10.1016/S1470-2045(11)70329-1.

9. Endlicher E, Schnoy E, Troppmann M, Rogler G, Messmann H, Klebl F, et al. Irinotecan plus gemcitabine and fluorouracil in advanced biliary tract cancer: a retrospective study. Digestion. 2016;93(3):229–33. https://doi.org/10.1159/000445187.

10. Chung MJ, Kim YJ, Park JY, Bang S, Song SY, Chung JB, et al. Prospective phase II trial of gemcitabine in combination with irinotecan as first-line chemotherapy in patients with advanced biliary tract cancer. Chemotherapy. 2011;57(3):236–43. https://doi.org/10.1159/000328021.

11. Williams TM, Majithia L, Wang SJ, Thomas CR Jr. Defining the role of adjuvant therapy: cholangiocarcinoma and gall bladder cancer. Semin Radiat Oncol. 2014;24(2):94–104. https://doi.org/10.1016/j.semradonc.2014.01.001.

12. Nakamura H, Arai Y, Totoki Y, Shirota T, Elzawahry A, Kato M, et al. Genomic spectra of biliary tract cancer. Nat Genet. 2015;47(9):1003–10. https://doi.org/10.1038/ng.3375.

13. Valle JW, Lamarca A, Goyal L, Barriuso J, Zhu AX. New horizons for precision medicine in biliary tract cancers. Cancer Discov. 2017;7(9):943–62. https://doi.org/10.1158/2159-8290.CD-17-0245.

14. Gandara DR, Lara PN Jr, Mack PC. Patient-derived xenografts for investigation of acquired resistance in oncogene-driven cancers: building a better mousetrap. J Clin Oncol. 2015;33(26):2839–40. https://doi.org/10.1200/JCO.2015.61.9692.

15. Bissig-Choisat B, Kettlun-Leyton C, Legras XD, Zorman B, Barzi M, Chen LL, et al. Novel patient-derived xenograft and cell line models for therapeutic testing of pediatric liver cancer. J Hepatol. 2016;65(2):325–33. https://doi.org/10.1016/j.jhep.2016.04.009.

16. Chapuy B, Cheng H, Watahiki A, Ducar MD, Tan Y, Chen L, et al. Diffuse large B-cell lymphoma patient-derived xenograft models capture the molecular and biological heterogeneity of the disease. Blood. 2016;127(18):2203–13. https://doi.org/10.1182/blood-2015-09-672352.

17. Nicolle D, Fabre M, Simon-Coma M, Gorse A, Kappler R, Nonell L, et al. Patient-derived mouse xenografts from pediatric liver cancer predict tumor recurrence and advise clinical management. Hepatology. 2016;64(4):1121–35. https://doi.org/10.1002/hep.28621.

18. Yang RM, Zhan M, Xu SW, Long MM, Yang LH, Chen W, et al. miR-3656 expression enhances the chemosensitivity of pancreatic cancer to gemcitabine through modulation of the RHOF/EMT axis. Cell Death Dis. 2017;8(10):e3129. https://doi.org/10.1038/cddis.2017.530.

19. Tentler JJ, Tan AC, Weekes CD, Jimeno A, Leong S, Pitts TM, et al. Patient-derived tumour xenografts as models for oncology drug development. Nat Rev Clin Oncol. 2012;9(6):338–50. https://doi.org/10.1038/nrclinonc.2012.61.

20. Hu X, Chen L, Du Y, Fan B, Bu Z, Wang X, et al. Postoperative chemotherapy with S-1 plus oxaliplatin versus S-1 alone in locally advanced gastric cancer (RESCUE-GC study): a protocol for a phase III randomized controlled trial. Chin J Cancer Res. 2017;29(2):144–8. https://doi.org/10.21147/j.issn.1000-9604.2017.02.07.

21. Hu X, Wang L, Lin L, Han X, Dou G, Meng Z, et al. A phase I trial of an oral subtype-selective histone deacetylase inhibitor, chidamide, in combination with paclitaxel and carboplatin in patients with advanced non-small cell lung cancer. Chin J Cancer Res. 2016;28(4):444–51. https://doi.org/10.21147/j.issn.1000-9604.2016.04.08.

22. Venditti JM, Wesley RA, Plowman J. Current NCI preclinical antitumor screening in vivo: results of tumor panel screening, 1976–1982, and future directions. Adv Pharmacol Chemother. 1984;20:1–20.

23. Zhou H, Song Y, Jiang J, Niu H, Zhao H, Liang J, et al. A pilot phase II study of neoadjuvant triplet chemotherapy regimen in patients with locally advanced resectable colon cancer. Chin J Cancer Res. 2016;28(6):598–605. https://doi.org/10.21147/j.issn.1000-9604.2016.06.06.

24. Choi SY, Lin D, Gout PW, Collins CC, Xu Y, Wang Y. Lessons from patient-derived xenografts for better in vitro modeling of human cancer. Adv Drug Deliv Rev. 2014;79–80:222–37. https://doi.org/10.1016/j.addr.2014.09.009.

25. Lai Y, Wei X, Lin S, Qin L, Cheng L, Li P. Current status and perspectives of patient-derived xenograft models in cancer research. J Hematol Oncol. 2017;10(1):106. https://doi.org/10.1186/s13045-017-0470-7.

26. Horgan AM, Amir E, Walter T, Knox JJ. Adjuvant therapy in the treatment of biliary tract cancer: a systematic review and meta-analysis. J Clin Oncol. 2012;30(16):1934–40. https://doi.org/10.1200/JCO.2011.40.5381.

27. Razumilava N, Gores GJ. Building a staircase to precision medicine for biliary tract cancer. Nat Genet. 2015;47(9):967–8. https://doi.org/10.1038/ng.3386.

28. Xue X, Liang XJ. Overcoming drug efflux-based multidrug resistance in cancer with nanotechnology. Chin J Cancer. 2012;31(2):100–9. https://doi.org/10.5732/cjc.011.10326.

29. Zhang JT. Use of arrays to investigate the contribution of ATP-binding cassette transporters to drug resistance in cancer chemotherapy and prediction of chemosensitivity. Cell Res. 2007;17(4):311–23. https://doi.org/10.1038/cr.2007.15.

14

Differential incidence trends of colon and rectal cancers in Hong Kong: an age-period-cohort analysis

Bo Zhang[1,2,4], Shao-Hua Xie[3,4*] and Ignatius Tak-sun Yu[4,5]

Abstract

Background: Colorectal cancer has been the second most common cancer among men and women in Hong Kong since 2012, but the underlying reasons for this increase remain unclear. We describe the incidence trend for colorectal cancer in Hong Kong to explore its etiology within this population.

Methods: The temporal trends in colorectal cancer incidence between 1983 and 2012 were analyzed with joinpoint regressions by sex, age groups, and anatomic sites among adults using data from the Hong Kong Cancer Registry. An age-period-cohort analysis was used to evaluate the effects of age, calendar periods, and birth cohorts on the observed temporal trends.

Results: The incidence of colon cancer among those aged 50 years and older in both sexes increased steadily from 1983 until the mid-1990s and was followed by a slight decrease thereafter, whereas the incidence among those aged 20–49 years decreased steadily from 1983 to 2012. In contrast, the incidence of rectal cancer steadily increased in men and remained stable in women throughout the study period. Significant period and birth cohort effects were observed for colon cancer, whereas period effects on the temporal trends were observed for male rectal cancer.

Conclusions: The incidences of colon and rectal cancers have exhibited divergent patterns between 1983 and 2012 in Hong Kong, indicating heterogeneous etiologies between these two types of cancers. Surveillance of the risk factors related to colon and rectal cancers in the Hong Kong population should be performed, and the increased rectal cancer incidence in males is worthy of extra attention.

Background

Colorectal cancer (CRC) is a commonly diagnosed cancer in both sexes worldwide [1]. The incidence of CRC varies significantly among countries [2, 3], and nearly 55% of the CRC cases worldwide occur in more-developed countries with Western lifestyles [1]. The incidence of CRC in Asia still ranks among the lowest in the world [2]. However, a number of Asian countries or regions, namely, mainland China, South Korea, Japan, Singapore, and Hong Kong, have experienced such a marked rise in

CRC incidence that the CRC incidence in East Asia has surpassed the global average in recent decades [1].

CRC has historically been considered a single type of cancer because the colon and rectum are situated at the end of digestive system and are contiguous in both anatomical position and physiological function. However, it is increasingly being recognized that CRC may not be homogenous in terms of morphological, molecular, and genetic characteristics at different anatomical sites [4]. In addition, notable divergent patterns in the incidence trends of colon and rectal cancers have been observed in many regions around the world [5–7], suggesting etiological heterogeneity of CRC according to anatomical site.

Hong Kong is a unique setting for epidemiological studies of CRC because of the special demographic history of the population, rapid economic development,

*Correspondence: shaohua.xie@ki.se
[3] Upper Gastrointestinal Surgery, Department of Molecular Medicine and Surgery, Karolinska Institute, Karolinska University Hospital, NS 67, 2nd Floor, 17176 Stockholm, Sweden
Full list of author information is available at the end of the article

and social transitions during the past few decades. CRC has been the second most common cancer among men and women since 2012 and is a leading cause of cancer deaths in both sexes in Hong Kong. A total of 4979 (2862 males and 2117 females) newly diagnosed CRC cases occurred in Hong Kong in 2014, with a crude incidence of 68.8 cases per 100,000 individuals; 2034 people died from CRC, which accounted for 28.0% of all cancer deaths in Hong Kong [8].

The temporal trend in CRC incidence in Hong Kong has not been recently updated. To better understand the changing epidemiology of CRC in Hong Kong and the underlying reasons for this change, we analyzed the time trends in the incidence of CRC by anatomic site in Hong Kong over the 30-year period of 1983–2012. We also performed an age-period-cohort analysis to address the effects of age, calendar periods, and birth cohorts on the observed trend. Etiological implications were further considered with reference to possible risk factors. Considering the probable heterogeneous etiologies of colon and rectal cancers, all analyses and interpretations were performed according to these two different anatomical sites.

Materials and methods
Data source
All newly diagnosed colon cancer and rectal cancer cases between 1983 and 2012 were identified from the Hong Kong Cancer Registry, a population-based cancer registry with over 95% coverage for most cancers [8]. The Hong Kong Cancer Registry is a member of the International Association of Cancer Registries (IACR) and has contributed regularly to the "Cancer Incidence in Five Continents" series since the 1970s. Mid-year population data for each calendar year were obtained from the Hong Kong Census and Statistics Department.

Joinpoint regression analysis
Age-standardized annual incidence was calculated by the direct method using the World Health Organization (WHO) 1966 World Standard Population as the reference. Temporal trends in the incidences of colon and rectal cancers were evaluated by sex using the Joinpoint Regression Program (version 4.5.0.0) developed by the US National Cancer Institute (NCI) [9]. The joinpoint regression attempted to identify potential changing points over time in the annual incidence and estimated the annual percent change (APC) in each trend segment under the assumption that the annual rate changed at a constant linear rate on a log scale.

Age-period-cohort analysis
We further performed age-period-cohort analyses for each gender to examine the effects of age, calendar periods, and birth cohorts on the incidence trends using a newly developed web tool from the US NCI [10]. In brief, age-period-cohort models delineate variance in disease trends over time according to age, period and cohort effects. Age at diagnosis is a surrogate for age-related biological factors and reflects the underlying natural history of the disease. Period effects are usually derived from factors that concurrently affect all age groups. In contrast, cohort effects are attributable to factors that influence specific generations (birth cohorts) and vary in prevalence by generation. A web tool that provided a suite of functions and parameters, including model-based estimators of cross-sectional and longitudinal age-specific rates, period and cohort rate ratios that incorporate the overall annual percent change (net drift), and estimators of the age-specific annual percent change (local drifts), was used for age-period-cohort analysis [10]. Particularly, net drift, which is an analog of the annual percent change in the incidence over the study period, estimates the average annual percentage change in the logarithm of the incidence with adjustment for a non-linear period and cohort effects. Local drift indicates the average annual percentage change in incidence over time across different age groups. Cohort (or period) deviations are orthogonal to the linear trend in the birth cohorts (or calendar periods) and reflect the non-linear cohort (or period) effects incorporated into cohort (or period) rate ratio and local drifts. An important implication of local drifts and/or cohort deviations is that a single-summary, age-standardized rate (ASR) curve and APC value or net drift cannot adequately describe the time trends across age groups. In this study, the incidence data were categorized into 14 5-year age groups (ages 20–24, 25–29, 30–34, 35–39, 40–44, ..., 80–84, and ≥ 85 years) and six 5-year calendar periods (1983–1987, 1988–1992, ..., and 2008–2012), spanning 19 partially overlapping 10-year birth cohorts indicated by the middle years (1898, 1903, ..., and 1988). The calendar period 1993–1997 and the 1938 birth cohort were used as reference categories for estimates of relative risk (RR).

Results
Incidence profiles of colon and rectal cancer
In general, the average age-standardized rates between 1983 and 2012 were 23.1 per 100,000 person-years for men and 17.8 per 100,000 person-years for women for colon cancer and 15.8 per 100,000 person-years for men and 9.7 per 100,000 person-years for women for rectal cancer among all age groups. Nearly all cases occurred in

individuals 20 years of age or older. A total of 54,984 incident cases of colon cancer and 33,308 cases of rectal cancer were recorded in Hong Kong from 1983 to 2012 for the 20-year+age group, among which nearly 90% of the cases were diagnosed at age 50 years or older, and 10% were diagnosed between the ages of 20 and 49 years.

Incidence trend of colon cancer

Figure 1 shows the age-standardized annual incidence of colon and rectal cancers by sex among individuals in the 20+ age group, 20–49 age group and 50+ age group, and the results from the joinpoint regression of the incidence trends are shown in Table 1. The temporal trends

were similar in men and women but differed between the 20–49 and 50+ age groups. Among people aged 50 years or older, the age-standardized incidence of colon cancer in men increased by 1.40% (95% confidence interval [CI] 1.16–1.64%) per year, from 86.3 per 100,000 in 1983 to 110.9 per 100,000 in 1996. This parameter then decreased by 0.44% on average (95% CI −0.57 to −0.31%) per year through 2012. Similarly, in women, the age-standardized incidence increased by 2.57% on average (95% CI 2.43–3.11%) per year from 1983 until it peaked in 1992, and then it decreased by 0.78% on average (95% CI −0.91 to −0.66%) per year through 2012. In contrast, for individuals in the 20–49 age group, the incidence of colon cancer

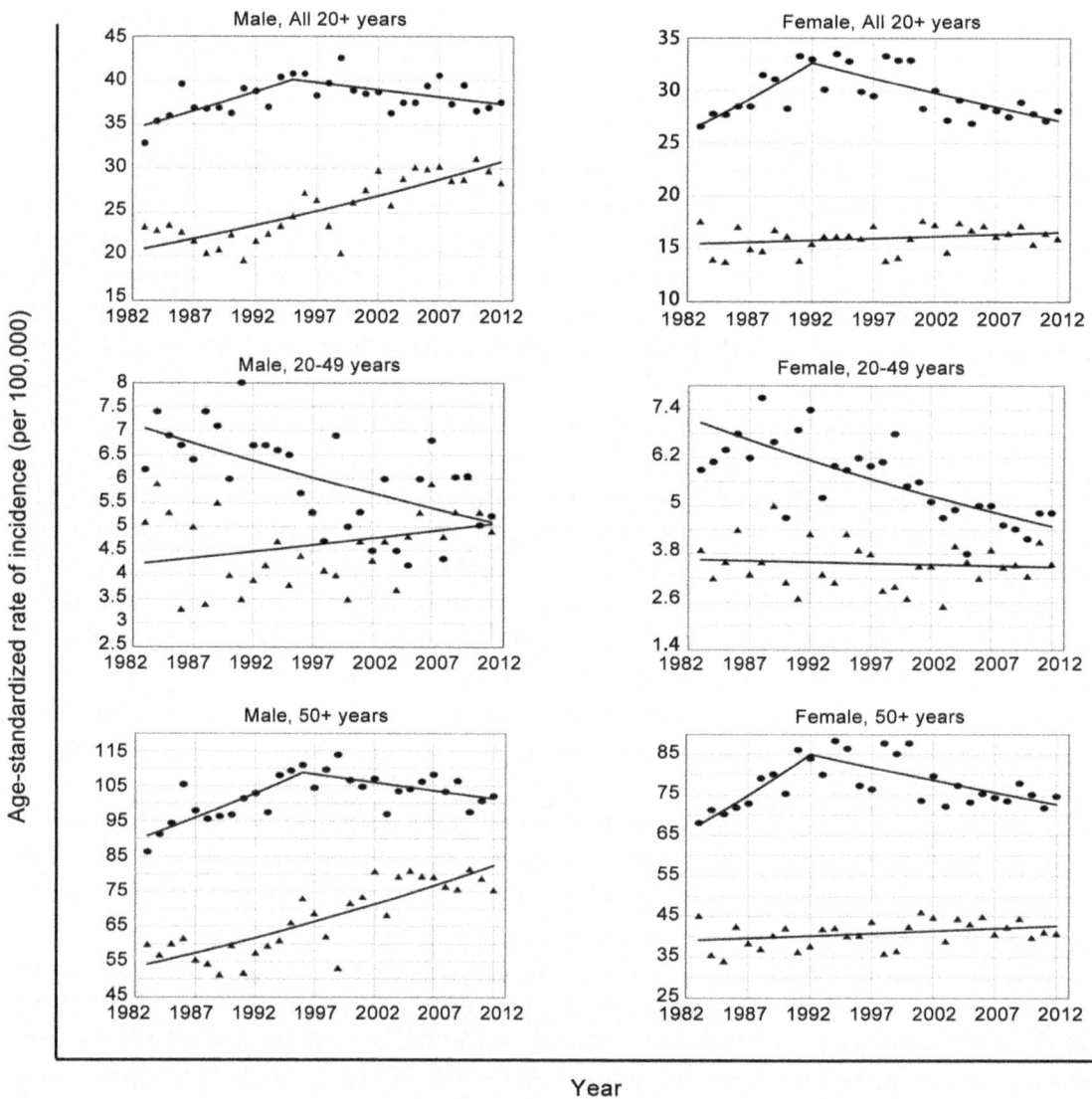

Fig. 1 Trends in colon and rectal cancer incidence among men and women by age group, 1983–2012. Rates are age-standardized to the 1966 world standard population. Scattered points are observed rates. Lines are fitted rates according to joinpoint regression, which allowed up to three joinpoints except for male rectal cancer in ages 20–49 years, with 0 joinpoints. Circles = colon cancer; triangles = rectal cancer

Table 1 Joinpoint analyses of colon and rectal cancer incidence by sex and age, 1983–2012, Hong Kong

Sex	Anatomic sites	Age	Calendar period	Average APC (95% CI)
Male	Colon cancer	All 20+	1983–1995	1.16 (0.88, 1.44)
			1995–2012	−0.42 (−0.54, −0.30)
			Full Period	0.05 (−0.02, 0.13)
		20–49	1983–2012	−1.11 (−1.32, −0.90)
		50+	1983–1996	1.40 (1.16, 1.64)
			1996–2012	−0.44 (−0.57, −0.31)
			Full Period	0.21 (0.13, 0.29)
	Rectal cancer	All 20+	1983–2012	1.35 (1.23, 1.46)
		20–49	1983–2012	0.60 (0.37, 0.84)
		50+	1983–2012	1.45 (1.32, 1.58)
Female	Colon cancer	All 20+	1983–1992	2.24 (1.68, 2.79)
			1992–2012	−0.91 (−1.04, −0.79)
			Full period	−0.33 (−0.43, −0.23)
		20–49	1983–2012	−1.56 (−1.73, −1.39)
		50+	1983–1992	2.57 (2.04, 3.11)
			1992–2012	−0.78 (−0.91, −0.66)
			Full period	−0.12 (−0.23, −0.01)
	Rectal cancer	All 20+	1983–2012	0.23 (0.13, 0.33)
		20–49	1983–2012	−0.17 (−0.40, 0.05)
		50+	1983–2012	0.29 (0.19, 0.39)

APC annual percent change

monotonically decreased in both men (APC = − 1.11%, 95% CI − 1.32 to − 0.90%) and women (APC = − 1.56%, 95% CI − 1.73 to − 1.39%) throughout the entire study period.

Incidence trend of rectal cancer

The temporal trends of rectal cancer differed in men and in women. The age-standardized incidence of rectal cancer in men increased at a steady rate of 1.35% (95% CI 1.23–1.46%) per year over the entire study period. The rate in women fluctuated between a low of 13.8 per 100,000 in 1985 and a high of 17.7 per 100,000 in 2001 and slightly increased over the study period (APC = 0.23%, 95% CI 0.13–0.33%). In both men and women, the rate increased more rapidly in people older than 50 years than in people aged 20–49 years (Table 1 and Fig. 1).

Age-period-cohort analysis

The fitted longitudinal age-specific incidences of colon cancer and rectal cancer adjusted for period deviations are illustrated in Fig. 2. The longitudinal age curves displayed generally identical patterns across different anatomical sites, indicating a monotonically increased risk with age in both sexes.

Local drifts, i.e., age-specific average APCs of the incidences of colon and rectal cancers over time, are illustrated by sex in Fig. 3. The age-specific average APC of colon cancer generally increased with age in both sexes. In contrast, irrespective of sex, no statistically significant differences in the APCs of the incidence of rectal cancer were observed across age groups, although there were seemingly large departures from the net drift for individuals below 40 years of age, with relatively wider 95% CIs compared with individuals over 40 years of age.

Figure 4 presents the rate ratios of colon and rectal cancers for each birth cohort by sex. We observed divergent birth cohort effects for colon and rectal cancers in both sexes. The risk of colon cancer in men increased from the early birth cohort until it peaked in the late-1930s cohort, plateaued in the following 15–20 years, and clearly decreased from 1963 forward. Colon cancer risk in women increased from the earliest cohort until the 1928 cohort and decreased steadily thereafter. The risk of rectal cancer generally increased in later birth cohorts for men. For women, the incidence ratio increased slowly until the 1968 birth cohort and decreased abruptly in the later cohorts, but these differences among different birth cohorts showed no statistical significance. The rate ratio plots for calendar periods showed patterns similar to those observed in the joinpoint analyses (Fig. 5).

The Wald test results for the age-period-cohort analyses are presented in Table 2. For the colon cancer incidence trends in both sexes, significant differences in local

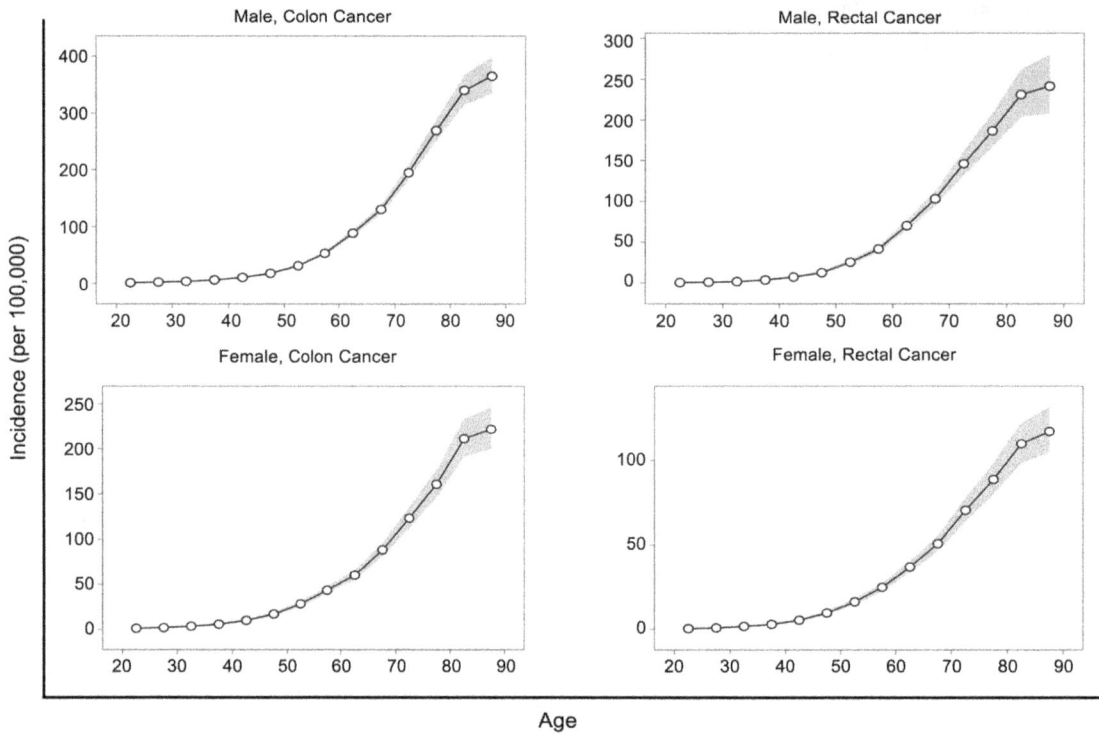

Fig. 2 Longitudinal age curves of incidence (1/100,000) for colon cancer and rectal cancer by sex. Shaded regions show pointwise 95% confidence intervals

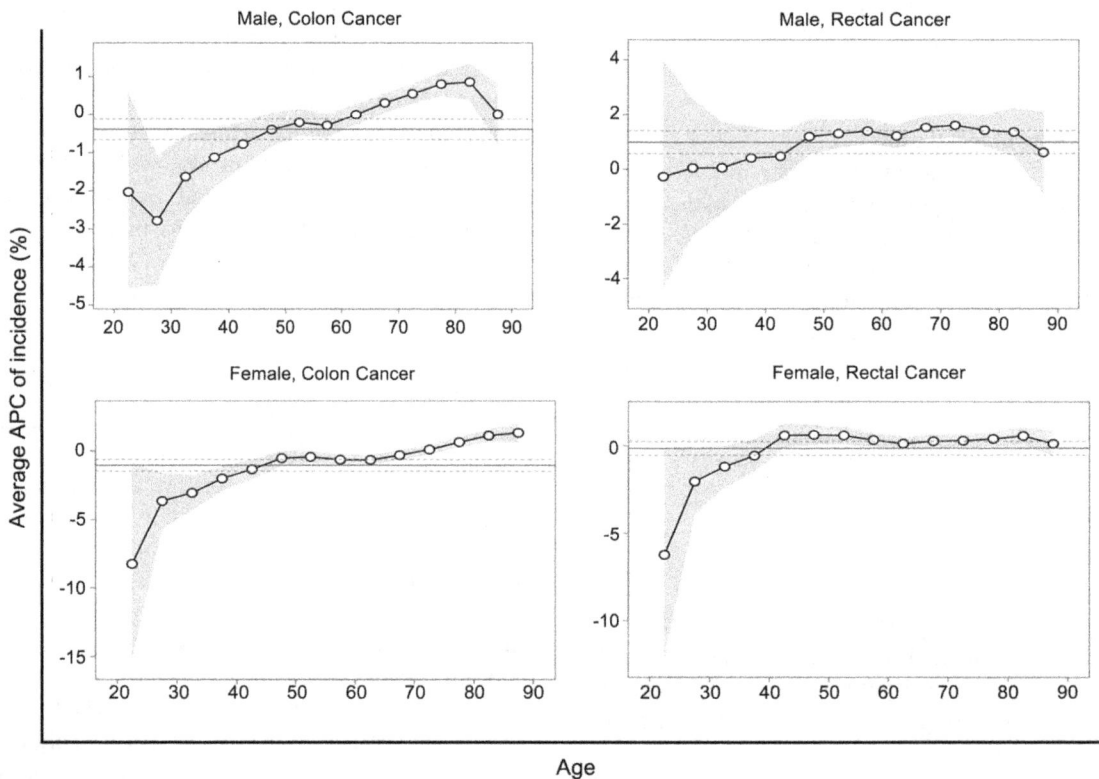

Fig. 3 Local drifts for colon and rectal cancer incidence by sex in 1983 and 2012. Shaded regions show pointwise 95% confidence intervals

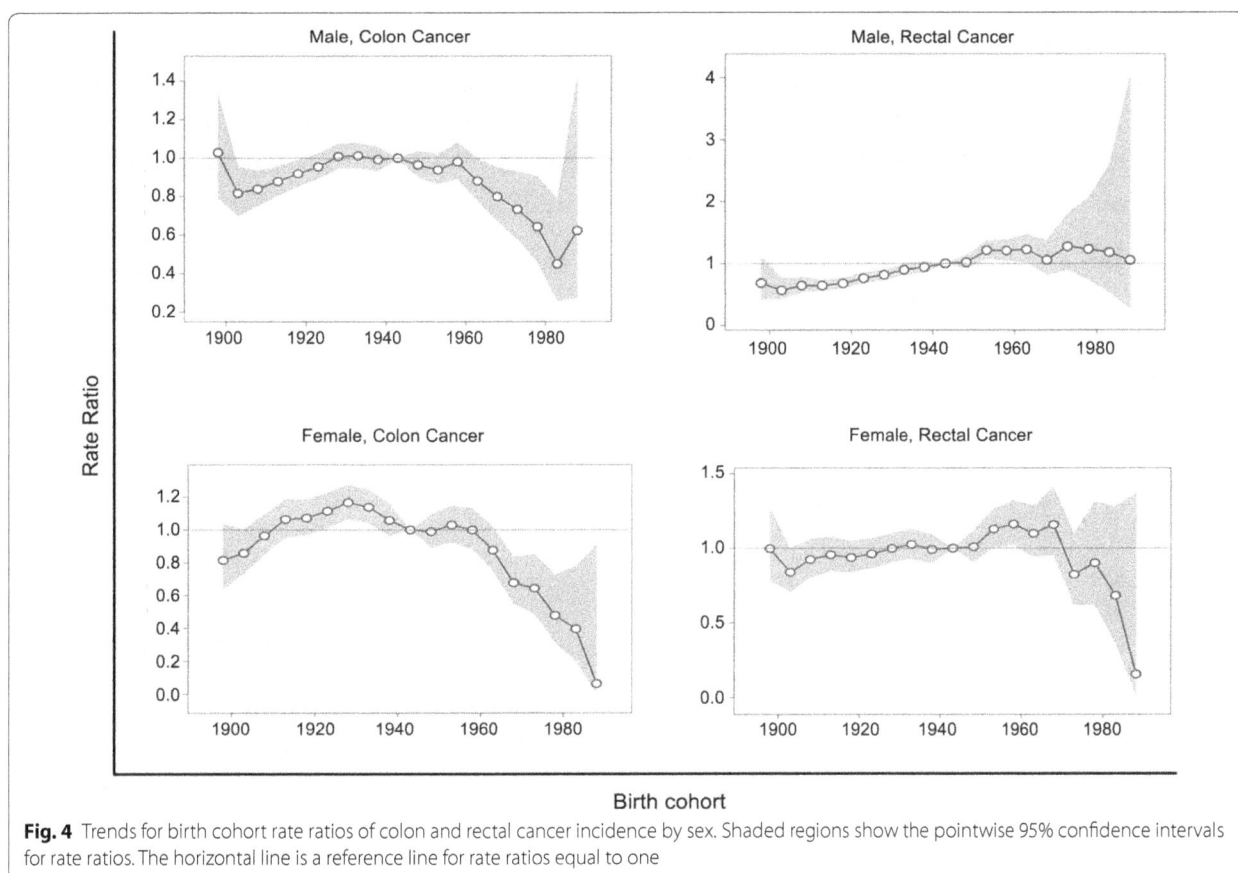

Fig. 4 Trends for birth cohort rate ratios of colon and rectal cancer incidence by sex. Shaded regions show the pointwise 95% confidence intervals for rate ratios. The horizontal line is a reference line for rate ratios equal to one

drifts and cohort deviations indicated potential cohort effects on the observed temporal trends, although period effects could not be ruled out. For rectal cancer, no significant local drifts and cohort deviations in the temporal trends were observed, indicating that there were no cohort effects. The temporal trends in male rectal cancer might be attributable to period effects.

Discussion

In this updated analysis of data from the 30-year period between 1983 and 2012, we observed divergent incidence trends for colon and rectal cancers in Hong Kong. Changes in the incidence of colon cancer showed similar patterns in both sexes, with increasing rates until the early 1990s followed by steady decreases thereafter among individuals in the 50+ age group. In addition, a steady decrease in colon cancer incidence between 1983 and 2012 was observed among individuals in the 20–49-year age group. In contrast, the incidence of rectal cancer increased steadily during the entire study period, and this increase was more pronounced in men.

The temporal trends in colon and rectal cancer incidences differ between Hong Kong and Japan, both of which have experienced similar socioeconomic

development and were high-income regions in the 1980s. The incidence trends for colorectal cancer in Japan began to differ according to anatomic sites in the early 1990s, when colorectal cancer screening was introduced nationwide [11]. At this time, the incidence of rectal cancer decreased, while that of distal colon cancer stabilized and that of proximal colon cancer continuously increased [11]. Because the Hong Kong government does not offer systematic population-based colorectal cancer screening programs for asymptomatic individuals in any defined age group, we speculated that the observed divergent incidence trends in colon and rectal cancers may be explained by anatomic site-specific environmental factors related to colorectal carcinogenesis. While the possibility of self-initiated screening could not be fully ruled out, it would have had limited influence on the observed incidence trends as it would only have occurred in people with relevant knowledge.

The protective role of dietary factors, such as fruit and vegetable consumption, on CRC has been identified but may be limited to colon cancer only. This is rational to some degree due to the short retention time of fruit and vegetables in the rectum. An earlier systematic review with meta-analysis reported an inverse association

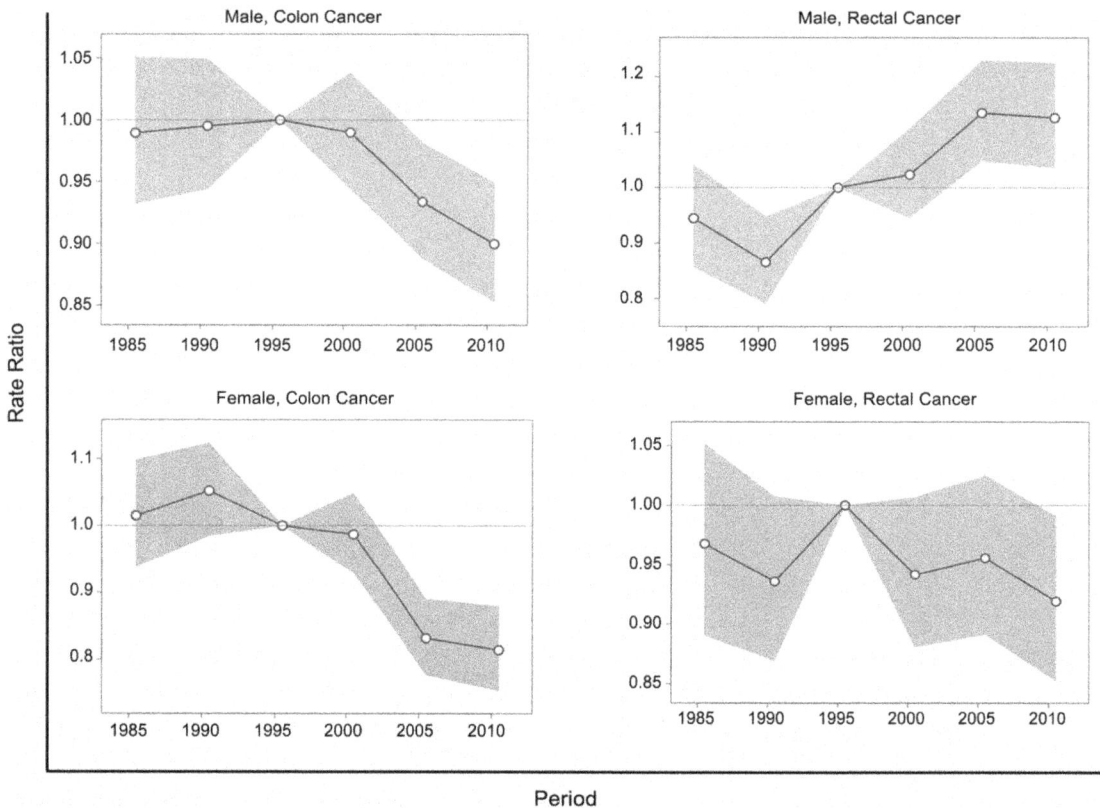

Fig. 5 Period effects on colon and rectal cancer incidence by sex. Shaded regions show the pointwise 95% confidence intervals for rate ratios

Table 2 Statistical parameters for overall and age-specific annual percent changes in age-period-cohort models

Sex	Cancer type	Net drift (% per year; 95% CI)	P value		
			All local drifts = net drift	All cohort deviations = 0	All period deviations = 0
Male	Colon	− 0.39 (− 0.66, − 0.12)	< 0.001	< 0.001	0.048
	Rectal	0.99 (0.57, 1.40)	0.562	0.636	0.018
Female	Colon	− 1.04 (− 1.46, − 0.61)	< 0.001	< 0.001	< 0.001
	Rectal	− 0.15 (− 0.54, 0.25)	0.098	0.107	0.210

between CRC risk and fruit and vegetable intake, which seemed to be restricted to colon cancer only (pooled RR for the highest versus the lowest intake level = 0.91, 95% CI 0.84–0.99) [12]. Another meta-analysis focusing on cruciferous vegetable consumption reported similar results only in terms of an inverse association between cruciferous vegetable intake and CRC risk that was restricted to colon cancer (pooled RR = 0.78, 95% CI 0.69–0.89) rather than rectal cancer (pooled RR = 0.91, 95% CI 0.74–1.13) [13]. Dietary fiber may be one explanation for the inverse association between fresh fruit and vegetable intake and colon cancer risk. Dietary fiber has

been hypothesized to reduce the risk of colorectal cancer, although it is unclear whether dietary fiber is independent from other CRC risk factors [14]. A prospective cohort study of Scandinavian populations observed a protective role of total and cereal fiber intake, particularly from cereal foods with a high fiber content, against colon cancer but not rectal cancer; a cereal fiber intake of 2 g per day was associated with a 6% reduced risk of colon cancer in men (incidence ratios = 0.94, 95% CI 0.90–0.98) and a 3% reduced risk in women (incidence ratio = 0.97, 95% CI 0.93–1.00) [15]. A case–control study nested within the European Prospective

Investigation into Cancer and Nutrition (EPIC) found an inverse association between plasma levels of alkylresorcinols, biomarkers of whole-grain rye and wheat intake [16, 17], and the risk of distal colon cancer but not rectal cancer [18]. In contrast, the protective role of fish intake against CRC seems more pronounced for rectal cancer (summary OR = 0.79, 95% CI 0.65–0.97) than for colon cancer (summary OR = 0.96, 95% CI 0.81–1.14) [19]. The decreasing age-standardized incidence of colon cancer since the 1990s may reflect the increasing intake of fresh fruit, vegetables and fish in the Hong Kong population [20]. However, this trend is contradicted by the increasing incidence of rectal cancer.

A recent systematic review and meta-analysis reported an increased risk of colon cancer associated with high red meat intake (RR = 1.22, 95% CI 1.06–1.39), but the association for rectal cancer was modestly statistically insignificant (RR = 1.13, 95% CI 0.96–1.34) [21]. How red meat intake influences CRC by anatomical sites and its potential effects on incidence trends for colon and rectal cancers require further research.

The protective effects of physical activity against colorectal cancer also differed by anatomical sites. Physical activity was inversely related to the risk of colon cancer in the proximal (RR = 0.76, 95% CI 0.70–0.83) and distal colon (RR = 0.77, 95% CI 0.71–0.83), but no such relationship could be established for the rectum (RR = 0.98, 95% CI 0.88–1.08) [22]. Due to a lack of surveillance data on physical activity among Hong Kong residents, the contribution of physical activity to the incidence trends of colon and rectal cancers could not be evaluated.

Some risk factors related to colorectal cancer showed a male predominance in either distribution (e.g., smoking and alcohol intake) or the magnitude of the association (e.g., red meat consumption), which might provide some clues to the sex- or anatomical site-specific incidence trends of colorectal cancer. Alcohol use is a well-established risk factor for CRC. A recent meta-analysis revealed a stronger association between heavy alcohol use and CRC risk in Asian populations (pooled RR = 1.81, 95% CI 1.33–2.46) than in Western populations [23], and the elevated CRC risk related to alcohol use does not seem to differ according to anatomical site [24]. A rising trend in alcohol use, in terms of both prevalence and patterns, has been noted in over the past few decades in Hong Kong [25], and this increase parallels the observed increase in the incidence of rectal cancer. However, this observation is not in line with the decreasing incidence of colon cancer over the last 2 decades. It has been suggested that cigarette smoking is associated with an increased risk of both colon cancer (current vs. never smokers, RR = 1.09, 95% CI 1.01–1.18) and rectal cancer (RR = 1.24, 95% CI 1.16–1.39) [26]. Since 1982, the Hong

Kong government has taken a progressive approach to tobacco control, raising tobacco taxes and imposing a comprehensive ban in 1999 on tobacco advertising and promotional activities [27]. Therefore, the prevalence of daily cigarette smokers aged 15 years or older decreased from 39.7% in 1982 to 19.1% in 2012 among males [28], which seems to be in line with the decreasing incidence of colon cancer in males over the last two decades. However, we cannot conclude a causal relationship between the decline in the prevalence of cigarette smoking and the decline in the age-standardized incidence of colon cancer because there should be a lag time between these two events, and the prevalence of cigarette smoking before 1980 was scarce. The prevalence of cigarette smoking is low among Hong Kong women, although an increasing trend emerged in 1990 [28]. The diverse temporal trends in the prevalence of cigarette smoking and colorectal cancer suggest that cigarette smoking does not play a major role in the etiology of colorectal cancer among Hong Kong women. The consumption of red meat has been modestly associated with an increased risk of CRC, but the positive association is limited for men. The summary RR estimates for high versus low intake of red meat among men and women were 1.21 (95% CI 1.04–1.42) and 1.01 (95% CI 0.87–1.17), respectively [29]. Therefore, the observed increasing incidence of rectal cancer in men may be, at least to some extent, attributable to the increased intake of red meat in the Hong Kong population [20].

Patients with long-standing inflammatory bowel disease (IBD), i.e., ulcerative colitis and Crohn's disease, have a 2- to 3-fold increased risk of developing colorectal cancer [30]. Although ulcerative colitis and Crohn's disease are still relatively rare, their age-adjusted prevalence in Hong Kong, increased from 0.49 to 0.05 per 100,000 in 1985–1989 to 21.14 and 14.17 per 100,000 in 2011–2014, respectively [31]. The dramatic increase in IBD cases in Hong Kong is alarming, however, both the risk factors driving the increase and the long-term consequences of these diseases, such as the risk of colorectal cancer, are unclear.

Diabetes mellitus (DM) is an independent risk factor for colon and rectal cancers with similar magnitudes of association. The association between DM and colon cancer incidence did not differ significantly by sex, but for rectal cancer, there was a significant association between DM and cancer risk for men (summary RR = 1.22, 95% CI 1.07–1.40), but not for women (summary RR = 1.09, 95% CI 0.99–1.19) [32]. The male-specific positive association between DM and rectal cancer is in line with the male-specific increase in the age-standardized incidence of rectal cancer, suggesting that DM may play an important role in etiology of male rectal cancer in Hong Kong. However, there is a lack of published data on long-term trends in the incidence of diabetes in Hong Kong, and therefore, we cannot confirm a causal relationship.

The present study has some strengths and limitations. The included data from the Hong Kong Cancer Registry were of high quality and had complete coverage. However, because proximal and distal colon cancers were not separately recorded in the Hong Kong Cancer Registry, we were unable to evaluate potential differences in incidence trends despite the increasing concerns regarding the etiological heterogeneity of cancers in these two anatomic subsites. Although we attempted to differentiate between the period and cohort effects on the observed incidence trends, all etiological explanations should be interpreted with caution because of the inherent limitations of age-period-cohort analysis, i.e., the collinearity among age, period, and cohort effects. Intuitively, period effects represent temporal variations in cancer incidence over time that affect all age groups simultaneously, and cohort effects represent differences across groups of individuals born in different eras. In our study, for colon cancer, it was difficult to distinguish between period and cohort effects because they varied in similar ways, while for rectal cancer, it seems that the period effect plays a role. However, the estimated period effects were probably a reflection of cohort effects due to the collinearity between period and cohort effects, instead of "true" period effects.

In summary, the incidences of colon and rectal cancers have changed in divergent patterns in Hong Kong between 1983 and 2012, supporting the belief that these two types of cancers have heterogeneous etiologies. The distinct changes in the epidemiology of colon and rectal cancers cannot be completely explained by current knowledge regarding the etiologies of these two types of cancers. Continuous monitoring of the incidence trends of CRC and research efforts aimed at understanding its etiology by anatomical site are warranted.

Authors' contributions
ZB, XSH and YIT conceived of the study and all participated in its design. ZB and XSH collected, analyzed and interpreted the data. All authors read and approved the final manuscript.

Author details
[1] Food Safety and Health Research Center, School of Public Health, Southern Medical University, Guangzhou 510515, Guangdong, P.R. China. [2] Department of Preventive Medicine, School of Public Health, Sun Yat-sen University, Guangzhou 510080, Guangdong, P.R. China. [3] Upper Gastrointestinal Surgery, Department of Molecular Medicine and Surgery, Karolinska Institute, Karolinska University Hospital, NS 67, 2nd Floor, 17176 Stockholm, Sweden. [4] JC School of Public Health and Primary Care, The Chinese University of Hong Kong, Hong Kong, SAR, China. [5] Hong Kong Occupational and Environmental Health Academy, Hong Kong, SAR, China.

Acknowledgements
Not applicable.

Competing interests
The authors declare that they have no competing interests.

Funding
No funding was received.

References

1. Ferlay J, Soerjomataram I, Dikshit R, et al. Cancer incidence and mortality worldwide: sources, methods and major patterns in globocan 2012. Int J Cancer. 2015;136:E359–86.
2. Center MM, Jemal A, Smith RA, et al. Worldwide variations in colorectal cancer. CA Cancer J Clin. 2009;59(6):366–78.
3. Center MM, Jemal A, Ward E. International trends in colorectal cancer incidence rates. Cancer Epidemiol Biomarkers Prev. 2009;18(6):1688–94.
4. Li FY, Lai MD. Colorectal cancer, one entity or three. J Zhejiang Univ Sci B. 2009;10(3):219–29.
5. Ji BT, Devesa SS, Chow WH, et al. Colorectal cancer incidence trends by subsite in urban shanghai, 1972–1994. Cancer Epidemiol Biomarkers Prev. 1998;7(8):661–6.
6. Wessler JD, Pashayan N, Greenberg DC, et al. Age-period-cohort analysis of colorectal cancer in east Anglia, 1971–2005. Cancer Epidemiol. 2010;34(3):232–7.
7. Siegel RL, Ward EM, Jemal A. Trends in colorectal cancer incidence rates in the united states by tumor location and stage, 1992–2008. Cancer Epidemiol Biomarkers Prev. 2012;21(3):411–6.
8. Authority H. Hospital authority: Hong kong cancer registry web site. www3.Ha.Org.Hk/cancereg/statistics.Html. Accessed July 2017.
9. Kim HJ, Fay MP, Feuer EJ, et al. Permutation tests for joinpoint regression with applications to cancer rates (correction: 2001;20:655). Stat Med. 2000;19(3):335–51.
10. Rosenberg PS, Check DP, Anderson WF. A web tool for age-period-cohort analysis of cancer incidence and mortality rates. Cancer Epidemiol Biomarkers Prev. 2014;23(11):2296–302.
11. Nakagawa H, Ito H, Hosono S, et al. Changes in trends in colorectal cancer incidence rate by anatomic site between 1978 and 2004 in Japan. Eur J Cancer Prev. 2017;26(4):269–76.
12. Aune D, Lau R, Chan DSM, et al. Nonlinear reduction in risk for colorectal cancer by fruit and vegetable intake based on meta-analysis of prospective studies. Gastroenterology. 2011;141(1):106–18.
13. Wu QJ, Yang Y, Vogtmann E, et al. Cruciferous vegetables intake and the risk of colorectal cancer: a meta-analysis of observational studies. Ann Oncol. 2013;24(4):1079–87.
14. Park Y, Hunter DJ, Spiegelman D, et al. Dietary fiber intake and risk of colorectal cancer: a pooled analysis of prospective cohort studies. JAMA. 2005;294(22):2849–57.
15. Hansen L, Skeie G, Landberg R, et al. Intake of dietary fiber, especially from cereal foods, is associated with lower incidence of colon cancer in the Helga cohort. Int J Cancer. 2012;131(2):469–78.
16. Landberg R, Kamal-Eldin A, Andersson A, et al. Alkylresorcinols as biomarkers of whole-grain wheat and rye intake: plasma concentration and intake estimated from dietary records. Am J Clin Nutr. 2008;87(4):832–8.
17. Landberg R, Aman P, Hallmans G, et al. Long-term reproducibility of plasma alkylresorcinols as biomarkers of whole-grain wheat and rye intake within northern Sweden health and disease study cohort. Eur J Clin Nutr. 2013;67(3):259–63.
18. Kyro C, Olsen A, Landberg R, et al. Plasma alkylresorcinols, biomarkers of whole-grain wheat and rye intake, and incidence of colorectal cancer. J Natl Cancer Inst. 2014;106(1):djt352.
19. Wu S, Feng B, Li K, et al. Fish consumption and colorectal cancer risk in humans: a systematic review and meta-analysis. Am J Med. 2012;125(6):551–9.
20. Koo LC, Mang OW, Ho JH. An ecological study of trends in cancer incidence and dietary changes in Hong kong. Nutr Cancer. 1997;28(3):289–301.
21. Vieira AR, Abar L, Chan DSM, et al. Foods and beverages and colorectal cancer risk: a systematic review and meta-analysis of cohort studies, an update of the evidence of the WCRF-AICR continuous update project. Ann Oncol. 2017;28(8):1788–802.

22. Robsahm TE, Aagnes B, Hjartaker A, et al. Body mass index, physical activity, and colorectal cancer by anatomical subsites: a systematic review and meta-analysis of cohort studies. Eur J Cancer Prev. 2013;22(6):492–505.

23. Fedirko V, Tramacere I, Bagnardi V, et al. Alcohol drinking and colorectal cancer risk: an overall and dose–response meta-analysis of published studies. Ann Oncol. 2011;22(9):1958–72.

24. Moskal A, Norat T, Ferrari P, et al. Alcohol intake and colorectal cancer risk: a dose–response meta-analysis of published cohort studies. Int J Cancer. 2007;120(3):664–71.

25. Yoon S, Lam TH. The alcohol industry lobby and Hong kong's zero wine and beer tax policy. BMC Public Health. 2012;12:717.

26. Cheng J, Chen Y, Wang X, et al. Meta-analysis of prospective cohort studies of cigarette smoking and the incidence of colon and rectal cancers. Eur J Cancer Prev. 2015;24(1):6–15.

27. Koplan JP, An WK, Lam RM. Hong kong: a model of successful tobacco control in China. Lancet. 2010;375(9723):1330–1.

28. Li HC, Chan SS, Lam TH. Smoking among Hong kong chinese women: behavior, attitudes and experience. BMC Public Health. 2015;15:183.

29. Alexander DD, Weed DL, Cushing CA, et al. Meta-analysis of prospective studies of red meat consumption and colorectal cancer. Eur J Cancer Prev. 2011;20(4):293–307.

30. Triantafillidis JK, Nasioulas G, Kosmidis PA. Colorectal cancer and inflammatory bowel disease: epidemiology, risk factors, mechanisms of carcinogenesis and prevention strategies. Anticancer Res. 2009;29(7):2727–37.

31. Ng SC, Leung WK, Shi HY, et al. Epidemiology of inflammatory bowel disease from 1981 to 2014: results from a territory-wide population-based registry in Hong kong. Inflamm Bowel Dis. 2016;22(8):1954–60.

32. Yuhara H, Steinmaus C, Cohen SE, et al. Is diabetes mellitus an independent risk factor for colon cancer and rectal cancer? Am J Gastroenterol. 2011;106(11):1911–21.

15

Development and validation of an endoscopic images-based deep learning model for detection with nasopharyngeal malignancies

Chaofeng Li[1,2,5,7†], Bingzhong Jing[1,2†], Liangru Ke[1,3], Bin Li[1,2], Weixiong Xia[1,4], Caisheng He[1,2], Chaonan Qian[1,4], Chong Zhao[1,4], Haiqiang Mai[1,4], Mingyuan Chen[1,4], Kajia Cao[1,4], Haoyuan Mo[1,4], Ling Guo[1,4], Qiuyan Chen[1,4], Linquan Tang[1,4], Wenze Qiu[1,4], Yahui Yu[1,4], Hu Liang[1,4], Xinjun Huang[1,4], Guoying Liu[1,4], Wangzhong Li[1,4], Lin Wang[1,4], Rui Sun[1,4], Xiong Zou[1,4], Shanshan Guo[1,4], Peiyu Huang[1,4], Donghua Luo[1,4], Fang Qiu[1,4], Yishan Wu[1,4], Yijun Hua[1,4], Kuiyuan Liu[1,4], Shuhui Lv[1,4], Jingjing Miao[1,4], Yanqun Xiang[1,4], Ying Sun[1,6], Xiang Guo[1,4,7*] and Xing Lv[1,4,7*]

Abstract

Background: Due to the occult anatomic location of the nasopharynx and frequent presence of adenoid hyperplasia, the positive rate for malignancy identification during biopsy is low, thus leading to delayed or missed diagnosis for nasopharyngeal malignancies upon initial attempt. Here, we aimed to develop an artificial intelligence tool to detect nasopharyngeal malignancies under endoscopic examination based on deep learning.

Methods: An endoscopic images-based nasopharyngeal malignancy detection model (eNPM-DM) consisting of a fully convolutional network based on the inception architecture was developed and fine-tuned using separate training and validation sets for both classification and segmentation. Briefly, a total of 28,966 qualified images were collected. Among these images, 27,536 biopsy-proven images from 7951 individuals obtained from January 1st, 2008, to December 31st, 2016, were split into the training, validation and test sets at a ratio of 7:1:2 using simple randomization. Additionally, 1430 images obtained from January 1st, 2017, to March 31st, 2017, were used as a prospective test set to compare the performance of the established model against oncologist evaluation. The dice similarity coefficient (DSC) was used to evaluate the efficiency of eNPM-DM in automatic segmentation of malignant area from the background of nasopharyngeal endoscopic images, by comparing automatic segmentation with manual segmentation performed by the experts.

Results: All images were histopathologically confirmed, and included 5713 (19.7%) normal control, 19,107 (66.0%) nasopharyngeal carcinoma (NPC), 335 (1.2%) NPC and 3811 (13.2%) benign diseases. The eNPM-DM attained an overall accuracy of 88.7% (95% confidence interval (CI) 87.8%–89.5%) in detecting malignancies in the test set. In the prospective comparison phase, eNPM-DM outperformed the experts: the overall accuracy was 88.0% (95% CI 86.1%–89.6%) vs. 80.5% (95% CI 77.0%–84.0%). The eNPM-DM required less time (40 s vs. 110.0±5.8 min) and exhibited encouraging performance in automatic segmentation of nasopharyngeal malignant area from the background, with an average DSC of 0.78±0.24 and 0.75±0.26 in the test and prospective test sets, respectively.

*Correspondence: guoxiang@sysucc.org.cn; lvxing@sysucc.org.cn
†Chaofeng Li and Bingzhong Jing contributed equally to this work
⁴ Department of Nasopharyngeal Carcinoma, Sun Yat-Sen University Cancer Center, Guangzhou 510060, P. R. China
Full list of author information is available at the end of the article

Conclusions: The eNPM-DM outperformed oncologist evaluation in diagnostic classification of nasopharyngeal mass into benign versus malignant, and realized automatic segmentation of malignant area from the background of nasopharyngeal endoscopic images.

Keywords: Nasopharyngeal malignancy, Deep learning, Differential diagnosis, Automatic segmentation

Introduction

A nasopharyngeal mass is a major sign of both malignancies and benign diseases, including nasopharyngeal carcinoma (NPC), lymphoma, melanoma, minor salivary gland tumour, fibroangioma, adenoids, and cysts. Among them, NPC accounts for 83.0% of all nasopharyngeal malignancies and 4.4% of all nasopharyngeal diseases [1, 2]. Guangdong province in southern China is a highly endemic area of NPC, with an age-standardized incidence rate of 10.38/100,000 in 2013 [3].

The majority of NPC patients are diagnosed at an advanced stage, contributing to the dismal prognosis of the disease [4]. The 10-year overall survival (OS) is 50%–70% for late stage NPC patients [4–6]. Given the rapid development of imaging techniques and radiotherapy, the local control rate of early NPC patients has increased up to 95% [7]. Thus, early detection is critical for improving the OS of NPC patients.

Non-specific symptoms and an occult anatomical location are prominent causes of delayed or missed detection of nasopharyngeal malignancies. Particularly, adenoidal hypertrophy and adenoid residue in the nasopharynx is very common in adolescents and adults, respectively. Histopathological diagnosis is the gold standard for diagnosing nasopharyngeal malignancies [8]. Currently, confirmation of NPC entails a nasopharyngeal endoscopy followed by an endoscopically directed biopsy at the site of an abnormality or sampling biopsies from an endoscopically normal nasopharynx. Clinically, NPC can coexist with adenoids or is concealed in adenoid tissues [9, 10]. In this situation, repeated biopsies of the inconspicuous lesion are required; anti-tumour treatment is delayed if a repeated biopsy is needed. Abu-Ghanem et al. reported an overall negative rate of 94.2% for malignancy among patients with suspicious nasopharyngeal malignancies [11]. Endoscopic biopsies may miss small nasopharyngeal carcinomas as they are typically submucosal or located at the lateral aspect of the pharyngeal recess, presenting a substantial diagnostic challenge in the era of NPC screening.

Driven by the high performance of computing power and the advent of massive amounts of labelled data supplemented by optimized algorithms, a machine learning technique referred to as deep learning has emerged and gradually drawn the attention of investigators [12]. In particular, deep learning has recently been shown to outperform experts in visual tasks, such as playing Atari games [13] and strategic board games, such as GO [14], object recognition [15], and biomedical image identification [16–19]. To increase the diagnostic yield in distinguishing nasopharynx abnormalities, especially malignancies, via endoscopic examination, we sought to develop tools to assist in the detection of nasopharyngeal malignancies and provide biopsy guidance using a pre-trained deep learning algorithm. Sun Yat-sen University Cancer Center is a tertiary care institution located in the highly endemic area of NPC in China and has a designated department focusing exclusively on NPC. More than 3000 newly diagnosed NPC cases are treated here every year. To take advantage of deep learning methods and abundant nasopharyngeal endoscopic images in our centre, in the current study, we developed a deep learning model to detect nasopharyngeal malignancies by applying a fully convolutional network, which we termed the endoscopic images-based nasopharyngeal malignancies detection model (eNPM-DM). We investigated the diagnostic performance of eNPM-DM versus oncologists in a training set and a test set of endoscopic images of persons who underwent routine clinical screening for nasopharyngeal malignancy. We further validated eNPM-DM in a prospective set. The current study demonstrated that eNPM-DM outperformed oncologists in nasopharyngeal malignancy detection and showed encouraging performance in malignant region segmentation. This artificial intelligence platform based on eNPM-DM could provide potential benefits, such as expanded coverage of screening programmes, higher malignancy detection, and thus lower rate of repeated biopsies.

Data and methods

Datasets of nasopharyngeal endoscopic images

We retrospectively reviewed the clinicopathologic data and nasopharyngeal endoscopic images of persons who underwent routine clinical screening for nasopharyngeal malignancy that retrospectively collected between January 1st, 2008, and December 31st, 2016 and prospectively collected between January 1st, 2017, and March 31st, 2017 at Sun Yat-sen University Cancer Center, Guangzhou, China.

The study protocol was approved by the Ethics Committee of the authors' affiliated institution. Consent to the study was not required because of the retrospective nature of the study. Patient data were anonymized. Furthermore, all images were de-identified and reorganized with randomized sequence disorganized in each dataset.

Endoscopic image acquisition

All endoscopic images were acquired from each person under local anaesthesia and mucous contraction with dicaine and ephedrine. All subjects provided written informed consent for endoscopy and biopsy before anaesthesia. Images were captured using an endoscope (Model No. Storz 1232AA, KARL STORZ-Endoskope, Tuttlingen, Germany) and endoscopy capture recorder (Model No. Storz 22201011U11O). Standard white light was used during examination and image capture.

Images of patients with pathologically proven malignancy other than NPC were considered indicative of other malignancies, including lymphoma, rhabdomyosarcoma, olfactory neuroblastoma, malignant melanoma and plasmacytoma. Images of patients with precancerous and/or atypical hyperplasia, fibroangioma, leiomyoma, meningioma, minor salivary gland tumor, fungal infection, tuberculosis, chronic inflammation, adenoids and/or lymphoid hyperplasia, nasopharyngeal cyst and foreign body were considered indicative of benign diseases. Endoscopic images were eligible for analysis if they met the following criteria: (1) an image had a resolution of a minimum of 500 pixels and 70 dpi; (2) an image had a maximum size of 300 kb; (3) an image was acquired during initial diagnosis. Eligible images were randomized to the training set, the validation set and the test set at a ratio of 7:1:2. Furthermore, 1430 additional images that were independent from the training set, the validation set and the test set were used as the prospective test set to validate the established model against oncologist evaluation.

Development and parameter tuning of the algorithm

A fully convolutional network was retrained, which could receive an input of arbitrary size and produce correspondingly sized output by deep learning [20]. The entire course of training and testing was implemented on a server with Intel® Xeon® CPU E5-2683/Memory: 128 GiB/GPU: GeForce GTX 1080 Ti. During training, we performed data augmentation as follows: rotation ± 30 degrees, shift $\pm 20\%$, shear 5%, zooming out/in 10% and channel shift 10%. The model was optimized for 100 epochs on the augmented training set with the initial learning rate at 0.001 and decreasing 0.1 time for each 40 epochs followed by best-model selection on the validation set.

Evaluation of eNPM-DM in detection and segmentation of nasopharyngeal malignancies

Experts delineated the malignant area in the images of patients with biopsy-proven malignancies in each dataset. eNPM-DM was trained to distinguish malignancies from benign diseases in the training set and output the probability map for all images in each dataset. An area with a probability greater than 0.5 in an image was considered a malignant area, and the corresponding image was considered indicative of malignancy. The performance of eNPM-DM in detecting nasopharyngeal malignancies was then assessed in the test set and the prospective test set, and compared with the performance of oncologists of different seniorities in the prospective test set. They included three experts, eight resident oncologists and three interns, with greater than 5 years, greater than 1 year, or less than 3 months of working experience at the Department of Nasopharyngeal Carcinoma of Sun Yat-sen University Cancer Center, respectively. In this evaluation, we measured the standard evaluation metrics of accuracy, sensitivity, specificity, positive predictive value (PPV), negative predictive value (NPV) and time-taken for test based on images, along with the corresponding 95% confidence interval (CI) for each metric. Specificity was defined by the percentage of truly negative images divided by all images correctly identified; sensitivity was defined by the percentage of truly positive images divided by all images correctly identified. Accuracy was defined by the proportion of images correctly identified divided by all images. PPV was defined by the percentage of truly positive images divided by all images labeled as "positive"; NPV was defined by the percentage of truly negative images divided by all images labeled as "negative". In addition, the area under curve (AUC) was calculated to assess the diagnostic efficacy of eNPM-DM in detection of nasopharyngeal malignancy using the receiver operating characteristic curve (ROC). Moreover, the combined performance of eNPM-DM and experts was assessed. An image was considered indicative of absence of malignancy if it was recognized to indicate a benign disease by either eNPM-DM or more than two experts. All analysis was performed using the Statistical Program for Social Sciences 22.0 (SPSS, Chicago, IL).

Moreover, the dice similarity coefficient (DSC) was used to evaluate the performance of eNPM-DM in automatic segmentation by measuring the overlapped ratio between expert-delineated area and eNPM-DM-defined malignant area. DSC was defined as:

$$s = \frac{2|S \cap F|}{|S| + |F|}$$

where S represents ground-truth segmentation and F stands for segmentation output.

Results

Demographic characteristics and disease categories of the study population

A total of 33,507 images were assessed for eligibility and 27,536 images from 7951 subjects were included for analysis. The study flowchart is shown in Fig. 1. In total, 5713 (19.7%) images came from histologically normal subjects, and 19,107 (66.0%), 335 (1.2%) and 3811 (13.2%) images came from patients with pathologically proven NPC, other malignancies and benign diseases, respectively. The training set included 19,576 images from 5557 patients, with 13,313 images from patients with biopsy-proven nasopharyngeal malignancies. The validation set was comprised of 2690 images, including 1771 images from patients with nasopharyngeal malignancies. The test set and prospective test set included 5270 images, with 3618 images from malignant cancer patients, and 1430 images, with 738 images from patients with malignancy, respectively. The demographic characteristics and disease categories of the study subjects in each dataset are shown in Table 1, and representative images of several types of nasopharyngeal masses are shown in Fig. 2.

Diagnostic performance of eNPM-DM

The overall accuracy of eNPM-DM for detecting malignancies in the test set was 88.7% (95% CI 87.8%–89.5%) with a sensitivity of 91.3% (95% CI 90.3%–92.2%) and a specificity of 83.1% (95% CI 81.1%–84.8%) (Table 2). We further compared the diagnostic performance of eNPM-DM with that of oncologists in nasopharyngeal malignancies in the prospective test set. eNPM-DM had an accuracy of 88.0% (95% CI 86.1%–89.6%) versus 80.5% (95% CI 77.0%–84.0%) for experts, 72.8% (95% CI 66.9%–78.6%) for residents and 66.5% (95% CI 48.0%–84.9%) for interns (Table 2). Moreover, eNPM-DM had higher specificity [85.5% (95% CI 82.7%–88.0%)] and similar sensitivity [90.2% (95% CI 87.8%–92.2%) versus experts: 70.8% (63.0%–78.6%) and 89.5% (87.4%–91.7%), respectively]. eNPM-DM also had higher PPV and NPV. eNPM-DM plus experts increased the specificity to 90.0% (95 CI 87.5%–92.1%) versus 85.5% (95% CI 82.7%–88.0%) for eNPM-DM. The AUC of eNPM-DM was 0.938 and 0.930 for nasopharyngeal malignancy in the test set and the prospective test set, respectively (Fig. 3). The training curve of eNPM-DM in nasopharyngeal malignancy detection revealed similar data loss in both the training set and the validation set, indicating no appreciable overfitting (Fig. 4) [18].

Moreover, it took eNPM-DM 40 s to render an opinion, which was considerably shorter versus experts [110.0 ± 5.8 min (95% CI 85.2–134.8)].

The performance of eNPM-DM in nasopharyngeal malignancy segmentation

Given that a high negative rate of malignancy is the most concerning issue during biopsy due to confounded adenoid/lymphoid hyperplasia in the nasopharynx, we sought to develop a deep learning-based tool for biopsy guidance for nasopharyngeal malignancies. To address that, automatic segmentation of the malignant area from the background of nasopharyngeal endoscopic images is the most important process. No malignant area was segmented for the normal nasopharynx as the original endoscopic image was recognized as non-malignant correctly by eNPM-DM (Fig. 5). In contrast, the suspicious malignant area in an image that was recognized as malignant was segmented by eNPM-DM. As noted, eNPM-DM could recognize and segment malignant areas based on the presence of a mass or mere rough surface (Fig. 5), yielding a mean DSC of 0.78 ± 0.24 and 0.75 ± 0.26 in the test set and the prospective test set, respectively.

Discussion

We developed an artificial intelligence model to assist physicians in the detection of nasopharyngeal malignancies and provide biopsy guidance by applying deep learning to nasopharyngeal endoscopy examination. We demonstrated that eNPM-DM was superior to oncological experts in detecting nasopharyngeal malignancies. Of note, eNPM-DM exhibited encouraging performance in nasopharyngeal malignancy segmentation.

Currently, the emerging field of machine learning, especially deep learning, has exerted significant impact on medical imaging. In general, deep learning algorithms recognize important features of images and properly giving weight to these features by modulating its inner parameters to make predictions for new data, thus accomplishing identification, classification or grading [21] and demonstrating strong processing ability and intact information retention [22], which is superior to previous machine learning methods [17]. Superiority of computer-aided diagnosis based on deep learning have recently been reported for a wide spectrum of diseases, including gastric cancer [23], diabetic retinopathy [16], cardiac arrhythmia [24], skin cancer [17] and colorectal polyp [25]. Notably, a wide variety of image types were explored in these studies, i.e., pathological slides [19, 23], electrocardiograms [24], radiological images [18, 26] and general pictures [17]. The deep learning method exhibited outstanding performance in most of the competitions between artificial intelligence and experts even

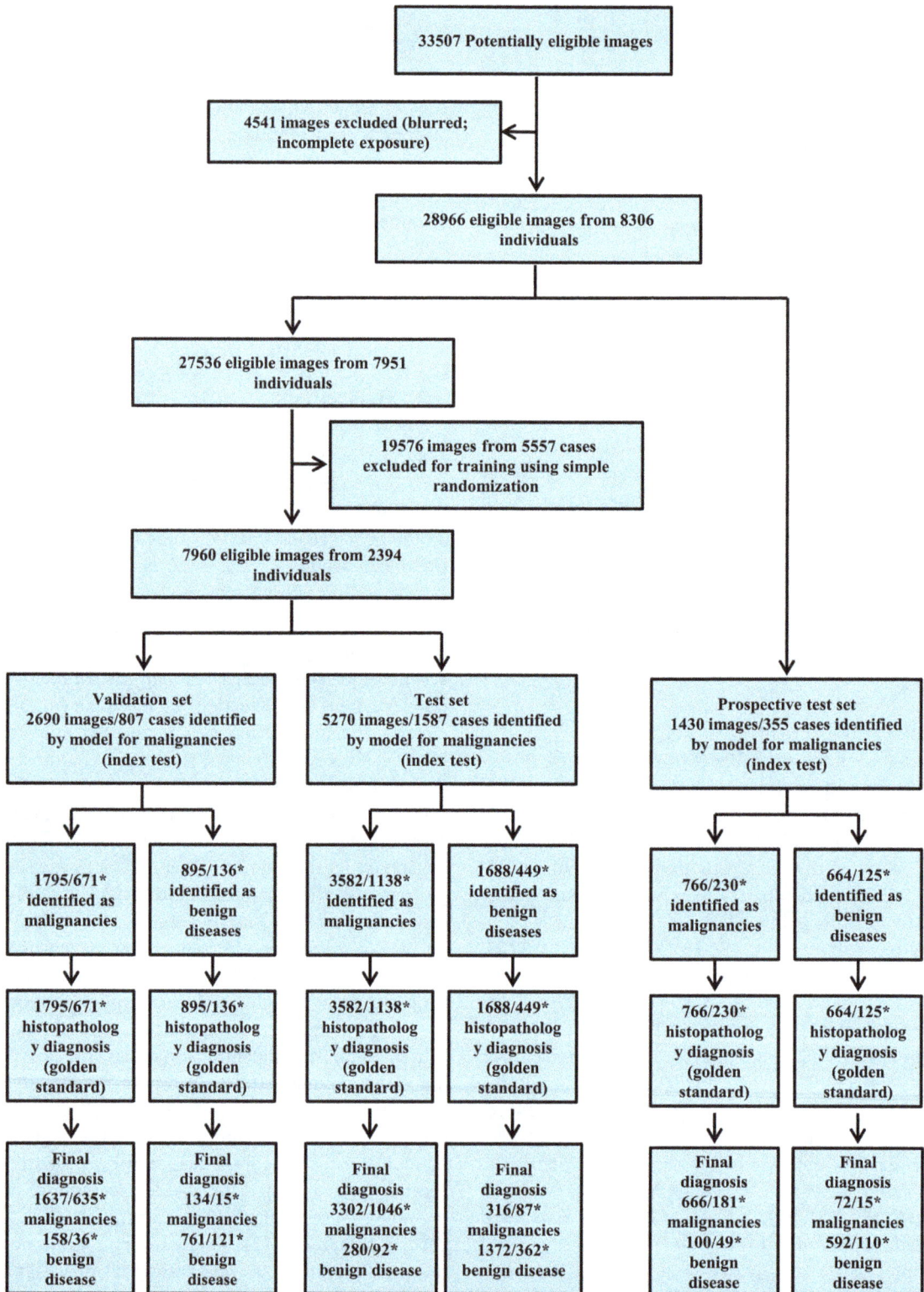

Fig. 1 The study flowchart. *The numbers of images and cases in each subset are presented

Table 1 Demographic characteristics and disease categories of the study subjects in different datasets

Characteristics	All	Training set	Validation set	Test set	Prospective test set
Subjects, n	8306	5557	807	1587	355
Mean ($\pm$ SD), years	45.9 $\pm$ 12.7	45.8 $\pm$ 12.7	45.9 $\pm$ 12.7	45.7 $\pm$ 12.7	47.8 $\pm$ 13.0
Sex, n(%)					
Female	2562 (30.9)	1681 (30.3)	250 (31.0)	507 (32.0)	124 (34.9)
Male	5612 (67.6)	3783 (68.1)	540 (66.9)	1058 (66.7)	231 (65.1)
N/A	132 (1.6)	93 (1.7)	17 (2.1)	22 (1.4)	0 (0.0)
Disease category, n(%)					
Normal	5713 (19.7)	3763 (19.2)	584 (21.7)	961 (18.2)	405 (28.3)
Malignancies					
NPC	19,107 (66.0)	13,061 (66.7)	1749 (65.0)	3564 (67.6)	731(51.1)
Others[a]	335 (1.2)	252 (1.3)	22 (0.8)	54 (1.0)	7 (0.4)
Benign diseases[b]	3811 (13.2)	2500 (12.8)	335 (12.5)	691 (13.1)	287(20.1)
Images, n(%)	28,966	19,576 (67.6)	2690 (9.3)	5270 (18.2)	1430 (4.9)

N/A not available, *NPC* nasopharyngeal carcinoma

[a] Lymphoma, rhabdomyosarcoma, olfactory neuroblastoma, malignant melanoma and plasmacytoma

[b] Precancerous/atypical hyperplasia, fibroangioma, leiomyoma, meningioma, minor salivary gland tumour, fungal infection, tuberculosis, chronic inflammation, adenoids/lymphoid hyperplasia, nasopharyngeal cyst and foreign bodies

though these medical images were captured by various types of equipment and presented in different forms, suggesting enormous potential of deep learning in auxiliary diagnoses. A well-trained algorithm for a specific disease can increase the accuracy of diagnosis and working efficiency of physicians, liberating them from repetitive tasks.

Recently, deep learning has been extensively used in the differential diagnosis of gastrointestinal disease in endoscopic images. Tomohiro et al. developed a convolutional neural network for detecting gastric cancer [27] and *Helicobacter pylori* infection based on endoscopic images [28]. Moreover, an artificial intelligence model was trained on endoscopic videos to differentiate diminutive adenomas from hyperplastic polyps, thus realizing real-time differential diagnosis [29]. Given that endoscopic examination is indispensable for biopsy and important for decision making in a clinical setting, developing tools for endoscopic auxiliary diagnosis can dramatically increase physicians' working efficiency via rapid recognition and biopsy guidance, especially in patients with multi-lesions or mixed lesions [30]. Given the illusive mass caused by adenoid/lymphoid hyperplasia, it is desirable to recognize nasopharyngeal malignancies using artificial intelligence tools. However, limited studies on deep learning methods in nasopharyngeal disease differentiation have been performed based on endoscopic images to date [31]. To this end, this study has taken advantage of the abundant resource of nasopharyngeal endoscopic images at our centre and the advanced methods to develop the targeted model.

Endoscopic examination is particularly indispensable for biopsy in participants at risk of nasopharyngeal malignancies. However, currently, no additional approaches are applied to the screening of nasopharyngeal malignancies except EBV serological test [32]. Our eNPM-DM outperformed experts in distinguishing nasopharyngeal malignancies from benign diseases using far less time with encouraging sensitivity and specificity. eNPM-DM was trained and fine-tuned on numerous images that covered patients diagnosed at our centre over 8 years and exhibited encouraging performance in a shorter learning period, suggesting that eNPM-DM 'learned' efficiently and was highly productive.

Over diagnosis is the major cause of misdiagnosis for both eNPM-DM and oncologists, suggesting that the model might learn object recognition in the same manner as a human. For example, both could distinguish different objects based on the texture, roughness, colour, size, and even vascularity on the surface of the lesion [17]. Moreover, given increased specificity eNPM-DM versus experts, eNPM-DM may also help achieve better heath economics in NPC screening [33], simultaneously improving diagnostic accuracy and screening productivity. Furthermore, the combination of eNPM-DM and experts further increased the accuracy rate and decreased the false positive rate of NPC, identifying as many cases of malignancies as possible with minimal health expenditure in NPC screening. Accordingly, the emerging deep learning could serve as a powerful assistant in clinical practice, increasing the accuracy of screening, reducing cognitive burden on

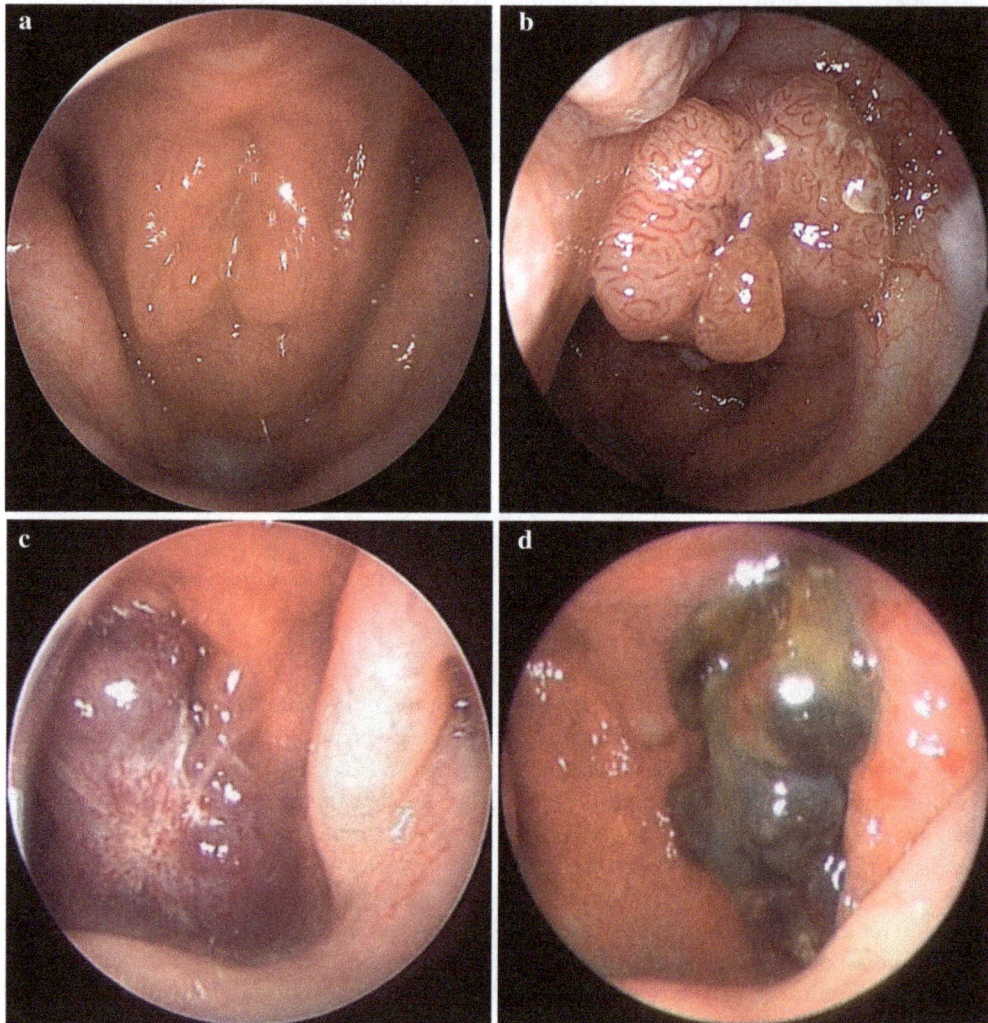

Fig. 2 Representative images of nasopharyngeal masses. **a** normal (adenoids hyperplasia); **b** Nasopharyngeal carcinoma; **c** fibroangioma; **d** malignant melanoma

Table 2 The diagnostic performance of eNPM-DM and/or oncologists in nasopharyngeal malignancy

Evaluation indicators	Test set[a]	Prospective test set[a]				eNPM-DM plus experts
	eNPM-DM		Oncologist level			
			Experts[b]	Residents[b]	Interns[b]	
Accuracy	88.7 (87.8, 89.5)	88.0 (86.1, 89.6)	80.5 ± 0.8 (77.0, 84.0)	72.8 ± 2.5 (66.9, 78.6)	66.5 ± 4.3 (48.0, 84.9)	89.0 (87.2, 90.5)
Sensitivity	91.3 (90.3, 92.2)	90.2 (87.8, 92.2)	89.5 ± 0.5 (87.4, 91.7)	88.8 ± 2.4 (83.1, 94.5)	92.2 ± 2.3 (82.1, 100.0)	87.9 (85.3, 90.2)
Specificity	83.1 (81.1, 84.8)	85.5 (82.7, 88.0)	70.8 ± 1.8 (63.0, 78.6)	55.5 ± 7.2 (38.6, 72.5)	38.9 ± 11.0 (8.5, 86.3)	90.0 (87.5, 92.1)
PPV	92.2 (91.2, 93.0)	86.9 (84.3, 89.2)	76.6 ± 1.1 (71.9, 81.3)	69.5 ± 3.1 (62.2, 76.8)	62.3 ± 3.9 (45.4, 79.2)	90.4 (87.9, 92.4)
NPV	81.3 (79.3, 83.1)	89.2 (86.5, 91.4)	86.4 ± 0.5 (84.0, 88.7)	83.2 ± 1.6 (79.4, 87.0)	82.2 ± 2.4 (71.9, 92.4)	87.5 (84.8, 90.0)
Time(min)		0.67 (~40 s)	110.0 ± 5.8 (85.2, 134.8)	99.3 ± 6.3 (84.3, 114.2)	106.7 ± 8.8 (68.7, 144.6)	

eNPM-DM endoscopic images-basednasopharyngeal malignancies detection model, *PPV* positive predictive value, *NPV* negative predictive value

[a] The numbers in parenthesis are the corresponding 95% confidence interval

[b] The performance of the oncologists is presented as mean ± standard error

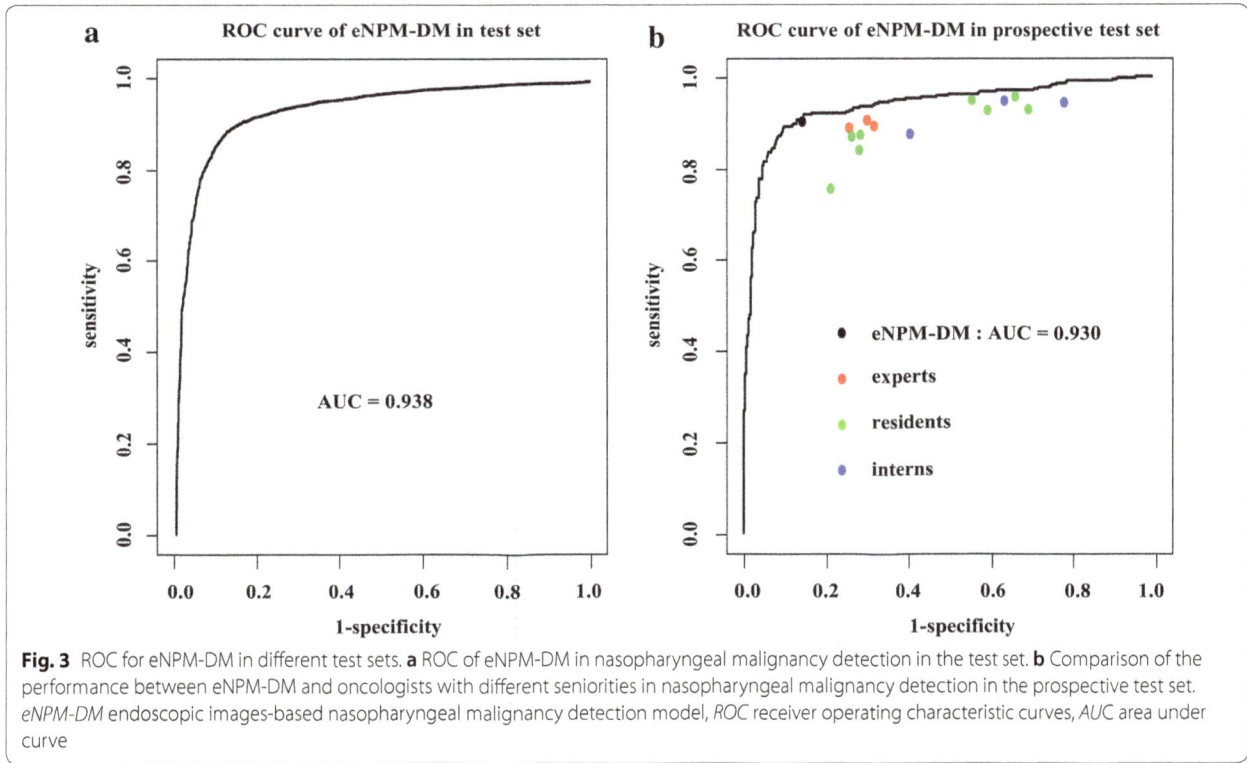

Fig. 3 ROC for eNPM-DM in different test sets. **a** ROC of eNPM-DM in nasopharyngeal malignancy detection in the test set. **b** Comparison of the performance between eNPM-DM and oncologists with different seniorities in nasopharyngeal malignancy detection in the prospective test set. *eNPM-DM* endoscopic images-based nasopharyngeal malignancy detection model, *ROC* receiver operating characteristic curves, *AUC* area under curve

clinicians, positively impacting patients' outcome and quality of life by fostering early intervention and reducing screening costs.

Additionally, our study offers a comprehensive method that is explicitly designed to develop a tool to segment nasopharyngeal malignancies in endoscopic images based on deep learning, which could be a promising biopsy guidance tool for nasopharyngeal malignancies, with the aim of increasing NPV of biopsy for malignancies. Here, eNPM-DM exhibited encouraging results in recognizing malignant areas in nasopharyngeal endoscopic images, which is consistent with the malignant lesion outlined by the experts. Accordingly, eNPM-DM could serve as a powerful biopsy guidance tool for resident oncologists or community physicians regardless of their limited experience in nasopharyngeal diseases.

To publicize our experience in nasopharyngeal malignancy detection and make full use of the advanced tool in clinical practice, we established an on-line platform (http://nasoai.sysucc.org.cn/). Both the patients and physicians may use this platform to assess the probability of malignancy in a certain image by uploading eligible nasopharyngeal endoscopic images to the artificial intelligence platform. If the lesion is recognized as malignant, the suggestive region for biopsy is provided.

There are limitations in this study. Given that all images were acquired from a single tertiary care

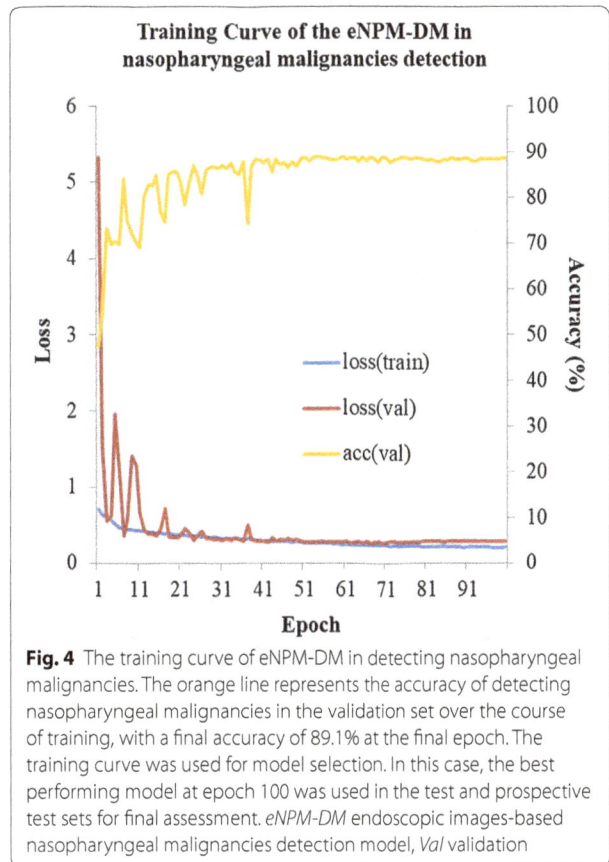

Fig. 4 The training curve of eNPM-DM in detecting nasopharyngeal malignancies. The orange line represents the accuracy of detecting nasopharyngeal malignancies in the validation set over the course of training, with a final accuracy of 89.1% at the final epoch. The training curve was used for model selection. In this case, the best performing model at epoch 100 was used in the test and prospective test sets for final assessment. *eNPM-DM* endoscopic images-based nasopharyngeal malignancies detection model, *Val* validation

centre in a highly endemic area of NPC, the diversity of nasopharyngeal diseases presented in this context might be reduced, subsequently resulting in overfitting. However, the training curve revealed that the loss of the training was similar to that of the validation, which is indicative of a well-fit curve. In addition, NPC was the most prominent malignancy in this study, which might reduce the detection efficiency for other malignancies. However, given that NPC is the most common malignancy in the nasopharynx [1, 2] and the sensitivity of eNPM-DM in detecting nasopharyngeal malignancies was 90.2%, we believe that eNPM-DM is the most powerful auxiliary diagnosis tool in nasopharyngeal malignancy detection to date.

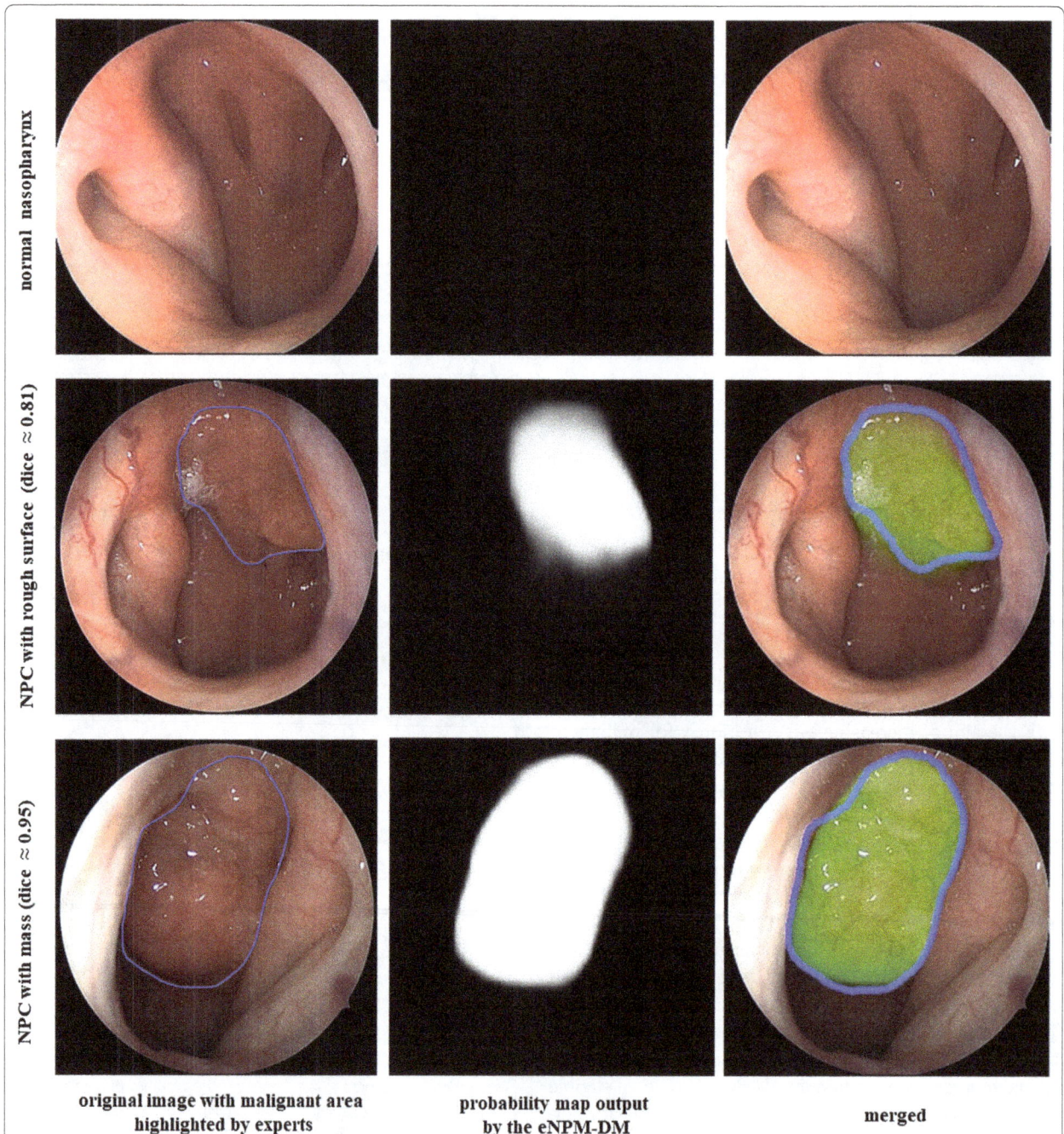

Fig. 5 Representative images of nasopharyngeal malignancies segmentation. Images from the left to the right in each row are the original endoscopic images with or without malignant area highlighted by the experts (blue), the probability map output by eNPM-DM and the merged images of the malignant area outlined by the experts (blue) and segmented by the eNPM-DM (green). *eNPM-DM* endoscopic images-based nasopharyngeal malignancy detection model, *NPC* nasopharyngeal carcinoma

One possible improvement could be a further increase in the spectrum of nasopharyngeal malignancies through collaboration with other centres in the future. Additionally, physical examination findings and laboratory test results, such as plasma antibody titters of EBV; and magnetic resonance imaging features of the nasopharynx and neck [9] can be taken into account during diagnosis in clinical practice. Therefore, integration of the endoscopic images, laboratory examination and radiologic images should be considered in nasopharyngeal malignancy detection based on deep learning. Similar to other deep leaning models, the exact features of eNPM-DM in malignancy detection remain unknown, and further investigation of detailed mechanisms is warranted. Particularly, since the model was trained on images, eNPM-DM could only render a diagnosis based on endoscopic images obtained in advance rather than real-time operation or video, and there is also a long and arduous way to combine eNPM-DM and the endoscopy system. Here, we manually selected 28,966 qualified images from numerous images and discarded the remaining images that are of poor quality or irrelevant. In future work, we plan to improve the performance of the model in image detection, identify the irrelevant images and evaluate image quality automatically. Finally, we plan to extend the developed deep learning image analysis framework to endoscopic image analysis and assessment in other types of cancers, such as gastric cancer, cervical cancer, and throat carcinoma.

Conclusion
The eNPM-DM outperformed experts in detecting nasopharyngeal malignancies. Moreover, the developed model could also conduct automatic segmentation of malignant area from the confusing background of nasopharyngeal endoscopic images efficiently, showing promising prospects in biopsy guidance for nasopharyngeal malignancies.

Abbreviations
eNPM-DM: endoscopic images-based nasopharyngeal malignancy detection model; NPC: nasopharyngeal carcinoma.

Authors' contributions
CL, XL, XG, YS, and YX designed the study. CL, BJ, BL, CH trained the model. WX, CQ, CZ, HM, MC, KC, HM, LG, QC, LT, WQ, YY, HL, XH, GL, WL, LW, RS, XZ, SG, PH, DL, FQ, YW, and YH collected the data. XG, YX, XL, WX, WQ, LK, YY, HL, XH, GL, WL, SL, KY, and JM participated in the competition. LK, BJ, and CL analysed and interpreted the data. LK, BJ, XL, CL, and YS prepared the manuscript. All authors read and approved the final manuscript.

Author details
[1] State Key Laboratory of Oncology in South China, Collaborative Innovation Center of Cancer Medicine, Guangzhou 510060, P. R. China. [2] Department of Information, Sun Yat-Sen University Cancer Center, Guangzhou 510060, P. R. China. [3] Department of Radiology, Sun Yat-Sen University Cancer Center, Guangzhou 510060, P. R. China. [4] Department of Nasopharyngeal Carcinoma, Sun Yat-Sen University Cancer Center, Guangzhou 510060, P. R. China. [5] Precision Medicine Center, Sun Yat-Sen University Cancer Center, Guangzhou 510060, P. R. China. [6] Department of Radiotherapy, Sun Yat-Sen University Cancer Center, Guangzhou 510060, P. R. China. [7] Guangdong Key Laboratory of Nasopharyngeal Carcinoma Diagnosis and Therapy, Guangzhou 510060, P. R. China.

Acknowledgements
Not applicable.

Competing interests
The authors declare that they have no competing interests.

Funding
This work was supported by the National Natural Science Foundation of China [Grant Nos. 81572665, 81672680, 81472525, 81702873]; the International Cooperation Project of Science and Technology Plan of Guangdong Province [Grant No. 2016A050502011]; the Health& Medical Collaborative Innovation Project of Guangzhou City, China (Grant No. 201604020003).

References
1. Berkiten G, Kumral TL, Yildirim G, Uyar Y, Atar Y, Salturk Z. Eight years of clinical findings and biopsy results of nasopharyngeal pathologies in 1647 adult patients: a retrospective study. B-ENT. 2014;10(4):279–84.
2. Stelow EB, Wenig BM. Update from the 4th edition of the World Health Organization classification of head and neck tumours: nasopharynx. Head Neck Pathol. 2017;11(1):16–22.
3. Wei KR, Zheng RS, Zhang SW, Liang ZH, Li ZM, Chen WQ. Nasopharyngeal carcinoma incidence and mortality in China, 2013. Chin J Cancer. 2017;36(1):90.
4. Liang H, Xiang YQ, Lv X, Xie CQ, Cao SM, Wang L, et al. Survival impact of waiting time for radical radiotherapy in nasopharyngeal carcinoma: a large institution-based cohort study from an endemic area. Eur J Cancer. 2017;73:48–60.
5. Yi JL, Gao L, Huang XD, Li SY, Luo JW, Cai WM, et al. Nasopharyngeal carcinoma treated by radical radiotherapy alone: ten-year experience of a single institution. Int J Radiat Oncol Biol Phys. 2006;65(1):161–8.
6. Su SF, Han F, Zhao C, Huang Y, Chen CY, Xiao WW, et al. Treatment outcomes for different subgroups of nasopharyngeal carcinoma patients treated with intensity-modulated radiation therapy. Chin J Cancer. 2011;30(8):565–73.
7. Lee N, Harris J, Garden AS, Straube W, Glisson B, Xia P, et al. Intensity-modulated radiation therapy with or without chemotherapy for nasopharyngeal carcinoma: radiation therapy oncology group phase II trial 0225. J Clin Oncol. 2009;27(22):3684–90.
8. Chan AT, Felip E. Nasopharyngeal cancer: ESMO clinical recommendations for diagnosis, treatment and follow-up. Ann Oncol. 2009;20(Suppl 4):123–5.
9. Cengiz K, Kumral TL, Yildirim G. Diagnosis of pediatric nasopharynx carcinoma after recurrent adenoidectomy. Case Rep Otolaryngol. 2013;2013:653963.
10. Wu YP, Cai PQ, Tian L, Xu JH, Mitteer RJ, Fan Y, et al. Hypertrophic adenoids in patients with nasopharyngeal carcinoma: appearance at magnetic resonance imaging before and after treatment. Chin J Cancer. 2015;34(3):130–6.
11. Abu-Ghanem S, Carmel NN, Horowitz G, Yehuda M, Leshno M, Abu-Ghanem Y, et al. Nasopharyngeal biopsy in adults: a large-scale study in a non endemic area. Rhinology. 2015;53(2):142–8.
12. Miotto R, Wang F, Wang S, Jiang X, Dudley JT. Deep learning for healthcare: review, opportunities and challenges. Brief Bioinform 2017.
13. Mnih V, Kavukcuoglu K, Silver D, Rusu AA, Veness J, Bellemare MG, et al. Human-level control through deep reinforcement learning. Nature. 2015;518(7540):529–33.
14. Silver D, Huang A, Maddison CJ, Guez A, Sifre L, van den Driessche G, et al. Mastering the game of Go with deep neural networks and tree search. Nature. 2016;529(7587):484–9.

15. Russakovsky O, Deng J, Su H, Krause J, Satheesh S, Ma S, et al. ImageNet large scale visual recognition challenge. Int J Comput Vision. 2015;115(3):211–52.

16. Gulshan V, Peng L, Coram M, Stumpe MC, Wu D, Narayanaswamy A, et al. Development and validation of a deep learning algorithm for detection of diabetic retinopathy in retinal fundus photographs. JAMA. 2016;316(22):2402–10.

17. Esteva A, Kuprel B, Novoa RA, Ko J, Swetter SM, Blau HM, et al. Dermatologist-level classification of skin cancer with deep neural networks. Nature. 2017;542(7639):115–8.

18. Lakhani P, Sundaram B. Deep learning at chest radiography: automated classification of pulmonary tuberculosis by using convolutional neural networks. Radiology. 2017;284(2):574–82.

19. Ertosun MG, Rubin DL. Automated grading of gliomas using deep learning in digital pathology images: a modular approach with ensemble of convolutional neural networks. AMIA Annu Symp Proc. 2015;2015:1899–908.

20. Shelhamer E, Long J, Darrell T. Fully convolutional networks for semantic segmentation. IEEE Trans Pattern Anal Mach Intell. 2017;39(4):640–51.

21. Korbar B, Olofson AM, Miraflor AP, Nicka CM, Suriawinata MA, Torresani L, et al. Deep learning for classification of colorectal polyps on whole-slide images. J Pathol Inf. 2017;8:30.

22. Suzuki K. Overview of deep learning in medical imaging. Radiol Phys Technol. 2017;10(3):257–73.

23. Sharma H, Zerbe N, Klempert I, Hellwich O, Hufnagl P. Deep convolutional neural networks for automatic classification of gastric carcinoma using whole slide images in digital histopathology. Comput Med Imaging Graph. 2017;61:2–13.

24. Schirrmeister RT, Springenberg JT, Fiederer L, Glasstetter M, Eggensperger K, Tangermann M, et al. Deep learning with convolutional neural networks for EEG decoding and visualization. Hum Brain Mapp. 2017;38:5391–420.

25. Komeda Y, Handa H, Watanabe T, Nomura T, Kitahashi M, Sakurai T, et al. Computer-aided diagnosis based on convolutional neural network system for colorectal polyp classification: preliminary experience. Oncology. 2017;93(Suppl 1):30–4.

26. van der Burgh HK, Schmidt R, Westeneng HJ, de Reus MA, van den Berg LH, van den Heuvel MP. Deep learning predictions of survival based on MRI in amyotrophic lateral sclerosis. Neuroimage Clin. 2017;13:361–9.

27. Hirasawa T, Aoyama K, Tanimoto T, Ishihara S, Shichijo S, Ozawa T, et al. Application of artificial intelligence using a convolutional neural network for detecting gastric cancer in endoscopic images. Gastric Cancer. 2018;21:653–60.

28. Shichijo S, Nomura S, Aoyama K, Nishikawa Y, Miura M, Shinagawa T, et al. application of convolutional neural networks in the diagnosis of helicobacter pylori infection based on endoscopic images. EBioMedicine. 2017;25:106–11.

29. Byrne MF, Chapados N, Soudan F, Oertel C, Linares PM, Kelly R, et al. Real-time differentiation of adenomatous and hyperplastic diminutive colorectal polyps during analysis of unaltered videos of standard colonoscopy using a deep learning model. Gut. 2017. https://doi.org/10.1136/gutjnl-2017-314547.

30. Mori H, Nishiyama N, Kobara H, Fujihara S, Kobayashi N, Nagase T, et al. The use of a detachable multiple polyp catcher to facilitate accurate location and pathological diagnosis of resected polyps in the proximal colon. Gastrointest Endosc. 2016;83(1):262–3.

31. Ribeiro E, Uhl A, Wimmer G, Hafner M. Exploring deep learning and transfer learning for colonic polyp classification. Comput Math Methods Med. 2016;2016:6584725.

32. Chan KC. Plasma Epstein-Barr virus DNA as a biomarker for nasopharyngeal carcinoma. Chin J Cancer. 2014;33(12):598–603.

33. Meng R, Wei K, Xia L, Xu Y, Chen W, Zheng R, et al. Cancer incidence and mortality in Guangdong province, 2012. Chin J Cancer Res. 2016;28(3):311–20.

16

DDIT4 promotes gastric cancer proliferation and tumorigenesis through the p53 and MAPK pathways

Feng Du[†], Lina Sun[†], Yi Chu[†], Tingyu Li, Chao Lei, Xin Wang, Mingzuo Jiang, Yali Min, Yuanyuan Lu[*], Xiaodi Zhao[*], Yongzhan Nie and Daiming Fan[*]

Abstract

Background: Gastric cancer (GC) is one of the most common malignancies worldwide, particularly in China. DNA damage-inducible transcript 4 (DDIT4) is a mammalian target of rapamycin inhibitor and is induced by various cellular stresses; however, its critical role in GC remains poorly understood. The present study aimed to investigate the potential relationship and the underlying mechanism between DDIT4 and GC development.

Methods: We used western blotting, real-time polymerase chain reaction, and immunohistochemical or immunofluorescence to determine DDIT4 expression in GC cells and tissues. High-content screening, cell counting kit-8 assays, colony formation, and in vivo tumorigenesis assays were performed to evaluate cell proliferation. Flow cytometry was used to investigate cell apoptosis and cell cycle distribution.

Results: DDIT4 was upregulated in GC cells and tissue. Furthermore, downregulating DDIT4 in GC cells inhibited proliferation both in vitro and in vivo and increased 5-fluorouracil-induced apoptosis and cell cycle arrest. In contrast, ectopic expression of DDIT4 in normal gastric epithelial cells promoted proliferation and attenuated chemosensitivity. Further analysis indicated that the mitogen-activated protein kinase and p53 signaling pathways were involved in the suppression of proliferation, and increased chemosensitivity upon DDIT4 downregulation.

Conclusion: DDIT4 promotes GC proliferation and tumorigenesis, providing new insights into the role of DDIT4 in the tumorigenesis of human GC.

Keywords: DNA damage-inducible transcript 4, Gastric cancer, Proliferation, Mitogen-activated protein kinase, p53

Background

Gastric cancer (GC) is one of the most common malignancies worldwide and remains the second leading cause of cancer-related death in China [1]. Despite the declining incidence of GC, the 5-year overall survival rate remains low at less than 30% [2]. Two of the major causes of the poor prognosis of GC are metastasis and multiple drug resistance, which greatly hamper the success of treatment modalities [1]. Genetic alterations are generally considered to drive cancer development and progression, and emerging evidence indicates that the complex molecular heterogeneity of GC underlies most, if not all, of the general ineffectiveness of current chemotherapeutics for GC [3]. Hence, improvements in the treatment of GC must be developed from a better understanding of its elaborate regulatory network because the underlying molecular mechanisms of GC tumorigenesis remain unclear.

DNA damage-inducible transcript 4 (DDIT4), also known as DNA damage response 1 (REDD1) and stress-triggered protein (RTP801), is induced by a variety of stress conditions, including oxidative stress, endoplasmic reticulum stress, hypoxia, and starvation [4]. DDIT4 protein inhibits mammalian target of rapamycin complex 1

*Correspondence: luyuandreamer@aliyun.com; leedyzhao@fmmu.edu.cn; daimingfan@fmmu.edu.cn
[†]Feng Du, Lina Sun and Yi Chu contributed equally to this work
State Key Laboratory of Cancer Biology, National Clinical Research Center for Digestive Diseases and Xijing Hospital of Digestive Diseases, Fourth Military Medical University, 127 Chang Le West Road, Xi'an 710032, China

(mTORC1) by stabilizing the tuberous sclerosis complex (TSC1–TSC2) [5]. Over the past decades, DDIT4 dysregulation has been observed in numerous human malignancies. In prostate cancer (PC) cells, DDIT4 enhances CCAAT/enhancer-binding protein beta (C/EBPbeta)-mediated autophagosome-lysosome fusion and desensitizes the cells to bortezomib [6]. Additionally, baicalein upregulates DDIT4 and inhibits mTORC1 and the proliferation of platinum-resistant cancer cells, indicating that DDIT4 expression has potential as a chemotherapeutic and chemoprevention agent [7]. Although mammalian target of rapamycin (mTOR) pathway inhibition is a current strategy for the treatment of cancer [8, 9], paradoxically, several in vitro and in vivo studies indicate that DDIT4 has a protective role against apoptosis [10–12]; *DDIT4* knockdown increases dexamethasone-induced cell death in murine lymphocytes [10]. Additionally, DDIT4 expression was significantly increased in serous adenocarcinoma compared with other histological types, and this increase was positively associated with ascites formation and late-stage disease in ovarian cancer (OC) [11]. A recent in silico evaluation of the online datasets Kaplan–Meier plotter and SurvExpress indicated that high DDIT4 levels were significantly associated with a worse prognosis in acute myeloid leukemia, glioblastoma multiforme, and breast, colon, skin and lung cancer [12]. However, in GC, the second most common type of cancer in Asia in terms of incidence and cancer mortality, the clinical significance and biological role of DDIT4 remain to be elucidated.

In the present study, we examined DDIT4 expression levels in GC tissue samples and cell lines, and investigated the role of DDIT4 and the mechanism by which it is dysregulated in gastric cancer.

Methods

Cell culture and tissue collection

The human GC cell lines SGC7901, BGC823, MKN45, and AGS, and the immortalized gastric epithelial cell line GES were purchased from the Cell Resource Center of the Chinese Academy of Sciences, Shanghai, China. Cells were maintained in Dulbecco's Modified Eagle's Medium (Thermo Scientific HyClone, Beijing, China) supplemented with 10% fetal bovine serum (HyClone), 100 U/mL penicillin, and 100 U/mL streptomycin (HyClone) in a 37 °C humidified incubator with a mixture of 95% air and 5% CO_2.

A total of 20 fresh primary GC samples and matched adjacent non-cancerous tissues were obtained from patients undergoing surgery at Xijing Hospital, Xi'an, China. All samples were confirmed by the Department of Pathology at Xijing Hospital and stored in a liquid nitrogen canister. All patients provided informed consent for excess specimens to be used for research purposes and all protocols employed in the present study were approved by the Medical Ethics Committee of Xijing Hospital.

Mice

Female BALB/c nude mice were provided by the Experimental Animal Center of the Fourth Military Medical University and were housed in pathogen-free conditions. All animal studies complied with the Fourth Military Medical University animal use guidelines, and the protocol was approved by the Fourth Military University Animal Care Committee.

Reagent and inhibitor

5-Fluorouracil was purchased from Sigma (Sigma-Aldrich Corporation, Los Angeles, CA, USA), and MAPK/ERK inhibitor (PD98059) and p53 inhibitor (A15201) were purchased from Invitrogen (Thermo Fisher Scientific, Cambridge, Massachusetts, USA); all were stored according to the manufacturer's instructions.

RNA extraction and real-time polymerase chain reaction (PCR)

Total RNA was extracted from cell lines using the RNeasy Plus Universal Tissue Mini Kit (Qiagen, Hilden, Germany) according to the manufacturer's instructions. The PCR primers for *DDIT4* and *ACTB* were synthesized by TaKaRa (Dalian, China). The sequences were as follows: *DDIT4*, 5′-GGACCAAGTGTGTTTGTTGTTTG-3′ (Forward) and 5′-CACCCACCCCTT CCTACTCTT-3′ (Reverse); *ACTB*, 5′-TCATGAAGTGTGACGTTGACA TCCGT- 3′ (Forward) and 5′-CCTAGAAGCATTTGC GGTGCACGATG-3′ (Reverse). cDNA was synthesized using the PrimeScript RT Reagent Kit (TaKaRa, Dalian, China). Real-time PCR was performed using SYBR Premix Ex Taq II (TaKaRa). Fluorescence was measured using a LightCycler 480 system (Roche, Basel, Switzerland). *ACTB* was used as an internal control for mRNA analysis. Each sample was run in triplicate.

Protein extraction and western blotting

Total proteins were prepared from fresh frozen tissue or cultured cells in radio immunoprecipitation assay (RIPA) lysis and extraction buffer (Beyotime Biotechnology, Shanghai, China) with protease and phosphatase inhibitors. Denatured proteins (20–50 mg) were separated by sodium dodecyl sulfate–polyacrylamide gel electrophoresis and transferred to polyvinylidene difluoride membranes. The following primary antibodies were used according to the manufacturer's instructions: anti-DDIT4 (Dilution 1:500, Abcam, Cambridge, MA, USA) and anti-β-actin (Dilution 1:2000), anti-Ki67 (Dilution 1:1000), anti-p53 (Dilution 1:1000), anti-p-p53 (p-Ser6) (Dilution

1:1000), anti-p-p53 (p-Ser315) (Dilution 1:1000), anti-p21^{Cip1} (Dilution 1:500), anti-p-p21^{Cip1} (p-Thr145) (Dilution 1:500), anti-MEK1 (Dilution 1:1000), anti-p-MEK1 (p-Ser221) (Dilution 1:1000), anti-p42/44MAPK (Dilution 1:1000), and anti-p-p42/44MAPK (p-Thr202 and p-Tyr204) (Dilution 1:1000) (Cell Signaling Technology, Beverly, MA, USA). Densitometry of specific blotted bands was analyzed by ImageJ 1.48 software (Image-Processing and Analysis in Java; National Institutes of Health, Bethesda, MD, USA; http://imagej.nih.gov/), and the intensity values were normalized against the β-actin loading control.

Tissue microarray immunohistochemistry

GC tissue microarrays were purchased from Superchip (Shanghai, China). Each array contained 90 cases of paired adjacent gastric tissues and primary GC tissues. Immunohistochemical (IHC) staining was performed using anti-DDIT4 and anti-Ki67 antibodies as per the manufacturer's instructions. IHC results were scored independently by two pathologists in a blinded manner. The scoring was based on the intensity and extent of staining. Staining intensity was graded as follows: 0, negative staining; 1, weak staining; 2, moderate staining; and 3, strong staining. The proportion of stained cells per specimen was determined semi-quantitatively as follows: 0, < 1%; 1, 1–25%; 2, 26–50%; 3, 51–75%; and 4, > 75%. The histological score (H-score) for each specimen was computed using the following formula: H-score = proportion score × intensity score. The samples were further characterized by H-score as negative (−, score: 0), weak (+, score: 1–4), moderate (++, score: 5–8), and strong (+++, score: 9–12). Samples with an H-score of > 4 were considered to exhibit high expression, and samples with an H-score of ≤ 4 were considered to exhibit low expression.

Immunofluorescence staining

Cells were plated onto glass coverslips, fixed with 4% paraformaldehyde for 20 min and permeabilized with 0.1% Triton X-100 in PBS for 15 min. Blocking solution was applied at room temperature for 1 h. Rabbit anti-human DDIT4 primary antibody (Abcam) was applied at 4 °C overnight. FITC-conjugated goat anti-rabbit and Cy3-conjugated goat anti-mouse secondary antibodies were incubated on the coverslips at room temperature for 2 h. Immunostaining signals and DAPI-stained nuclei were visualized at room temperature using a confocal microscope (FV10i; Olympus, Tokyo, Japan) equipped with a 10×/0.30 numerical aperture objective lens (Olympus) and Fluoview software (version 4.3; Olympus). No imaging medium was used. For better visualization, the images were adjusted using the level and brightness/

contrast tools in Photoshop according to the guidelines for the presentation of digital data.

Lentivirus infection

DDIT4-overexpression or sh-DDIT4 lentivirus infection was conducted by GeneChem (Shanghai, China). Target cells (1×10^5) were infected with 1×10^7 lentivirus-transducing units in the presence of 5 mg/mL polybrene. An empty lentiviral vector was used as a negative control. After transfection and antibiotic selection for 6 weeks, cells were collected for further investigation.

High-content screening assay

Cells transfected with lentivirus stably expressing green fluorescent protein (GFP) were seeded into 96-well plates and treated with increasing doses of 5-FU (0, 10, 20 μg/mL for GC cells or 0, 2, 4 μg/mL for GES cells). Cells were imaged every 4 h for 48 h using the Thermo Scientific CellInsight CX7 High Content Analysis Platform (0, 10, 20 μg/mL for GC cells or 0, 2, 4 μg/mL for GES cells; Thermo Fisher Scientific, Cambridge, Massachusetts, USA). Proliferation curves were plotted and analyzed using HCS Studio Software (Thermo Fisher Scientific).

Colony formation assays

Transfected cells were seeded in six-well plates (1000 cells/well). After 14–18 days of incubation to establish stable clones, cells were fixed with 70% ethanol and stained with crystal violet solution. Colonies containing greater than 50 cells were counted. The experiment was conducted with three independent triplicates.

Cell cycle and apoptosis assays

For cell cycle analysis, target cells were selected with antibiotics (penicillin–streptomycin solution) for 48 h after transfection as indicated, fixed in 75% ethanol, and stained with propidium iodide supplemented with RNase A (Roche, Mannheim, Germany) for 30 min at 22 °C. The Annexin V-FITC Apoptosis Detection Kit (Cell Signaling Technology, Beverly, MA, USA) was used for apoptosis assays. Cells (1×10^4) were stained according to the manufacturer's protocol and sorted using a fluorescence-activated cell sorting sorter (BD Biosciences, La Jolla, CA, USA). Data were analyzed using ModFit software (BD Biosciences).

In vivo tumorigenicity

BGC823 cells (5×10^5 cells in 0.2 mL of PBS) transfected with pCMV-DDIT4 or empty pCMV were injected subcutaneously into the dorsal flank of 5-week-old female Balb/c nude mice (five mice per group). Tumor diameter was measured every 3 days for 30 days. Tumor volume (mm^3) was calculated based on the longest and shortest diameters as follows: volume = (shortest diameter)^2 × (longest diameter) × 0.5. Thirty days after injection, all mice were killed, and the tumor xenografts were isolated for further analysis. All experimental animals were supplied by the Experimental Animal Center of the Fourth Military Medical University. All protocols for animal studies were approved by the Fourth Military Medical University Animal Care Committee.

Cell counting kit-8 (CCK8) assay

For cell counting kit 8 assays, cells were seeded into 96-well plates at a density of 1000 cells in 100 μL of complete culture medium per well. At the indicated time points, the medium was replaced with a kit solution (TransDetect cell counting kit, Transgene, Beijing, China) and complete culture medium at a ratio of 1:9, and the samples were incubated for 2 h at 37 °C. The absorbance of each sample was analyzed at 450 nm using a microtiter plate reader (Tecan, Switzerland). The assay was repeated in triplicate.

Phospho-specific protein microarray analysis

Phospho-array detection was performed in cooperation with Wayen Biotechnology (Shanghai, China). At 48 h post-transfection, all treated cells were collected for protein extraction. Protein samples of 50 mg each were tagged with biotin reagent and hybridized on a Phosphorylation ProArray (Full Moon BioSystems, USA) using an Antibody Array Kit (FullMoon BioSystems, USA) for the detection of 248 site-specific cancer signaling phospho-antibody profiles. Finally, fluorescence intensity was scanned by GenePix 4000B (Axon Instruments, Houston, USA) using GenePix Pro 6.0. The raw data were manipulated using Grubbs' method. The phosphorylation ratio was calculated as follows: phosphorylation ratio ¼ phospho value/unphospho value.

Statistical analyses

SPSS software (version 19.0, SPSS Inc., Chicago, IL, USA) was used for statistical analyses. Continuous data are presented as the mean ± standard deviation (SD), and Student's unpaired t-test was utilized for comparisons between two groups. Frequencies of categorical variables were compared using the χ^2 test. A P value of less than 0.05 was considered significant.

Results

DDIT4 was upregulated in GC tissues

To determine the expression pattern of DDIT4 in GC, we measured DDIT4 expression in 20 pairs of GC and adjacent normal tissue specimens using real-time PCR and western blotting. DDIT4 expression was upregulated in 13 of 20 GC tissues compared with matched adjacent normal tissues (Fig. 1a). Similar to DDIT4 mRNA levels, DDIT4 protein levels were increased in GC samples compared with their normal counterparts (Fig. 1b). Furthermore, we performed IHC using a GC tissue microarray containing 90 pairs of primary GC tissues and paired adjacent normal tissues. The IHC analysis revealed clear elevation of DDIT4 levels in GC tissues compared with the corresponding normal tissues, and DDIT4 expression was primarily located in the cytoplasm (Fig. 1c, d). Univariate survival analysis demonstrated that tumor size ($P = 0.013$), invasion depth ($P = 0.015$), lymphatic metastasis ($P = 0.018$), distant metastasis ($P < 0.001$), AJCC stage ($P < 0.001$), and pathological grade ($P < 0.001$) exhibit statistically significant associations with GC patient survival (Table 1). Taken together, DDIT4 expression was increased in GC tissues.

Increased DDIT4 in GC cells promotes proliferation and colony formation

To validate the expression pattern of DDIT4, we detected DDIT4 protein and mRNA levels in four GC cell lines (MKN45, AGS, SGC7901, and BGC823) and an immortalized gastric epithelial cell line, GES. Similar to the GC tissues, DDIT4 levels were significantly increased at both the protein and mRNA level in GC cells compared with GES cells (Fig. 2a, b). Moreover, immunofluorescence revealed that DDIT4 was mainly localized to the cytoplasm (Fig. 2c). To analyze biological function, we silenced DDIT4 in SGC7901 and BGC823 cells with a lentiviral vector and upregulated DDIT4 levels in GES cells using a DDIT4-overexpressing lentiviral vector. After cell transfection and antibiotic screening for 6 weeks, the lentiviral transfection efficiency was confirmed by real-time PCR and western blotting. Among three shDDIT4 vectors, shDDIT4-2 was the most effective at silencing DDIT4 in SGC7901 and BGC823 cells (Fig. 2d, e). In contrast, transfection of the DDIT4-overexpressing lentiviral vector significantly upregulated DDIT4 levels in GES cells (Fig. 2f). Therefore, shDDIT4-2 and the DDIT4-overexpressing lentiviral vector were employed in the subsequent experiments.

Given that DDIT4 has been implicated in oncogene- and stress-induced DNA damage [4], we hypothesized that DDIT4 upregulation might be involved in the initiation and development of GC. To test this hypothesis, we conducted high-content screening assays and colony formation assays to determine whether DDIT4 regulates GC cell proliferation. The high-content screening assays revealed that cell proliferation was significantly inhibited by DDIT4 silencing in SGC7901 cells compared with the lentiviral control (Fig. 3a). Given that chemotherapeutics cause cytotoxic effects and DNA damage, we assessed whether DDIT4 was involved in the response of GC cells to these agents.

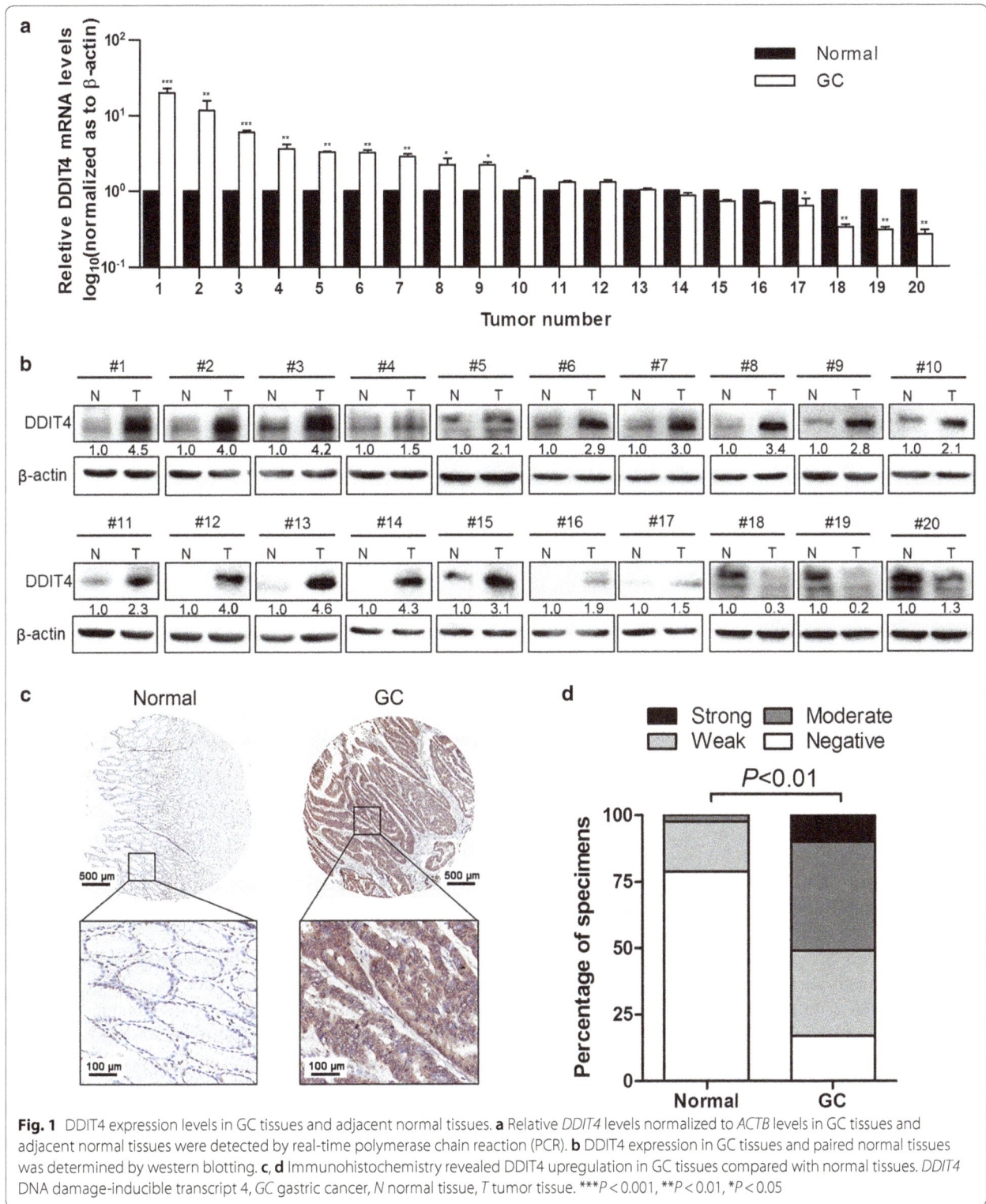

Fig. 1 DDIT4 expression levels in GC tissues and adjacent normal tissues. **a** Relative *DDIT4* levels normalized to *ACTB* levels in GC tissues and adjacent normal tissues were detected by real-time polymerase chain reaction (PCR). **b** DDIT4 expression in GC tissues and paired normal tissues was determined by western blotting. **c, d** Immunohistochemistry revealed DDIT4 upregulation in GC tissues compared with normal tissues. *DDIT4* DNA damage-inducible transcript 4, *GC* gastric cancer, *N* normal tissue, *T* tumor tissue. ***P < 0.001, **P < 0.01, *P < 0.05

Thus, we monitored SGC7901 cell proliferation after treatment with 5-FU (10 or 20 μg/mL) and found that *DDIT4* downregulation suppressed proliferation in the presence of 5-FU (Fig. 3b, c). Consistently, colony formation assays revealed that *DDIT4* downregulation inhibited SGC7901 colony formation with or without 5-FU (Fig. 3d). Similar

Table 1 Univariate and multivariate survival analysis of 90 GC patients

Variable	Univariate log rank survival analysis			Multivariate Cox survival analysis		
	RR	95% CI	P value	RR	95% CI	P value
Age (years)						
< 60	1.000					
≥ 60	1.085	0.832–1.413	0.547			
Gender						
Male	1.000					
Female	1.091	0.797–1.494	0.588			
Tumor size (cm)						
< 5	1.000					
≥ 5	1.182	1.036–1.349	0.013	1.387	0.827–2.325	0.215
Invasion depth						
T1/2	1.000					
T3/4	1.610	1.098–2.360	0.015	1.496	0.696–3.216	0.302
Lymphatic metastasis						
N0	1.000					
N1–3	1.369	1.056–1.774	0.018	1.093	0.456–2.621	0.842
Distant metastasis						
M0	1.000					
M1	1.468	1.268–1.299	< 0.001	4.364	1.830–10.409	0.001
AJCC stage						
I/II	1.000					
III/IV	1.500	1.214–1.853	< 0.001	1.755	0.768–4.011	0.183
Pathological grade						
I/II	1.000					
III/IV	1.912	1.125–3.250	0.017	2.077	0.863–4.996	0.103
DDIT4 expression						
Low	1.000					
High	3.583	2.345–4.271	0.146			

RR risk ratio, *95% CI* 95% confidence interval, *AJCC* American Joint Committee on Cancer

to SGC7901 cells, *DDIT4* downregulation in BGC823 cells reduced cell proliferation (Fig. 3e–g) and increased sensitivity to 5-FU (Fig. 3h). In contrast, ectopic expression of *DDIT4* promoted GES cell proliferation and colony formation (Fig. 3i, l) and attenuated the sensitivity of GES cells to 5-FU (Fig. 3j–l). In addition, we performed Transwell assays to determine whether DDIT4 regulates GC cell migration and invasion, but no significant difference was observed in cells transfected with shDDIT4 lentivirus compared with the control group (Additional file 1: Figure S1). Taken together, these observations indicated that *DDIT4* acts as an oncogene that promotes GC cell proliferation and reduces chemosensitivity.

Downregulation of *DDIT4* increases 5-FU-induced apoptosis but decreases 5-FU-induced S phase arrest in GC cells

Beneath the complexity and idiopathy of cancer lies a limited number of critical events that propel the tumor cell and its progeny into uncontrolled expansion and invasion [13]. Two such events are deregulation of apoptosis and the cell cycle, which together with the obligatory compensatory dysregulation of proliferation provide a minimal "platform" necessary to support further neoplastic progression [13]. Thus, we performed flow cytometry to determine whether DDIT4 modulates apoptosis and the cell cycle, which contribute to gastric carcinogenesis. *DDIT4* downregulation promoted apoptosis of SGC7901 cells treated with 0, 10 or 20 μg/mL 5-FU compared with the negative controls (Fig. 3m). In addition, *DDIT4* silencing in SGC7901 cells attenuated gastric cancer cell S phase arrest (Fig. 3n). Similarly, in BGC823 cells, *DDIT4* downregulation significantly increased GC cell apoptosis and reduced S phase arrest compared with the control (Fig. 3m, n). In contrast, *DDIT4* overexpression in GES cells significantly reduced apoptosis in the absence and presence of 5-FU (10 or 20 μg/mL) (Fig. 3m). Moreover, as demonstrated by cell cycle analysis, ectopic

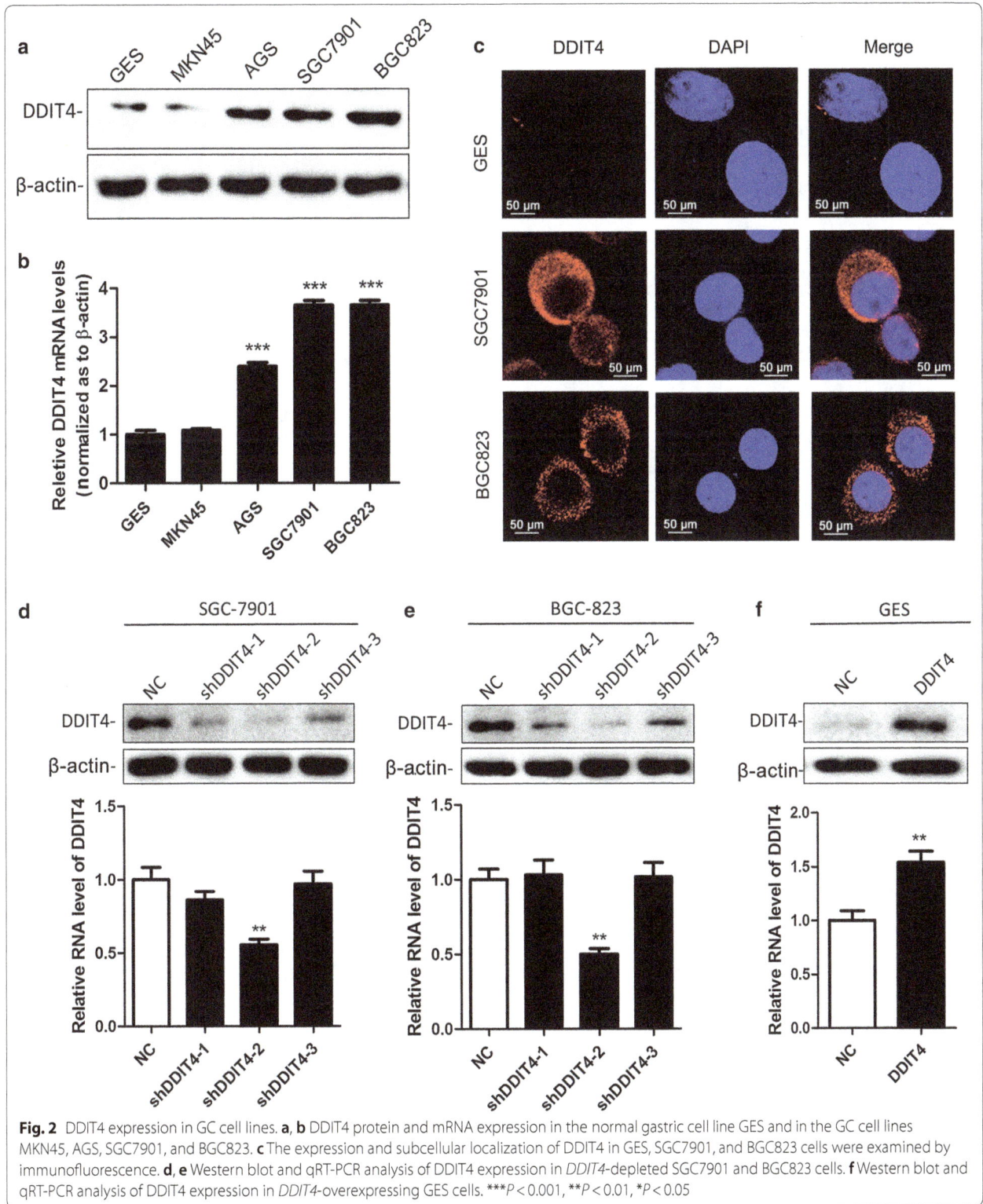

Fig. 2 DDIT4 expression in GC cell lines. **a, b** DDIT4 protein and mRNA expression in the normal gastric cell line GES and in the GC cell lines MKN45, AGS, SGC7901, and BGC823. **c** The expression and subcellular localization of DDIT4 in GES, SGC7901, and BGC823 cells were examined by immunofluorescence. **d, e** Western blot and qRT-PCR analysis of DDIT4 expression in *DDIT4*-depleted SGC7901 and BGC823 cells. **f** Western blot and qRT-PCR analysis of DDIT4 expression in *DDIT4*-overexpressing GES cells. ***$P < 0.001$, **$P < 0.01$, *$P < 0.05$

expression of *DDIT4* in GES cells drove the cell cycle into S phase and G_2/M phase and reduced the population of cells in G_1 phase compared with the control (Fig. 3n).

Taken together, these findings indicated that DDIT4 is associated with 5-FU-induced apoptosis and cell cycle progression in GC cells in a dose-dependent manner.

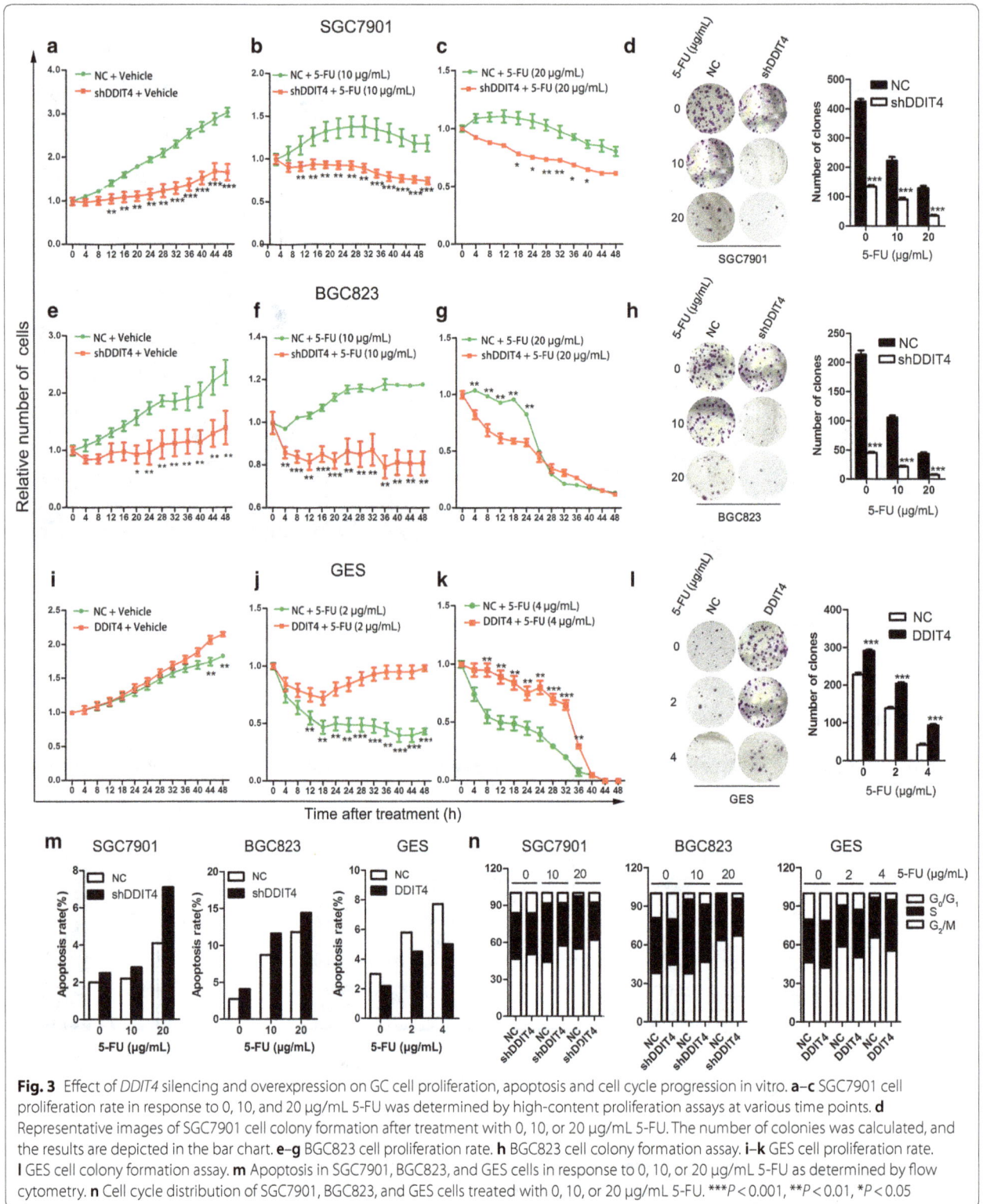

Fig. 3 Effect of *DDIT4* silencing and overexpression on GC cell proliferation, apoptosis and cell cycle progression in vitro. **a–c** SGC7901 cell proliferation rate in response to 0, 10, and 20 µg/mL 5-FU was determined by high-content proliferation assays at various time points. **d** Representative images of SGC7901 cell colony formation after treatment with 0, 10, or 20 µg/mL 5-FU. The number of colonies was calculated, and the results are depicted in the bar chart. **e–g** BGC823 cell proliferation rate. **h** BGC823 cell colony formation assay. **i–k** GES cell proliferation rate. **l** GES cell colony formation assay. **m** Apoptosis in SGC7901, BGC823, and GES cells in response to 0, 10, or 20 µg/mL 5-FU as determined by flow cytometry. **n** Cell cycle distribution of SGC7901, BGC823, and GES cells treated with 0, 10, or 20 µg/mL 5-FU. ***$P < 0.001$, **$P < 0.01$, *$P < 0.05$

DDIT4 silencing inhibits GC cell tumorigenesis in vivo

To investigate the effect of DDIT4 on GC tumorigenic behavior in vivo, we conducted tumorigenicity assays in nude mice by subcutaneously injecting BGC823 cells stably expressing shDDIT4 or scrambled control shRNA into the dorsal flank of several mice. *DDIT4* depletion resulted in a significant reduction in tumor growth (Fig. 4a). *DDIT4*-knockdown tumors grew significantly slower (Fig. 4b) and weighed significantly less on average (Fig. 4c, d) compared with control tumors. Furthermore, we used western blotting and IHC to detect DDIT4 expression in xenografts and validated the lower DDIT4 levels in *DDIT4*-knockdown tumors compared with control tumors (Fig. 4e, f). Finally, we observed a reduced Ki67 (proliferation marker)-positivity rate in tumor tissues in the *DDIT4*-knockdown group compared with the control group (Fig. 4f). Taken together, these observations indicated that DDIT4 promotes GC growth in vivo and might function as an oncogene in gastric carcinogenesis.

DDIT4 downregulation inhibits GC cell proliferation through the MAPK and p53 pathways

To understand the molecular mechanism underlying GC growth regulation by DDIT4, we utilized phospho-array assays that detect 131 phosphorylation sites in 12 critical cancer signaling molecules (Additional file 2: Table S1). Given that DDIT4 acts as a negative regulator of mTOR, we first examined the activity of the phosphatidylinositol-4,5-bisphosphate 3-kinase (PI3K)/ AKTkt/mTOR pathway in GC cells upon *DDIT4* downregulation. Phospho-array assays revealed that the PI3K/ AKT/mTOR pathway did not exhibit significant changes in *DDIT4*-knockdown cells (data not shown). Western blotting assays confirmed this observation (Fig. 5a), indicating that DDIT4 might activate other signaling pathways in GC cells. To uncover the molecular mechanism underlying GC growth regulation by DDIT4, we assessed MAPK and p53 signaling pathways in *DDIT4*-downregulated GC cells. In contrast to the PI3K/AKT/mTOR pathway, obvious alterations in the MAPK and p53 signaling pathways were observed (Fig. 5b). Anti-apoptotic BCL-2 levels were reduced, whereas pro-apoptotic BAD and proliferation-suppressive p21^{Cip1} levels were increased in *DDIT4*-downregulated cells (Fig. 5b). To further examine the effect of blocking the MAPK and p53 signaling pathways on gastric cancer cell proliferation following *DDIT4* knockdown, we performed rescue experiments by blocking the MAPK and p53 signaling pathways using a MAPK/ERK inhibitor (PD98059) and a p53 inhibitor (A15201) in *DDIT4*-knockdown cells. MAPK and p53 inhibition abolished the BCL-2 suppression and p21^{Cip1} elevation that was induced by *DDIT4* downregulation (Fig. 5c). Consistent with western blot assays, the CCK8 assays indicated that MAPK and p53 inhibition restored GC cell proliferation, which was suppressed by *DDIT4* knockdown (Fig. 5d). Taken together, these findings indicated that the MAPK and p53 signaling pathways

might play a critical role in DDIT4-mediated GC cell proliferation.

Discussion

Our study suggests that DDIT4 is an important regulator that is markedly upregulated in GC tissues and cells, and that knockdown of *DDIT4* suppresses the proliferation and tumorigenicity of GC cells both in vitro and in vivo. In addition, DDIT4 is attributed to chemotherapy-induced apoptosis and S phase arrest in GC cells. Mechanically, the proliferation-suppressive and chemosensitive effect of DDIT4 downregulation might be associated with activation of the p53 and MAPK signaling pathways.

GC currently poses a tremendous health burden on communities worldwide and is thought to result from a combined attack of environmental factors and genetic alterations [14, 15]. Among these factors, oncogene activation triggers replication stress and DNA damage, thereby increasing genome instability [16]. Additionally, the transient and long-term lack of nutrients, oxygen, and growth factors causes GC cells to be subject to frequent metabolic stress [17]. Thus, most GC cells display oncogene- or adverse environment-induced DNA damage [18]. DDIT4, a DNA damage-inducible transcript, is transcriptionally upregulated in multiple settings of DNA damage [4]. Notably, recent studies highlighted the important roles of DDIT4 in various types of human cancer [6, 19, 20]. In breast cancer, DDIT4 acts as a tumor-suppressor to regulate miR-495-mediated oncogenesis and hypoxia resistance [19]. Friedman et al. reported that DDIT4 enhances C/EBPbeta mediated autophagosome-lysosome fusion and desensitized PC cells to bortezomib [6]. In contrast, a positive correlation between DDIT4 and p-AKT was identified in ovarian cancer (OC), and DDIT4 expression in OC tissues was significantly increased in patients with serous adenocarcinoma and late FIGO stage [11], indicating that DDIT4 might be a tumor promotor in OC. These above findings demonstrated context-dependent regulation of DDIT4 in tumorigenesis and progression. However, whether and how DDIT4 plays critical roles in GC, which is characterized by frequent DNA damage, remains largely unknown. In the present study, we detected DDIT4 expression in GC tissues and cell lines, and found that DDIT4 was significantly upregulated in GC tissues and cell lines. In subsequent loss- and gain-of-function analyses, we observed that overexpression of *DDIT4* promoted GES cell proliferation, whereas knockdown of *DDIT4* suppressed GC cell proliferation both in vitro and in vivo. Therefore, our results demonstrated that DDIT4 is a proliferation-promoting and oncogenic protein in GC cells. Moreover, several lines of evidence demonstrate that DDIT4

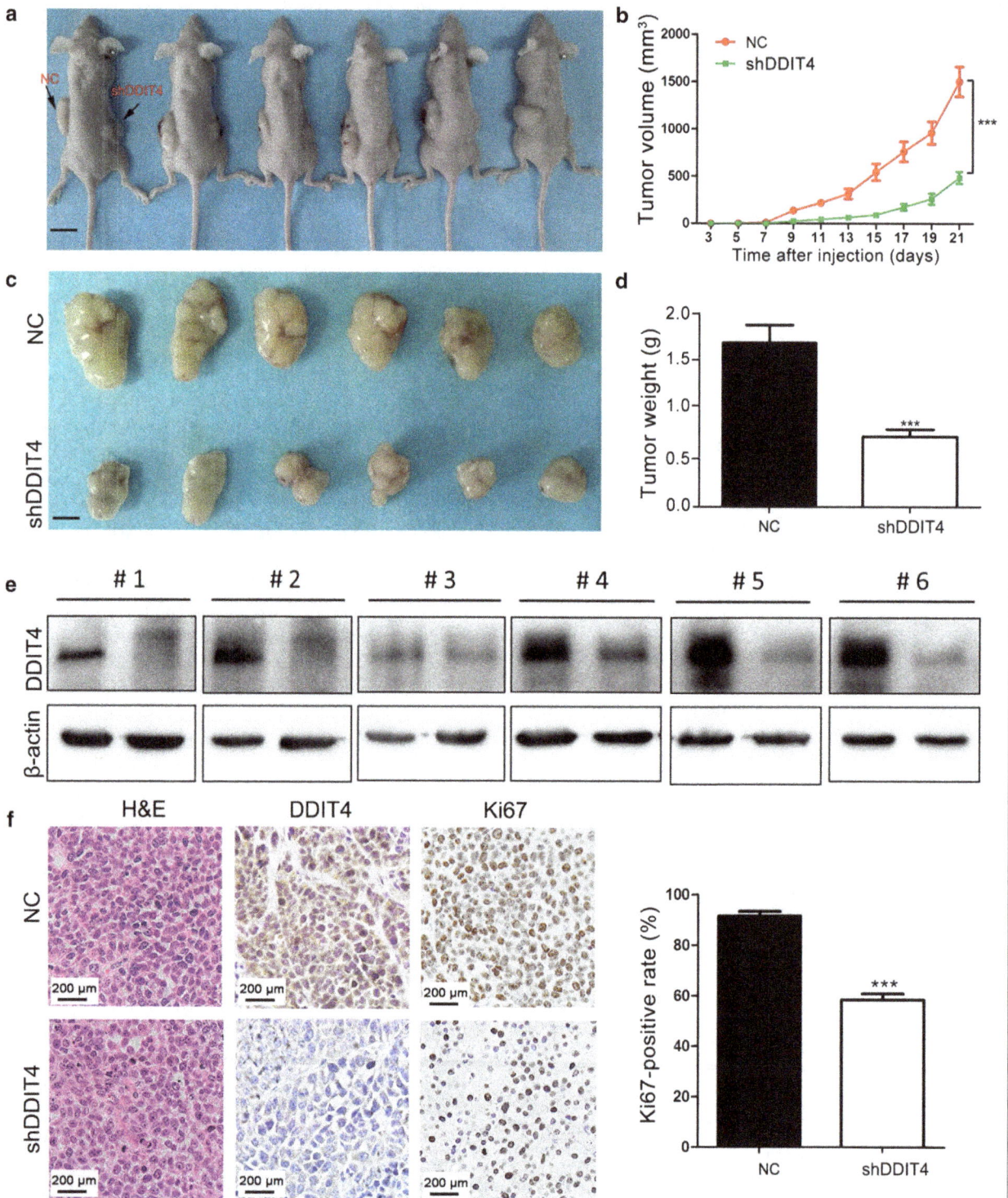

Fig. 4 *DDIT4* depletion inhibited GC xenograft tumor growth in vivo. **a** BGC823 cells stably expressing si-DDIT4 or scrambled control siRNA were subcutaneously injected into nude mice. *DDIT4*-silenced BGC823 cells formed smaller tumors compared with cells expressing the scrambled control after 4 weeks. **b** Tumor growth curves. **c** Representative images of xenograft tumors. **d** Tumor weight. **e** DDIT4 expression in xenograft tumors was determined by western blot. **f** HE and immunohistochemical staining for DDIT4 and Ki67 in xenograft tumors. ***$P < 0.001$, **$P < 0.01$, *$P < 0.05$

(See figure on next page.)
Fig. 5 Downregulation of *DDIT4* activates the mitogen-activated protein kinase (MAPK) and p53 pathways in GC cells. **a** The total and phosphorylated levels of AKT, mTOR and 4EBP1 in *DDIT4*-silenced and *DDIT4*-overexpressing cells were examined by western blot. **b** The total and phosphorylated levels of MEK1, P42/44-MAPK, BCL-1, BAD, p53, and p21^{Cip1} in *DDIT4*-silenced and *DDIT4*-overexpressing cells were examined by western blot. **c, d** SGC7901 and BGC823 cells were infected shDDIT4 lentivirus and then were treated with inhibitors specific to p53 (A15201) or MAPK (PD98059). **c** The protein expression levels of phosphorylated and total ERK, BCL-2, p53 and p21^{Cip1} were analyzed by western blot. **d** Cell proliferation was analyzed by CCK8 assay

is involved in anti-tumor chemotherapeutic treatment. For example, baicalein upregulates DDIT4 and causes mTORC1 and growth inhibition in platinum-resistant cancer cells [7]. Melatonin enhances arsenic trioxide-induced cell death via sustained upregulation of DDIT4 expression in breast cancer cells [21]. DDIT4 expression is an independent prognostic factor for triple-negative breast cancer resistant to neoadjuvant chemotherapy [12]. Here, we investigated the role of DDIT4 in response to increasing concentrations of 5-FU. We found that DDIT4 did not alter apoptosis and the cell cycle of GC cells in the absence of 5-FU but reduced apoptotic rate and S phase arrest in GES cells. In contrast, downregulation of *DDIT4* in GC cells increased cell apoptosis and S phase arrest. Collectively, our findings indicated that DDIT4 might contribute to GC development and chemosensitivity, suggesting that inhibiting DDIT4-mediated apoptosis and cell cycle arrest can lead to a greater apoptotic response and retard the cell cycle, thereby potentiating the efficacy of the chemotherapeutic agents against cancer.

Pinto et al. [12] demonstrated with an analysis in KM-Plotter that DDIT4 expression over the median is a protective factor for time to first progression (HR = 0.62; 95% CI 0.5–0.75, $P = 1.7 \times 10^{-6}$). However, analysis of the data downloaded from The Cancer Genome Atlas (TCGA) for gastric adenocarcinoma did not reveal differences in survival when comparing two groups with low and high DDIT4 expression (*P*-value in the log rank test of 0.999) [12]. In our study, we found that DDIT4 expression was increased in GC and that it functioned as an oncogene. In addition, univariate survival analysis revealed that DDIT4 did not exhibit statistically significant associations with GC patient survival, which is consistent with TCGA analysis for gastric adenocarcinoma. The inconsistencies of the evaluation of DDIT4 implied that the prognostic value of DDIT4 requires further investigation.

Reversible protein phosphorylation is one of the most important biological mechanisms for signal transduction, which is tightly regulated by protein kinases and phosphatases to maintain the balance of the protein's phosphorylation status and control its biological functions [22]. Accumulating evidence indicates that perturbation of this balance contributes to the origin and pathogenesis of several human diseases. In cigarette

smoke-induced pulmonary injury and emphysema, DDIT4 is necessary and sufficient for nuclear factor-kappaB (NF-kappaB) activation, and promoted alveolar inflammation, oxidative stress and apoptosis in alveolar septal cells [23]. DDIT4 promotes protein phosphatase 2A (PP2A)-dependent de-phosphorylation of AKT on Thr (308) but not on Ser (473) for phosphorylation of TSC2 [24]. Moreover, DDIT4 displays critical roles in hypoxia-inducible factor-1 (HIF-1) and p53 pathway crosstalk [4, 25]. However, the specific oncogenic pathway regulated by DDIT4 under different conditions remains unclear. In our study, we explored the mechanistic basis for DDIT4-mediated regulation of GC cells using phospho-antibody microarray-based proteomic analysis and found that the proliferation-suppressive and chemosensitive effect of *DDIT4* downregulation might be associated with activation of the MAPK signaling pathway, resulting in subsequent phosphorylation of BCL-2 (p-Ser70), which inhibits cell proliferation and induces apoptosis. Consistent with previous studies, we demonstrated that the MAPK pathway is frequently activated in human cancers, leading to malignant phenotypes such as autonomous cellular proliferation [26]. In addition to the MAPK signaling pathway, extensive studies have demonstrated that the p53 tumor suppressor protein preserves genome integrity by regulating growth arrest and apoptosis in response to DNA damage [27–29]. This notion is further supported by our data demonstrating that DDIT4 regulated the activation of multiple pro-apoptotic and growth-suppressive proteins, including p53. The p53 protein displayed a dual change in its phosphorylation state in *DDIT4*-knockdown cells compared with negative controls, as follows: (1) downregulation of phosphorylation at Ser6, which induces apoptosis; and (2) upregulation of phosphorylation at Ser315, leading to phosphorylation of p21^{Cis1} (p-Thr145), which rescues cells from apoptosis. Thus, in our study, we identified multiple pro-apoptotic and growth-suppressive proteins of which the phosphorylation and activation levels were regulated by DDIT4 in GC cells.

Conclusions

In summary, our results demonstrated that DDIT4 promoted the tumorigenicity of gastric cancer cells by facilitating proliferation and colony formation and alleviating

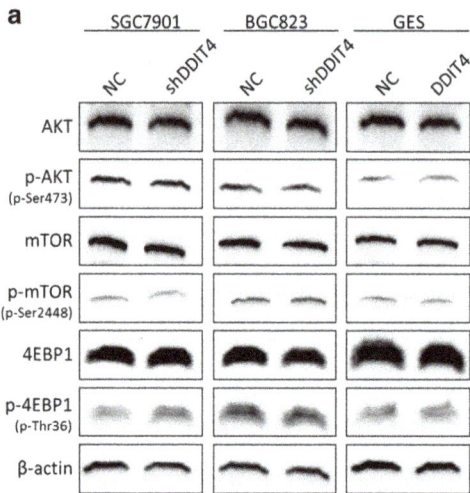

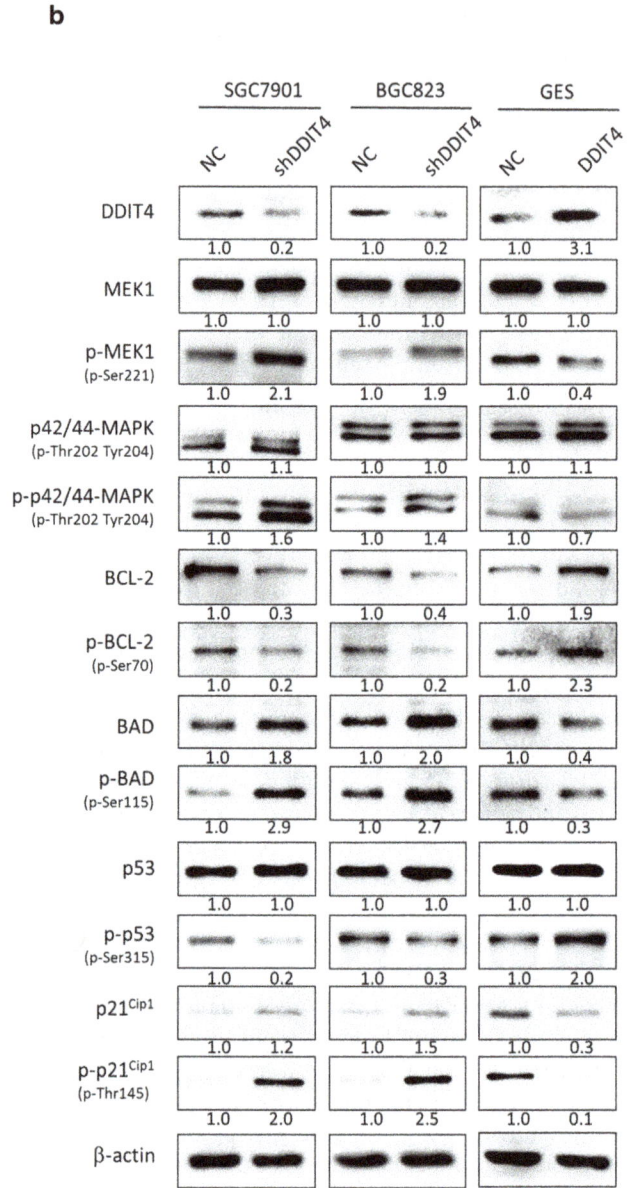

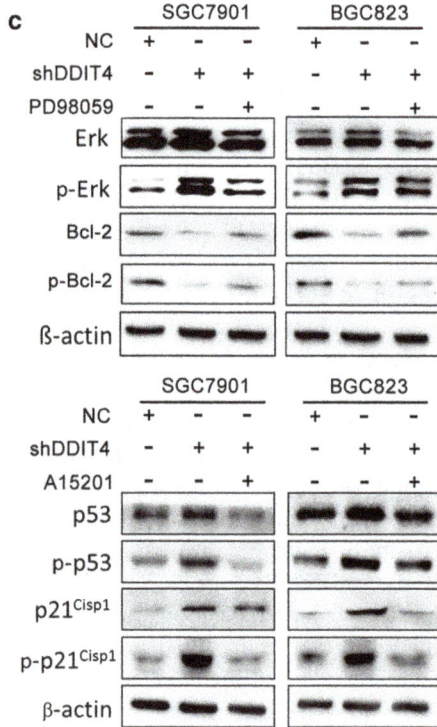

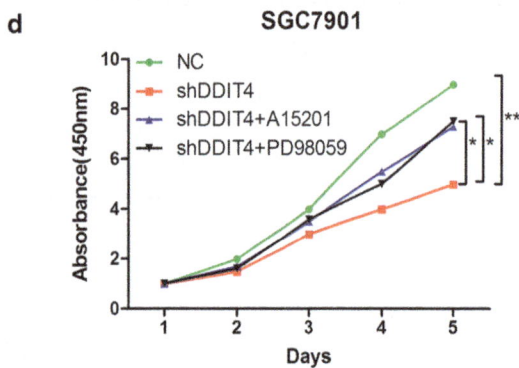

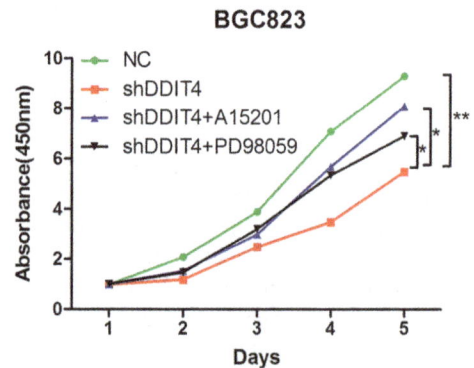

5-FU-induced apoptosis through the p53 and MAPK pathways. The mouse model experiment further demonstrated that *DDIT4* downregulation significantly inhibited tumor growth in vivo. Taken together, our results suggest that DDIT4 may function as an oncogene in gastric cancer, providing a promising therapeutic strategy for GC treatment.

Abbreviations
DDIT4: DNA-damage-inducible transcript 4; GC: gastric cancer; MAPK: mitogen-activated protein kinase; PC: prostate cancer; OC: ovarian cancer; NF-kappaB: nuclear factor-kappaB; PP2A: protein phosphatase 2A.

Authors' contributions
XZ, YL, YN and DF conceived and directed the projects. FD, XZ and YL designed experiments. FD, LS and YT performed experiments, FD, TL, CL, MJ, XW, and YM conducted data analysis and interpreted the results. FD and XZ wrote and edited the manuscript. All authors read and approved the final manuscript.

Acknowledgements
We acknowledge Lei Geng, Fenli Zhou, Jianhua Dou and Guangbo Tang for their generous help to the present study.

Competing interests
The authors declare that they have no competing interests.

Funding
The present study was supported by the National Natural Science Foundation of China (Nos. 81430072, 81421003, 81602641, 81572929).

References
1. Sun W, Yan L. Gastric cancer: current and evolving treatment landscape. Chin J Cancer. 2016;35(1):83.
2. Crew KD, Neugut AI. Epidemiology of gastric cancer. World J Gastroenterol. 2006;12(3):354–62.
3. Bass AJ, Thorsson V, Shmulevich I, Reynolds SM, Miller M, Bernard B, et al. Comprehensive molecular characterization of gastric adenocarcinoma. Nature. 2014;513(7517):202–9.
4. Ellisen LW, Ramsayer KD, Johannessen CM, Yang A, Beppu H, Minda K, et al. REDD1, a developmentally regulated transcriptional target of p63 and p53, links p63 to regulation of reactive oxygen species. Mol Cell. 2002;10(5):995–1005.
5. DeYoung MP, Horak P, Sofer A, Sgroi D, Ellisen LW. Hypoxia regulates TSC1/2-mTOR signaling and tumor suppression through REDD1-mediated 14-3-3 shuttling. Genes Dev. 2008;22(2):239–51.
6. Barakat DJ, Mendonca J, Barberi T, Zhang J, Kachhap SK, Paz-Priel I, et al. C/EBPbeta regulates sensitivity to bortezomib in prostate cancer cells by inducing REDD1 and autophagosome-lysosome fusion. Cancer Lett. 2016;375(1):152–61.
7. Wang Y, Han E, Xing Q, Yan J, Arrington A, Wang C, et al. Baicalein upregulates DDIT4 expression which mediates mTOR inhibition and growth inhibition in cancer cells. Cancer Lett. 2015;358(2):170–9.
8. Gordon MA, D'Amato NC, Gu H, Babbs B, Wulfkuhle J, Petricoin EF, et al. Synergy between androgen receptor antagonism and inhibition of mTOR and HER2 in breast cancer. Mol Cancer Ther. 2017;16:1389–400.
9. Rehan M. An anti-cancer drug candidate OSI-027 and its analog as inhibitors of mTOR: computational insights into the inhibitory mechanisms. J Cell Biochem. 2017;118:4558–67.
10. Molitoris JK, McColl KS, Swerdlow S, Matsuyama M, Lam M, Finkel TH, et al. Glucocorticoid elevation of dexamethasone-induced gene 2 (Dig2/RTP801/REDD1) protein mediates autophagy in lymphocytes. J Biol Chem. 2011;286(34):30181–9.
11. Jia W, Chang B, Sun L, Zhu H, Pang L, Tao L, et al. REDD1 and p-AKT overexpression may predict poor prognosis in ovarian cancer. Int J Clin Exp Pathol. 2014;7(9):5940–9.
12. Pinto JA, Rolfo C, Raez LE, Prado A, Araujo JM, Bravo L, et al. In silico evaluation of DNA damage inducible transcript 4 gene (DDIT4) as prognostic biomarker in several malignancies. Sci Rep. 2017;7(1):1526.
13. Evan GI, Vousden KH. Proliferation, cell cycle and apoptosis in cancer. Nature. 2001;411(6835):342–8.
14. Kalisperati P, Spanou E, Pateras IS, Korkolopoulou P, Varvarigou A, Karavokyros I, et al. Inflammation, DNA damage, *Helicobacter pylori* and gastric tumorigenesis. Front Genet. 2017;8:20.
15. Coussens LM, Werb Z. Inflammation and cancer. Nature. 2002;420(6917):860–7.
16. Negrini S, Gorgoulis VG, Halazonetis TD. Genomic instability—an evolving hallmark of cancer. Nat Rev Mol Cell Biol. 2010;11(3):220–8.
17. Luo J, Solimini NL, Elledge SJ. Principles of cancer therapy: oncogene and non-oncogene addiction. Cell. 2009;136(5):823–37.
18. Zhou X, Liu W, Hu X, Dorrance A, Garzon R, Houghton PJ, et al. Regulation of CHK1 by mTOR contributes to the evasion of DNA damage barrier of cancer cells. Sci Rep. 2017;7(1):1535.
19. Hwang-Verslues WW, Chang PH, Wei PC, Yang CY, Huang CK, Kuo WH, et al. miR-495 is upregulated by E12/E47 in breast cancer stem cells, and promotes oncogenesis and hypoxia resistance via downregulation of E-cadherin and REDD1. Oncogene. 2011;30(21):2463–74.
20. Jin HO, Seo SK, Woo SH, Kim YS, Hong SE, Yi JY, et al. Redd1 inhibits the invasiveness of non-small cell lung cancer cells. Biochem Biophys Res Commun. 2011;407(3):507–11.
21. Yun SM, Woo SH, Oh ST, Hong SE, Choe TB, Ye SK, et al. Melatonin enhances arsenic trioxide-induced cell death via sustained upregulation of Redd1 expression in breast cancer cells. Mol Cell Endocrinol. 2016;422:64–73.
22. Iakoucheva LM, Radivojac P, Brown CJ, O'Connor TR, Sikes JG, Obradovic Z, et al. The importance of intrinsic disorder for protein phosphorylation. Nucleic Acids Res. 2004;32(3):1037–49.
23. Yoshida T, Mett I, Bhunia AK, Bowman J, Perez M, Zhang L, et al. Rtp801, a suppressor of mTOR signaling, is an essential mediator of cigarette smoke-induced pulmonary injury and emphysema. Nat Med. 2010;16(7):767–73.
24. Dennis MD, Coleman CS, Berg A, Jefferson LS, Kimball SR. REDD1 enhances protein phosphatase 2A-mediated dephosphorylation of Akt to repress mTORC1 signaling. Sci Signal. 2014;7(335):a68.
25. Horak P, Crawford AV, Vadysirisack DD, Nash ZM, DeYoung MP, Sgroi D, et al. Negative feedback control of HIF-1 through REDD1-regulated ROS suppresses tumorigenesis. Proc Natl Acad Sci USA. 2010;107(10):4675–80.
26. Wagner EF, Nebreda AR. Signal integration by JNK and p38 MAPK pathways in cancer development. Nat Rev Cancer. 2009;9(8):537–49.
27. Deng C, Zhang P, Harper JW, Elledge SJ, Leder P. Mice lacking p21CIP1/WAF1 undergo normal development, but are defective in G1 checkpoint control. Cell. 1995;82(4):675–84.
28. Tibbetts RS, Brumbaugh KM, Williams JM, Sarkaria JN, Cliby WA, Shieh SY, et al. A role for ATR in the DNA damage-induced phosphorylation of p53. Genes Dev. 1999;13(2):152–7.
29. Miyashita T, Reed JC. Tumor suppressor p53 is a direct transcriptional activator of the human bax gene. Cell. 1995;80(2):293–9.

17

Adjuvant transcatheter arterial chemoembolization after curative resection for hepatocellular carcinoma patients with solitary tumor and microvascular invasion

Wei Wei[1,2†], Pei-En Jian[1,2†], Shao-Hua Li[1,2†], Zhi-Xing Guo[1,2†], Yong-Fa Zhang[1,2], Yi-Hong Ling[1,3], Xiao-Jun Lin[1,2], Li Xu[1,2], Ming Shi[1,2], Lie Zheng[1,4], Min-Shan Chen[1,2] and Rong-Ping Guo[1,2*]

Abstract

Background: The optimal strategy for adjuvant therapy after curative resection for hepatocellular carcinoma (HCC) patients with solitary tumor and microvascular invasion (MVI) is controversial. This trial evaluated the efficacy and safety of adjuvant transcatheter arterial chemoembolization (TACE) after hepatectomy versus hepatectomy alone in HCC patients with a solitary tumor $\geq$ 5 cm and MVI.

Methods: In this randomized, open-labeled, phase III trial, HCC patients with a solitary tumor $\geq$ 5 cm and MVI were randomly assigned (1:1) to receive either 1–2 cycles of adjuvant TACE after hepatectomy (Hepatectomy-TACE) or hepatectomy alone (Hepatectomy Alone). The primary endpoint was disease-free survival (DFS); the secondary endpoints included overall survival (OS) and adverse events.

Results: Between June 1, 2009, and December 31, 2012, 250 patients were enrolled and randomly assigned to the Hepatectomy-TACE group ($n = 125$) or the Hepatectomy Alone group ($n = 125$). Clinicopathological characteristics were balanced between the two groups. The median follow-up time from randomization was 37.5 months [interquartile range 18.3–48.2 months]. The median DFS was significantly longer in the Hepatectomy-TACE group than in the Hepatectomy Alone group [17.45 months (95% confidence interval [CI] 11.99–29.14) vs. 9.27 months (95% CI 6.05–13.70), hazard ratio [HR] = 0.70 (95% CI 0.52–0.95), $P = 0.020$], respectively. The median OS was also significantly longer in the Hepatectomy-TACE group than in the Hepatectomy Alone group [44.29 months (95% CI 25.99–62.58) vs. 22.37 months (95% CI 10.84–33.91), HR = 0.68 (95% CI 0.48–0.97), $P = 0.029$]. Treatment-related adverse events were more frequently observed in the Hepatectomy-TACE group, although these were generally mild and manageable. The most common grade 3 or 4 adverse events in both groups were neutropenia and liver dysfunction.

Conclusion: Hepatectomy followed by adjuvant TACE is an appropriate option after radical resection in HCC patients with solitary tumor $\geq$ 5 cm and MVI, with acceptable toxicity.

Keywords: Solitary tumor, Hepatocellular carcinoma, Adjuvant therapy, Transcatheter arterial chemoembolization, Hepatectomy alone, Microvascular invasion

*Correspondence: guorp@sysucc.org.cn
†Wei Wei, Pei-En Jian, Shao-Hua Li and Zhi-Xing Guo contributed equally to this work
2 Department of Hepatobiliary and Pancreatic Surgery, Sun Yat-sen University Cancer Center, Guangzhou 510060, Guangdong, P. R. China
Full list of author information is available at the end of the article

Introduction

Hepatocellular carcinoma (HCC) is the sixth most common malignancy worldwide [1] and the second leading cause of cancer-related death in China [2]. An estimated 466,100 new HCC cases and 422,100 deaths occurred in China in 2015 [3]. Surgical resection remains the main radical treatment for HCC, although the recurrence rate after hepatectomy is high and hampers further improvement in the prognosis of HCC patients [4, 5]. The conventional risk factors for recurrence include tumor size, multiple lesions, vascular invasion, poor differentiation, and tumor rupture [6–8]. Over the past decade, microvascular invasion (MVI) has been proposed as a potential risk factor for recurrence after hepatectomy [9, 10]. Recent studies have confirmed the significance of MVI in postoperative recurrence [11–13]. A previous study by our research group also showed that the recurrence rate was over 50% for HCC patients with solitary tumor ≥ 5 cm and MVI, where MVI was confirmed as the only independent risk factor for overall survival (OS) and disease-free survival (DFS) among that cohort [14].

Different therapeutic agents and/or approaches have been evaluated as adjuvant therapy for HCC after curative resection, including interferon [15], oral chemotherapeutic agents (1-hexylcarbamoyl-5-fluorouracil (HCFU) [16] and capecitabine [17]), hepatic arterial infusion chemotherapy [18], and targeted therapy (sorafenib) [19]. Unfortunately, it has been shown that most of these approaches did not reduce the risk of recurrence or were poorly tolerated, and, most importantly, these strategies were not associated with significant survival benefits [20]. As such, an optimal adjuvant therapy with respect to efficacy, safety, and cost-effectiveness remains to be defined. Our previous phase III randomized clinical study indicated that transcatheter arterial chemoembolization (TACE) may be an appropriate adjuvant therapy option for stage IIIA HCC patients [21]. Therefore, this present phase III clinical trial was designed to evaluate the efficacy and safety of radical hepatectomy plus adjuvant TACE (Hepatectomy-TACE), compared with radical hepatectomy alone (Hepatectomy Alone), in HCC patients with solitary tumor ≥ 5 cm and MVI after curative resection.

Methods

Trial design

This study was an open-labeled, randomized, phase III trial conducted at the Sun Yat-sen University Cancer Center (Guangzhou, China), designed to evaluate the efficacy and safety of radical hepatectomy plus adjuvant TACE versus radical hepatectomy alone among HCC patients with solitary tumor ≥ 5 cm and MVI after curative resection. The protocol and all modifications were

approved by the Institutional Review Board and Ethics Committee of our cancer center. This study complied with the Declaration of Helsinki and the Good Clinical Practice Guidelines (International Conference on Harmonisation of Technical Requirements for Registration of Pharmaceuticals for Human Use (ICH), Version E6) [22]. All patients provided written informed consents. This study was registered in ClinicalTrials.gov (http://ClinicalTrials.gov, trial number NCT02788526) on March 23, 2016.

Eligibility criteria

The eligibility criteria for inclusion were as follows: 18–75 years of age; histologically confirmed HCC with MVI (MVI was defined by the presence of tumor emboli within either the central hepatic vein, the portal, or the large capsular vessels [23]); Eastern Cooperative Oncology Group performance score (ECOG PS) ≤ 2; no previous treatment for HCC; solitary tumor ≥ 5 cm before surgery confirmed by 2 radiological examinations (ultrasonography with computer tomography or magnetic resonance imaging); R0 resection; no evidence of recurrence at radiological follow-up at 3–5 weeks after surgery; adequate hematologic, hepatic, and renal functions. The exclusion criteria included histologically positive resection margin (R1 resection); evidence of recurrence at radiological follow-up 3–5 weeks after surgery; history of organ transplantation; active uncontrolled infection; allergy to any TACE agent; other malignancies over the preceding 5 years before the HCC diagnosis, except for adequately treated carcinoma in situ of the cervix and squamous or basal cell carcinoma of the skin; pregnancy, breastfeeding, or lack of use of adequate contraception among women of childbearing potential; neurological or psychiatric disorders that may affect cognitive assessment and inform consent; concomitant antitumor therapy or participation in other interventional clinical trials.

Hepatectomy

All surgical resection procedures were performed following the techniques described in our previous study [10]. Briefly, routine abdominal exploration was carefully performed to evaluate the extent of the tumor and to exclude extrahepatic metastases. After adequate mobilization of the liver, we used intraoperative ultrasound (ALOKA SSD-5500, Tokyo, Japan) to assess the number of lesions and tumor size, the presence of MVI, and the extent of resection. During tumor removal, the liver parenchyma was separated using the Cavitron Ultrasonic Surgical Aspirator (Integra LifeSciences CUSA Excel, Plainsboro, NJ, USA), and the involved vessels were ligated. The Pringle maneuver was also applied to occlude blood inflow to the liver.

Randomization

All patients were screened for enrollment at the first follow-up (3–5 weeks after hepatectomy). Full patient assessment, including demographic characteristics, medical history, physical examination, routine blood analysis (hematology and biochemistry), and radiological examinations [computed tomography (CT) or magnetic resonance imaging (MRI)], were performed within 1 week of the study enrollment. The patients with evidence of recurrence during the screening for enrollment were excluded. Then the eligible patients were randomly assigned (at a 1:1 ratio) to receive either 1–2 cycles of adjuvant TACE (Hepatectomy-TACE group) or routine follow-up without adjuvant treatment (Hepatectomy Alone group). Randomization was performed using a sealed envelope system according to a predesigned random number.

Adjuvant TACE

The patients in the Hepatectomy-TACE group underwent TACE 4–6 weeks after hepatectomy according to liver function and performance status. TACE was performed using the techniques we have described previously [24]. In brief, a catheter was placed into the proper hepatic artery through the femoral artery using the Seldinger technique, hepatic arterial angiography was performed, and 200 mg/m^2 carboplatin (Carboplatin, Bristol-Myers Squibb, New York, NY, USA) and 6 mg/m^2 mitomycin (Mitomycin, Hisun, Taizhou, China) were infused followed by 4–5 mL of the emulsion of iodized oil (lipiodol, Andre Guerbet, Aulnay-sous-Bois, France) and 40 mg/m^2 epirubicin (Epirubicin Hydrochloride, Pfizer, New York, NY, USA). After 4–6 weeks, these patients underwent a complete assessment consisting of physical examination, routine blood analysis, and CT scan. The second cycle of TACE was performed according to the decision of investigators based on the patients' conditions and the assessment results.

Follow-up

All patients were followed-up at an interval of 2–3 months. To avoid the potential effect of hepatitis B virus (HBV) reactivation on recurrence, all patients with positive serum hepatitis B surface antigen (HBsAg) were administered with routine antiviral therapy with lamivudine (GlaxoSmithKline, Brentford, UK; 100 mg, once daily) or entecavir (Bristol-Myers Squibb, New York, USA; 0.5 mg, once daily). At each follow-up visit, physical examination, blood test (serum alpha-fetoprotein [AFP] and liver function), and enhanced abdominal CT or MRI scan were performed. Once suspicious recurrence/metastasis was detected, further examinations

including hepatic angiography or biopsy were conducted. Recurrence/metastasis was confirmed based on the cytologic/histologic evidence or on the non-invasive diagnostic criteria for HCC by the European Association for the Study of Liver [7]. Patients with recurrence in both groups received subsequent treatment according to the decision of the multi-disciplinary team of our cancer center. Adverse events (AEs) were recorded from the day of randomization to the last day of follow-up. Toxicity was evaluated according to the National Cancer Institute Common Terminology Criteria for Adverse Events (version 3.0). The study was censored on March 31, 2016.

Statistical analyses

The primary endpoint was DFS and was defined as from the time of randomization to the diagnosis of recurrence or death from any cause. The secondary endpoints included OS, which was defined as from the time of randomization to the date of the last follow-up or death, and AEs.

Assuming an increase in median DFS of 6 months between the Hepatectomy-TACE group (18.0 months) and Hepatectomy Alone group (12.0 months) [hazard ratio (HR) 0.66], it was estimated that 176 events and a total of 210 patients (105 in each group) were required for randomization to achieve a statistical power of 85% with a significance level of 0.05 for a one-sided error. All analyses were performed according to the per-protocol principle. Survival curves were estimated using the Kaplan–Meier method and compared using the log-rank test. The median survival with 95% confidence interval (CI) was calculated. Cox proportional analyses were performed to estimate HRs with 95% CIs. The t-test was used for group comparisons of AEs. We also performed subgroup analyses for sex (male vs. female), age (< 60 years vs. ≥ 60 years), ECOG PS (0 vs. 1–2), tumor size (5–10 cm vs. > 10 cm), cirrhosis (present vs. absent), and resection margin (< 2 cm vs. ≥ 2 cm). All statistical tests were performed with the Statistical Package for the Social Sciences (SPSS) (version 23, Chicago, IL, USA), Stata (version 13, College Station, TX, USA), and Medcalc (version 16.1, Acacialaan, Belgium) statistical software, and P values < 0.05 were considered significant.

Results

Patient characteristics and treatment administration

Between June 1, 2009, and December 31, 2012, 250 patients were enrolled and randomly assigned to receive 1–2 cycles of adjuvant TACE after radical hepatectomy (the Hepatectomy-TACE group, $n = 125$) or hepatectomy alone (the Hepatectomy Alone group, $n = 125$). In the Hepatectomy-TACE group, 2 patients withdrew consent because of the potential toxicity of TACE, 3 patients had antitumor Chinese herbal prescriptions with HCC indications, and 4 patients were lost to follow-up. These patients were therefore excluded from the analysis. In the Hepatectomy Alone group, 4 patients had antitumor Chinese herbal prescriptions, and 3 patients were lost to follow-up and were also excluded from the analysis (Fig. 1).

Baseline demographic and clinical characteristics were well balanced between the two groups (Table 1). The median follow-up time for the entire cohort was 37.5 months from randomization [interquartile range (IQR), 18.3–48.2 months]. In the Hepatectomy-TACE group, 55 patients underwent 1 cycle of TACE, and 61 patients underwent 2 cycles of TACE.

Operative variables and postoperative outcomes

The operative variables and postoperative outcomes observed from the first day after hepatectomy till the date of discharge are summarized in Table 2. Twenty-four and 23 complications occurred in the Hepatectomy-TACE and Hepatectomy Alone group, respectively, including grade 1–2 fever, ascites, transient jaundice, pleural effusion, and hypoalbuminemia. One patient in the Hepatectomy-TACE group and 2 patients in the Hepatectomy Alone group experienced grade 3 liver bleeding. No patient died of complications during hospitalization.

Efficacy of treatment

The median DFS was 17.45 months (95% CI 11.99–29.14) in the Hepatectomy-TACE group and 9.27 months

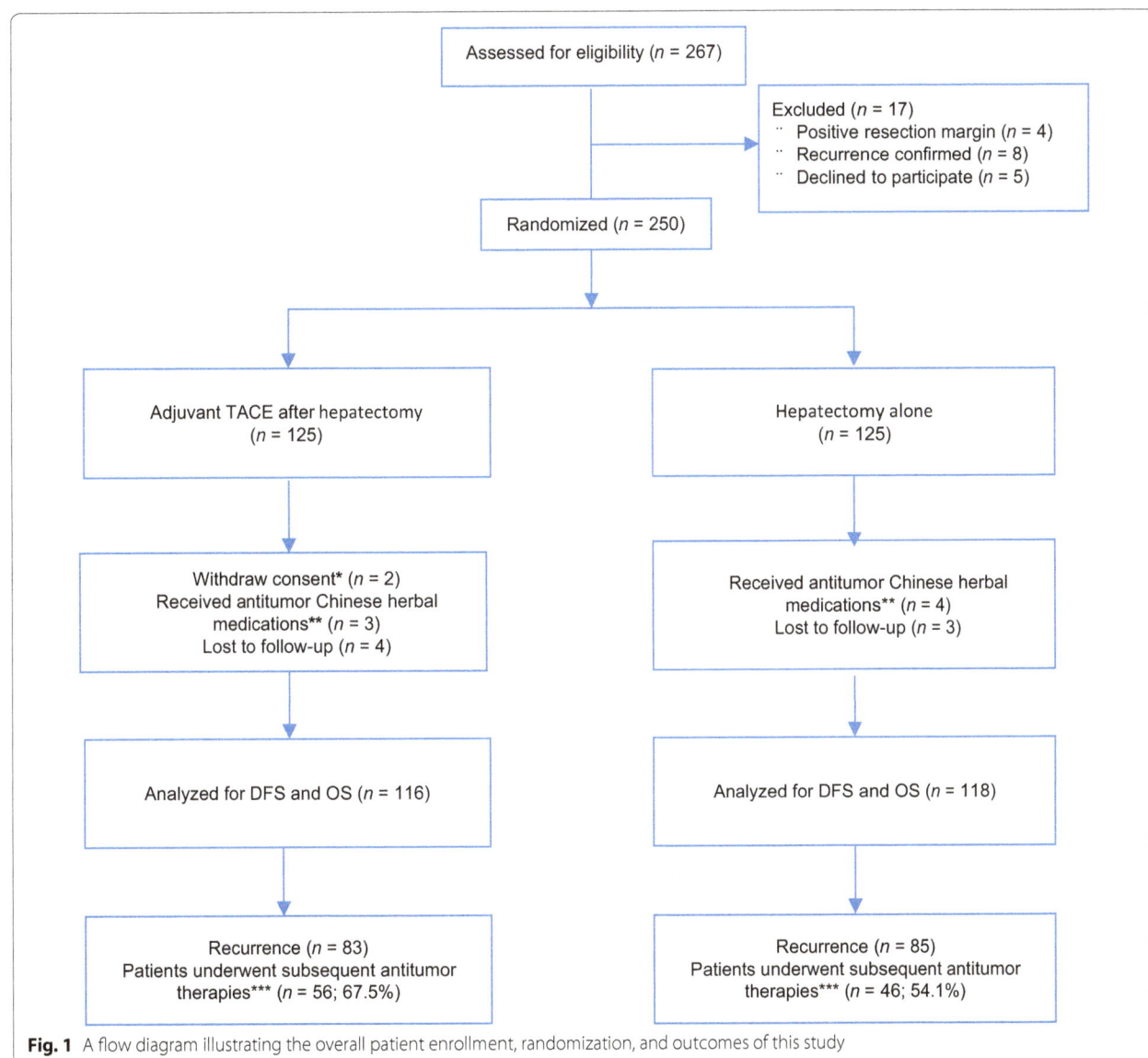

Fig. 1 A flow diagram illustrating the overall patient enrollment, randomization, and outcomes of this study

Table 1 Baseline characteristics of the investigated hepatocellular carcinoma patients

Characteristic	Hepatectomy-TACE group (n = 116)	Hepatectomy Alone group (n = 118)	P-value
Age [years; median (range)]	44.0 (18–75)	48.5 (18–74)	0.112
Gender [cases (%)]			
Male	106 (91.4)	106 (89.8)	0.824
Female	10 (8.6)	12 (10.2)	
ECOG performance status [cases (%)]			
0	48 (41.4)	53 (44.9)	0.794
1	65 (56.0)	63 (53.4)	
2	3 (2.6)	2 (1.7)	
Serum HBsAg [cases (%)]			
Positive	94 (81.0)	101 (85.6)	0.384
Negative	22 (19.0)	17 (14.4)	
Preoperative serum AFP [cases (%)]			
< 25 ng/mL	37 (31.9)	36 (30.5)	0.888
≥ 25 ng/mL	79 (68.1)	82 (69.5)	
Hemoglobin (g/L; mean ± SD)	142.3 ± 23.7	141.2 ± 24.4	0.711
Platelet ($\times 10^9$/L; mean ± SD)	205.2 ± 79.1	178.6 ± 80.0	0.119
Alanine aminotransferase (U/L; mean ± SD)	55.3 ± 57.4	45.1 ± 27.9	0.086
Serum albumin (g/L; mean ± SD)	41.4 ± 5.7	41.6 ± 3.4	0.741
Serum total bilirubin (mol/L; mean ± SD)	14.4 ± 5.8	17.3 ± 24.6	0.212
Prothrombin time (s; mean ± SD)	12.2 ± 1.2	12.2 ± 1.1	0.725
Child–Pugh grade [cases (%)]			
Class A	116 (100.0)	116 (98.3)	0.498
Class B	0 (0.0)	2 (1.7)	
Serum urea (mmol/L; mean ± SD)	5.0 ± 1.6	5.2 ± 1.3	0.378
Serum creatinine (μmol/L; mean ± SD)	78.1 ± 24.4	73.8 ± 15.5	0.114

Continuous variables were compared by Student t-test; categorical variables are compared by the χ^2 test or the Fisher's exact test

Hepatectomy-TACE: radical hepatectomy followed by adjuvant transcatheter arterial chemoembolization; Hepatectomy Alone: had undergone only radical hepatectomy; HBsAg: hepatitis B surface antigen; AFP: alpha-fetal protein; SD: standard deviation

(95% CI 6.05–13.70) in the Hepatectomy Alone group (HR = 0.70, 95% CI 0.52–0.95, P = 0.020; Fig. 2a). By March 31, 2016, 168 (71.8%) of the 234 patients had experienced recurrence (83 in the Hepatectomy-TACE group and 85 in the Hepatectomy Alone group). The 1-, 2-, 3-, and 5-year DFS rates for the Hepatectomy-TACE group were 58.6%, 44.7%, 38.4%, and 26.7% and were 43.5%, 30.6%, 26.5%, and 22.6% for the Hepatectomy Alone group, respectively.

The median OS for the Hepatectomy-TACE group was 44.29 months (95% CI 25.99–62.58) and was 22.37 months (95% CI 10.84–33.91) in the Hepatectomy Alone group (HR = 0.68, 95% CI 0.48–0.97, P = 0.029; Fig. 2b). By March 31, 2016, 128 (54.7%) of the 234 enrolled patients had died (62 in the Hepatectomy-TACE group and 66 in the Hepatectomy Alone group). The 1-, 2-, 3-, and 5-year OS rates for the Hepatectomy-TACE group were 87.8%, 64.3%, 53.5%, and 40.2% and were 67.2%, 49.8%, 43.6%, and 28.8% for the Hepatectomy Alone group, respectively.

The results of subgroup analyses were generally consistent with those of the primary analyses. It indicated that male patients, age < 60 years, presence of cirrhosis, tumor > 10 cm, and resection margin < 2 cm were associated with a greater DFS (Fig. 3a) and OS benefits (Fig. 3b) from adjuvant TACE.

After recurrence, 56 patients (67.5%) in the Hepatectomy-TACE group and 46 patients (54.1%) in the Hepatectomy Alone group underwent subsequent antitumor therapies, including locoregional ablation, hepatectomy, systemic chemotherapy, sorafenib, and TACE (summarized in Table 3).

Safety of treatment

Grade 3–4 AEs from the time of randomization to the last day of follow-up were reported in 25 patients (21.6%) from the Hepatectomy-TACE group and 10 patients (8.5%) in the Hepatectomy Alone group (Table 4). Fever, nausea/vomiting, and liver dysfunction were the most common AEs in the Hepatectomy-TACE group. The

Table 2 Operative variables and postoperative outcomes of the enrolled patients upon undergoing radical hepatectomy

Characteristic	Hepatectomy-TACE group (n = 116)	Hepatectomy alone group (n = 118)	P-value
Cirrhosis [cases (%)]			
Present	50 (43.1)	42 (35.6)	0.285
Absent	66 (56.9)	76 (64.4)	
Tumor size [cases (%)]			
5–10 cm	82 (70.7)	97 (82.2)	0.055
> 10 cm	34 (29.3)	21 (17.8)	
Operation time (min)	173.2 ± 48.6	182.3 ± 65.2	0.225
Operation blood loss (mL)	518.9 ± 441.6	421.6 ± 353.3	0.064
Blood transfusion [cases (%)]	26 (22.4)	18 (15.3)	0.183
Extent of liver resection [cases (%)]			
Major	45 (38.8)	46 (39.0)	1.000
Minor	71 (61.2)	72 (61.0)	
Resection margin [cases (%)]			
< 2 cm	91 (78.4)	92 (78.0)	1.000
≥ 2 cm	25 (21.6)	26 (22.0)	
Postoperative complications [cases (%)]	24 (20.7)	23 (19.5)	0.871
Grade 1			
Fever	5 (4.3)	3 (2.5)	0.497
Grade 2			
Fever	2 (1.7)	1 (0.8)	0.620
Ascites	5 (4.3)	3 (2.5)	0.497
Transient jaundice	5 (4.3)	6 (5.1)	1.000
Pleural effusion	3 (2.6)	3 (2.5)	1.000
Hypoalbuminemia	3 (2.6)	5 (4.2)	0.722
Grade 3			
Liver bleeding	1 (0.9)	2 (1.7)	1.000

Continuous variables are compared by Student t-test; categorical variables are compared by the χ^2 test or the Fisher's exact test

Hepatectomy-TACE: radical hepatectomy followed by adjuvant transcatheter arterial chemoembolization; Hepatectomy Alone: had undergone only radical hepatectomy

most common grade 3 or 4 adverse events in both groups were neutropenia and liver dysfunction. However, most AEs were mild and manageable and no toxicity-associated deaths occurred in this study.

Discussion

In this open-labeled, randomized, phase III trial, we evaluated the efficacy and safety of adjuvant TACE versus hepatectomy alone among HCC patients with solitary tumor ≥ 5 cm and MVI after curative resection. The results showed that, compared with the Hepatectomy Alone group, the Hepatectomy-TACE group had significantly both prolonged median DFS (17.45 vs.

9.27 months, HR = 0.70, $P = 0.020$) and OS (44.29 vs. 22.37 months, HR = 0.68, $P = 0.029$) from randomization. In subgroup analyses, we found that male patients, age < 60 years, presence of cirrhosis, tumor > 10 cm, and resection margin < 2 cm may derive a greater survival benefit from adjuvant TACE and that these factors should be considered in the selection process for future clinical trials.

MVI is a recognized risk factor for recurrence after hepatectomy in HCC patients. The presence of MVI is associated with multiple factors including tumor size. In an international multicenter study which enrolled 1073 HCC patients, Pawlik et al. [25] reported that the rate of MVI increased with tumor size (≤ 3.0 cm, 25%;

(See figure on next page.)

Fig. 2 Kaplan-Meier estimates illustrating the differences in **a** disease-free survival (DFS) and **b** overall survival (OS) of the enrolled patients who underwent radical hepatectomy alone against those who had radical hepatectomy and adjuvant TACE. TACE: transcatheter arterial chemoembolization; HR: hazard ratio; CI: confidence interval

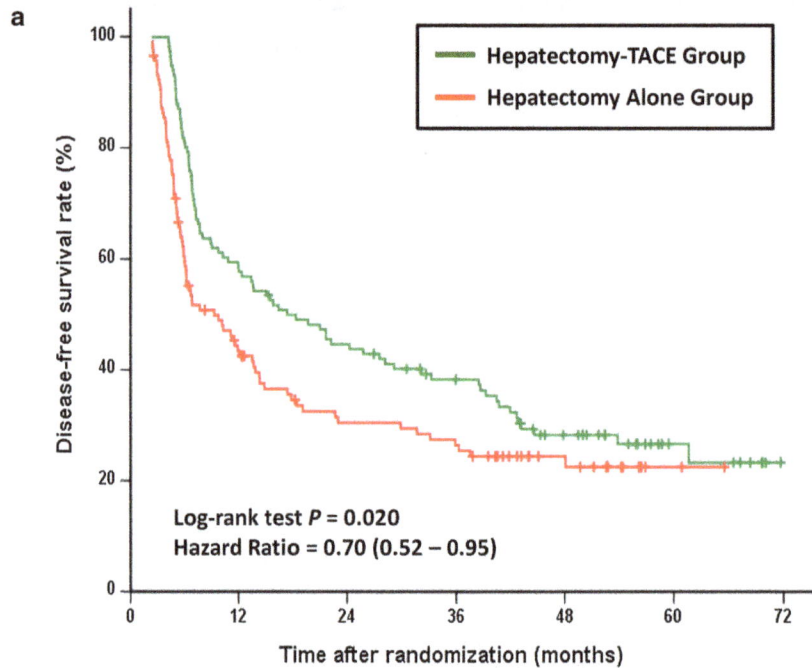

a

Log-rank test *P* = 0.020
Hazard Ratio = 0.70 (0.52 – 0.95)

Time after randomization (months)

Number of patients at risk from each group

Hepatectomy-TACE	116	68	51	39	23	8	0
Hepatectomy Alone	118	47	30	26	13	2	0

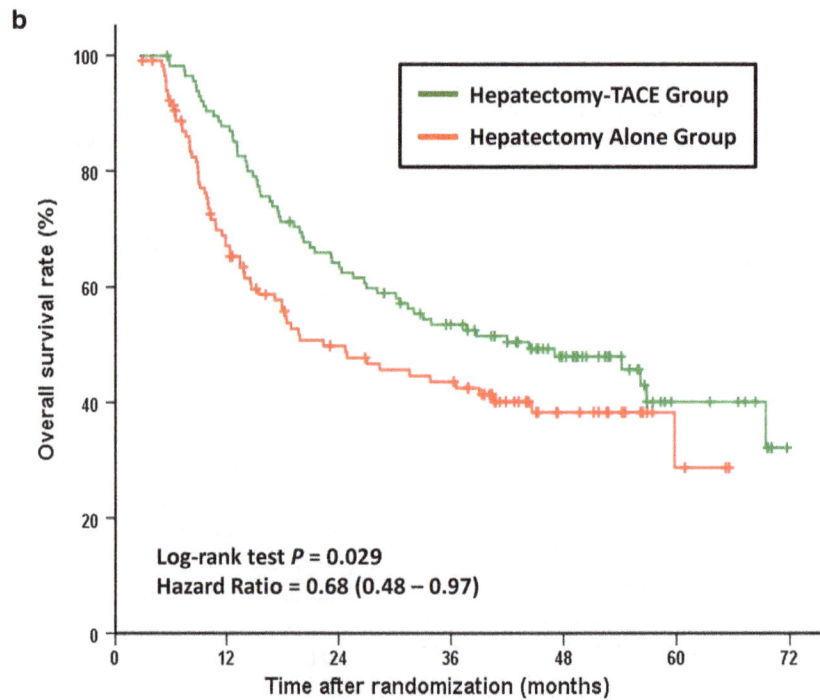

b

Log-rank test *P* = 0.029
Hazard Ratio = 0.68 (0.48 – 0.97)

Time after randomization (months)

Number of patients at risk from each group

Hepatectomy-TACE	116	101	73	56	33	9	0
Hepatectomy Alone	118	74	49	42	17	3	0

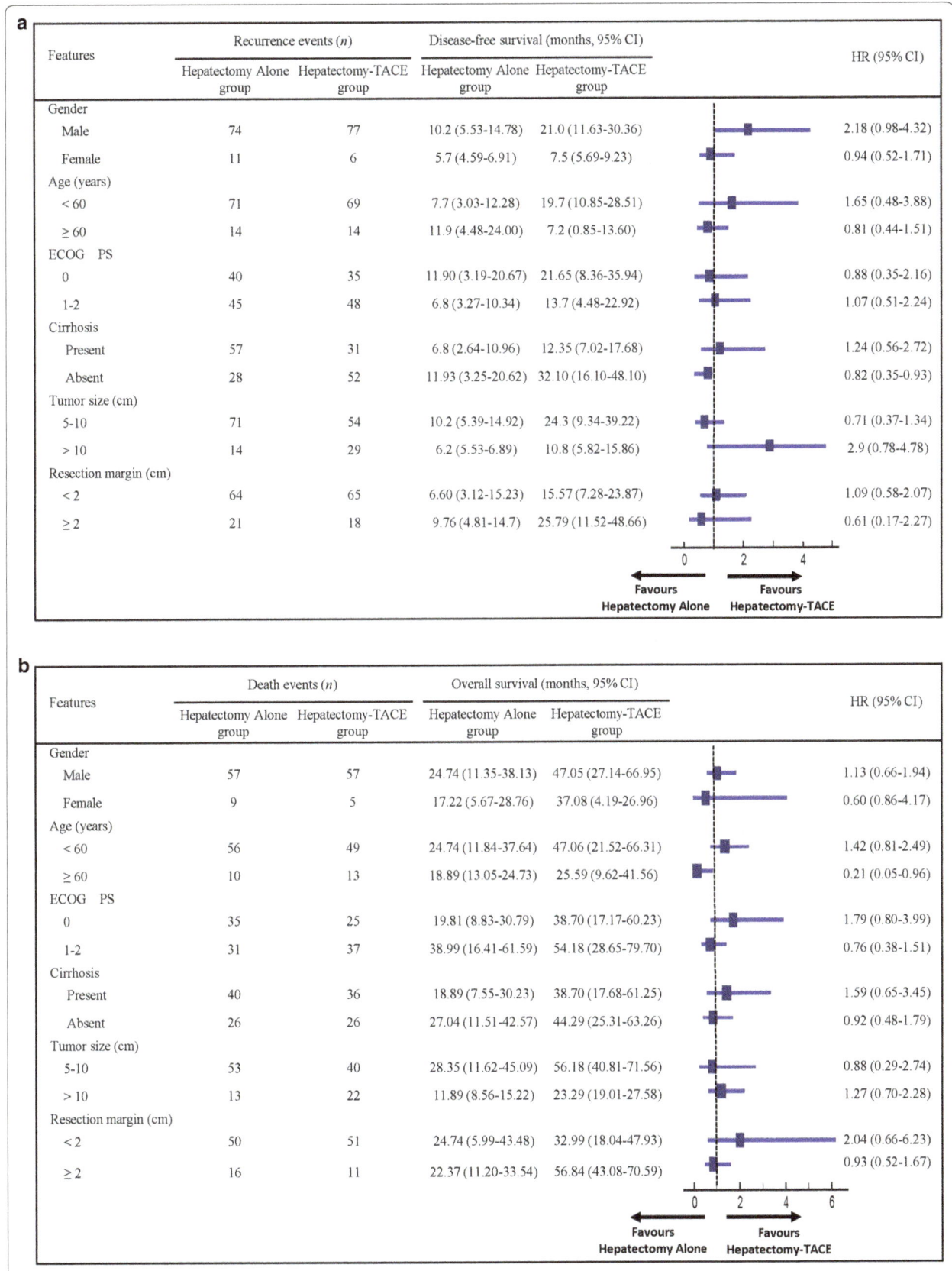

a

Features	Recurrence events (n) Hepatectomy Alone group	Recurrence events (n) Hepatectomy-TACE group	Disease-free survival (months, 95% CI) Hepatectomy Alone group	Disease-free survival (months, 95% CI) Hepatectomy-TACE group		HR (95% CI)
Gender						
Male	74	77	10.2 (5.53-14.78)	21.0 (11.63-30.36)		2.18 (0.98-4.32)
Female	11	6	5.7 (4.59-6.91)	7.5 (5.69-9.23)		0.94 (0.52-1.71)
Age (years)						
< 60	71	69	7.7 (3.03-12.28)	19.7 (10.85-28.51)		1.65 (0.48-3.88)
≥ 60	14	14	11.9 (4.48-24.00)	7.2 (0.85-13.60)		0.81 (0.44-1.51)
ECOG PS						
0	40	35	11.90 (3.19-20.67)	21.65 (8.36-35.94)		0.88 (0.35-2.16)
1-2	45	48	6.8 (3.27-10.34)	13.7 (4.48-22.92)		1.07 (0.51-2.24)
Cirrhosis						
Present	57	31	6.8 (2.64-10.96)	12.35 (7.02-17.68)		1.24 (0.56-2.72)
Absent	28	52	11.93 (3.25-20.62)	32.10 (16.10-48.10)		0.82 (0.35-0.93)
Tumor size (cm)						
5-10	71	54	10.2 (5.39-14.92)	24.3 (9.34-39.22)		0.71 (0.37-1.34)
> 10	14	29	6.2 (5.53-6.89)	10.8 (5.82-15.86)		2.9 (0.78-4.78)
Resection margin (cm)						
< 2	64	65	6.60 (3.12-15.23)	15.57 (7.28-23.87)		1.09 (0.58-2.07)
≥ 2	21	18	9.76 (4.81-14.7)	25.79 (11.52-48.66)		0.61 (0.17-2.27)

Favours Hepatectomy Alone — Favours Hepatectomy-TACE

b

Features	Death events (n) Hepatectomy Alone group	Death events (n) Hepatectomy-TACE group	Overall survival (months, 95% CI) Hepatectomy Alone group	Overall survival (months, 95% CI) Hepatectomy-TACE group		HR (95% CI)
Gender						
Male	57	57	24.74 (11.35-38.13)	47.05 (27.14-66.95)		1.13 (0.66-1.94)
Female	9	5	17.22 (5.67-28.76)	37.08 (4.19-26.96)		0.60 (0.86-4.17)
Age (years)						
< 60	56	49	24.74 (11.84-37.64)	47.06 (21.52-66.31)		1.42 (0.81-2.49)
≥ 60	10	13	18.89 (13.05-24.73)	25.59 (9.62-41.56)		0.21 (0.05-0.96)
ECOG PS						
0	35	25	19.81 (8.83-30.79)	38.70 (17.17-60.23)		1.79 (0.80-3.99)
1-2	31	37	38.99 (16.41-61.59)	54.18 (28.65-79.70)		0.76 (0.38-1.51)
Cirrhosis						
Present	40	36	18.89 (7.55-30.23)	38.70 (17.68-61.25)		1.59 (0.65-3.45)
Absent	26	26	27.04 (11.51-42.57)	44.29 (25.31-63.26)		0.92 (0.48-1.79)
Tumor size (cm)						
5-10	53	40	28.35 (11.62-45.09)	56.18 (40.81-71.56)		0.88 (0.29-2.74)
> 10	13	22	11.89 (8.56-15.22)	23.29 (19.01-27.58)		1.27 (0.70-2.28)
Resection margin (cm)						
< 2	50	51	24.74 (5.99-43.48)	32.99 (18.04-47.93)		2.04 (0.66-6.23)
≥ 2	16	11	22.37 (11.20-33.54)	56.84 (43.08-70.59)		0.93 (0.52-1.67)

Favours Hepatectomy Alone — Favours Hepatectomy-TACE

Table 3 The subsequent antitumor therapies prescribed to the enrolled hepatocellular carcinoma patients after diagnosis of tumor recurrence

Antitumor therapy	Hepatectomy-TACE group (n = 56)	Hepatectomy Alone group (n = 46)	P-value
Locoregional ablation	27	8	< 0.001
Hepatectomy[a]	2	2	1.000
Systemic chemotherapy	1	5	0.210
Sorafenib	14	5	0.029
TACE	12	26	0.016

Hepatectomy-TACE: radical hepatectomy followed by adjuvant transcatheter arterial chemoembolization; Hepatectomy Alone: had undergone only radical hepatectomy

[a] Resection of the recurrent lesion(s) in the liver

3.1–5.0 cm, 40%; 5.1–6.5 cm, 55%; and > 6.5 cm, 63%) ($P < 0.005$). Among patients with solitary tumor only, MVI occurred more frequently with tumors measuring 5.1–6.5 cm (41%) than for those with tumors measuring ≤ 5.0 cm (27%) ($P < 0.003$). Although wide resection margins may decrease the postoperative recurrence rate and improve survival outcomes [10], however, adequate resection margins were often unachievable due to the cumbersome tumor location and concomitant cirrhosis. Also, MVI beyond the resection margin may become the origin of recurrence. Also, in this study, we excluded patients with solitary tumors < 5 cm because they had a relatively low risk of recurrence due to the low rate

of MVI and the high achievability of wide resection margins.

Unfortunately, there is no universally accepted adjuvant therapy for HCC patients with MVI in which efficacy, safety, and cost-effectiveness are conclusive. Some studies have evaluated TACE as a single adjuvant approach or in combination with other therapies (including antiviral therapy and interferon-α) for HCC patients with high risks of recurrence after resection [26–29]. In addition, a recent retrospective study also showed that postoperative adjuvant TACE could prolong the recurrence-free survival (RFS) and OS among HCC patients with MVI [30]. As such, these studies provided the rational evidence to select TACE as an adjuvant therapy in this present study.

Compared with the participants in the above studies, who showed high heterogeneity in tumor stage, the participants were relatively homogeneous in our present study. Solitary HCC is considered as a curable disease, and patients usually undergo more aggressive surgical treatment, although there is no recommended adjuvant therapy in the current official guidelines for these patients with solitary HCC and MVI. To our knowledge, this is the first study to report the value of adjuvant TACE in this specific population.

Interestingly, adjuvant TACE significantly reduced early recurrence rate (within 2 years) after hepatectomy. The 1- and 2-year DFS rates were 58.6% and 44.7% for the Hepatectomy-TACE group and 43.5% and 30.6% for the Hepatectomy Alone group, respectively. However, this difference was less obvious when comparing

Table 4 Adverse events of the enrolled patients after hepatectomy from the day of randomization to the last day of follow-up

Adverse events	Hepatectomy-TACE group (n = 116)		Hepatectomy Alone group (n = 118)		P-value
	Grade 1–2	Grade 3–4	Grade 1–2	Grade 3–4	
Neutropenia	16	6	6	2	0.006
Anemia	8	2	4	2	0.312
Thrombocytopenia	15	4	3	1	< 0.001
Fever	29	3	4	0	< 0.001
Pain	16	2	5	1	0.010
Nausea/vomiting	26	1	2	0	< 0.001
Liver dysfunction	39	5	6	3	< 0.001
Fatigue	12	2	4	1	0.032

Hepatectomy-TACE: radical hepatectomy followed by adjuvant transcatheter arterial chemoembolization; Hepatectomy Alone: had undergone only radical hepatectomy

the 5-year DFS rate between the two groups (26.7% in Hepatectomy-TACE group vs. 22.6% in Hepatectomy Alone group). MVI was found to be the only independent risk factor for early recurrence, which is consistent with our previous study [31]. With the stimulation of multiple growth factors after hepatectomy, occult tumor cells proliferate rapidly and form visible recurrences as the remnant liver regenerates. The high sensitivity of actively proliferating tumor cells to chemotherapeutic agents may be an important reason for the decreased in early recurrence rate in the Hepatectomy-TACE group. Conversely, adjuvant TACE could increase the local concentration of chemotherapeutic agents in the liver, potentially avoiding the undesirable adverse events of systemic chemotherapy.

We also analyzed the underlying reasons for the considerably prolonged OS in the Hepatectomy-TACE group. After diagnosis of tumor recurrence, only 46 patients (54.1%) in the Hepatectomy Alone group underwent subsequent antitumor therapies (such as locoregional ablation, hepatectomy, systemic chemotherapy, sorafenib, and TACE; Table 3), which were less than those in the Hepatectomy-TACE group where greater proportion of patients, 67.5% (56 patients) had antitumor therapies and therefore may have resulted in a shorter OS in the Hepatectomy Alone group. Furthermore, as shown in Table 3, a greater number of patients with recurrence in the Hepatectomy-TACE group underwent locoregional ablation and were prescribed with sorafenib as a subsequent antitumor therapy. This may reflect the fact that recurrence was often localized and controllable. Conversely, more patients with recurrence in the Hepatectomy Alone group underwent relative palliative TACE, which may be associated with more extensive recurrence, as well as unfavorable factors, such as macrovascular tumor thrombus and extrahepatic metastases. However, our results should be interpreted with caution since the impact of adjuvant TACE on recurrence patterns, together with the direct therapeutic effects of adjuvant TACE itself, might collectively contribute to the survival benefits in the Hepatectomy-TACE groups.

As an important trial, the adjuvant sorafenib for hepatocellular carcinoma after resection or ablation (STORM) trial did not reach its primary endpoint of prolonging RFS [19]. The negative results of the STORM trial suggested that antitumor activity against existing or advanced HCC is not necessarily associated with efficacy in the adjuvant setting against micro-metastatic disease. In the absence of established predictive biomarkers of response to sorafenib in patients with advanced HCC, a population potential benefit from adjuvant sorafenib cannot be defined [32]. Besides, the STORM trial underscored the importance of selecting appropriate candidates with a high recurrence risk in such adjuvant settings.

Despite the results of this study demonstrating the superiority of adjuvant TACE over radical hepatectomy alone, there are still some limitations worth mentioning in this study. First, this is a single-center study. To validate the significance of adjuvant TACE in this specific population, a prospective, well-designed, multicenter, and randomized trial is necessary. Second, recent studies have reported that not only the presence of MVI but also the grade of MVI can impact the recurrence and survival of HCC patients [33, 34]. However, we did not investigate the grade of MVI due to the early design of this study protocol. Third, the optimal adjuvant TACE protocol (including chemotherapeutic agents, dosage, and interval) remains to be elucidated and further studies are required.

Conclusions

Our findings demonstrate the survival and safety benefits of adjuvant TACE in HCC patients with solitary tumor ≥ 5 cm and MVI after curative resection. However, future prospective, multicenter, randomized clinical trials are necessary to evaluate the optimal TACE regimens (including drugs and dosages) and the feasibility of combination with other antitumor therapies.

Authors' contributions
RPG designed and conducted this study and contributed to manuscript drafting. WW, PEJ, SHL and ZXG contributed equally to the data collection, analysis and interpretation, and manuscript drafting. YFZ, YHL, XJL, LX, MS, LZ, and MSC contributed to participant enrollment, clinical treatment, follow-up, data interpretation, and critical manuscript revision. All authors read and approved the final manuscript.

Author details
[1] State Key Laboratory of Oncology in South China, Collaborative Innovation Center for Cancer Medicine, Sun Yat-sen University Cancer Center, Guangzhou 510060, Guangdong, P. R. China. [2] Department of Hepatobiliary and Pancreatic Surgery, Sun Yat-sen University Cancer Center, Guangzhou 510060, Guangdong, P. R. China. [3] Department of Pathology, Sun Yat-sen University Cancer Center, Guangzhou 510060, Guangdong, P. R. China. [4] Department of Medical Imaging, Sun Yat-sen University Cancer Center, Guangzhou 510060, Guangdong, P. R. China.

Acknowledgements
We acknowledge all the staffs of the Department of Hepatobiliary and Pancreatic Surgery in Sun Yat-sen University Cancer Center for their assistance and collaboration in this work. We would like to thank Editage (http://www.editage.com) for their assistance in the English language editing.

Competing interests
The authors declare that they have no competing interests.
Requirements for Registration of Pharmaceuticals for Human Use (ICH), Version E6). The protocol and all modifications have been approved by the Institutional Review Board and Ethics Committee of Sun Yat-Sen University Cancer Center (Approval No: YB 2005-06-08). All patients provided written informed consents to participate.

Funding
This study was supported by the National Natural Science Foundation of China (No. 81172037); Science and Technology Program of Guangdong Province, China (No. 2013B021800159); and Clinical Trials Project (308 Project) of Sun Yat-sen University Cancer Center (No. 308-2015-014).

References

1. Torre LA, Bray F, Siegel RL, Ferlay J, Lortet-Tieulent J, Jemal A. Global cancer statistics, 2012. CA Cancer J Clin. 2015;65(2):87–108. https://doi.org/10.3322/caac.21262.

2. He MK, Le Y, Li QJ, Yu ZS, Li SH, Wei W, et al. Hepatic artery infusion chemotherapy using mFOLFOX versus transarterial chemoembolization for massive unresectable hepatocellular carcinoma: a prospective non-randomized study. Chin J Cancer. 2017;36(1):83. https://doi.org/10.1186/s40880-017-0251-2.

3. Chen W, Zheng R, Baade PD, Zhang S, Zeng H, Bray F, et al. Cancer statistics in China, 2015. CA Cancer J Clin. 2016;66(2):115–32. https://doi.org/10.3322/caac.21338.

4. Llovet JM, Bruix J. Novel advancements in the management of hepatocellular carcinoma in 2008. J Hepatol. 2008;48(Suppl 1):S20–37. https://doi.org/10.1016/j.jhep.2008.01.022.

5. de Lope CR, Tremosini S, Forner A, Reig M, Bruix J. Management of HCC. J Hepatol. 2012;56(Suppl 1):S75–87. https://doi.org/10.1016/S0168-8278(12)60009-9.

6. Bruix J, Sherman M, American Association for the Study of Liver D. Management of hepatocellular carcinoma: an update. Hepatology. 2011;53(3):1020–2. https://doi.org/10.1002/hep.24199.

7. European Association For The Study Of The L, European Organisation For R, Treatment Of C. EASL-EORTC clinical practice guidelines: management of hepatocellular carcinoma. J Hepatol. 2012;56(4):908–43. https://doi.org/10.1016/j.jhep.2011.12.001.

8. Imamura H, Matsuyama Y, Tanaka E, Ohkubo T, Hasegawa K, Miyagawa S, et al. Risk factors contributing to early and late phase intrahepatic recurrence of hepatocellular carcinoma after hepatectomy. J Hepatol. 2003;38(2):200–7.

9. Shi M, Zhang CQ, Zhang YQ, Liang XM, Li JQ. Micrometastases of solitary hepatocellular carcinoma and appropriate resection margin. World J Surg. 2004;28(4):376–81. https://doi.org/10.1007/s00268-003-7308-x.

10. Shi M, Guo RP, Lin XJ, Zhang YQ, Chen MS, Zhang CQ, et al. Partial hepatectomy with wide versus narrow resection margin for solitary hepatocellular carcinoma: a prospective randomized trial. Ann Surg. 2007;245(1):36–43. https://doi.org/10.1097/01.sla.0000231758.07868.71.

11. Lim KC, Chow PK, Allen JC, Chia GS, Lim M, Cheow PC, et al. Microvascular invasion is a better predictor of tumor recurrence and overall survival following surgical resection for hepatocellular carcinoma compared to the Milan criteria. Ann Surg. 2011;254(1):108–13. https://doi.org/10.1097/SLA.0b013e31821ad884.

12. Hung HH, Lei HJ, Chau GY, Su CW, Hsia CY, Kao WY, et al. Milan criteria, multi-nodularity, and microvascular invasion predict the recurrence patterns of hepatocellular carcinoma after resection. J Gastrointest Surg. 2013;17(4):702–11. https://doi.org/10.1007/s11605-012-2087-z.

13. Du M, Chen L, Zhao J, Tian F, Zeng H, Tan Y, et al. Microvascular invasion (MVI) is a poorer prognostic predictor for small hepatocellular carcinoma. BMC Cancer. 2014;14:38. https://doi.org/10.1186/1471-2407-14-38.

14. Li SH, Wei W, Guo RP, Shi M, Guo ZX, Chen ZY, et al. Long-term outcomes after curative resection for patients with macroscopically solitary hepatocellular carcinoma without macrovascular invasion and an analysis of prognostic factors. Med Oncol. 2013;30(4):696. https://doi.org/10.1007/s12032-013-0696-3.

15. Chen LT, Chen MF, Li LA, Lee PH, Jeng LB, Lin DY, et al. Long-term results of a randomized, observation-controlled, phase III trial of adjuvant interferon Alfa-2b in hepatocellular carcinoma after curative resection. Ann Surg. 2012;255(1):8–17. https://doi.org/10.1097/SLA.0b013e3182363ff9.

16. Yamamoto M, Arii S, Sugahara K, Tobe T. Adjuvant oral chemotherapy to prevent recurrence after curative resection for hepatocellular carcinoma. Br J Surg. 1996;83(3):336–40.

17. Xia Y, Qiu Y, Li J, Shi L, Wang K, Xi T, et al. Adjuvant therapy with capecitabine postpones recurrence of hepatocellular carcinoma after curative resection: a randomized controlled trial. Ann Surg Oncol. 2010;17(12):3137–44. https://doi.org/10.1245/s10434-010-1148-3

18. Nitta H, Beppu T, Imai K, Hayashi H, Chikamoto A, Baba H. Adjuvant hepatic arterial infusion chemotherapy after hepatic resection of hepa-

tocellular carcinoma with macroscopic vascular invasion. World J Surg. 2013;37(5):1034–42. https://doi.org/10.1007/s00268-013-1957-1.

19. Bruix J, Takayama T, Mazzaferro V, Chau GY, Yang J, Kudo M, et al. Adjuvant sorafenib for hepatocellular carcinoma after resection or ablation (STORM): a phase 3, randomised, double-blind, placebo-controlled trial. Lancet Oncol. 2015;16(13):1344–54. https://doi.org/10.1016/S1470-2045(15)00198-9.

20. Kuczynski EA, Kerbel RS. Implications of vessel co-option in sorafenib-resistant hepatocellular carcinoma. Chin J Cancer. 2016;35(1):97. https://doi.org/10.1186/s40880-016-0162-7.

21. Zhong C, Guo RP, Li JQ, Shi M, Wei W, Chen MS, et al. A randomized controlled trial of hepatectomy with adjuvant transcatheter arterial chemoembolization versus hepatectomy alone for Stage III A hepatocellular carcinoma. J Cancer Res Clin Oncol. 2009;135(10):1437–45. https://doi.org/10.1007/s00432-009-0588-2.

22. Group ICoHEW. ICH harmonised tripartite—guideline for good clinical practice E6 (R1). Buckinghamshire: Institute of Clinical Research Marlow; 1996.

23. Vauthey JN, Lauwers GY, Esnaola NF, Do KA, Belghiti J, Mirza N, et al. Simplified staging for hepatocellular carcinoma. J Clin Oncol. 2002;20(6):1527–36.

24. Shi M, Chen JA, Lin XJ, Guo RP, Yuan YF, Chen MS, et al. Transarterial chemoembolization as initial treatment for unresectable hepatocellular carcinoma in southern China. World J Gastroenterol. 2010;16(2):264–9.

25. Pawlik TM, Delman KA, Vauthey JN, Nagorney DM, Ng IO, Ikai I, et al. Tumor size predicts vascular invasion and histologic grade: implications for selection of surgical treatment for hepatocellular carcinoma. Liver Transpl. 2005;11(9):1086–92. https://doi.org/10.1002/lt.20472.

26. Zhu SL, Zhong JH, Ke Y, Xiao HM, Ma L, Chen J, et al. Comparative efficacy of postoperative transarterial chemoembolization with or without antiviral therapy for hepatitis B virus-related hepatocellular carcinoma. Tumour Biol. 2015;36(8):6277–84. https://doi.org/10.1007/s13277-015-3313-6.

27. Zuo CH, Xia M, Liu JS, Qiu XX, Lei X, Xu RC, et al. Transcatheter arterial chemoembolization combined with interferon-alpha is safe and effective for patients with hepatocellular carcinoma after curative resection. Asian Pac J Cancer Prev. 2015;16(1):245–51.

28. Liu C, Sun L, Xu J, Zhao Y. Clinical efficacy of postoperative adjuvant transcatheter arterial chemoembolization on hepatocellular carcinoma. World J Surg Oncol. 2016;14(1):100. https://doi.org/10.1186/s12957-016-0855-z.

29. Peng BG, He Q, Li JP, Zhou F. Adjuvant transcatheter arterial chemoembolization improves efficacy of hepatectomy for patients with hepatocellular carcinoma and portal vein tumor thrombus. Am J Surg. 2009;198(3):313–8. https://doi.org/10.1016/j.amjsurg.2008.09.026.

30. Sun JJ, Wang K, Zhang CZ, Guo WX, Shi J, Cong WM, et al. Postoperative adjuvant transcatheter arterial chemoembolization after R0 hepatectomy improves outcomes of patients who have hepatocellular carcinoma with microvascular invasion. Ann Surg Oncol. 2016;23(4):1344–51. https://doi.org/10.1245/s10434-015-5008-z.

31. Li SH, Guo ZX, Xiao CZ, Wei W, Shi M, Chen ZY, et al. Risk factors for early and late intrahepatic recurrence in patients with single hepatocellular carcinoma without macrovascular invasion after curative resection. Asian Pac J Cancer Prev. 2013;14(8):4759–63.

32. Kelley RK. Adjuvant sorafenib for liver cancer: wrong stage, wrong dose. Lancet Oncol. 2015;16(13):1279–81. https://doi.org/10.1016/S1470-2045(15)00296-X.

33. Iguchi T, Shirabe K, Aishima S, Wang H, Fujita N, Ninomiya M, et al. New pathologic stratification of microvascular invasion in hepatocellular carcinoma: predicting prognosis after living-donor liver transplantation. Transplantation. 2015;99(6):1236–42. https://doi.org/10.1097/TP.0000000000000489.

34. Sumie S, Nakashima O, Okuda K, Kuromatsu R, Kawaguchi A, Nakano M, et al. The significance of classifying microvascular invasion in patients with hepatocellular carcinoma. Ann Surg Oncol. 2014;21(3):1002–9. https://doi.org/10.1245/s10434-013-3376-9.

18

Proposal and validation of a modified staging system to improve the prognosis predictive performance of the 8th AJCC/UICC pTNM staging system for gastric adenocarcinoma: a multicenter study with external validation

Cheng Fang[1†], Wei Wang[1†], Jing-Yu Deng[2†], Zhe Sun[3], Sharvesh Raj Seeruttun[1], Zhen-Ning Wang[3], Hui-Mian Xu[3*], Han Liang[2*] and Zhi-Wei Zhou[1*] (ID)

Abstract

Background: The 8th edition of the American Joint Committee on Cancer/Union for International Cancer Control (AJCC/UICC) pathological tumor-node-metastasis (pTNM) staging system may have increased accuracy in predicting prognosis of gastric cancer due to its important modifications from previous editions. However, the homogeneity in prognosis within each subgroup classified according to the 8th edition may still exist. This study aimed to compare and analyze the prognosis prediction abilities of the 8th and 7th editions of AJCC/UICC pTNM staging system for gastric cancer and propose a modified pTNM staging system with external validation.

Methods: In total, clinical data of 7911 patients from three high-capacity institutions in China and 10,208 cases from the Surveillance, Epidemiology, and End Results (SEER) Program Registry were analyzed. The homogeneity, discriminatory ability, and monotonicity of the gradient assessments of the 8th and 7th editions of AJCC/UICC pTNM staging system were compared using log-rank x^2, linear-trend x^2, likelihood-ratio x^2 statistics and Akaike information criterion (AIC) calculations, on which a modified pTNM classification with external validation using the SEER database was proposed.

Results: Considerable stage migration, mainly for stage III, between the 8th and 7th editions was observed in both cohorts. The survival rates of subgroups of patients within stage IIIA, IIIB, or IIIC classified according to both editions were significantly different, demonstrating poor homogeneity for patient stratification. A modified pTNM staging

*Correspondence: xuhuimian@126.com; tjlianghan@126.com; zhouzhw@sysucc.org.cn
†Cheng Fang, Wei Wang and Jing-Yu Deng contributed equally to this work
[1] Department of Gastric Surgery, Sun Yat-sen University Cancer Center, State Key Laboratory of Oncology in South China, Collaborative Innovation Center for Cancer Medicine, 651 Dongfeng Road East, Guangzhou, Guangdong 510060, P. R. China
[2] Department of Gastric Cancer Surgery, Tianjin Medical University Cancer Institute & Hospital, Tianjin 300000, P. R. China
[3] Department of Surgical Oncology, The First Hospital of China Medical University, Shenyang 110000, P. R. China

system using data from the Chinese cohort was then formulated and demonstrated an improved homogeneity in these abovementioned subgroups. This staging system was further validated using data from the SEER cohort, and similar promising results were obtained. Compared with the 8th and 7th editions, the modified pTNM staging system displayed the highest log-rank χ^2, linear-trend χ^2, likelihood-ratio χ^2, and lowest AIC values, indicating its superior discriminatory ability, monotonicity, homogeneity and prognosis prediction ability in both populations.

Conclusions: The 8th edition of AJCC/UICC pTNM staging system is superior to the 7th edition, but still results in homogeneity in prognosis prediction. Our modified pTNM staging system demonstrated the optimal stratification and prognosis prediction ability in two large cohorts of different gastric cancer populations.

Keywords: Pathological TNM staging system, Gastric cancer, Akaike information criterion (AIC), Prognosis prediction, SEER, Chinese

Background

Gastric cancer (GC) remains both the second most prevalent cancer [1] and the most frequent cause of cancer-related death in China [2]. Nearly half of the global total new GC diagnoses each year occur in China [3, 4]. Although current practice includes chemotherapy, irradiation, and/or targeted therapy in the treatment protocol, surgical resection remains the only means for cure [5]. Regarding the prognostic markers for patients undergoing surgical treatment, the American Joint Committee on Cancer (AJCC)/International Union against Cancer (UICC) pathological tumor-node-metastasis (pTNM) staging system is currently used as the most important and basic tool for patient stratification. The AJCC/UICC has published the 8th edition of pTNM staging system for GC and has introduced some changes on the basis of the 7th edition [6, 7]. Among those changes, the most important one is the subdivision of the category N3ab into N3a and N3b, which affects consequent staging, especially for stage III. Thus, the prediction of survival probability of stage III patients are believed to be considerably affected, and this latest edition may have implications on treatment. To date, although the prognosis prediction ability of the 8th AJCC/UICC pTNM staging system for GC has already been addressed, its accuracy remains unclear.

In this retrospective study, we compared the prognosis prediction abilities of the 8th and 7th editions of AJCC/UICC pTNM staging system using a large Chinese multicenter database of GC as a training cohort. We then proposed a modified pTNM staging system for better prognosis prediction of advanced GC and performed external validation in a large cohort of Western GC patients.

Patients and methods

Patients

Between January 1, 2000 and December 31, 2012, a consecutive cohort of GC patients who underwent radical gastrectomy at the Department of Gastric Surgery at the Sun Yat-sen University Cancer Center (SYSUCC),

Department of Gastric Cancer Surgery at Tianjin Medical University Cancer Institute & Hospital (TJMU), and Department of Surgical Oncology at the First Hospital of China Medical University (CMU) were selected. The eligibility criteria were as follows: (1) pathologically confirmed primary gastric adenocarcinoma; (2) no synchronous malignancy; (3) no distant metastasis; (4) no preoperative chemotherapy; (5) patients having undergone gastrectomy plus lymphadenectomy (limited or extended) according to the Japanese Gastric Cancer Treatment Guidelines 2014 (version 3) [8]; (6) R0 resection (i.e., no residual macroscopic or microscopic tumor); (7) postoperative survival of at least 3 months; and (8) patients with no missing data regarding the analyzed clinicopathological characteristics.

From 18 registries of the Surveillance, Epidemiology, and End Results Program (SEER), a retrospective review of clinical records of all GC patients who underwent gastrectomy between January 1998 and December 2012 was performed. The patients were excluded if they had incomplete/missing information regarding their age, tumor size, tumor location, Lauren type, depth of invasion, lymph node status, non-radical resection, and/or status of distant metastasis. This study protocol was approved by the institutional review boards of SYSU, TJMU, and CMU.

Follow-up

A strict disease-monitoring program with outpatient records, telephonic interviews, and electronic messages was conducted and included clinical and laboratory examinations every 3 months for the first 2 years, every 6 months from the 3rd to the 5th years, and annually thereafter until at least 5 years after the operation or until the patient died, whichever came first. The last date of follow-up was December 31, 2016. The endpoint of this study was overall survival (OS), which was defined as the date from surgery until the date of death or the last date of follow up. Patients who were still alive after the completion of follow-up were all censored.

Statistical analyses

All patients were restaged according to the 8th and 7th AJCC/UICC GC pTNM staging systems. Survival curves were plotted using the Kaplan–Meier method, and the log-rank test was used to determine the relationships between the investigated clinicopathological factors and OS. Factors deemed having potential significance ($P<0.05$) on univariate analysis were included in multivariate analyses. Multivariate analysis of OS was performed using the Cox proportional hazards model with the forward logistic regression (LR) stepwise procedure for variable selection.

The prognosis prediction performance of the 8th and 7th AJCC/UICC GC staging systems was investigated in terms of discriminatory ability (differences in the survival among patients in different stages), monotonicity (patients at earlier stages with longer survival than those in later stages), homogeneity (small differences in the survival among patients within the same stage) [9]. The log-rank χ^2 test, linear-trend χ^2 test, likelihood-ratio χ^2 test, and Akaike information criterion (AIC) within the Cox regression model were used to compare the stratification and prognosis prediction performance between the two editions of staging systems. The discriminatory ability and monotonicity of gradient assessments were measured using the log-rank χ^2 test and the linear-trend χ^2 test. Homogeneity was measured using the likelihood-ratio χ^2 test, and AIC was used to measure the prognostic stratifications. Higher log-rank χ^2 and linear-trend χ^2 scores indicated better discriminatory ability and monotonicity, higher likelihood-ratio χ^2 scores indicated greater homogeneity, and smaller AIC values represented better prognostic stratification. Hazard ratios (HR) and 95% confidence intervals (95% CI) were also generated. All calculations were performed using SPSS 20.0 software (SPSS Inc., Chicago, IL, USA), and a P value <0.05 was considered statistically significant.

Results

Patient clinicopathological features, univariate and multivariate analyses

After screening of all the patients to be investigated, 7911 patients from the Chinese database were identified as being eligible (median age, 59 years; age range, 15–89 years) and were defined as the training cohort (Fig. 1). Among 31,988 cases from 18 SEER registries, 10,208 were eligible (median age, 67 years; age range, 14–100 years) and were defined as the external validation cohort. The median follow-up was 74 months (range, 1–182 months). The proportions of patients with ≤ 15 and > 15 retrieved lymph nodes (LNs) were 30.5% and 69.5%, respectively, in the training cohort and 53.2% and 46.8%, respectively, in the external validation cohort. Table 1 illustrates the association of

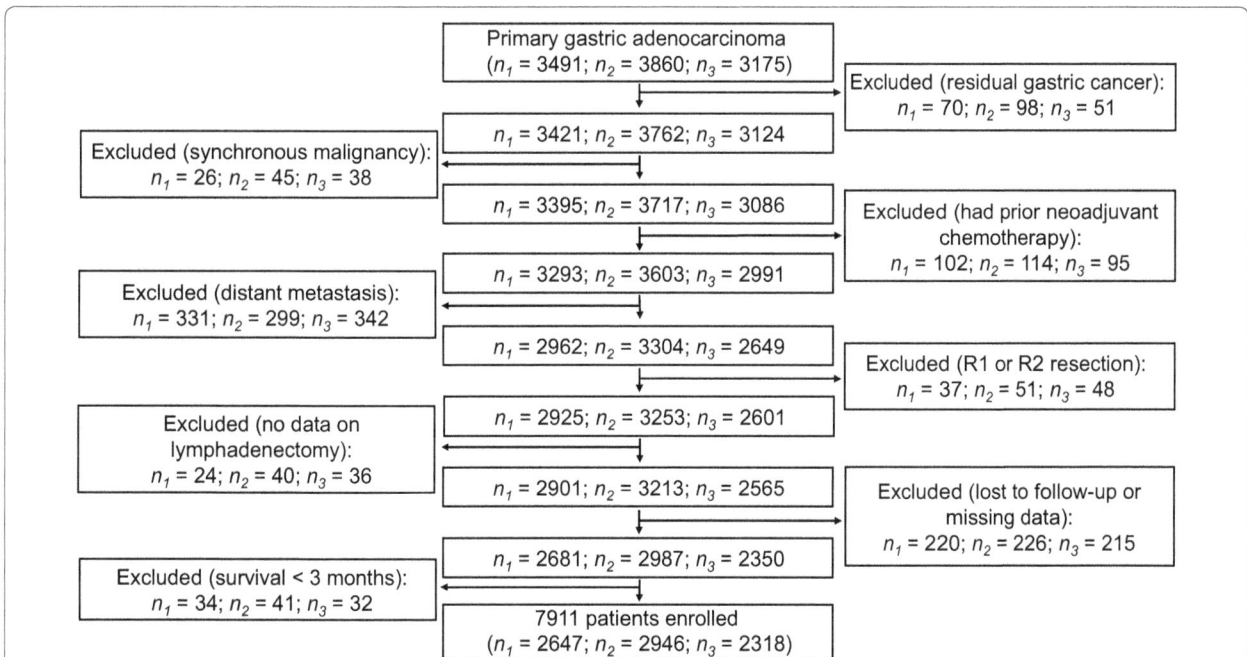

Fig. 1 A flow diagram illustrating the selection process for the training cohort of gastric cancer from 3 Chinese institutions. n_1 the number of patients from Sun Yat-sen University Cancer Center, n_2 the number of patients from the First Hospital of China Medical University, n_3 the number of patients from Tianjin Medical University Cancer Institute and Hospital, *R0 resection* complete resection of the tumor with microscopically negative surgical margins

Table 1 Clinicopathologic variables and univariate analysis of the Chinese training cohort and SEER external validation cohort of gastric cancer patients

Variable	Training cohort ($n = 7911$)			External validation cohort ($n = 10,208$)		
	No. of patients [cases (%)]	5-year OS rate (%)	P value	No. of patients [cases (%)]	5-year OS rate (%)	P value
Age (years)			< 0.001			< 0.001
≤ 59	4117 (52.0)	57.6		5142 (50.4)	47.1	
> 59	3794 (48.0)	48.0		5066 (49.6)	34.9	
Gender			0.108			0.082
Male	5586 (70.6)	52.5		6360 (62.3)	40.1	
Female	2325 (29.4)	54.3		3848 (37.7)	42.3	
Tumor location			< 0.001			< 0.001
Antrum	3578 (45.2)	61.4		3382 (33.1)	43.2	
Body	1523 (19.3)	50.5		2701 (26.5)	47.2	
Cardia/fundus	2144 (27.1)	47.7		3694 (36.2)	36.9	
Whole stomach	666 (8.4)	30.7		431 (4.2)	19.1	
Tumor size (cm)			< 0.001			< 0.001
≤ 4.5	4081 (51.6)	65.5		5086 (49.8)	51.4	
> 4.5	3830 (48.4)	39.9		5122 (50.2)	31.1	
Lauren type			< 0.001			< 0.001
Intestinal	3329 (42.1)	59.7		4062 (39.8)	47.7	
Diffuse	4582 (57.9)	48.2		6146 (60.2)	36.6	
pT stage			< 0.001			< 0.001
T1	954 (12.1)	95.6		2172 (21.3)	72.3	
T2	1447 (18.3)	66.4		1402 (13.7)	55.0	
T3	1291 (16.3)	53.2		3901 (38.2)	33.4	
T4a	3675 (46.5)	40.6		2061 (20.2)	22.5	
T4b	544 (6.9)	26.8		672 (6.6)	18.4	
pN stage			< 0.001			< 0.001
N0	2870 (36.3)	79.6		4014 (39.3)	62.3	
N1	1403 (17.7)	57.6		2069 (20.3)	40.4	
N2	1547 (19.6)	44.0		1849 (18.1)	30.0	
N3a	1407 (17.8)	24.2		1654 (16.2)	16.4	
N3b	684 (8.6)	14.1		622 (6.1)	8.9	
pTNM stage (7th ed.)			< 0.001			< 0.001
IA	801 (10.1)	96.6		1718 (16.8)	76.6	
IB	735 (9.3)	84.4		1048 (10.3)	62.5	
IIA	699 (8.8)	75.5		1507 (14.8)	51.3	
IIB	1499 (18.9)	63.0		1512 (14.8)	38.1	
IIIA	1248 (15.8)	46.6		1410 (13.8)	29.6	
IIIB	1352 (17.1)	35.8		1777 (17.4)	20.9	
IIIC	1577 (19.9)	17.4		1236 (12.1)	10.9	
pTNM stage (8th ed.)			< 0.001			< 0.001
IA	801 (10.1)	96.6		1718 (16.8)	76.6	
IB	735 (9.3)	84.4		1048 (10.3)	62.5	
IIA	699 (8.8)	75.5		1507 (14.8)	51.3	
IIB	1499 (18.9)	63.0		1507 (14.8)	38.2	
IIIA	2076 (26.2)	44.5		2012 (19.7)	28.5	
IIIB	1340 (16.9)	23.2		1643 (16.1)	16.9	
IIIC	761 (9.6)	13.6		773 (7.6)	8.1	

Table 1 (continued)

Variable	Training cohort ($n = 7911$)			External validation cohort ($n = 10,208$)		
	No. of patients [cases (%)]	5-year OS rate (%)	P value	No. of patients [cases (%)]	5-year OS rate (%)	P value
pTNM stage (modified)			< 0.001			< 0.001
IA	801 (10.1)	96.6		1718 (16.8)	76.6	
IB	735 (9.3)	84.4		1048 (10.3)	62.5	
IIA	699 (8.8)	75.5		1507 (14.8)	51.3	
IIB	1499 (18.9)	63.0		1507 (14.8)	38.2	
IIIA	1078 (13.6)	50.9		1420 (13.9)	30.3	
IIIB	1447 (18.3)	36.9		1668 (16.3)	21.7	
IIIC	1652 (20.9)	16.0		1340 (13.1)	9.7	

p pathological, *TNM* tumor-node-metastasis, *ed.* edition

the investigated clinicopathological features with the 5-year OS rates of GC patients. The median tumor size was 4.5 cm (range, 0.1–35.0 cm), and the median number of LNs retrieved was 21 (range, 1–118) in the training cohort. For the external validation cohort, the median tumor size was 4.1 cm (range, 0.1–30.0 cm), and the median number of LNs retrieved was 15 (range, 1–90). In the univariate analyses of both cohorts, age, tumor location, tumor size, Lauren type, pT stage, pN stage, and pTNM stage classified according to the 7th and 8th editions of AJCC/UICC staging system were significantly associated with the 5-year OS rates (all P < 0.001).

In multivariate analyses, age, tumor size, tumor location, Lauren type, and pTNM stage classified according to the 7th and 8th editions of AJCC/UICC staging system were identified as independent prognostic factors (all P < 0.001; Table 2).

Stage migration

Figure 2 illustrates the stage migration between the 7th and 8th AJCC/UICC staging systems for both cohorts. The migration was mainly observed in stage III patients. In the training cohort, 197 (2.5%) and 1841 (23.2%) patients were observed to be upstaged and downstaged, respectively, as classified according to the 8th edition over the 7th edition of AJCC/UICC staging system. The external validation cohort similarly demonstrated that 260 patients (2.5%) were upstaged, and 1320 patients (12.9%) were downstaged.

Discriminatory ability and monotonicity of the 7th and 8th AJCC/UICC staging systems

The OS curves of patients grouped according to the two editions of AJCC/UICC staging system are displayed in Fig. 3a, b, d, e. The 5-year OS rates of the training and external validation cohorts were 53.0% and 41.0%,

Table 2 Multivariate survival analyses of the training and external validation cohorts of gastric cancer patients

Variable	The 7th AJCC/UICC staging system			The 8th AJCC/UICC staging system			The modified staging system		
	P value	HR	95% CI	P value	HR	95% CI	P value	HR	95% CI
Training cohort									
Age	< 0.001	1.017	1.014–1.020	< 0.001	1.018	1.015–1.021	< 0.001	1.017	1.014–1.020
Tumor size	< 0.001	1.058	1.045–1.071	< 0.001	1.055	1.042–1.068	< 0.001	1.056	1.043–1.069
Tumor location	< 0.001	1.093	1.058–1.129	< 0.001	1.105	1.070–1.141	< 0.001	1.105	1.070–1.142
Lauren type	< 0.001	1.178	1.098–1.265	< 0.001	1.183	1.102–1.270	< 0.001	1.170	1.090–1.256
pTNM stage	< 0.001	1.547	1.511–1.584	< 0.001	1.644	1.601–1.687	< 0.001	1.575	1.538–1.612
External validation cohort									
Age	< 0.001	1.030	1.028–1.032	< 0.001	1.030	1.028–1.033	< 0.001	1.030	1.028–1.032
Tumor size	0.037	1.001	1.000–1.002	0.067			0.020	1.001	1.000–1.002
Tumor location	< 0.001	1.106	1.072–1.141	< 0.001	1.109	1.076–1.143	< 0.001	1.105	1.071–1.140
Lauren type	< 0.001	1.182	1.113–1.255	< 0.001	1.189	1.120–1.262	< 0.001	1.169	1.101–1.241
pTNM stage	< 0.001	1.387	1.364–1.411	< 0.001	1.432	1.408–1.456	< 0.001	1.387	1.363–1.410

HR hazard ratio, *CI* confidence interval, *p* pathological classification, *TNM* tumor-node-metastasis staging system

a

The training cohort [cases (%)] — 7th ed. / 8th ed. / Modified

T \ N	N0	N1	N2	N3a	N3b
T1	801 (10.1) IA/IA/IA	84 (1.1) IB/IB/IB	51 (0.6) IIA/IIA/IIA	18 (0.2) IIB/IIB/IIB	0 (0.0) IIB/IIIB/IIIB
T2	651 (8.2) IB/IB/IB	271 (3.4) IIA/IIA/IIA	266 (3.4) IIB/IIB/IIB	182 (2.3) IIIA/IIIA/IIIB	77 (1.0) IIIA/IIIB/IIIC
T3	377 (4.8) IIA/IIA/IIA	263 (3.3) IIB/IIB/IIB	292 (3.9) IIIA/IIIA/IIIA	239 (3.0) IIIB/IIIB/IIIB	120 (1.5) IIIB/IIIC/IIIC
T4a	952 (12.0) IIB/IIB/IIB	697 (8.8) IIIA/IIIA/IIIA	816 (10.3) IIIB/IIIB/IIIB	814 (10.3) IIIC/IIIC/IIIC	396 (5.0) IIIC/IIIC/IIIC
T4b	89 (1.1) IIIB/IIIB/IIIA	88 (1.1) IIIB/IIIB/IIIB	122 (1.5) IIIC/IIIC/IIIB	154 (1.9) IIIC/IIIC/IIIC	91 (1.2) IIIC/IIIC/IIIC

b

The external validation cohort [cases (%)] — 7th ed. / 8th ed. / Modified

T \ N	N0	N1	N2	N3a	N3b
T1	1718 (16.8) IA/IA/IA	304 (3.0) IB/IB/IB	106 (1.0) IIA/IIA/IIA	39 (0.4) IIB/IIB/IIB	5 (0.05) IIB/IIIB/IIIB
T2	744 (7.3) IB/IB/IB	347 (3.4) IIA/IIA/IIA	190 (1.9) IIB/IIB/IIB	100 (1.0) IIIA/IIIA/IIIB	21 (0.2) IIIA/IIIB/IIIC
T3	1054 (10.3) IIA/IIA/IIA	911 (8.9) IIB/IIB/IIB	905 (8.9) IIIA/IIIA/IIIA	797 (7.8) IIIB/IIIB/IIIB	234 (2.3) IIIB/IIIC/IIIC
T4a	367 (3.6) IIB/IIB/IIB	384 (3.8) IIIA/IIIA/IIIA	492 (4.8) IIIB/IIIB/IIIB	541 (5.3) IIIC/IIIC/IIIC	277 (2.7) IIIC/IIIC/IIIC
T4b	131 (1.3) IIIB/IIIA/IIIA	123 (1.2) IIIB/IIIB/IIIB	156 (1.5) IIIC/IIIB/IIIB	177 (1.7) IIIC/IIIC/IIIC	85 (0.8) IIIC/IIIC/IIIC

c

The training cohort — pTNM staging system

Stage	7th edition	8th edition	Modified
Stage I	1536 (19.4)	1536 (19.4)	1536 (19.4)
I A	801 (10.1)	801 (10.1)	801 (10.1)
I B	735 (9.3)	735 (9.3)	735 (9.3)
Stage II	2198 (27.8)	2198 (27.7)	2198 (27.7)
II A	699 (8.8)	699 (8.8)	699 (8.8)
II B	1499 (18.9)	1499 (18.9)	1499 (18.9)
Stage III	4177 (52.8)	4177 (52.8)	4177 (52.8)
III A	1248 (15.8)	2076 (26.2)	1078 (13.6)
III B	1352 (17.1)	1340 (16.9)	1447 (18.3)
III C	1577 (19.9)	761 (9.6)	1652 (20.9)

d

The external validation cohort — pTNM staging system

Stage	7th edition	8th edition	Modified
Stage I	2766 (27.1)	2766 (27.1)	2766 (27.1)
I A	1718 (16.8)	1718 (16.8)	1718 (16.8)
I B	1048 (10.3)	1048 (10.3)	1048 (10.3)
Stage II	3019 (29.6)	3014 (29.5)	3014 (29.5)
II A	1507 (14.8)	1507 (14.8)	1507 (14.8)
II B	1512 (14.8)	1507 (14.8)	1507 (14.8)
Stage III	4423 (43.3)	4428 (43.4)	4428 (43.4)
III A	1410 (13.8)	2012 (19.7)	1420 (13.9)
III B	1777 (17.4)	1643 (16.1)	1668 (16.3)
III C	1236 (12.1)	773 (7.6)	1340 (13.1)

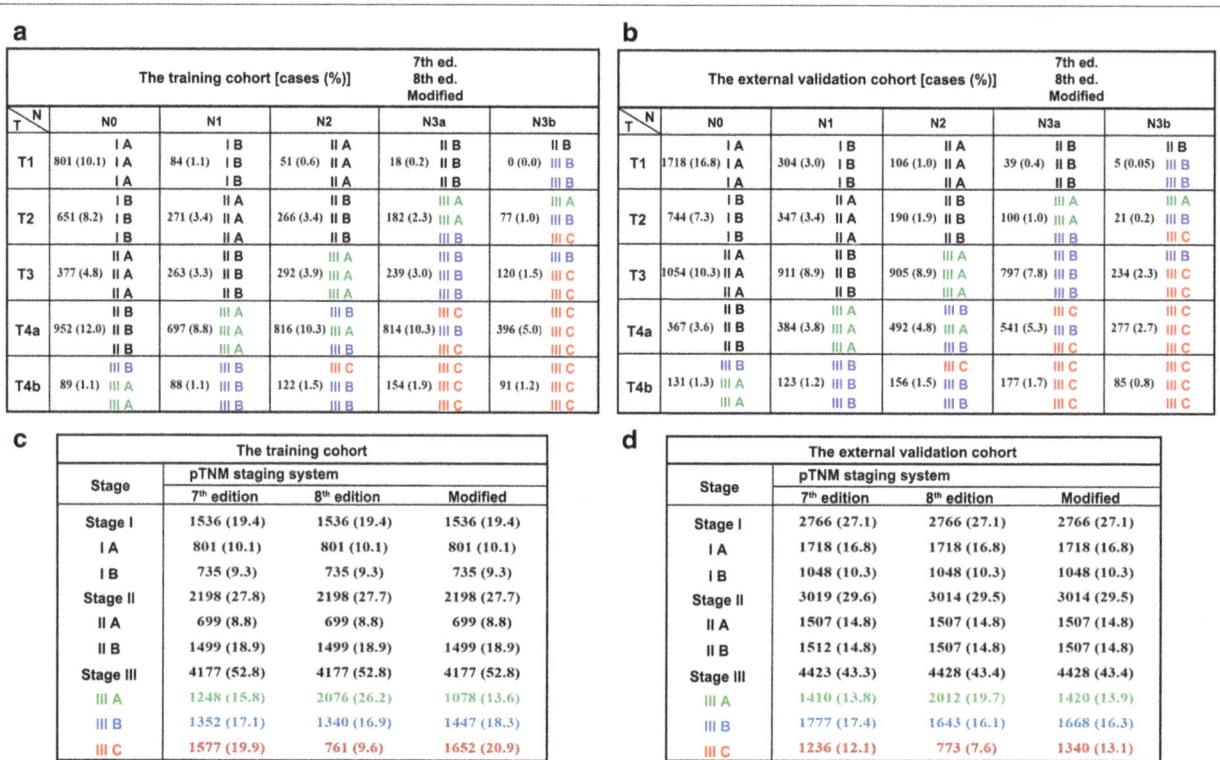

Fig. 2 Stage migration between the 7th and 8th editions of AJCC/UICC staging system as well as the modified pTNM staging system for both the training and external validation cohorts. **a** Classification illustrated in the training cohort; **b** classification illustrated in the external validation cohort; **c** patient grouping in the training cohort; **d** patient grouping in the external validation cohort. Stage migration was mainly observed for patients with stage III disease; therefore, for better contrast among patients at this specific stage, its sub-stages IIIA, IIIB, and IIIC were colored green, blue, and red, respectively. Abbreviations: AJCC/UICC, American Joint Committee on Cancer/Union for International Cancer Control; ed., edition of the tumor-node-metastasis (TNM) staging system

respectively. For the training cohort, the OS curves showed significant differences between every two groups classified according to either the 7th (all $P < 0.001$; Fig. 3a) or the 8th AJCC/UICC staging system (all $P < 0.001$; Fig. 3b). Similar results were observed in the external validation cohort (all $P < 0.001$; Fig. 3d, e). The observed survival differences among the groups represented satisfactory discriminatory ability and monotonicity of both staging editions.

Homogeneity of the 7th and 8th AJCC/UICC staging systems

In the training cohort, the 7th AJCC/UICC staging system demonstrated poor homogeneity in stage IIIA-C because the survival rates of subgroups of patients within stage IIIA, IIIB, or IIIC were significantly different (all $P < 0.001$; Fig. 4a–c). When classified according to the 8th AJCC/UICC staging system, subgroups of patients within stage IIIA or IIIB still showed significant differences in survival (both $P < 0.001$; Fig. 4d, e), but those within stage IIIC did not show such differences ($P = 0.364$; Fig. 4f).

In the external validation cohort, the 7th AJCC/UICC staging system demonstrated good homogeneity in stage IIIA ($P = 0.397$; Fig. 4j), but not in stages IIIB and IIIC ($P = 0.034$ and $P = 0.005$; Fig. 4k, l); the 8th AJCC/UICC staging system demonstrated good homogeneity in stages IIIA and IIIC ($P = 0.085$ and 0.060; Fig. 4m, o), but not in stage IIIB ($P = 0.002$; Fig. 4n).

Proposal of a modified pTNM staging system

To improve the homogeneity in stage III classification, a modified pTNM staging system was proposed according to the best log-rank χ^2 values in the training cohort. In the modified pTNM staging system, with the best-observed homogeneity (Fig. 5, upper part), stage IIIA was composed T3N2, T4aN1, and T4bN0; stage IIIB was composed of T2N3a, T3N3a, T4aN2, T4bN1, and T4bN2; and stage IIIC was composed of T2N3b, T3N3b, T4aN3a, T4aN3b, T4bN3a, and T4bN3b (Fig. 5, lower part). Stage I and II classifications remained unchanged. The modified pTNM staging system demonstrated optimal discriminatory ability and monotonicity in both the training and external validation cohorts as supported by

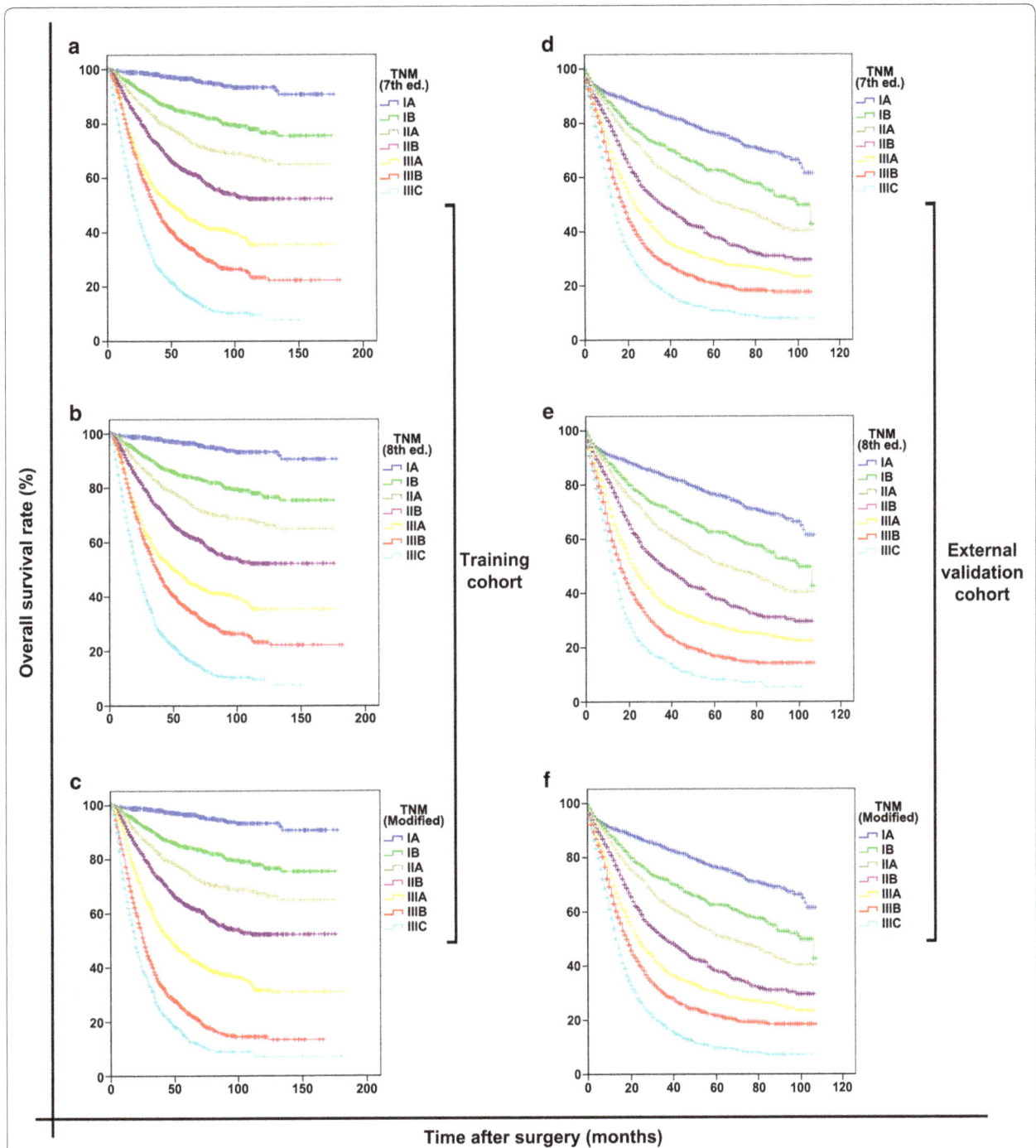

Fig. 3 Discriminatory ability and monotonicity of the 7th and 8th AJCC/UICC staging systems and the modified pTNM staging system for both the training and external validation cohorts. **a–c** The training cohort grouped according to the 7th, 8th, and modified pTNM staging systems, respectively; **d–f** the external validation cohort grouped according to the 7th, 8th, and modified pTNM staging systems, respectively. *AJCC/UICC* American Joint Committee on Cancer/Union for International Cancer Control, *ed.* edition of the TNM staging system

mild differences in survival (Fig. 3c, f). When classified according to the modified pTNM staging system, subgroups of patients within stage IIIA, IIIB, or IIIC showed no significant differences in survival in either the training cohort (all *P* > 0.05; Fig. 4g–i) or the external validation cohort (all *P* > 0.05; Fig. 4p–r).

Prognosis prediction performances of the 7th and 8th AJCC/UICC staging systems against the modified pTNM staging system

The performance results of the competing staging systems are displayed in Table 3. Compared with the 7th and 8th AJCC/UICC staging systems, the modified pTNM staging system demonstrated the best homogeneity (the highest likelihood-ratio χ^2 score), discriminatory ability, gradient monotonicity (the highest log-rank χ^2 and linear-trend χ^2 scores), and the lowest AIC value, displaying an optimal prognostic stratification ability in both the training and external validation cohorts.

Discussion

In the present study, both the 7th and 8th AJCC/UICC staging systems demonstrated poor homogeneity in the training and external validation cohorts, particularly for stages IIIA, IIIB, and IIIC, an observation that was not mentioned by the International Gastric Cancer Association (IGCA). Thus, a modified pTNM staging system was proposed. For convenience in the clinical application of the proposed modified pTNM staging system, the classifications of "T" and "N" categories were not altered, and, based on our statistics, we focused on a more homogenized re-classification approach to improve the subgroup classification. The Kaplan–Meier OS curves demonstrated similarity among the subgroups of patients within stage IIIA, IIIB, or IIIC classified according to the modified pTNM staging system and revealed optimal homogeneity. Furthermore, compared with the 7th and 8th AJCC/UICC staging systems, the modified pTNM staging system also displayed the best homogeneity, discriminatory ability, and monotonicity of gradients both in the training and external validation cohorts.

The TNM staging system is the common "language of cancer" [10, 11], enabling comparisons between different populations irrespective of country and ethnicity. With the improvement of surgical techniques, the number of retrieved LNs is increased dramatically, and the definition of the category N3ab as the presence of more than 6 metastatic LNs is too broad. In the 8th AJCC/UICC pTNM staging system for GC, the category N3ab is subdivided into N3a and N3b to improve the accuracy of staging and prognosis prediction. Our results have shown

that, with this subdivision, the 8th AJCC/UICC pTNM staging system (comprised of 25 subgroups of the T, N, and M categories) provided a more precise classification than those the 7th edition (comprised of 20 subgroups), emphasizing personalized treatment. However, among the recently published studies that had compared the prognosis prediction performance between the 8th and 7th editions, none focused on the homogeneity of both editions [12–15].

In the present study, 197 (2.5%) patients were upstaged and 1841 (23.2%) were downstaged as classified according to the 8th edition over the 7th edition of AJCC/UICC pTNM staging system in the training cohort, whereas 260 (2.5%) were upstaged and 1320 (12.9%) were downstaged in the external validation cohort. We also observed that the majority of stage migration occurred for stage III patients (99%, data not shown) in both cohorts, whereas only 1% was observed for stage II patients (T1N3b and T2N3b). As such, the present study was mainly focused on patients with stage III disease.

Furthermore, our analyses revealed that the 8th edition had better discriminatory ability and monotonicity than did the 7th edition in both cohorts, which was consistent with the results reported by IGCA [16]. However, Kaplan–Meier analyses indicated significant differences in OS among the subgroups of patients within stage IIIA, IIIB, or IIIC classified according to either of the two staging editions. This poor homogeneity was significantly improved in our modified pTNM staging system.

Although our proposed modified pTNM staging system was shown to be superior to the 7th and 8th AJCC/UICC pTNM staging systems, there are certain limitations worth mentioning. First, our training cohort was based on a Chinese population database. Whether this proposed modified pTNM staging system is suitable for populations from other countries has yet to be verified. However, the treatment protocol for locally advanced GC of the same TNM category differs in Asian and Western cancer centers and may explain the observed lower 5-year OS rate in the external validation cohort as compared with that in the training cohort. Neoadjuvant therapies followed by radical resection (including D1 or D1+ lymphadenectomy) are conventionally opted in the west; however, in Asian cancer centers, radical surgery (D2

(See figure on next page.)

Fig. 4 Homogeneity in stage classifications using the 7th and 8th AJCC/UICC staging systems and the modified pTNM staging system for both the training and external validation cohorts. **a–c** Stages IIIA, IIIB, and IIIC classified according to the 7th edition, respectively; **d–f** stages IIIA, IIIB, and IIIC classified according to the 8th edition, respectively; **g–i** stages IIIA, IIIB, and IIIC classified according to the modified pTNM staging system, respectively. **j–l** Stages IIIA, IIIB, and IIIC classified according to the 7th edition, respectively; **m–o** stage IIIA, IIIB, and IIIC classified according to the 8th edition, respectively; **p–r** stage IIIA, IIIB, and IIIC classified according to the modified pTNM staging system, respectively. The homogeneity of the proposed modified pTNM staging system is higher, supporting by mild differences in survival curves, than those of the 7th and 8th AJCC/UICC staging systems

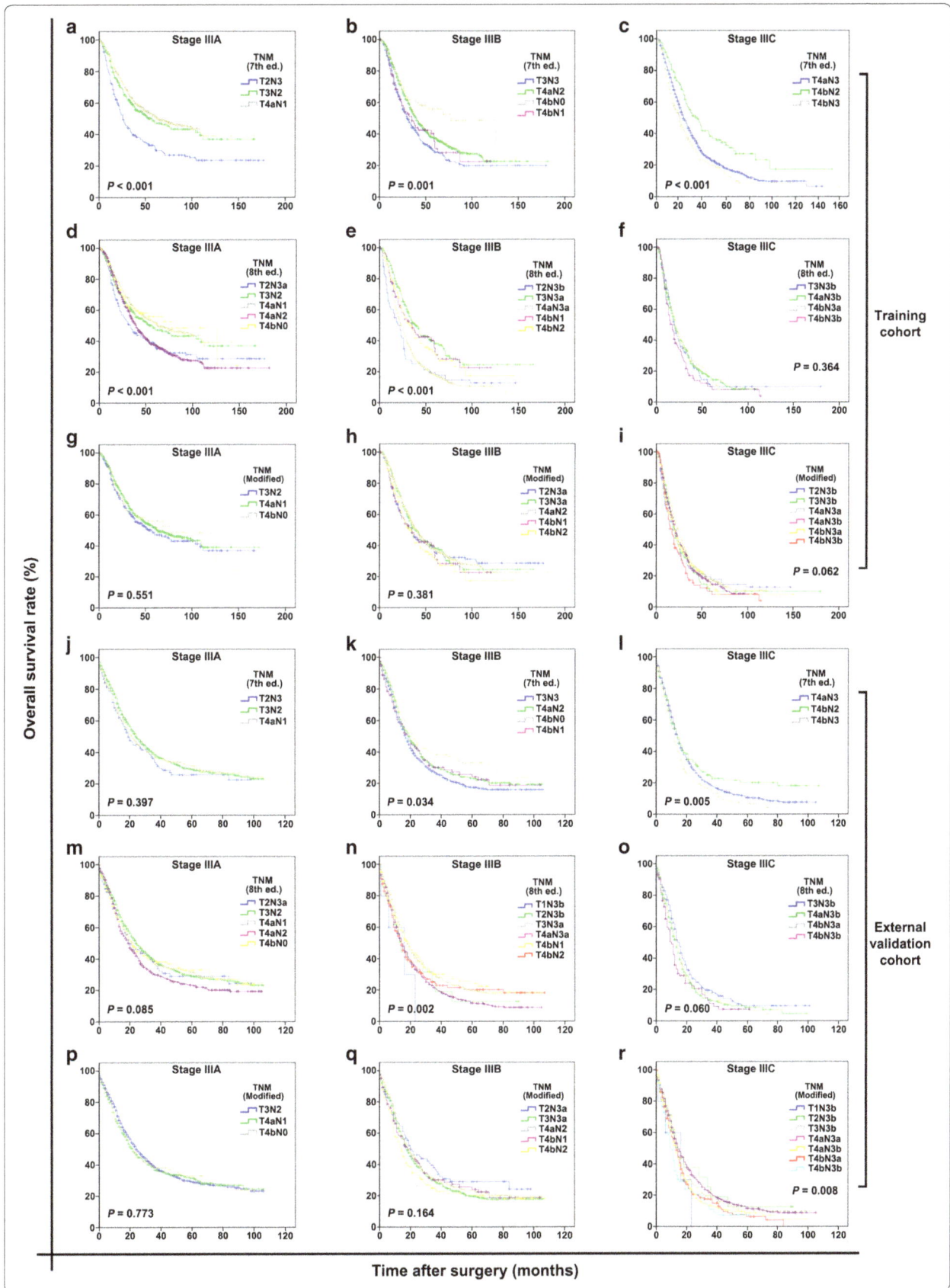

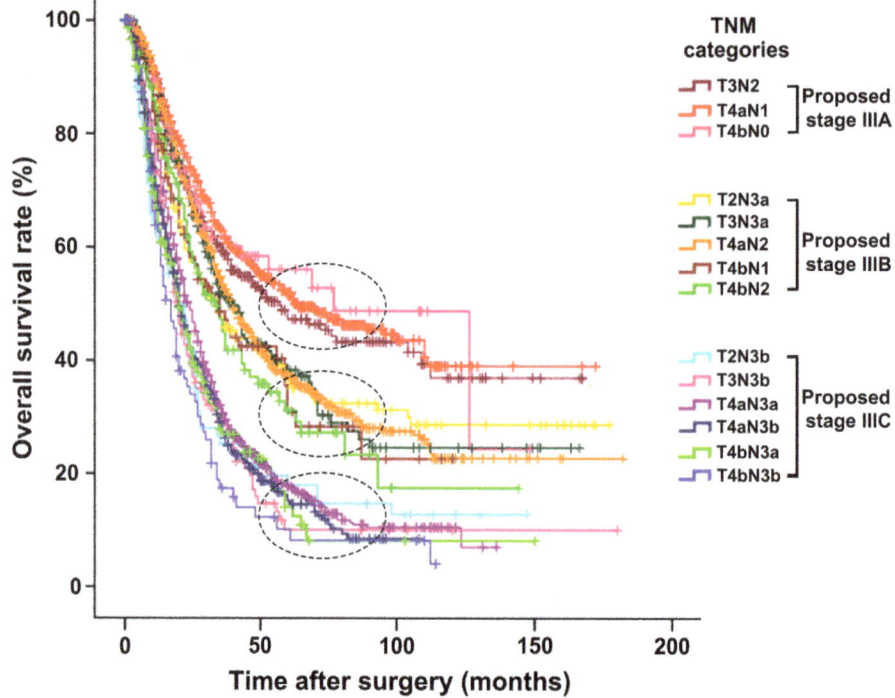

Stage III category	T2N3a		T2N3b		T3N2	
	Chi-square	P value	Chi-square	P value	Chi-square	P value
T2N3a			13.654	<0.001	6.331	<0.001
T2N3b	13.654	<0.001			36.549	<0.001
T3N2	6.331	0.012	36.549	<0.001		
T3N3a	0.454	0.500	20.277	<0.001	3.813	0.049
T3N3b	18.938	<0.001	0.015	0.903	50.374	<0.001
T4aN1	16.108	<0.001	60.745	<0.001	1.232	0.267
T4aN2	0.514	0.474	27.806	<0.001	6.003	0.014
T4aN3a	24.885	<0.001	0.581	0.446	79.435	<0.001
T4aN3b	29.390	<0.001	0.000	0.990	82.581	<0.001
T4bN0	5.347	0.021	24.320	<0.001	0.353	0.553
T4bN1	0.090	0.764	8.182	0.004	5.410	0.020
T4bN2	0.496	0.481	7.987	0.005	9.214	0.002
T4bN3a	20.590	<0.001	0.021	0.885	54.938	<0.001
T4bN3b	28.072	<0.001	1.020	0.312	62.881	<0.001

Fig. 5 Proposal of a modified pTNM staging system according to the best log-rank χ^2 values in the training cohort. In the modified pTNM staging system, stage IIIA was composed of T3N2, T4aN1, and T4bN0; stage IIIB was composed of T2N3a, T3N3a, T4aN2, T4bN1, and T4bN2; and stage IIIC was composed of T2N3b, T3N3b, T4aN3a, T4aN3b, T4bN3a, and T4bN3b. The M classification was not considered since all patients underwent R0 resection and had no distant metastasis

lymphadenectomy) followed by adjuvant therapy are primarily considered. Therefore, to extend the possible use of our proposed modified pTNM staging system, we used the SEER database for external validation. Additionally, to the best of our knowledge, the sample size of the training cohort, came from three highest-capacity GC centers across North and South China, is the largest among all such studies. This further supports the reliability of the results of the present study. Additionally, despite the difference in OS between the training and external validation cohorts that may have been caused by distinct demographic features, different lymphadenectomy types

Table 3 Comparison of prognosis prediction performances of the 7th and 8th AJCC/UICC staging systems with the modified pTNM staging system

pTNM staging system	Figure	Log-rank χ^2	Linear-trend χ^2	Likelihood-ratio χ^2	AIC
Training cohort					
7th edition	3A	2236	1595	2251	56781
8th edition	3B	2295	1636	2283	56749
Modified	3C	2425	1727	2360	56672
External validation cohort					
7th edition	3D	1917	1643	1870	84973
8th edition	3E	1941	1662	1884	84959
Modified	3F	1957	1674	1894	84949

AJCC/UICC American Joint Committee on Cancer/Union for International Cancer Control, *pTNM* pathological tumor-node-metastasis staging system, *AIC* Akaike information criterion

and pathological variables, the proposed modified pTNM staging system can still be universally applied in the West because it was successfully validated in a large external validation cohort from the SEER database. Second, the sample sizes of some subgroups classified according to the 8th AJCC/UICC pTNM staging system were relatively small [for instance, T1N3b (0% in the training cohort and 0.05% in the external validation cohort) and T2N3b (1.0% in the training cohort and 0.2% in the external validation cohort)], possibly due to the low rate of LN metastasis in patients at stage T1 or T2, and may have influenced the efficiency of comparison. Therefore, a study with a much larger sample size is required to further confirm the findings of the present study. Third, due to the retrospective nature of the present study, tumors involving the esophagogastric junction (EGJ) were not included in our analysis because the distances of their epicenters from the EGJ were not specifically mentioned in the retrieved Chinese and SEER databases.

Conclusions
Using large cohorts of patients from Chinese cancer centers and the SEER database, our results identified that both the 7th and 8th AJCC/UICC pTNM staging systems still possess poor homogeneity, particularly for stage III GC patients, although the homogeneity, discriminatory ability, and monotonicity of gradients are improved in the 8th edition. A modified pTNM staging system for GC was thereby proposed and validated, demonstrating superior stratification and prognosis prediction ability and suggesting high potential for clinical application in different populations.

Authors' contributions
Conception and design: CF, ZW, HX, HL, and ZZ. Collection and assembly of data: WW, SRS, JD, and ZS. Data analysis and interpretation: WW. Manuscript writing: CF, WW, and SRS. All authors read and approved the final manuscript.

Acknowledgements
The authors thank Medbanks (Beijing) Network Technology Co. Ltd for facilitating data collection, entry, and management.

Competing interests
The authors declare that they have no competing interests.

Funding
This work was supported by the Major Program of Collaborative Innovation of Guangzhou (No. 201508030042), the Natural Science Foundation of Guangdong Province (No. 2015A030313089, 2018A030313631), Guangdong Provincial Scientific and Technology Project (No. 2014A020232331), Guangzhou Medical, Health Science and Technology Project (No. 20151A011077), China Postdoctoral Science Foundation Grant (No. 2017M622879), and National Natural Science Foundation of China (No. 81802451).

References
1. Torre LA, Bray F, Siegel RL, Ferlay J, Lortet-Tieulent J, Jemal A. Global cancer statistics, 2012. CA Cancer J Clin. 2015;65(2):87–108. https://doi.org/10.3322/caac.21262.
2. Zheng R, Zeng H, Zhang S, Chen W. Estimates of cancer incidence and mortality in China, 2013. Chin J Cancer. 2017;36(1):66. https://doi.org/10.1186/s40880-017-0234-3.
3. Chen W, Zheng R, Baade PD, Zhang S, Zeng H, Bray F, et al. Cancer statistics in China, 2015. CA Cancer J Clin. 2016;66(2):115–32. https://doi.org/10.3322/caac.21338.
4. Chen W, Zheng R, Zeng H, Zhang S. The incidence and mortality of major cancers in China, 2012. Chin J Cancer. 2016;35(1):73. https://doi.org/10.1186/s40880-016-0137-8.
5. Ajani JA, D'Amico TA, Almhanna K, Bentrem DJ, Chao J, Das P, et al. Gastric cancer version 3.2016, NCCN clinical practice guidelines in oncology. J Natl Compr Cancer Netw. 2016;14(10):1286–312.
6. Amin MB, Edge S, Greene F, Byrd DR, Brookland RK, Washington MK, Gershenwald JE, Compton CC, Hess KR, Sullivan DC, Jessup JM, Brierley JD, Gaspar LE, Schilsky RL, Balch CM, Winchester DP, Asare EA, Madera M, Gress DM, Meyer LR. The 8th edition of the AJCC cancer staging manual. New York: Springer; 2017.
7. Edge S, Byrd DR, Compton CC, Fritz AG, Greene F, Trotti A. The 7th AJCC cancer staging handbook. New York: Springer; 2010.
8. Japanese Gastric Cancer A. Japanese gastric cancer treatment guidelines 2014 (ver. 4). Gastric Cancer. 2017;20(1):1–19.
9. Wang W, Sun XW, Li CF, Lv L, Li YF, Chen YB, et al. Comparison of the 6th and 7th editions of the UICC TNM staging system for gastric cancer: results of a Chinese single-institution study of 1,503 patients. Ann Surg Oncol. 2011;18(4):1060–7. https://doi.org/10.1245/s10434-010-1424-2.
10. Greene FL, Sobin LH. The staging of cancer: a retrospective and prospective appraisal. CA Cancer J Clin. 2008;58(3):180–90. https://doi.org/10.3322/CA.2008.0001

11. Wang W, Sun Z, Deng JY, Qi XL, Feng XY, Fang C, et al. A novel nomogram individually predicting disease-specific survival after D2 gastrectomy for advanced gastric cancer. Cancer Commun. 2018;38(1):23. https://doi.org/10.1186/s40880-018-0293-0.

12. In H, Solsky I, Palis B, Langdon-Embry M, Ajani J, Sano T. Validation of the 8th edition of the AJCC TNM staging system for gastric cancer using the national cancer database. Ann Surg Oncol. 2017;24(12):3683–91. https://doi.org/10.1245/s10434-017-6078-x.

13. Ji X, Bu ZD, Yan Y, Li ZY, Wu AW, Zhang LH, et al. The 8th edition of the American joint committee on cancer tumor-node-metastasis staging system for gastric cancer is superior to the 7th edition: results from a Chinese mono-institutional study of 1663 patients. Gastric Cancer. 2017. https://doi.org/10.1007/s10120-017-0779-5.

14. Lu J, Zheng CH, Cao LL, Ling SW, Li P, Xie JW, et al. Validation of the American joint commission on cancer (8th edition) changes for patients with stage III gastric cancer: survival analysis of a large series from a specialized eastern center. Cancer Med. 2017;6(10):2179–87. https://doi.org/10.1002/cam4.1118.

15. Seeruttun SR, Yuan S, Qiu H, Huang Y, Li Y, Liang Y, et al. A comprehensive analysis comparing the eighth AJCC gastric cancer pathological classification to the seventh, sixth, and fifth editions. Cancer Med. 2017;6(12):2804–13. https://doi.org/10.1002/cam4.1230.

16. Sano T, Coit DG, Kim HH, Roviello F, Kassab P, Wittekind C, et al. Proposal of a new stage grouping of gastric cancer for TNM classification: international gastric cancer association staging project. Gastric Cancer. 2017;20(2):217–25. https://doi.org/10.1007/s10120-016-0601-9.

Permissions

The contributors of this book come from diverse backgrounds, making this book a truly international effort. This book will bring forth new frontiers with its revolutionizing research information and detailed analysis of the nascent developments around the world.

We would like to thank all the contributing authors for lending their expertise to make the book truly unique. They have played a crucial role in the development of this book. Without their invaluable contributions this book wouldn't have been possible. They have made vital efforts to compile up to date information on the varied aspects of this subject to make this book a valuable addition to the collection of many professionals and students.

This book was conceptualized with the vision of imparting up-to-date information and advanced data in this field. To ensure the same, a matchless editorial board was set up. Every individual on the board went through rigorous rounds of assessment to prove their worth. After which they invested a large part of their time researching and compiling the most relevant data for our readers.

The editorial board has been involved in producing this book since its inception. They have spent rigorous hours researching and exploring the diverse topics which have resulted in the successful publishing of this book. They have passed on their knowledge of decades through this book. To expedite this challenging task, the publisher supported the team at every step. A small team of assistant editors was also appointed to further simplify the editing procedure and attain best results for the readers.

Apart from the editorial board, the designing team has also invested a significant amount of their time in understanding the subject and creating the most relevant covers. They scrutinized every image to scout for the most suitable representation of the subject and create an appropriate cover for the book.

The publishing team has been an ardent support to the editorial, designing and production team. Their endless efforts to recruit the best for this project, has resulted in the accomplishment of this book. They are a veteran in the field of academics and their pool of knowledge is as vast as their experience in printing. Their expertise and guidance has proved useful at every step. Their uncompromising quality standards have made this book an exceptional effort. Their encouragement from time to time has been an inspiration for everyone.

The publisher and the editorial board hope that this book will prove to be a valuable piece of knowledge for researchers, students, practitioners and scholars across the globe.

List of Contributors

Xiuying Gu
Cancer Research Institute, Cancer Hospital, Xinjiang Medical University, Urumqi 830011, P. R. China

Rongshou Zheng, Changfa Xia, Hongmei Zeng, Siwei Zhang, Xiaonong Zou, Zhixun Yang, He Li and Wanqing Chen
National Office for Cancer Prevention and Control, National Cancer Center/Cancer Hospital, Chinese Academy of Medical Sciences and Peking Union Medical College, Beijing 100021, P. R. China

Mengying Tong,Mengying Yang, Chang Xu, Xiaolong Zhang, Qingzheng Zhang, Yuwei Liao, Xiaodi Deng, Dekang Lv, Xuehong Zhang, Yu Zhang, Peiying Li, Luyao Song, Aisha Al-Dherasi and Zhiguang Li
Center of Genome and Personalized Medicine, Institute of Cancer Stem Cell, Dalian Medical University, Dalian 116044, Liaoning, P. R. China

Ziqian Deng and Quentin Liu
Center of Genome and Personalized Medicine, Institute of Cancer Stem Cell, Dalian Medical University, Dalian 116044, Liaoning, P. R. China
State Key Laboratory of Oncology in South China, Collaborative Innovation Center of Cancer Medicine, Sun Yat-sen University Cancer Center, Guangzhou, Guangdong 510060, P. R. China

Bicheng Wang
State Key Laboratory of Oncology in South China, Collaborative Innovation Center of Cancer Medicine, Sun Yat-sen University Cancer Center, Guangzhou, Guangdong 510060, P. R. China Cancer Center, Union Hospital, Tongji Medical College, Huazhong University of Science and Technology, Wuhan, Hubei 430022, P. R. China

Edina Bugyik, Vanessza Szabó, Katalin Dezső, András Rókusz, Armanda Szücs and Péter Nagy
First Department of Pathology and Experimental Cancer Research, Semmelweis University, Budapest, Üllői út 26, 1085, Hungary

Sándor Paku
First Department of Pathology and Experimental Cancer Research, Semmelweis University, Budapest, Üllői út 26, 1085, Hungary

Tumor Progression Research Group, Hungarian Academy of Sciences-Semmelweis University, Budapest 1085, Hungary

József Tóvári
Department of Experimental Pharmacology, National Institute of Oncology, Budapest 1122, Hungary

Balázs Döme
Department of Thoracic Surgery, Semmelweis University-National Institute of Oncology, Budapest 1122, Hungary
Department of Thoracic Surgery, Medical University of Vienna, Waehringer Guertel 18-20, 1090 Vienna, Austria
Department of Biomedical Imaging and Image-guided Therapy, Medical University of Vienna, 1090 Vienna, Austria
National Koranyi Institute of Pulmonology, Budapest 1122, Hungary

Viktória László
Department of Thoracic Surgery, Medical University of Vienna, Waehringer Guertel 18-20, 1090 Vienna, Austria
Department of Biomedical Imaging and Image-guided Therapy, Medical University of Vienna, 1090 Vienna, Austria

Yanjun Huang, Sichun Zhou, Caimei He, Jun Deng, Ting Tao, Qiongli Su, Kwame Oteng Darko and Xiaoping Yang
Key Laboratory of Study and Discovery of Targeted Small Molecules of Hunan Province and Department of Pharmacy in the School of Medicine and Laboratory of Animal Nutrition and Human Health, Hunan Normal University, Changsha 410013, Hunan, P. R. China

Mei Peng
Key Laboratory of Study and Discovery of Targeted Small Molecules of Hunan Province and Department of Pharmacy in the School of Medicine and Laboratory of Animal Nutrition and Human Health, Hunan Normal University, Changsha 410013, Hunan, P. R. China

Department of Pharmacy, Xiangya Hospital, Central South University, Changsha 410008, Hunan, P. R. China

Xiangyang Yu, Yongbin Lin, Yingsheng Wen, Yongqiang Chen, Weidong Wang and Lanjun Zhang
State Key Laboratory of Oncology in South China, Collaborative Innovation Center for Cancer Medicine, Guangzhou 510060, Guangdong, China
Department of Thoracic Surgery, Sun Yat-sen University Cancer Center, 651 Dongfeng Road East, Guangzhou 510060, Guangdong, China

Xuewen Zhang
State Key Laboratory of Oncology in South China, Collaborative Innovation Center for Cancer Medicine, Guangzhou 510060, Guangdong, China
Department of Medical Oncology, Sun Yat-sen University Cancer Center, Guangzhou 510060, Guangdong, China

Zichen Zhang
State Key Laboratory of Oncology in South China, Collaborative Innovation Center for Cancer Medicine, Guangzhou 510060, Guangdong, China
Department of Molecular Pathology, Sun Yat-sen University Cancer Center, Guangzhou 510060, Guangdong, China

Fuh Yong Wong, Wei Ying Tham, Wen Long Nei and Cindy Lim
Division of Radiation Oncology, National Cancer Centre Singapore, 11 Hospital Drive, Singapore 169610, Singapore

Hui Miao
Saw Swee Hock School of Public Health, National University of Singapore, Singapore, Singapore

Yi-Xin Zeng and Tiebang Kang
State Key Laboratory of Oncology in South China, Collaborative Innovation Center for Cancer Medicine, Sun Yat-sen University Cancer Center, No. 651 Dongfeng East Road, Guangzhou 510060, People's Republic of China

Yi Sang
State Key Laboratory of Oncology in South China, Collaborative Innovation Center for Cancer Medicine, Sun Yat-sen University Cancer Center, No. 651 Dongfeng East Road, Guangzhou 510060, People's Republic of China

Department of Center Laboratory, The Eighth Affiliated Hospital of Sun Yat-Sen University, No. 3025 Shennan Middle Road, Shenzhen 518033, People's Republic of China
Jiangxi Key Laboratory of Cancer Metastasis and Precision Treatment, The Third Affiliated Hospital of Nanchang University, No.128 Xianshan North Road, Nanchang 330008, People's Republic of China

Chun Cheng
Jiangxi Key Laboratory of Cancer Metastasis and Precision Treatment, The Third Affiliated Hospital of Nanchang University, No.128 Xianshan North Road, Nanchang 330008, People's Republic of China

Haixia Deng, Jiewei Chen, Binkui Li, Chenyuan Wang and Dan Xie
The State Key Laboratory of Oncology in South China, Collaborative Innovation Center for Cancer Medicine, Sun Yat-Sen University Cancer Center, No. 651, Dongfeng Road East, Guangzhou 510060, China

Liru He, Shiliang Liu and Mengzhong Liu
The State Key Laboratory of Oncology in South China, Collaborative Innovation Center for Cancer Medicine, Sun Yat-Sen University Cancer Center, No. 651, Dongfeng Road East, Guangzhou 510060, China
Department of Radiation Oncology, Sun Yat-Sen University Cancer Center, Guangzhou, China

Xin Wang
The State Key Laboratory of Oncology in South China, Collaborative Innovation Center for Cancer Medicine, Sun Yat-Sen University Cancer Center, No. 651, Dongfeng Road East, Guangzhou 510060, China
Department of Thoracic Oncology, Sun Yat-Sen University Cancer Center, Guangzhou, China

Yiguo Jiang
The State Key Laboratory of Respiratory Disease, Guangzhou Medical University, Guangzhou, China

Ningfang Ma
Key Laboratory of Protein Modification and Degradation, School of Basic Medical Sciences, Affiliated Cancer Hospital & Institute of Guangzhou Medical University, Guangzhou, China

Feifei Zhang, Wenjie Wang, Yuan Long, Hui Liu, Jijun Cheng, Lin Guo, Rongyu Li, Chao Meng, Shan Yu and Danyi Wen
Shanghai LIDE Biotech Co.,LTD, Shanghai 201203, P. R. China

Qingchuan Zhao
Department of Surgery, Xijing Hospital, The Fourth Military Medical University, Xi'an 710032, P. R. China

Shun Lu
Department of Oncology, Shanghai Chest Hospital Affiliated to Shanghai Jiao Tong University, Shanghai 200030, P. R. China

Lili Wang and Haitao Wang
The Second Hospital of Tianjin Medical University, Tianjin Key Laboratory of Urology, Tianjin 300211, P. R. China

Ching-Ying Kuo
Department of Clinical Laboratory Sciences and Medical Biotechnology, College of Medicine, National Taiwan University, Taipei 10048, Taiwan, China

David K. Ann
Department of Diabetes Complications and Metabolism, Diabetes and Metabolism Research Institute, Beckman Research Institute, City of Hope, Duarte, CA 91010, USA
Irell and Manella Graduate School of Biological Sciences, City of Hope, Duarte, CA 91010, USA

Xinran Qiao, Xiaofei Wang, Yue Shang, Yi Li and Shu-zhen Chen
Institute of Medicinal Biotechnology, Chinese Academy of Medical Sciences & Peking Union Medical College, Beijing 100050, P. R. China

Na Liu, Yingqin Li, Qingmei He, Xiaoqun Yang and Musheng Zeng
State Key Laboratory of Oncology in South China, Collaborative Innovation Center for Cancer Medicine, Guangdong Key Laboratory of Nasopharyngeal Carcinoma Diagnosis and Therapy, Sun Yat-sen University Cancer Center, Guangzhou 510060, P. R. China

Qiuyan Chen, Linquan Tang, Ling Guo, Shanshan Guo, Liting Liu, Pan Wang, Qingnan Tang, Yang Li, YuJing Liang, XueSong Sun, Rui Sun, Haoyuan Mo, Kajia Cao, Xiang Guo and Haiqiang Mai
State Key Laboratory of Oncology in South China, Collaborative Innovation Center for Cancer Medicine, Guangdong Key Laboratory of Nasopharyngeal Carcinoma Diagnosis and Therapy, Sun Yat-sen University Cancer Center, Guangzhou 510060, P. R. China
Department of Nasopharyngeal Carcinoma, Sun Yat-sen University Cancer Center, Guangzhou 510060, P. R. China

Feng Han and Jianwei Wang
State Key Laboratory of Oncology in South China, Collaborative Innovation Center for Cancer Medicine, Guangdong Key Laboratory of Nasopharyngeal Carcinoma Diagnosis and Therapy, Sun Yat-sen University Cancer Center, Guangzhou 510060, P. R. China
Department of Ultrasound, Sun Yat-sen University Cancer Center, Guangzhou 510060, P.R China

Chuanmiao Xie and Yunxian Mo
State Key Laboratory of Oncology in South China, Collaborative Innovation Center for Cancer Medicine, Guangdong Key Laboratory of Nasopharyngeal Carcinoma Diagnosis and Therapy, Sun Yat-sen University Cancer Center, Guangzhou 510060, P. R. China
Department of Imaging, Sun Yat-sen University Cancer Center, Guangzhou 510060, P. R. China

Ying Guo
State Key Laboratory of Oncology in South China, Collaborative Innovation Center for Cancer Medicine, Guangdong Key Laboratory of Nasopharyngeal Carcinoma Diagnosis and Therapy, Sun Yat-sen University Cancer Center, Guangzhou 510060, P. R. China
Department of Clinical Trial Center, Sun Yat-sen University Cancer Center, Guangzhou 510060, P. R. China

Jun Ma
State Key Laboratory of Oncology in South China, Collaborative Innovation Center for Cancer Medicine, Guangdong Key Laboratory of Nasopharyngeal Carcinoma Diagnosis and Therapy, Sun Yat-sen University Cancer Center, Guangzhou 510060, P. R. China

Department of Radiation Oncology, Sun Yat-sen University Cancer Center, Guangzhou 510060, P. R. China

Huai Liu
Department of Radiation Oncology, Key Laboratory of Translational Radiation Oncology, Hunan Cancer Hospital and The Affiliated Cancer Hospital of Xiangya School of Medicine, Central South University, Changsha 410013, P. R. China

Yanfang Ye
Department of Science and Education, Sun Yat-sen Memorial Hospital, Guangzhou 510120, P. R. China

Lu Zhang
Department of Radiation Oncology, The First Affiliated Hospital of Guangzhou Medical University, Guangzhou 510120, P. R. China

Ming Zhan, Rui-meng Yang, Hui Wang, Min He, Wei Chen, Sun-wang Xu, Lin-hua Yang and Jian Wang
Department of Biliary-Pancreatic Surgery, Renji Hospital, School of Medicine, Shanghai Jiao Tong University, 160 Pujian Road, Shanghai 200127, P. R. China

Qiang Liu
Department of Pathology, Renji Hospital, School of Medicine, Shanghai Jiao Tong University, Shanghai 200127, P. R. China

Man-mei Long
Department of Pathology, Shanghai Ninth People's Hospital, School of Medicine, Shanghai Jiao Tong University, Shanghai 200011, P. R. China

Bo Zhang
Food Safety and Health Research Center, School of Public Health, Southern Medical University, Guangzhou 510515, Guangdong, P. R. China
Department of Preventive Medicine, School of Public Health, Sun Yat-sen University, Guangzhou 510080, Guangdong, P. R. China
JC School of Public Health and Primary Care, The Chinese University of Hong Kong, Hong Kong, SAR, China

Shao-Hua Xie
Upper Gastrointestinal Surgery, Department of Molecular Medicine and Surgery, Karolinska Institute, Karolinska University Hospital, NS 67, 2nd Floor, 17176 Stockholm, Sweden

JC School of Public Health and Primary Care, The Chinese University of Hong Kong, Hong Kong, SAR, China

Ignatius Tak-sun Yu
JC School of Public Health and Primary Care, The Chinese University of Hong Kong, Hong Kong, SAR, China
Hong Kong Occupational and Environmental Health Academy, Hong Kong, SAR, China

Bingzhong Jing, Bin Li and Caisheng He
State Key Laboratory of Oncology in South China, Collaborative Innovation Center of Cancer Medicine, Guangzhou 510060, P. R. China
Department of Information, Sun Yat-Sen University Cancer Center, Guangzhou 510060, P. R. China

Chaofeng Li
State Key Laboratory of Oncology in South China, Collaborative Innovation Center of Cancer Medicine, Guangzhou 510060, P. R. China
Department of Information, Sun Yat-Sen University Cancer Center, Guangzhou 510060, P. R. China
Precision Medicine Center, Sun Yat-Sen University Cancer Center, Guangzhou 510060, P. R. China
Guangdong Key Laboratory of Nasopharyngeal Carcinoma Diagnosis and Therapy, Guangzhou 510060, P. R. China

Liangru Ke
State Key Laboratory of Oncology in South China, Collaborative Innovation Center of Cancer Medicine, Guangzhou 510060, P. R. China
Department of Radiology, Sun Yat-Sen University Cancer Center, Guangzhou 510060, P. R. China

Weixiong Xia, Chaonan Qian, Chong Zhao, Haiqiang Mai, Mingyuan Chen, Kajia Cao, Haoyuan Mo, Ling Guo, Qiuyan Chen, Linquan Tang, Wenze Qiu, Yahui Yu, Hu Liang, Xinjun Huang, Guoying Liu, Wangzhong Li, Lin Wang, Rui Sun, Xiong Zou, Shanshan Guo, Peiyu Huang, Donghua Luo, Fang Qiu, Yishan Wu, Yijun Hua, Kuiyuan Liu, Shuhui Lv, Jingjing Miao and Yanqun Xiang
State Key Laboratory of Oncology in South China, Collaborative Innovation Center of Cancer Medicine, Guangzhou 510060, P. R. China
Department of Nasopharyngeal Carcinoma, Sun Yat-Sen University Cancer Center, Guangzhou 510060, P. R. China

Xiang Guo and Xing Lv
State Key Laboratory of Oncology in South China, Collaborative Innovation Center of Cancer Medicine, Guangzhou 510060, P. R. China
Department of Nasopharyngeal Carcinoma, Sun Yat-Sen University Cancer Center, Guangzhou 510060, P. R. China
Guangdong Key Laboratory of Nasopharyngeal Carcinoma Diagnosis and Therapy, Guangzhou 510060, P. R. China

Ying Sun
State Key Laboratory of Oncology in South China, Collaborative Innovation Center of Cancer Medicine, Guangzhou 510060, P. R. China
Department of Radiotherapy, Sun Yat-Sen University Cancer Center, Guangzhou 510060, P. R. China

Feng Du, Lina Sun, Yi Chu, Tingyu Li, Chao Lei, Xin Wang, Mingzuo Jiang, Yali Min, Yuanyuan Lu, Xiaodi Zhao, Yongzhan Nie and Daiming Fan
State Key Laboratory of Cancer Biology, National Clinical Research Center for Digestive Diseases and Xijing Hospital of Digestive Diseases, Fourth Military Medical University, 127 Chang Le West Road, Xi'an 710032, China

Wei Wei, Pei-En Jian, Shao-Hua Li, Zhi-Xing Guo, Yong-Fa Zhang, Xiao-Jun Lin, Li Xu, Ming Shi, Min-Shan Chen and Rong-Ping Guo
State Key Laboratory of Oncology in South China, Collaborative Innovation Center for Cancer Medicine, Sun Yat-sen University Cancer Center, Guangzhou 510060, Guangdong, P. R. China
Department of Hepatobiliary and Pancreatic Surgery, Sun Yat-sen University Cancer Center, Guangzhou 510060, Guangdong, P. R. China

Yi-Hong Ling
State Key Laboratory of Oncology in South China, Collaborative Innovation Center for Cancer Medicine, Sun Yat-sen University Cancer Center, Guangzhou 510060, Guangdong, P. R. China
Department of Pathology, Sun Yat-sen University Cancer Center, Guangzhou 510060, Guangdong, P. R. China

Lie Zheng
State Key Laboratory of Oncology in South China, Collaborative Innovation Center for Cancer Medicine, Sun Yat-sen University Cancer Center, Guangzhou 510060, Guangdong, P. R. China

Department of Medical Imaging, Sun Yat-sen University Cancer Center, Guangzhou 510060, Guangdong, P. R. China

Cheng Fang, Wei Wang, Sharvesh Raj Seeruttun and Zhi-Wei Zhou
Department of Gastric Surgery, Sun Yat-sen University Cancer Center, State Key Laboratory of Oncology in South China, Collaborative Innovation Center for Cancer Medicine, 651 Dongfeng Road East, Guangzhou, Guangdong 510060, P. R. China

Jing-Yu Deng and Han Liang
Department of Gastric Cancer Surgery, Tianjin Medical University Cancer Institute & Hospital, Tianjin 300000, P. R. China

Zhe Sun, Zhen-Ning Wang and Hui-Mian Xu
Department of Surgical Oncology, The First Hospital of China Medical University, Shenyang 110000, P. R. China

Index